PAINLESS

CANCER
CURES

& PREVENTIONS
Your Doctor May Not Be Aware Of

Teresa Moreno
9421 Canter Ct
Riverside, CA 92509

Deanna K. Loftis, R.N. B.B.A.

JADA

PAINLESS CANCER CURES & PREVENTIONS
Your Doctor May Not Be Aware Of

Published in 2005 by JADA Press
Jacksonville, Florida
www.JadaPress.com

Cover and interior design by www.bookmakersink.com

ISBN: 0-9771343-1-8
LCCN: 2005906688

Printed in the United States of America

Credits

****

DEDICATION

Dedicated to "the high and lofty One that inhabiteth
eternity, whose name is Holy;" and to His Son,
The Lord Jesus Christ, "In whom are hid all the
treasures of wisdom and knowledge."
(ISA 57:15 & COL 2:3 KJV)

ACKNOWLEDGEMENTS

I wish to extend my deepest appreciation and thanks to the many people who were helpful to me during the time that I was compiling this book and even years before I had the opportunity to make it a reality:

- My dear twin sister, Chris, for her endless encouragement during the many long hours I worked far into the night on this book, as well as for her many prayers. No one could ever ask for a kinder, more tender-hearted, caring person to enrich their lives as she has mine.

- My sisters, Shelby and Patsy, for their encouragement and confidence in me.

- My mother-in-law, Nolaine, for her time, patience, and helpful input while she was reading through so many of the chapters at all hours of the day (and night!)

- My dear friends: Dee Underwood, Mary Fisher, Antionette Judkins, Carol Woodworth, Ann Tino, and Tina Reed, who shared many happy and sad times with me, back when I was going through some of the experiences that would later prompt me to write this book.

- My good friend, Gwen Nichols, who encouraged me way before the first draft was ever finished.

DISCLAIMER

This book is neither a medical guide, nor a manual for self-treatment. It is for informational purposes only and is not intended as a substitute for medical diagnosis, treatment or competent health care, nor should it be construed as practicing medicine. Nutrients given herein are dosage suggestions and are for your information only. You should always check with your physician for your own individual needs regarding any supplements. Anyone with a serious disease or illness should consult a physician before initiating a change in treatment or before beginning any new treatment or if you have health questions regarding the use of any information in this book. The author and publisher do not prescribe and assume no liability for any adverse effects or consequences resulting from the use of any of the suggestions, preparations, recipes, or procedures discussed in this book, nor for the reliance thereon, nor for interpretation errors or transcription errors.

Many of the statements made regarding various nutrients herein have not been thoroughly evaluated by the FDA. It is also noted that some people are allergic to, or may have allergic responses to herbs, vitamins, minerals, and their preparations, so caution is advised. If you ever develop breathing problems after taking any herb, nutrient, food or medicine, you should seek immediate help as this can be an indication of a potentially life-threatening reaction. The publisher and author are not affiliated with the websites mentioned herein, nor their products, nor do the author and publisher of this book attest to the reliability of any of those products, unless it is those items the author herself has used and highly recommends (such as those marketed by Maureen Kennedy Salaman and Dee Simmons). What you choose to do with that information is up to you. The publisher and author of this book assume no liability for those decisions. Should you use products from those websites, you do so at your own discretion and risk.

TABLE OF CONTENTS

INTRODUCTION

In this book, you will find new information, old information and, if you are already ill, perhaps a new hope in getting well! If you are ill, there is no time to lose, because it is very possible that the information in this book could save or extend your life or the life of someone you love!

Note that some of the alternative treatments in this book are not painless, since they may be given by injection, but they are mentioned for informational purposes and because they have achieved commendable results without the use of toxic chemo or radiation! This book is by no means an exhaustive work on alternative cancer therapies. There are many alternative therapies that you can find on the internet that I have chosen not to include in this book such as: Cancell, Anvirzel, Carnivore, DMSO, GEIPE, Sun Farms Soup, Urea, the Ayurvedic treatments, Alsihum, Aveloz, Dries Cancer Diet, IAT, Issels Treatment, Wiedbrande Treatment, Osiecki Treatment, Yuccalive, Glyconutrition, TVZ-7, and many others too numerous to list here. Neither does this book discuss in detail BCG, monoclonal antibodies, cryosurgery, or growth factor/toxins.

If you or someone you know has already been diagnosed with cancer (for example a brain tumor), and told that it is inoperable and your situation hopeless, read chapter 13 of this book immediately! Do not let a physician tell you that there is no cure out there for the type of cancer you have, and that the only choice you have is maybe extending your life another six months with chemo or radiation! (There are many people with so-called "terminal" brain cancers who were initially sent home to die, who have been cured without chemo or radiation, and several of them are described in chapter 13 of this book!)

Some of the treatments in this book would come under the heading of *immunotherapy,* or giving the body substances to boost the immune system to enable it to fight disease off by itself. You may also hear it referred *to as biological response modifier therapy* or *biotherapy.*

There is probably no illness or disease in the last or current century that has evoked more horror, dread, and fear than the scourge of cancer. We have been told now for many decades that there is a *war on cancer*. However, the frightening truth is that the so-called *war on cancer* is being lost in a very big way. As a matter of fact, the statistics are now so dismal that you can be sure if cancer does not strike you, it will strike someone very close to you, if it has not already done so!

In spite of all the tragic loss of life (and limb) associated with cancer, it may grieve you to know that the awful truth is that the cancer establishment (e.g. FDA, AMA, American Cancer Society, Pharmaceutical Companies, etc.) appears to be in no rush to win the war on cancer, though there is much media hype that would try to convince you otherwise! The first chapter of this book deals with the *cancer establishment* and why it is to their benefit that research continues indefinitely, but a *cure* is never found. Lest you think this is an exaggeration, you have never seriously contemplated the billions of dollars in profit that are generated every year in the United States alone by the thousands of cancer victims who go from treatment to treatment in a desperate search to find a cure for their disease! If the war on cancer is being won, why are there entire medical complexes today that did not exist twenty-thirty years ago just for the treatment of cancer? The truth of the matter is that there already are **cancer cures** out there, but you will seldom read or hear of them in the mainstream media or medicine. The reason you will rarely hear of them is because much of this information is routinely suppressed. Anyone who has ever come even remotely close to proposing a cancer *cure* has been systematically attacked, ridiculed, harassed, and in many cases, run out of the country as you will see in reading this book.

If you are diagnosed with cancer tomorrow, your physician will tell you that there are three primary, acceptable, recommended treatments available for you, depending on the type of cancer that you have: surgery, chemotherapy or radiation. You will be told that the only way to treat your cancer is to cut you, burn you or poison you, and you will be led to believe that unless you accept one (or all three) of these treatments, you will die, and that submitting to these accepted treatments may prolong your life. What most oncologists will not tell you is that the surgery, radiation and chemotherapy may kill you anyway, and that chemotherapy and radiation especially, may shorten your life span. I have been involved in the lives and case histories of many cancer victims. As a nurse, I have seen cancer patients struggle from one treatment to the next, hoping to extend their life.

During the time that I worked as an R.N. Transplant Coordinator for a major insurance company, I followed cancer patients telephonically as they underwent bone marrow (or stem cell) transplants as well as various solid organ transplants. I was especially appalled at what happened with the bone marrow cases. I knew about the dreadful side effects from massive doses of chemotherapy used to obliterate their immune systems. I have watched loved ones from my own family let their physicians talk them into taking round after round of radiation and chemotherapy, only to die an agonizing, slow and torturous death. The cancer did not kill them; the side effects of the chemotherapy and radiation they received killed them! If you gain nothing else from reading this book except to know that there is hope out there for cancer patients (apart from the cut, poison and burn route), then it will have accomplished its purpose.

While working on a med-surg floor, I have had many patients going through various cancer treatments, and I have seen the side of the medical establishment that fights a rigorous battle to treat cancer victims with mutilating (and often unnecessary) surgeries, medications that poison and destroy the immune system, and radiation that burns beyond belief. Many times I have stood at the bedside of patients dying with breast cancer, pancreatic cancer, colon cancer, liver cancer, brain cancer or other types of cancer, unable to do a thing for them other than palliative nursing care. Looking back, I am appalled at how many of those patients were not actually dying from their cancers as much as they were dying from the surgery, radiation, or chemo they had received!

Though some surgeries are unwarranted, I do believe that in certain instances, surgery may be the best choice for cancer. A surgical removal can often bring about total remission in certain types of cancer, and sometimes surgery (for example in the case of a bowel being obstructed by a large tumor) is needed immediately. However, if a lifetime of bad habits and poor choices resulted in cancer, unless you change those habits, the cancer may likely return. If you have a cancerous tumor growing (for example, in your lung), you have a *sys-*

temic disease, not an isolated problem in one organ. Your entire immune system is ill, or you wouldn't have cancer in the first place. (There are many cancers that are not described in detail in this book, such as: germ cell tumors, Wilm's tumors, LCH, spindle cell carcinomas, GISTs, desmoid tumors, acral and lentigo maligna melanomas, rhabdomyosarcomas, MPNSTs, MALT tumors, pNETs, and others, however, most of the alternative therapies described herein have been used for all types of cancers, even those considered very rare!)

As far as chemo and radiation are concerned, in my own personal opinion, I believe it is best to seek alternative therapies before allowing oneself to be subjected to damaging radiation and chemotherapy, however, if you are diagnosed with cancer, whether or not you choose to go the conventional medicine route, or alternative route, will ultimately have to be **YOUR** decision. It is a decision that I cannot make for you. You will hear of an occasional remission due to chemo and radiation, but remember that both are a double-edged sword! The cancers often return twice as deadly as they were before, and they inflict an enormous blow to an immune system that is already ill! The purpose of this book is to give you enough information so that you will know what is available in alternative therapies, as well as how to use preventative measures to assist your immune system in getting you well and keeping you well! It will also tell you about the cancer CURES that multitudes of people have experienced without ever undergoing surgery, chemo or radiation! I feel certain that in the next few decades, humanity will look back on our current conventional system of treating cancer victims and marvel at the barbarity to which we have subjected our loved ones in the name of disease management!

I believe there is a God who never slumbers. I believe that one day He will demand an account from those who are practicing atrocities against humanity in the name of medicine, while their true vested interest lies in padding their own wallets. Before you even finish the first few chapters of this book, I believe you will agree.

Deanna K. Loftis, R.N, B.B.A.

CHAPTER I

WHO PROFITS WHEN YOU'RE ILL?

"In the 1970s America's undeclared war in Vietnam ended in spectacular defeat. In the 1980s its highly touted war against cancer simply disappeared into the night."

(Ralph W. Moss, Ph.D., from his book: *The Cancer Industry)*[1]

Cancer Politics

Cancer has become such a big business that, as pointed out by Maureen Kennedy Salaman in her book, *Nutrition: The Cancer Answer II,* searching for a cure is extremely profitable, however, there appears to be little incentive to finding one![2] Despite what you are currently being told by the cancer establishment and the mass media, there really are alternative therapies that countless people are using to CURE their cancers! Cures apart from the triune *god* of the cancer establishment: chemotherapy, radiation and surgery. This book has many examples of people **cured from cancer** without using chemo, radiation or surgery!

What exactly is the "cancer establishment?" Dr. Robert Willner, M.D., Ph.D., writer of *The Cancer Solution & Deadly Deception,* describes them:

> The "cancer establishment" is a network of extremely powerful and wealthy companies whose members sit on the boards of many non-profit organizations. They literally control and direct all cancer research within the USA and throughout the world. Although these centers are non-profit they serve their masters by suppressing most, if not all, non-patentable treatments in favor of the expensive treatment therapies that have wrought havoc with patients while losing the war against cancer.[2a]

Are you aware that in the U.S. if you are given a diagnosis of cancer, you will be told that you have three choices for treatment? Those three choices are: surgery, chemotherapy or radiation. The SCR, scar or scare treatments! You will be told that you can choose between being cut, poisoned or burned, but the choices will be dressed up in formal technical language to make you think you are going to be CURED by one of them, when in reality, the chances of a cure by any of the SCR treatments is statistically dismal. (Some cancers are initially cured with surgery, but they often return.) In essence, you will be frightened to death by your physician. You will be told that unless you submit to one of these *choices,* you will die. Or you may be told that your life could be extended another six months if you submit to this treatment. What you will NOT be told is that chemo, radiation or both, may destroy your immune system and kill you anyway, and you will die quicker and much more miserably! Many patients agree to surgery then refuse to have chemo or radiation afterwards.

I am not against surgery for cancer, especially in a case like bowel cancer where an obstruction has occurred, or an isolated tumor that can be completely removed, or a hysterectomy in the case of cervical or uterine cancer. However, as stated earlier, cancer is a systemic disease. When you have cancer, your entire body is ill, not just the organ or section where the tumor has manifested. Though surgery by itself may successfully eradicate a primary cancer, the results are often temporary, because the cancer may return. If your cancer is the result of a lifestyle of bad choices (e.g. smoking, alcohol, junk food, lack of exercise, lack of sufficient water, fresh air, etc.), unless you make better choices, the cancer will likely return.

Patients often develop a desperate dependency on their physicians when they are confronted with a terminal illness, blindly following their doctor's advice, desperately hoping that they will be cured, without doing any of their own research into alternative treatments available.

Many times, it is not until patients have become so ill and debilitated from chemo or radiation that they suddenly realize they are little more than guinea pigs. Then they begin a desperate search for help, going from one specialist to another, frantically hoping for a cure!

Dr. Ralph Moss in his book, *The Cancer Industry,* describes a comment by Dr. "Andrew P. Morley...chairman of the American Academy of Family Physicians," to give you some idea of the megabucks generated by the cancer establishment: "It's a win-win-win situation...Cancer physicians use a great many diagnostic procedures, and the cancer victim and the insurance companies must pay for them."[2b]

Though most physicians and other medical practitioners sincerely want to see their patients recover from disease and are dedicated to that end, when a physician tells a patient that their only hope for recovery is chemotherapy, radiation or surgery, in most cases, they believe they are telling them the truth. They are merely parroting what they have been told and led to believe either in medical school or through the brainwashing of the conventional cancer media, whose priority is pushing chemotherapy drugs and radiation.

If you are unconvinced that cancer generates megabucks for the medical profession, consider just the diagnostic tools such as MRIs. Costs of these machines are very high, but Dr. Moss explains that they generate hundreds of thousands of dollars per year for those "who manufacture the machines," and the professionals who use them.[3] He further describes what happened with the cancer war:

> By 1974 the public, which had enthusiastically hoped a cure for cancer was in the offing, was beginning to feel it had been betrayed. The cancer war was Nixon's "other war," and when Nixon resigned over Watergate, this only fueled public suspicion of a double-cross.[4]

What Went Wrong?

The war on cancer disappeared because the FDA, the pharmaceutical companies, the American Cancer Society, and many members of the AMA and prominent research facilities jumped in bed together, and they've been warm and cozy ever since!

Dr. Moss further explains in *The Cancer Industry*, that many physicians hold influential positions of leadership on pharmaceutical boards and in medical colleges and universities as well as positions in the FDA. Some members of the FDA own thousands of dollars in stock in the drug companies that apply to them for drug approvals! Though this should be considered a major "conflict of interest," it is never addressed.[5]

Medical school graduates do not focus on healing. They are taught how to alleviate and treat *symptoms*, and which drugs to prescribe for which illness.

If you go to your doctor and tell him or her that you are having abdominal pain, you will often be scheduled for diagnostic testing. By the time you leave the office, you may very well have in hand several FREE drug *samples* (left by pharmaceutical sales reps), or a written prescription to treat your *symptoms* until your follow-up visit. Forget about alternative therapies. Your insurance company, working with beaurocrats in Washington, D.C. as well as leaders in the medical establishment, can guarantee that your treatment options won't include alternative medication and cancer treatments by classifying them as *experimental* and *unconventional*. This is because many alternative treatments involve natural products and natural products can not be patented!

Pharmaceutical companies can not make a profit from a naturally occurring herb or nutrient because the FDA will not allow them to patent natural substances, thus it is not considered an accepted treatment, and not a *covered benefit,* so you are denied coverage! Do you see how the *system* works? If you still doubt the sincerity of the FDA and the pharmaceutical companies in allowing you access to the best cancer treatments available for cancer, read chapter five in this book about colon cancer and the herb, *Graviola*.

Believe me, the AMA wants as little competition from alternative medicine as possible. As noted by Barry Lynes in his book *Helping the Cancer Victim*:

> The AMA was found guilty by a U.S. Court of Appeals in 1980 of "conspiracy to restrain competition." The Federal Trade Commission had made the original ruling in 1979. The Court of Appeals recognized that, as a result of pressure from the AMA, "new methods of health care have been discouraged, restricted, and in some instances, eliminated."[6]

Mr. Lynes details the desperate struggle one such patient describes in an attempt to get alternative therapies that might be life-saving:

> I felt like I was drowning in the ocean and someone in a boat had a life preserver. They'd wave the life preserver at me and say this could save your life but you can't have it. I've been taking chemotherapy over one year without success....I know from my own experience cancer is a money maker. I see the bills I have and I can't believe the costs....[7]

Many of these potentially "lifesaving" alternative therapies that have proven successful in treating cancer are not easily accessible. Dr. Robert Willner, M.D., Ph.D., who wrote *The Cancer Solution & Deadly Deception,* explains why:

> You may have difficulty in obtaining some of these therapies...because the FDA has literally pressured Congress, under the guise of protecting the public, to keep time-honoured cultural and natural therapies out of the hands of the general public. If you look at the record of the FDA, it becomes obvious they are serving interessts (sic) other than yours and mine[8].

Dr. Abram Hoffer, M.D., Ph.D., FRCP(C) has had tremendous success with cure rates in treating cancer patients using Orthomolecular Medicine (high dose vitamin-mineral therapy), yet in his book *Healing Cancer – Complementary Vitamin & Drug Treatments*, he says that "In California, for example, it was considered malpractice to advise patients to take vitamin C if they had cancer." Dr. Hoffer explains:

> No one was allowed to tell their patients to take vitamin C if they had cancer. No one was allowed to tell their patients that the vitamin could be therapeutic...Therefore doses above those recommended by food-and-drug administrations, the so-called RDA (Recommended Dietary Allowance) doses,

are contra-indicated and even considered dangerous. Often where there is no toxicity, it is invented – for example, the false belief that vitamin C will cause pernicious anemia because it destroys vitamin B12 (it does not) or that vitamin C will cause kidney stones when it does not....Vitamins, even in large doses, are safe, especially the water soluble ones. The toxicity of vitamins has been grossly exaggerated. Very few people eat diets so well balanced they obtain adequate quantities of many of the vitamins, even when they are well.[8a]

Dr. Hoffer further describes how the cancer establishment has tried to suppress the use of Orthomolecular Medicine treatments (e.g. high dose vitamin C) in spite of its value in fighting cancer:

Among the various attempts to suppress or discredit research studies showing the efficacy of vitamin C, a study led by C. G. Moertel at The Mayo Clinic, published in 1985 in The New England Journal of Medicine, provides a good example of how the cancer establishment works. Every physician seems to know about this study, at least enough to say to the patient, "The Mayo Clinic showed that vitamin C has no value against cancer." This statement is false, however, because the study was so flawed as to make it quite unreliable. In this study, 50 patients with advanced colorectal cancer were given vitamin C, 10 g per day. They were given the vitamin for a median time of only 75 days. During the first 75 days, only 1 patient died. After being taken off [the] vitamin, the patients then began to die rapidly, about half of them dying during the next 75 days. We had previously pointed out that there is a potential rebound effect when high-dose vitamin C is suddenly stopped, and that it might be dangerous for cancer patients to do so. (We repeat the recommendation that the intake of high doses of vitamin C and other nutrients not to be suddenly stopped.)[8b]

See chapter twenty-six for more information on Orthomolecular Medicine. There are also other chapters in this book describing cancer cures that came about due to megadose vitamin or mineral therapy.

The SCR Treatment – How Effective Is It?

Nothing in the SCR treatment (surgery, chemo, or radiation) has been particularly successful at eradicating the scourge of cancer. The history of surgery for cancer treatment doesn't exactly get rave reviews as a means of curing the disease. As further explained by Barry Lynes, surgery itself "has a cure rate of less than 50% according to specialists who are sympathetic to conventional treatments….*Often only the surgeon benefits!*"[9] Chemotherapy is even more grim, and "…is recognized by many qualified researchers and physicians as a dismal failure despite the cost and the agony produced by it."[10]

If chemotherapy is failing so miserably, why do physicians keep using it? Well, for one thing, it is generating an enormous profit for the drug companies pushing their products! In the early part of the 90s, over 3.5 billion dollars worth of chemo drugs were being prescribed, and within a four year period of time, this amount had increased to nearly 8 billion! Strangely enough, as the amount of money spent on chemo increased, so did the cancer death statistics!

According to Dr. Abram Hoffer in his book, *Healing Cancer – Complementary Vitamin & Drug Treatments,* "Chemotherapy has little value in the treatment of breast cancer although oncologists continue to administer new combinations of chemotherapeutic drugs to breast cancer patients in the effort to find a useful therapy."[11]

With a record like this, why do consumers keep using chemo when common sense should tell us otherwise? *Wellness Directory of Minnesota™,* website explains this strange human phenomenon:

> We choose chemotherapy because doctors are authorities. It doesn't matter that your doctor (probably) knows less about how the human body heals than your average cab driver. Your doctor is an authority on "medicine" and upwards of 70% of us will choose to put this toxic poison in our bodies, simply because of the authority she or he stands for…[12]

The track record for radiation is even more dismal! Although it "...is the most common treatment for breast cancer following surgery," according to Dr. John R. Lee, David Zava, Ph.D., and Virginia Hopkins in their book, *What Your Doctor May Not Tell You About Breast Cancer,* radiation [also] "is not working:"

> [W]hile using local radiation to treat breast cancer reduces deaths from this disease by 13.2 percent, it increases death from other causes, mostly heart disease, by 21.2 percent. The obvious conclusion of this study: "The treatment was a success but the patient died."[13]

Just to note a few of the complications from radiation for breast cancer, Barry Lynes in his book, *Helping the Cancer Victim*, quotes Dr. Robert Jones from the *Seattle Times*, (July 27, 1980):

> [F]ibrous shrunken breasts, rib fractures...nerve damage...suppression of all blood cells, immune suppression....Many radiation complications do not occur for several years after treatment, giving the therapist and the patient a false sense of security for a year or two following therapy...[14]

How Trusting Are You?

Before you set your hopes on a cancer cure by taking a chemo drug, you need to know that the major hope you have of getting well is boosting your depressed immune system and the intervention of God's help in your behalf! If your immune system were functioning properly you would not have cancer. The job of the immune system is to destroy defective cells and cancer cells are *defective* cells. (See the last chapter in this book*, What To Do If You Are Already Ill!*) Chemotherapy is destructive to the immune system, and most chemotherapy drugs are proven failures! It is not unusual for patients who faithfully adhere to a prescribed chemo or radiation regimen for one type of cancer, to discover a year or two later (when they think they are in remission) that a second, even more sinister cancer than the one they started with, has invaded their system – just one of the *little* side effects of their toxic treatment! I would recommend strongly that you read the rest of this book and the book by Dr. Ray D. Strand, M.D., *Death By Prescription,* if your physician wants to give you chemotherapy!

Even if you opt for chemo, there is no guarantee that you will be given exactly what the doctor ordered! In a story at Karl Loren's website *(www.karlloren.com)*, "an award winning health columnist...died on December 3, 1994. She died of chemotherapy." The patient had been diagnosed with "breast cancer," and she allowed the medical establishment to convince her that chemotherapy was her best chance of recovery! This "39-year-old mother of two" received "a lethal dose of chemotherapy which was overlooked by at least a dozen physicians, nurses and pharmacists for over four days." It was eventually revealed that she "died of heart failure after she was given four times the maximum safe dosage of a highly toxic drug during her chemotherapy treatment."[15] This unfortunate patient had "horrendous symptoms" that everyone overlooked. "She was vomiting sheets of tissue....The whole lining of her gut from one end to the other was shedding. They said it was the worst they had ever seen. But the doctors said this was all normal, according to" her husband. This is not an isolated occurrence. "Just two days before her death [another patient] a 52-year-old woman was the victim of the same mistake..."[16]

An article appearing at website *www.molocure.com,* discussed a May 2002 report from the *Journal of the American Medical Association (JAMA),* which stated that "20% of new drugs will be labeled 'Dangerous' or Withdrawn from Market."[17] The website goes on to warn: "taking the findings of this study to heart, perhaps patients should also be warned against taking a prescription for a drug released within the last seven years..."[18]

In chapter five of this book (on colon cancer), you will read how a pharmaceutical company attempted to take a naturally occurring substance and alter its molecular structure, only to find that it no longer worked at curing colon cancer. This naturally occurring herb was found to be comparable at curing colon cancer (in studies on laboratory animals) to the chemotherapy drug, Adriamycin, but without the toxic side effects of Adriamycin, however, it could not be patented in its natural state, so there was no way for the drug company to profit from the herb. They hushed the research! According to website *http://www.hsibaltimore.com*, it was never published![19]

In chapter 21 of this book (on Prescription HRT), you will discover that for decades physicians have been prescribing a synthetic form of progesterone and estrogen to their female patients. This synthetic hormone replacement was developed by a pharmaceutical company because they could not patent the NATURAL form of the hormones. They changed molecules in the natural hormones, patented the end result and created a new drug. There was, however, one very BIG problem with their new creation! It was foreign to the human body! Progesterone and estrogen in their natural forms do NOT have the **toxic side effects of the synthetic formulas!**

The synthetic hormones that the pharmaceutical companies had created caused major side effects that physicians were supposed to warn their patients about. Why did they create these hybrid mutants? Because they could not make a profit from natural estrogen and progesterone, since natural products cannot be patented. If they can not corner the market with a product, they are not interested in promoting it!

Have YOU ever been on hormone replacement therapy (HRT)? Did your physician tell you about all the potential deadly side effects of taking them? Did your physician ever tell you that there are NATURAL forms of estrogen and progesterone and that you can walk into your local health food store and purchase these naturally occurring hormones? They are applied topically to your skin in a cream form and absorbed through the skin, and when used in normal dosages, there are **no toxic side effects!** Of course, you were never told this! Because your physician is trained to dispense prescriptions, synthetic forms of the hormones created by multi-billion dollar drug conglomerates that make millions from the creation and distribution of these drugs! See chapter 21 of this book for more information on natural progesterone and the problems associated with synthetic HRT.

On website *www.Molo-Cure.com*, a writer complains:

> What has happened to the integrity of the medical profession? Why do traditional doctors (MD's) often loosely prescribe toxic drugs without reserve and yet exhibit little interest in providing the patient with information for harmless and effective natural healing solutions?[20]

The web page goes on to discuss a news article describing how the pharmaceutical companies "wine and dine" physicians to gain their favor to prescribe their drugs:

> During the past six months, Dr. Eugene Fierman and his two colleagues were showered with offers worth thousands of dollars. At least once a week, the nation's pharmaceutical firms invited them for "educational evenings" at some of the city's priciest restaurants, including cocktail and dinner at Radius paid for by Pfizer, an insomnia discussion at Locke-Ober, and a depression talk at Maison Robert – both on Wyeth's tab…[21]

In his book, *Death By Prescription*, Dr. Ray D. Strand, M.D. pulls no punches when it comes to his assessment of the condition of our current drug testing and approval program. At one time it took years for a drug to be approved by the FDA. Now, approval can be done in as little as six months. Dr. Strand explains how this process was accelerated:

> Congress passed the Prescription Drug User Free Act (PDUFA) in 1992, an act impacting us heavily today. This act allowed the FDA to collect a "user's fee" from pharmaceutical companies to help cover the expense of getting new drugs approved.[22]

It was supposed to be a temporary thing, but not so. Dr. Strand described it as:

The Deadly Partnership – Congress had formed a partnership between the FDA and the pharmaceutical companies, and our "great protector" would now receive a significant amount of its funding from the industry it was intended to regulate.[23]

It wasn't long before this nefarious relationship became more and more corrupt. You won't get very far into *Death By Prescription* without becoming extremely appalled at the flagrant disregard that the FDA (in conjunction with the pharmaceutical industry) has for human life!

If you have any doubts about the flippancy with which the FDA treats our safety, all you have to do is research what happens with their drug approval system! Below is a typical horror story:

Propulsid

When the drug Propulsid was undergoing review in 1993, FDA medical officers knew of 48 patients participating in clinical trials who had experienced changes in their heart rates and rhythms. The reviewers did not, however, consider the problems important. As a result, on July 29, 1993 Populsid was approved for general use. By the time Propulsid was ordered off the market on March 23, 2000 some 301 deaths including those of several infants had been linked to the drug.[24]

Baycol

The drug Baycol was linked "to at least 31 deaths involving a fatal muscle disorder called rhabdomyolysis," as noted in the article "FDA Opens Baycol Probe" at website: *www.consumeraffairs.com/news04/vioxx_baycol_fda.html:*

One article written by University of Washington medical professor Bruce Psaty alleged that Bayer was aware of the risks of Baycol within months of its launch in February 1998, more than three years before it was withdrawn. By the time Baycol was removed from the market, the estimated number of cases of rhabdomyolysis had reached the tens of thousands, one of the JAMA articles said. As of this fall, Bayer has settled 2,861 lawsuits involving Baycol.[25]

In chapter five of his book, *Death By Prescription*, Dr. Ray Strand explains that before Rezulin (another drug that caused dozens of deaths) ever came out on the market, Warner-Lambert had a checkered past! They were:

Scrambling for a recovery in sales, compromises were made, and by November of 1995 *Warner-Lambert pleaded guilty to a felony of concealing deficiencies from the FDA* in its manufacturing of several other drugs. Lack of integrity is disturbing news, but in the world of business, progress marches on.[26]

How many people taking Rezulin ever knew this, I wonder!? Dr. Strand commented that "Putting blind faith in the system that has gone wrong could cost you or your loved ones a life."[27]

The Horror Stories Continue

Just recently, I watched a live report on national news warning that the pharmaceutical manufacturer of yet another drug has come forth to admit that taking their drug can increase your risk of developing lymphatic cancers.

Then again a short while later, the news hit the airwaves that the manufacturer of *Vioxx* knew their drug could cause fatal heart attacks, but the information had been suppressed.[28]

The *Wall Street Journal* reported that thousands died from cardiac problems after taking Vioxx.[29] Has the FDA moved in to close MERCK down and confiscate all their records? Where is the outcry at? Do you know what would have happened if this had been a natural, alternative herbal supplement not owned by a billion-dollar drug conglomerate? Those who manufactured the natural supplement would be in jail facing prison terms, their records would be in the hands of the FDA, and the story would be making headline news every single day for weeks before it would finally die down! And of course, the FDA would be screaming about the need to place all vitamins, herbs, and supplements under their direct control! (To protect you and I, of course! The same way they protected us from Propulsid, Vioxx and Celebrex?) Yes, not only Vioxx, but Celebrex is also being implicated as increasing user's risks of heart attacks! Some of these drugs have been on the market for years! Why has it taken so long for this *news* to be made public?

The Vaccination Controversy

Are you aware that there are many health issues related to vaccinations? Childhood vaccinations have been suspected in Crohn's disease, autism, juvenile diabetes, other autoimmune disorders, and many other illnesses, yet your school officials will tell you that you MUST have your child vaccinated, when in reality you can always request a *waiver* from your school to opt out of the vaccination. Most public officials will not tell you this. If vaccinations are effective, *why are booster shots needed for some vaccines?* You may wish to read the book by Neil Z. Miller, *Vaccines: Are They Really Safe & Effective,* before you take that next flu shot or take your child for their next vaccination! There are many recent news articles circulating regarding a preservative in vaccines causing autism in children, and many websites have information about the dangers associated with flu shots. This is all being ignored by the CDC. For example see *www.whale.to/v/flu4.html.* If you have a child who has recently been diagnosed with autism, Crohn's disease, type I diabetes, meningitis, Guillian-Barre' syndrome, or you've lost a child to SIDS (sudden infant death syndrome), ask yourself this question: *when was the last time they were vaccinated, and what was it for?*

Did you know that in "253 infant death cases [the families were] awarded more than $61 million by the U.S. Court of Federal Claims under the compensation program? 224, or 86 percent, were attributed to vaccinations with DPT, the diptheria, pertussis (whooping cough), tetanus shot." These were just the cases filed by parents during the 90's. Before it was determined that the DPT caused the deaths, "40 percent" of them had first been blamed on SIDS![30] (When it comes to SIDS, many proponents of Orthomolecular Medicine agree that SIDS cases would drop drastically if more mothers would breastfeed their infants and they also believe that SIDS can be prevented by ascorbate acid (vitamin C). Check with your pediatrician regarding infant vitamin supplements! Be aware that I am **not** telling you **that you should NOT take** vaccines or flu shots. As for taking vaccines (or flu shots) for yourself or your children, that is a decision **you will have to make and live with!** I am giving you resources that you can check for yourself to make a more informed decision about them!

In their August 2001 newsletter, *Wellness Directory of Minnesota™* website had this to say of vaccinations: "In 1972, one of the heads of the FDA, Bernice Eddy, stood in front of Congress and predicted a cancer epidemic because of the contaminated vaccines."[31] This same website gives their simple solution for finding a cure for cancer in their article: *Everyone Gets Rich When You Get Sick*:

> Now, if you really want to find a cure for cancer, cut the funding to cancer research. Yup, cut the funding. There is no incentive to find a cure…If we want to find a cure for cancer, we have to offer an incentive to finding a cure. So, let's cut all funding and offer a reward. Then sit back and watch all the breakthroughs come flying in.[32]

The next time you go to your physician's office, you may be loaded down with *free* samples of the latest *new* drug on the market, or pressured into taking that promising new vaccine someone just developed! Don't be surprised if your doctor sends you merrily on your way with no advice about side effects to these new drugs, except maybe a printed phamphlet with microscopic-sized warnings on line 135 of the drug label! Do you know how the FDA and the pharmaceutical companies will determine the extent of serious side effects involved with the new drug? If **you** don't have serious side effects from taking it and it doesn't kill **you**, then it stays on the market, and even if it does kill you, or a loved one, or make you deathly ill, it could still stay on the market for years before it is forced off!

The drug companies depend on your physician to contact them if you have a serious side effect to a medication you are taking. You, your spouse, or your child may be the next guinea pig for the latest new drug! Still think that the FDA is a staunch advocate for the safety of the public? The name of the game is *profit,* and the FDA, as stated previously, is not concerned about you, your family, your friends or your neighbors! Neither are the pharmaceutical companies. They are in it for the money, folks, and human life and misery is immaterial to them. It does not matter whether the drug is for high blood pressure, kidney disease or a chemo drug for cancer. The bottom line is bucks, and **you**, dear reader, are the guinea pig!

Conflicts of Interest in the FDA

Maureen Kennedy Salaman, in her book, *Nutrition: The Cancer Answer II*, has this to say about the current pharmaceutical disaster in America:

> Major institutions of medical learning in the U.S. are, without exception, subsidized by the foundations and grants of a multi-billion-dollar drug industry. This industry is repaid for its largesse with countless prescriptions written by its student protégés....The result is a medical community that thrives on sickness.[33]

I watched a story that aired live on national news during 2004, describing a case where another pharmaceutical company was paying millions of dollars in fines for promoting off-label usage of one of their drugs.

Now, do you feel that you can trust that chemotherapy drug your physician wants to try out on **you**? Do you feel secure taking it simply because it was approved by the FDA? What about those *freebies* your doctor dispenses at your next visit? Are you going to eagerly accept them without question, simply because they are free? What might they ultimately cost you? A kidney? Your liver? Your life?

CHAPTER 2

A SAFE, NATURAL INGREDIENT USED TO CURE ABDOMINAL, BRAIN, BREAST, & OVARIAN CANCER

"Every new idea goes through three phases: Phase I: It is ignored...Phase II: It is ridiculed...Phase III: The establishment claims it as their own discovery."

(Maureen Kennedy Salaman, from her book,
Nutrition: The Cancer Answer II)[1]

A Forgotten Blessing for America?

In her book, *The Grape Cure*, Johanna Brandt said that she came to America from South Africa in "July, 1927." She came with the intention of blessing America with her "discovery," an astounding cancer cure. Her story was first published on "January 21, 1928" in the "*New York Evening Graphic.*"[2] In recounting her story, she describes how she was first diagnosed with abdominal cancer:

[I] was persuaded by my doctor to go into the General Hospital in Johannesburg for an x-ray examination. Many plates were taken, and a noted surgeon pronounced his verdict – the stomach was being divided in two by a vicious fibrous growth. An immediate operation was recommended as the only means of prolonging my life. This I refused.[2a]

Johanna began a cleansing, fasting diet, drinking only water for three weeks and taking in fresh air and sunshine. Six months later, the x-rays were repeated and no trace of the growth was found! However, she still experienced abdominal pain and was fearful that the cancer was not completely gone and she might relapse. She began a search for a food that would "destroy the growth effectually, eliminate the poison and build new tissue."[3]

As time went by, Johanna embarked on a trial and error "fasting and dieting program." At the end of a long period of trying various diets and cleansing fasts, she claims a remarkable discovery:

[I]n 1925, after a seven-day fast, I accidentally discovered a food that had the miraculous effect of healing me completely within six weeks...A METHOD THAT MAY CURE CANCER, MAY CURE ALMOST ANY OTHER DISEASE. WHAT IS MORE, IT MAY PREVENT CANCER AND ALMOST EVERY OTHER DISEASE.[4]

What was this amazing food with the miraculous healing effect? None other than the lowly **grape!** Johanna experienced a complete cure from her abdominal cancer by consuming fresh grapes and drinking fresh grape juice, as well as a total raw foods diet. It did not seem to matter what type of grape she consumed, the more the variety the better. She healed herself completely without surgery, radiation or chemotherapy!

In her book, *The Grape Cure*, Johanna discussed several "test cases" of cancer patients in the final stages of life, all of them brought back to health merely through using her *Grape Cure* diet! In what she refers to as the "first stage" of the diet, she advises fasting for "two or three days, drinking plenty of pure, cold water" during the fast (and the use of "a quart of lukewarm water daily with the strained juice of one lemon" as a cleansing enema).[5] "After the fast, the patient drinks one or two glasses of pure, cold water the first thing in the morning... [then] starting at 8 a.m." in the morning until "8 p.m." at night, a small meal of grapes "every two hours," or a total of "seven meals daily" is eaten.[6]

If fresh grapes are not available, it is okay to substitute grape juice or even raisins. This diet is recommended for one to two weeks.[7] Johanna suggests a "minimum quantity of one pound" of grapes and a "maximum [per day] should not exceed four pounds...small quantities" are best.[8]

In the "second stage" of *The Grape Cure*, "the gradual introduction of other fresh fruits" and vegetables begins, plus, the diet allows for "sour milk" and "cottage cheese," so it is not a complete vegan diet as recommended by Ann Wigmore and Eydie Mae Hunsberger. (See their stories in chapter three of this book!)[9]

The "third stage" allows for the incorporation of all manner of raw foods into the diet: "vegetables, salads, fruits, nuts, raisins, dates, figs…," and again, some dairy products can be included: "butter, cottage cheese, sour milk, yogurt and buttermilk…."[10]

The "fourth stage" of *The Grape Cure* is what Johanna refers to as *"the mixed diet,"* allowing "one cooked meal a day," though she is reluctant to even say so, because she believes that once you start cooking foods again, the "old" problems may return. Raw is better![11]

It is interesting that Johanna Brandt came up with what she called "The Seven Doctors of Nature: (1) Fasting, (2) Air, (3) Water, (4) Sunlight, (5) Exercise, (6) Food, (7) Mind," with "Mind" being "the most important."[12] These are many of the same ingredients used by other cancer survivors described in this book, who healed their immune systems.

Johanna learned (after her own discovery) that a cure using common table grapes was, in fact, "nothing new." Europeans had been using grapes for curative purposes more than 400 years ago, and again more recently, as she explains: "Over a hundred years ago Dr. Lambe, a pioneer reformer and dietitian, treated cancer in England with grapes…"[13]

Detailed specifics of Johanna's grape cure diet can be found in her book, *The Grape Cure,* which is available from Ehret Literature Publishing Co., Inc. (for $4.95) website *www.arnoldehret.org,* P. O. Box 24, Dobbs Ferry, N. Y. 10522. This book, though written more than 70 years ago, is still very relevant today!

Even though there was much less pollution of dairy products with pesticides, herbicides, antibiotics, and hormones during Johanna's day, you may want to read chapter 25 in this book before you incorporate dairy products into your diet! In the new millennium, I would not recommend dairy products to anyone, unless soy based, and then only moderate amounts! If you insist on them, use certified *organic* only, to ensure that you will not be ingesting hormones and other toxins. Fermented soy products, such as Haelan, can help remove harmful estrogens from the body in estrogen-receptor positive cancers.

What Gives Grapes Their Punch?

During her day, many people adopted Johanna's grape cure, but others were critical, disbelieving that something this simple could affect disease so profoundly. Modern researchers, however, have isolated an amazing ingredient in grapes, known as ***resveratrol!*** It is a very powerful antioxidant that not only inhibits the growth of cancer cells, but contains healing and blood-thinning properties. Johanna Brandt's remarkable cure from abdominal cancer certainly proved that she was ahead of her time, and that there is indeed something miraculous in the healing power of fasting, detoxification and the lowly grape!

If you are wondering about resveratrol content in fresh grapes as opposed to wine, according to Reese Dubin in his book, *Miracle Food Cures From The Bible:* "It takes a pound of home-grown grapes to get as much resveratrol as there is in 2 cups of red wine," and apparently there is very little resveratrol in white wine, "because in making white wine, the resveratrol-rich skins are discarded…in making red wine, the crushed grapes are left to sit in the skins to ferment."[13a]

In *The Super Anti-Oxidants,* by James Balch, M.D., he discusses yet another antioxidant known as "grape seed extract," a potent "pycnogenol" extracted from "both the seeds and the skins of grapes." He believes that this particular antioxidant has marvelous rejuvenation properties for the entire human body, and it occurs in many plants, "including purple, white, red, and green grapes, as well as pine bark, lemon tree bark, hazelnut tree leaves, blueberries, cherries, cranberries, and others. The most concentrated of these is in the seeds of the white and green grapes."[14]

Most of us are familiar with recent health studies showing the lack of heart disease and lack of harmful cholesterol levels found in the French (known as the *"French paradox"*), yet they enjoy "rich foods" and consume wine with most of their meals.[15] According to Reese Dubin in his book *Miracle Food Cures From The Bible*, this *"paradox"* has been attributed to the wine, which has the effect of boosting HDL, the "good…cholesterol." It appears to dissolve harmful layers of fat from arteries and transport it "off to the liver where it is broken down – in effect destroyed – and sent out of the body."[16] However, you don't need alcohol-containing wine to do this! Fasting, juicing and a detox regimen can do the same thing!

Mr. Dubin further points out that "during the cholera epidemic of Paris in the late 1800s," drinking wine saved the lives of thousands of people. The wine was shown to "kill cholera germs," and it did not seem to matter whether the wine was "red or white…full strength or mixed half and half with water. Mothers began soaking fish and fruit in wine, in order to kill the bacteria in them."[17] He explains that "…unlike antibiotics, which can kill bacteria but can't touch viruses, red wine stops them dead." However, it isn't necessary to drink wine to get this benefit, says Mr. Dubin, because the grape extract does the same thing![18] He also reveals that during the 1970's, viruses were tested against grape extract. "None of the viruses tested survived 24 hours' contact with [the] grape extract."[19] Be aware that any drink containing alcohol is damaging to the liver, not to mention what it does to the brain! Grape extract also kills viruses and bacteria without harming the liver or the brain and it inhibits cancer rather than increasing its risks!

No adverse side effects have been reported from taking grape seed extract. It has been useful in the treatment of many disorders including, "varicose veins…diabetic retinopathy, and macular degeneration…"[20]

More Abdominal Cancer Cures

Reese Dubin also describes a dramatic cure for abdominal cancer, much like the one experienced by Johanna Brandt: "Ogden K., a retired photographer, had been diagnosed with a malignant tumor in his abdomen. The doctors wanted to do surgery and give him massive doses of chemotherapy and radiation, but he refused." (He opted for alternative treatment.) "Instead, he went on a fast for several months, subsisting mostly on grape juice and a fruit-and-vegetable diet."[21]

Ogden's tumor began responding "within a week after" he began the "grape juice and raw-fruits-and-vegetable diet." He remained on the diet "until x-rays showed that the cancer was totally gone."[22]

In her book, *The Food Pharmacy – Dramatic New Evidence That Food Is Your Best Medicine,* author Jean Carper has this to say of grapes:

The fruit also possesses extraordinarily high levels of caffeic acid, a polyphenol compound with strong powers to prevent cancer in animals. In a recent study, raisins (dried grapes) were linked to lower rates of cancer deaths in a group of elderly Americans.[23]

Grapes are also rich in ellagic acid. So are raspberries, strawberries, and cherries! According to Dr. Earl Mindell, in *Earl Mindell's Food As Medicine*, ellagic acid appears to block "carcinogens, thus preventing them from turning healthy cells into cancerous ones."[24] Pomegranates are also a good source of this nutrient.

Remember this: it isn't necessary to get your resveratrol from wine because, as Dr. Mindell points out: "red grape juice has as much resveratrol as many wines...in some cases, even more. Better yet, grape juice won't get you drunk and it's safe for children."[25]

Brain Cancer and Breast Cancer Cured

In 1989, Johanna Brandt's grape cure book was published under the title: *How to Conquer Cancer, Naturally,* by Tree of Life Publications in Joshua Tree, California. This edition included several pages of testimonials in the back of the book from grateful followers of *The Grape Cure,* who had experienced miraculous cures from following the grape diet. Here are just two of those many remarkable testimonials:

[1] "I suffered from a tumor on the brain for four years, but I am happy to say it is gone, due to grapes. I was operated on by one of the best brain specialists in the U.S., only to be sent home to die. I took the grape cure with sun baths and water treatment. The tumor is entirely gone and I am so happy I want to tell everyone..."[26]

[2] "The most remarkable case I have had, beginning last August, was a lady operated on and sewed up to die with cancer of the stomach. I used no other therapy (until she was able to be up) except the transitional diet leading to grape juice. When I first took the case, she could not lift her hand. It has been a 'miracle case' and has excited much interest in the GRAPE CURE." (Dr. G. McD.)[27]

Grapes & Alkalinity

The healthiest state for the human body is one of moderate alkalinity. The ideal pH of the body is 7.35 – 7.45. The lower the number, the more acid your body is; the higher the number, the more alkaline. If you keep your body in a state of alkalinity, rather than acidity, you will drastically slash your risks for getting cancer and other diseases, because diseases thrive when the body is maintained in a state of acidity. A diet high in meat, dairy products, and cooked foods keeps the body in a state of constant acidity, increasing the risk for cancer and all chronic diseases.

Raw fruits and vegetables contribute to the body's alkalinity. Any cooking of foods immediately reduces their alkalinity and makes them more acid. Meat, dairy products, refined sugar, cooked foods, and processed foods are acid forming. Grapes alkalize the blood. As described by Dr. T. A. Baroody, N.D., D.C., Ph.d, in his book, *Alkalize or Die,* "The sweeter Thompson seedless" grapes, for example, are 7.0. "More sour are 6.0 to 6.5."[28]

See chapter 29, later in this book, for more information on the acid/alkaline balance and what those numbers represent. Diets that promote acidity cause large amounts of free radicals to circulate in the human body. Free radicals are a type of aberrant electron, and though some are good for us, most are toxic. Those that are harmful have the capacity to cause chaos within a cell's DNA, leading to mutations that can result in cancer and chronic diseases.

According to Dr. Baroody, when the body has a high acidity, waste acids, instead of being excreted are often "reabsorbed from the colon into the liver" where they are "put back into general circulation," only to be returned to "the tissues. *It is these tissue residues that determine sickness or health!"*[29]

(This is one reason I feel that the low carb diet is unhealthy. The body is kept in a state of acidity rather than alkalinity, not to mention the fact that it's high intake of fat and low intake of fresh fruits and vegetables increases the risk for developing cancer.)

Those who criticized Johanna Brandt during her lifetime did so out of ignorance. They knew nothing of free radicals, proanthocyanidins, carotenoids, or super antioxidants. As time goes by, more and more amazing properties of Johanna's miracle grapes are being discovered!

Concord Grape Extract Slows Tumor Growth

As described at website: *http://www.compassionateacupuncture.com/cancer.htm,* a recent research report said that a substance found within concord grapes could repress the growth of tumors as effectively as a common chemo drug.[30]

More Kudos for Resveratrol

Research on this compound has shown that resveratrol can inhibit the cancer process in any of its three stages of development from beginning to end! It also has anti-inflammatory properties similar to some chemo drugs, but without their damaging effects to normal cells!

Grapes Toxic to Ovarian Cancer Cells

Resveratrol also demonstrated the ability to destroy ovarian cancer cells in a laboratory study recently completed. It was noted that resveratrol had the ability to inhibit the proliferation of (and destroy) human ovarian cancer cells. Resveratrol, even in large doses is not toxic. Animal research revealed that there were no adverse side effects even when animals were given massive doses many times greater than you or I would ever ingest. They suffered no ill effects.

Prevention for Prostate Cancer & Skin Cancers

Resveratrol has also been touted as a potent protection against prostate cancer, according to Life Extension website at *www.lef.org.* Researchers from the "University of Wisconsin" listed "six criteria for a good anticancer agent," and resveratrol met every single one: "It should: a) have no toxic effects in healthy cells; b) work against different types of cancers; c) be administered orally; d) have known mechanisms of action; e) be inexpensive; and f) be acceptable to humans."[31] Since the 1990's, "resveratrol has been the subject of hundreds of scientific papers, making it one of the most intensely studied supplements on the market today."[32]

In a CNN interactive article from their "Health Story Page" at *www.cnn.com,* entitled, "Study: Grapes inhibit cancer growth," more benefits to eating grapes were discussed:

> More good news for grape lovers: The fruit of the vine may fight cancer: The study, published in this week's journal Science, found that the substance called resveratrol can block cancer during three major stages of development before a tumor appears...in an 18-week study of mice, doses of resveratrol reduced the number of skin tumors by up to 98 percent compared with skin cancers on control mice.[33]

Other Health Benefits of Eating Grapes

Organically grown grapes should be purchased whenever possible. Grapes are one of the most highly sprayed fruits in production. Organically grown grapes are certified to be free of pesticides and herbicides. Grapes are a rich source of quercetin, a potent antioxidant and they also contain the important anti-inflammatory, antioxidant, pycnogenol. Pycnogenol helps with debilitative disorders such as cardiac and circulatory problems, arthritis, stress, and even inhibits allergies and cancerous growths.

A research group recently reported that resveratrol protects against both liver and breast cancer. But don't look for resveratrol in white wine, because it is found only in the pulp and seeds which are excluded when white wine is processed from the juice. However, as stated earlier, alcohol consumption in itself can increase the risk of certain cancers. The cancer fighting chemicals are found in grapes before they are ever fermented into wine! Why not consume them the way our Creator gave them to us? In their healthiest and most natural state! Resveratrol supplements are available in health food stores. If taking resveratrol, consult with your physician first, especially if you are on prescription meds or are pregnant or lactating.

Another Healing Ingredient Discovered in Grapes

In our annuals of modern medicine, every single day seems to bring more amazing discoveries about the healing properties of natural foods such as grapes and their cancer fighting nutrients! Yet another compound has recently been discovered in grapes that may not only fight cancer, but diabetes as well. The compound is known as *pterostilbene*. It is supposed to work much like resveratrol, but also lowers blood sugar and cholesterol. One researcher noted that the compound could prevent the cellular mutations that carcinogens generally cause, especially against malignant breast cells. For some reason, this particular nutrient, though found in blue, red and black grapeskins, is destroyed when the juice is made into wine. Another reason to consume the grape in its most natural form, the way our Creator intended!

Grapes Effective Against Lung Cancer, Colon Cancer, Breast Cancer, Liver Cancer, & Leukemia

This isn't the end of the miraculous grape and resveratrol. According to an article on website, *CancerProject.org*:

> [S]tudies show that resveratrol may slow tumor growth in the lungs by preventing the replication of DNA, prevent tumors from forming both in the lungs and the colon by destroying potential carcinogens, prevent liver cancer because of its antioxidant activity, prevent breast cancer by protecting cells from the harmful effects of linoleic acid, a type of fatty acid implicated in breast cancer, and arrest the growth of leukemia cells.[34]

Is it any wonder that Johanna Brandt's grape cure diet was such a potent enemy against so many forms of cancer? She was considered a *genius* by some in her day while others scoffed at her. Modern scientific studies are proving that resveratrol and other compounds in grapes are effective against breast, prostate, skin, colon, abdominal, lung, and liver cancer, as well as leukemia and other cancers. It appears that where the scientific community is concerned, Johanna Brandt has had the last laugh! (It is, however, very unfortunate that her *Grape Cure* "blessing" never reached the majority of Americans for which it was intended! How many people have ever heard of it before now? **Have you?**)

Another rich source of resveratrol is the root of the Japanese knotweed plant known as *Hu Zhang*. Some resveratrol supplements are taken from Hu Zhang, others use ground up purple grape skin.

Which Grapes Are Best?

Though many nutritionists favor the red and purple grapes for their antioxidants, for higher OPC content, Dr. James F. Balch, M.D., recommends "green and white grapes rather than the red grape..."[35]

I believe the best advice, as given by Johanna Brandt, is to eat a **variety**, because you will get more **resveratrol** in the red and purple grapes, yet more **OPC's** in the green and white grapes, and **you need both**!

CHAPTER 3

PAINLESS CURES & PREVENTIONS
FOR BREAST CANCER

"There is not one, but many cures for cancer available. But they are all being systematically suppressed by the ACS, the NCI and the major oncology centers. They have too much of an interest in the status quo."

—Dr Robert Atkins, M.D.[1]

This chapter has some amazing cases of complete breast cancer cures, most of them without surgery, chemo or radiation. Many are finding that switching to a raw foods, vegan diet can help begin the healing process for the body's immune system!

In her web article, *Take Two Carrots And Call Me In The Morning*, Connie Guttersen, R.D., Ph.D., states of diet and breast cancer, "the accumulated evidence of hundreds of research studies all point in the same direction: eating large amounts of fruits and vegetables lowers your chance of developing cancer."[2]

I. A Simple, Non-Toxic Breast Cancer Cure

Eydie Mae Hunsberger Cured Naturally
of Breast Cancer!

Eydie Mae Hunsberger was given up by the medical establishment when she developed breast cancer. However, within one year of changing her diet and lifestyle, her cancer was in remission and has not returned since. She has been cancer free for many years. When she was first diagnosed with right breast cancer and a "radical mastectomy" was recommended, one of her first impulses was to hang onto the hope of a cure. In her book, *How I Conquered Cancer Naturally*, she writes: "I saw our government pouring millions of dollars into research grants to find a cure for cancer. With all that money working for me, I figured they just might find a cure within the next year." She was hoping that "If I could stretch my luck that long, maybe I could buy a pill to cure cancer over the drugstore counter by this time next year. That was one of my biggest hopes."[2a]

Many cancer victims find themselves clinging to this "big hope." The hope that the American Cancer Society will actually come out and announce to the world that *Yes, there IS finally a cure for cancer! All those millions and millions that have poured into our coffers finally did it! The research is back! The cure is available!* (Don't pin your hopes on this event happening any time soon!)

Eydie Mae chose an alternative cancer treatment much to the dismay of the surgeon who recommended her radical surgery. Was the surgeon happy for Eydie that she had opted out of conventional treatment for her breast cancer? Hardly! Her husband, Arn, called the surgeon to announce that Eydie was refusing the mastectomy and she describes what happened: "Arn took a tongue lashing like he had never taken before or since." She says that "Irritated to the point of disgust, the surgeon reprimanded Arn saying there should be laws against people like him…he chastised Arn, telling him that he could hold himself directly responsible for my ensuing death."[3]

But there was no "ensuing death!" Though she decided to have a simple lumpectomy, Eydie struggled to find a physician who would agree to do the lumpectomy. Most refused to have anything to do with any surgery less than a mastectomy, but she did eventually find someone to do the lumpectomy. She then began a natural raw foods and juicing diet that caused her breast cancer to go into total remission. She followed the diet popularized by Ann Wigmore, the *Hippocrates Diet,* as described in Ann's books: *The Wheatgrass Book* and *The Hippocrates Diet and Health Program.* At first Eydie admits that she wasn't totally enthusiastic about this new approach to diet and health. She explains: "Believe me, we had to do some mind-stretching when we started considering the idea of drinking wheatgrass juice and eating only live raw foods to bring about a reversal of my malignant breast cancer." She also revealed that "Within the next year, the doctor's research uncovered the unknown ingredient that could reverse the growth of a cancerous tumor…it is the abscisic acid in the wheatgrass that reverses the growth."[4]

Eydie traveled to Ann Wigmore's mansion and spent several days there learning the basics of the raw foods diet. She describes her feel-ings of happiness not long after she started the diet: "I was so filled with joy one morning. My thoughts just tumbled over one another. How unbelievable! Here I am, a cancer patient, not long ago given an eighty percent chance to live one year."[5]

It is interesting to note that Ann Wigmore and Eydie Mae both followed a raw foods vegan diet, as did most of the other breast cancer survivors discussed in this chapter.

Wheat grass is very detoxifying to the body. It can only be tolerated in small amounts when first beginning the raw foods diet. During her stay at Ann Wigmore's mansion, Eydie was consuming two ounces of wheat grass juice up to four times a day, besides using wheat grass implants rectally (directions for which can be found in her book).

Dee Simmons' Breast Cancer Cured

Dee Simmons was a successful business woman in 1987 when she was terrified with an unexpected diagnosis of breast cancer. When her doctor recommended a modified radical mastectomy, she underwent the surgery. Dee began a search that resulted in the formation of a whole foods company, *Ultimate Living*. Using a natural approach to health, Dee began developing nutritional supplements that she herself took for maintaining good health and well-being. Dee has remained cancer free for many years, and currently travels the world lecturing on the importance of nutrition and healthy lifestyle in cancer prevention and wellness. Information on her excellent nutritional products is available at her website *http://ultimateliving.com,* as well as in her book, *Ultimate Living,* which describes her story and her products.

Dr. Kristine Nolfi's Breast Cancer Cured Naturally

Kristine Nolfi, M.D., a physician in Denmark for over 50 years, discovered the advantage of a raw food treatment for breast cancer when she herself developed the disease, which began as a "node the size of a hen's egg." She describes her initial reaction to the diagnosis:

> As a physician I had seen enough to be unwilling to submit to the treatment of cancer generally employed....I felt it as quite a natural thing that I would have to carry through a one hundred percent raw vegetable diet.[6]

Dr. Nolfi successfully cured her own breast cancer on a raw foods diet. It is interesting that before Dr. Nolfi developed breast cancer, her attitude was much like that of all other physicians: "to treat the symptoms of the disease without thinking of preventing it."[7]

As soon as Dr. Nolfi tried to return to a diet of cooked food, she relapsed. She immediately went back to a total raw (vegetarian) food diet and, again, her cancer disappeared. She opened up a health resort, *"Humlegaarden"* (much like Ann Wigmore had done), and treated cancer patients (who came to her over the years) with a strict raw foods diet. In her book, *Raw Food Treatment of Cancer,* Dr. Nolfi discusses a few of her patients and their recovery from cancer. One of her patients was a "thirty-eight-year-old woman" with a small, palpable, cancerous breast growth. A week-and-a-half before she was to have a radical mastectomy, she stayed with Dr. Nolfi, subsisting completely on a raw foods, vegan diet. When she returned to her physician, it was found that the cancer had shriveled to "the size of a grain of rice..." Needless to say, she cancelled the surgery![8]

Dr. Nolfi also describes a "49-year-old" woman with a "nut" sized breast tumor. After "two weeks" on a strict raw food diet, the growth was "the size of a pin-head."[9]

In addition to the raw foods diet, Dr. Nolfi also recommends sunlight exposure, fresh outdoor air, and putting in your own garden.[10] (Home gardening will provide you with exercise, fresh air, sunshine and fresh organic vegetables!)

Rita Myers Cures Her Stage IV Breast Cancer

When Rita Myers was told that she had Stage IV invasive "ductal cell carcinoma," which had metastasized to her bone, physicians gave her six months to two years to live. She began to prepare to die. Her doctors recommended surgery, radiation, and chemotherapy. She started on chemotherapy until her husband, Leon, discovered the *Hallelujah Acres* diet. Rita realized that she did not want her "lymph nodes" taken out, that she needed them for "her immune system to function properly." She stopped chemo abruptly, "refused the radiation," and started on the *Hallelujah Acres* program of biblical nutrition. Rita believes that it was prayer and the *Hallelujah Acres* program that saved her life and healed her completely! Four-and-a-half years later, she is still cancer free and following a raw foods program, juicing about "50 pounds of carrots..." a week. In Rita's words:

> People who hear my story have rarely heard of anyone with stage IV cancer surviving. They are in wonder and amazement. They realize the traditional way is not working and want the same kind of miracle in their life that I experienced.[11]

The *Hallelujah Acres* diet can be found at their *website www.hacres.com,* and is discussed in more detail in this book in chapter five. It is mainly a raw food, vegan diet, much like that advocated by Dr. Kristine Nolfi, Eydie Mae, Ann Wigmore, and Johanna Brandt.

Ann Marie Baker Cured of Breast Cancer

Anne-Marie Baker a "registered nurse" from "Ft. Meyers, Florida," described her colleagues as being "mortified" when she opted out of conventional treatment for her breast cancer and chose alternative nutritional therapy. She refused the "radical mastectomy ...chemotherapy and radiation" her doctor recommended. Instead, she chose "a nutritional program that included wheatgrass, raw vegetable juices, supplements, exercise, and detox," to completely cure her breast cancer. At one point, she was drinking up to "6-9 oz." of wheat grass juice per day.[12]

The Raw Foods Diet & Oxalates

A note on the raw foods diet: be aware that there are many raw foods such as kiwi, spinach, and berries that are considered high-oxalate* foods which should not be used in large amounts by those who may be prone to develop gallstones or kidney stones.[13] Many times this could be avoided by simply increasing fluid intake and making sure that you are taking sufficient amounts of magnesium and B vitamins every day, but there will always be some folks who get stones, no matter what they do! Also, if you are taking "calcium supplements," wait "2-3 hours before or after" ingesting oxalate foods, since oxalates can inhibit calcium's assimilation by the body.[14] The majority of people have no problem with oxalate foods, especially if they consume sufficient fluids. (This information is not repeated everywhere in this book where these type foods are mentioned.) There are many websites that give complete lists of all the foods that contain oxalates. (*Oxalates are a type of acid that can form crystals which sometimes aggregate into kidney stones or gallstones. The acids can also irritate joints such as in the case of gout or rheumatoid arthritis.)

Burzynski's Antineoplastons

See chapter 13 of this book for amazing cases of cancer patients completely cured of "terminal" cancers; people who were basically sent home to die, then chose non-toxic antineoplastons from the Burzynski Clinic in Houston, Texas. Also see many of the patient's own stories about their success in fighting cancer with antineoplastons at website: *http://burzynskipatientgroup.org/stories.html*. Many of these cases were breast cancer patients. Many were "hopeless," very aggressive brain tumors. The main Burzynski Clinic website is at *www.cancermed.com*.

Curing Breast Cancer by Eliminating
Dairy Products

See information in chapter 25 of this book about a physician who cured her breast cancer simply by removing all dairy products from her diet!

Do Unto Others, But Not Unto Thyself

Many physicians will recommend chemo, radiation or surgery to their patients, but often refuse it if they *themselves* are diagnosed with cancer, and with good reason. They know the failure record for radiation and chemotherapy, and the toxic side effects. I have read surveys done on physicians who prescribe radiation and chemotherapy. Many of these oncologists admitted that they would never take the radiation or the chemo drugs **themselves** that they give to their own patients (nor would they recommend or prescribe them to a loved one)! Dr. Ralph Moss even said in an interview once, that an oncologist sat right in front of him and admitted that he would never take the chemotherapy himself that he was prescribing for his cancer patients!

For more information on how you can use diet, juicing, and prayer if you are fighting cancer, see chapter 35 in this book entitled, *What To Do If You Are Already Ill.*

The Raw Food Vegan Diet & Vitamin B-12 Concerns

A note about vegetarians and B-12 deficiencies: vegetarians are often told that they will suffer a vitamin B-12 deficiency without consuming meats. B-12 can be destroyed by gastric acid in the stomach, though some amounts of B-12 are created by *friendly* bacteria in the intestines. For concern about gastric acid destruction of vitamin B-12, this vitamin is available in **sublingual** tablets at most health food stores. You simply put the small tablet under your tongue and it is dissolved and absorbed directly into the rich supply of blood vessels there, completely bypassing the stomach acid.

I do make an exception in the raw food diet when it comes to hard-boiled eggs, but they must be certified ORGANIC! Eggs contain many nutrients! However, if you are battling cancer, you may want to exclude eggs and go with completely raw foods as many of the survivors in this chapter were able to do!

Chlorella alga is vitamin and mineral rich, and for those concerned about protein (in a vegetarian diet) it is high in protein as well. It is discussed in more detail later in chapter eight of this book. Also, don't forget that you don't need meat to get complete proteins in your diet. Combining grains and legumes gives complete proteins!

In animal research with chlorella, tumor masses completely vanished in half the subjects receiving chlorella. All of the animals not on the extract worsened as their cancers continued to grow. All those not given chlorella died.

II. Hormones Can Cure – Or Kill

One of the most important ingredients for breast cancer prevention in women is the right balance of hormones in the body. See chapter 21 in this book entitled, *Prescription HRT – The Great Tragedy of the 20th Century*. It explains how millions of women were prescribed hormone replacement therapy in the last forty plus years that have had deadly side effects, because they were given SYNTHETIC hormones, created by pharmaceutical companies. Their physicians never told them that there are NATURAL hormones (estrogen as well as progesterone) that are available to them without **TOXIC side effects**! What was the reason for this very blatant cover-up? The natural hormones can be bought at any natural health food store and they can not be PATENTED, so the huge drug companies could not make a profit from selling them. Instead, they pushed their synthetic versions of the hormones onto the unwitting public, and thousands have paid the price with their health and their lives due to the deadly side effects of these drugs; effects like blood clots, strokes, uterine cancer, and breast cancer! This same chapter will also tell you how a simple and safe natural hormone found at your local health food store may reduce your risk for uterine and breast cancers, fibroids, endometriosis, and may even cure problems with cystic breasts, irregular periods, and infertility!

III. Nutrients That Prevent & Treat Breast Cancer

CoQ10 & Selenium

CoQ10, though not a vitamin, has often been referred to as a vitamin because it is so essential to every cell in our body. All cells have some amounts of CoQ10, but unfortunately, as we grow older, our bodies manufacture less and less of this nutrient. How healthy you are can often be determined by how much CoQ10 is in your body.

Stephen T. Sinatra, M.D., tells in his informative book, *The Coenzyme Q10 Phenomenon,* how super antioxidant **CoQ10** affects breast cancer: "In humans, anecdotal reports have demonstrated that high dose CoQ10 supplementation (i.e., 390 mg. per day) has been associated with **complete remission**, even for patients with **metastatic breast cancer**."[15]

Do you realize that Dr. Sinatra isn't talking about **animal testing** reports? He is talking about reports of **COMPLETE REMISSION in <u>humans</u>** taking CoQ10! Have you been diagnosed with breast cancer? Has your physician recommended CoQ10 supplements for you? If not, <u>why</u>? (See pp. 193-194.)

This amazing antioxidant isn't just for breast cancer! Dr. Sinatra further elaborates by pointing out the studies done by the late Dr. "Karl Folkers," a highly regarded scientist and primary researcher of CoQ10. Dr. Folkers believed that insufficient amounts of "coenzymes B6 and Q10…" were a major cause of cancer in humans. These deficiencies resulted in an "abnormal pairing of bases of DNA" which causes "mutations and diverse cancers" as described by Dr. Sinatra:

> In one unpublished study, he found deficiencies in CoQ10 in the blood of 83 patients in the United States who had cancer of the breast, lung, prostate, pancreas, colon, stomach, rectum and other sites. The incidence of CoQ10 deficiency was higher for breast cancer…[16]

For optimum health, CoQ10 should be taken in conjunction with selenium, because, according to Dr. R. W. Moss, in *Antioxidants against Cancer,* being deficient in selenium (in animal testing), caused a reduction of CoQ10 by half in "the liver" and by "15 percent in the hearts" of animals tested. An adequate amount for most adults is "200 **micrograms** of selenium" per day. You can get this much by simply eating an "ounce per day of fresh Brazil nuts."[17] Other natural "food sources" of this mineral are: "garlic, onions, wheat germ, broccoli, and egg yolks," but remember that having adequate supplies of this mineral in foods that you grow will largely depend on the selenium-richness of the soil.[18]

Dr. Moss says that selenium is so important that Chinese scientists have discovered it has the ability "to cure Keshan's disease," a viral disease that "attacks the heart. Vitamin E is similarly effective. These nutrients suppress the genes that are essential for the virus to spread."[19] Selenium in excessive amounts can be toxic. "The Recommended Daily Allowance (RDA) is 50 to 100 micrograms (not milligrams!) but few people get even that much."[20] (There is more information on selenium later in this chapter.) Note that the amount of minerals and vitamins listed as the RDA (recommended daily allowance) is generally much lower than most physicians feel are needed by the general populace, as you will read later in this book.

D.I.M. & Breast Cancer

As described at website *www.cancertutor.com,* "Researchers from the University of California at Berkeley looked at the effects of broccoli on human breast cancer cells." They explained that "indoles [from broccoli] are digested and broken down in the stomach to a compound called I3C diindolylmethane (DIM). This compound may be the key to keeping cancer at bay."[20a] DIM is able to eliminate harmful estrogens from the body, a very important health attribute, especially considering the fact that most women have excessive amounts of estrogen! It may also contribute to lowering one's risk for prostate cancer. It is found in all the cruciferous vegetables, not just broccoli.

Grape Seed Extract

See chapter two for more information on the ingredient in grapes *(resveratrol)* that has a history of curative properties for many types of cancers. Though grape seeds should be consumed with the grapes, the actual grape seed extract has become world famous for its super antioxidant properties!

Dr. Ralph Moss in *Antioxidants against Cancer*, discussed earlier, says that "Pycnogenol®...the proprietary name of a product derived from the bark of the French maritime pine tree..." is rich in "bioflavonoids."[21] These bioflavonoids are also found in the seeds of grapes and are sold as supplements. He calls them *super antioxidants*, important in prevention of disease and boosting the immune system, and says that they are "20 times as potent...as vitamin C and 50 times more potent than vitamin E," and apparently, the only thing stronger at zapping "free radicals is green tea extract."[22] It is best to take decaffeinated green tea, since caffeine acts as a diuretic, stripping your body of water.

If you are fighting cancer – grape seed extract, CoQ10, resveratrol, and green tea should be in your nutritional arsenal for healing your immune system!

Selenium & Iodine Deficiencies Linked To Breast Cancer

Besides the work of super antioxidants in preventing and curing cancers such as breast cancer, the fact that our soils have been leached of minerals is the focus of much attention on mineral supplements for cancer prevention. Maureen Kennedy Salaman, a popular nutrition author and advocate warns in her excellent book, *Nutrition: The Cancer Answer II,* of the disastrous consequences we face as a nation due to the lack of vital minerals in our soils. She discusses the studies done by "Dr. Bernard Eskin, Director of Endocrinology, Department of Obstetrics and Gynecology, Medical College of Philadelphia," studies of thousands of laboratory rats and **human beings**:

Dr. Eskin learned that the highest incidence of breast cancer, and deaths from it, are in the goiter belts of Austria, Poland, Switzerland and the United States....Breast cancer death rates in the United States are the highest in the Great Lakes area. The breast cancer death rate in Japan, where iodine is liberally supplied in seafood and seaweed eaten daily, is just **one-fifth** that of the United States.[23]

Not only are our soils depleted of iodine, but other minerals as well, minerals like selenium. Ms. Salaman calls selenium, the "secret weapon" to prevent "breast cancer," and she described in her above book, how levels of this mineral were "mapped...across the United States," then another "map of cancer cases in each state" was placed on top of it. She says that those states with very low amounts of selenium in their soil had "the highest incidence of cancer cases."[24] The state with the greatest levels of selenium and subsequent lowest cancer rate was "South Dakota," while "Ohio" with the "lowest amount of soil selenium," had a **"200% greater"** rate of cancer than "South Dakota."[25] [Emphasis mine.]

Critics of the study claimed that the cancer itself caused the low levels of selenium, however, Ms. Salaman further explained that a second study was done involving thousands of Americans. Blood tests of participants were obtained, "frozen and stored over the years." When a patient in the study "developed cancer," their lab sample was "thawed out for analysis." Ms. Salaman said that it was very obvious that individuals who had cancer were "the ones who, at the start of the study, had the lowest blood selenium levels." In fact, "low blood selenium doubled the chance of developing cancer."[26]

Ms. Salaman also noted that "Gerhard N. Schrauzer, Ph.D.," of the "University of California," discovered the importance of selenium in breast cancer prevention when he found that adding a trace amount of selenium to the drinking water of test animals prone to develop "breast cancer decreased their incidence of such cancer...From 82 percent to 10 percent."[27]

Many Americans are even more mineral deficient than they are vitamin deficient. Maureen Kennedy Salaman has an excellent line of health products, including a super, easily absorbable mineral drink that I recommend and use myself called *Mineral Rich®,* high in essential minerals, including selenium! (It tastes great too!) You can find it, along with her other great products at her website: *www.mksalaman.com.* Her health products are also available at many health food stores.

A Word About Nutrients & Breast Health

This chapter does not have an all-inclusive list of minerals or vitamins needed for breast cancer prevention or treatment. There are many minerals and vitamins needed for optimum health and recovery! If you are juicing every day, eating a nutritious diet, and taking vitamin-mineral supplements, you will obtain the many important vitamins, minerals, and enzymes needed for optimal health. I do recommend, if you are taking supplements, whenever possible, take **organic whole food supplements,** for example Dee Simmons' excellent *Green Miracle* powdered drink (available at her website: *http://www.ultimateliving.com/DeeSimmons.asp.),* and other drinks such as kamut and barley green powdered drinks. For easily assimilated minerals, I recommend and use *Mineral Rich®,* available from Maureen Kennedy Salaman's website *www.mksalaman.com.*

There are many other very rich nutrient-dense drink mixes coming on the market. One in particular, is *Exsula,* available at website *www.exsula.com.* Also see *www.life-enthusiast.com/exsula/exsula_main-htm.* Exsula comes in different strengths. Their top of the line product "Iridesca" contains 240 nutrient ingredients, including coral calcium, extracts of purple cabbage, tomato, ellagic acid from red raspberry seed, broccoli, kale, cracked-cell chlorella, golden flax seed, cat's claw, chuchuhuasi, Reishi, Coriolus, Maitake, Shiitake, bee pollen, ginger, aloe vera, turmeric, citrus pectin, CoQ10, astragalus, ginkgo, bilberry, and garlic, to name a **few**![27a]

See chapters 9 and 13 for information on an amazing nutrient called Poly-MVA that many cancer survivors are crediting with curing their "terminal" cancers!

Vitamins Important for Breast Cancer Prevention & Treatment

As described at *www.alternativehealth.com.au*, scientific research has shown that **vitamin A** "helps to prevent and inhibit the further development of Breast Cancer," and **vitamin C** has been used for cancer prevention (and treatment) in large doses due to its antioxidant effects.[27b] Dr. Abram Hoffer, in his book, *Healing Cancer – Complementary Vitamin & Drug Treatments,* discusses how vitamin C megadosing brought about a remarkable healing of breast cancer for the very first doctor who began using it:

> Dr. Paul Klenner was the first physician to use ascorbic acid [vitamin C] in large doses. He found it very effective in healing a large variety of diseases, whether given by mouth or given intravenously....He described the response of a patient with breast cancer. She had a large mass in her breast and she had refused to take standard therapy. Instead, he gave her 100 grams of ascorbic acid intravenously daily. After several months, the tumor had stopped growing and was extruded by the normal breast tissue and the breast healed.[28]

There are many other nutrients and vitamins important in breast cancer prevention. "A **vitamin D** deficiency" can cause breast cancer,[28a] and **Vitamin E** is such an important super antioxidant, it should be included on a daily basis for anyone fighting breast cancer or just for overall health maintenance. *Alternativehealth.com.au* says that "Vitamin E helps to prevent the development of breast cancer (by optimizing the body's Progesterone: Oestradiol ratio)...600 U of supplemental Vitamin E restores the body's Progesterone: Oestradiol ratio in 86% of persons."[29]

Algae & Breast Cancer

There are several different algae important in breast cancer prevention and treatment. As described at *http://www.alternativehealth.com.au,*

Chlorella has been shown to "prolong survival time in persons afflicted with Breast cancer..." In animal testing, chlorella was able to increase lifespan "an average of 300%..."[30] The website also says that "**Dunaliella** retards the progression of Breast Cancer (due to its Beta-Carotene and other constituents)...**Kelp** *(Laminaria species)* helps to prevent breast cancer (due to its content of fucoidan) [scientific research – rats],"[31] and **Spirulina** is also important as a breast cancer preventative with its high chlorophyll and nutrient content. A blue-green algae known as **Aphanizomenon flos-aquae**, harvested from Klamath Lake in Klamath Falls, Oregon, is also very rich in chlorophyll, beta-carotene and many other vitamins and minerals. (It is best to take algae supplements on an empty stomach.)

Essiac Tea

See Chapter five in this book for the story of a Canadian nurse who healed hundreds of her cancer patients with a super-antioxidant tea mixture containing four herbs known as *Essiac Tea*. Many of those she healed were diagnosed as terminally ill cancer patients. Several brands of *Essiac* tea are available in health food stores, or it can be brewed by purchasing the herbs in bulk. See chapter five for more details.

Ginger and Breast Cancer Testing

See chapter four for more information on studies conducted by scientist, Dr. Laura Murphy on the effects of ginger against breast cancer cells in laboratory and animal tests (as well as its effects on prostate cancer cells).

Graviola Supplement & Breast Cancer Cures

See Chapter five of this book for information on the herb, *Graviola,* and its preventative and curative properties. According to Health Sciences Institute, "[S]ince the early 1990s, extensive independent research – including research by one of today's leading drug companies and by the National Cancer Institute confirms that the [Graviola] tree's chemical extracts attack and destroy cancer cells with lethal precision.[32] It has even been noted, in laboratory testing that Graviola has greater capacity at killing colon and breast cancer cells than Adriamycin, a common chemo drug. HSI explains that the chemicals in Graviola "selectively hunt down and kill cancer cells without harming healthy cells, unlike chemotherapy."[33] Research at "Purdue University...recently found that leaves from the Graviola tree killed cancer cells 'among six human-cell lines' and were especially effective against **prostate and pancreatic** cancer cells."[34] (See chapter four in this book for the story of a cancer patient who used Graviola to cure his prostate cancer, and chapter five for the patient who used it to cure abdominal cancer!)

IV. Fruits That Can Save Your Life!

Limonene Destroys Breast Cancer Cells

Research has revealed that an ingredient found in citrus fruits (as well as the skin of oranges, limes, and grapefruits) can block the formation of breast and lung cancers. Selene Yeager, author of *Doctors Book of FOOD REMEDIES,* describes one particular animal study from "Duke University Medical Center, Durham, North Carolina...[where] 10% limonene" was added to the diets of the animals, resulting in a "70% reduction in cancerous tumors," and of "the tumors that remained, 20 percent shrank to less than half their former size."[35] She explains further:

> "The way that limonene acts on tumor cells or lesions is really interesting and unique," says Michael Gould, Ph.D., professor of human oncology at the University of Wisconsin Medical School in Madison. Essentially, the compound gets cancer cells to self-destruct. It assists them in their own suicides.[36]

Limonene is available as a supplement at natural health food stores. You should know that before you start grating raw citrus peelings for this nutrient, take caution. Raw fruit peelings such as lemons, limes, and grapefruits are fine in small amounts, but they do have chemicals that can be toxic if ingested in excessively large quantities. (I can't imagine anyone wanting to eat a lot of lemon peel!)

Cherries Prevent & Treat Cancer

According to Ms. Yeager, "perillyl alcohol" is "a monoterpene that is found in cherries..," which can inhibit the formation of "breast, lung, stomach, liver and skin" cancers as discovered in animal testing at the "University School of Medicine in Indianapolis."[37]

She says that studies were also done at the "University of Wisconsin" by "Charles Elson, Ph.D...professor of nutritional sciences," who reported that the compound in cherries doesn't just "fight cancer" by zapping the toxins that promote cancer, but it was found to work in test "animals with existing tumors."[38] The monoterpene found in cherries is even more potent than limonene against cancer!

Always try to get organic cherries if possible. Conventionally grown cherries are often heavily sprayed with pesticides and herbicides. (Cherries, especially sour cherries, have long been used to relieve the symptoms of gout.)

In her book *How To Renew You*, Maureen Kennedy Salaman says of "malic acid" found in "apples, cherries, and other fruits," that it works as a natural chelating agent, and that according to lab studies, it "effectively removed aluminum from the brains of aluminum-poisoned mice."[39] Ms. Salaman also notes that sulfur containing foods ("onions, garlic, chives, red pepper...egg yolks...asparagus, legumes...sesame, pumpkin...sunflower seeds, and English walnuts") are good chelating agents, removing toxic metals from the human body.[40] (Cilantro works much the same way.)

(You can get some very potent cherry and blueberry supplements at website: *http://www.flavonoidsciences.com/research/c3.htm.*)

Lifesaving Berries

Researchers have discovered that compounds taken from fruits inhibited not only cancer of the cervix, but two types of breast cancers. The fruits tested were blueberries and strawberries.

Cranberries & Breast Cancer

Animal studies done at Western Ontario University demonstrated that ingesting cranberries on a regular basis may be important in preventing breast cancers.[41]

Ellagic Acid & Tangeretin Against Breast Cancer

Ellagic acid (most abundant in grapes and berries), according to Dr. Don Colbert in his book, *Walking in Divine Health*, "neutralizes cancer and the toxins that cause cancer. They also protect against damage to our chromosomes."[42] One of the richest sources of ellagic acid is raspberries! (Pomegranates also have ellagic acid.)[43]

Dr. Colbert says that tangerines contain a powerful antioxidant known as "tangeretin" that "inhibits the invasiveness of cancer.[44] Research is also being conducted regarding its ability to help slow the spread of breast cancer...." Tangerines are one of the few fruits that are not sprayed with "pesticides..."[45]

Papaya for Breast Cancer

According to Harald Tietze in *Papaya The Healing Fruit*, papaya can "inhibit the growth of human breast cancer cells."[46] It "detoxifies the body, speeds metabolic processes and increases elimination of toxins...and has become recognized as one of the major medicinal plants in tropical countries."[47] See Chapter 20 of this book for more information on papaya and cancer. Also note that papaya enzymes may have blood-thinning properties.

Resveratrol – How Grapes May Save Your Life

Refer to chapter two for information on this amazing ingredient in grapes that has shown the ability to not only suppress the growth of cancer cells, but in many cases, even destroy them once they have already developed!

Mangosteen Fruit for Breast Cancer

According to a study described at the *Cancer Tutor*™ website, when mangosteen fruit's *"(Garcinia mangostana L)"* potent antioxidant plant nutrients were tested against a "human breast cancer cell line," it was discovered that they had the ability to cause the cells to self-destruct, making it a candidate for breast cancer prevention. This fruit is grown and harvested in several countries.[48]

V. Life-Saving Vegetables

Anti-Cancer Nutrients in the Cabbage Family

Cruciferous vegetables such as broccoli, cauliflower, cabbage and brussel sprouts are receiving a great deal of publicity in the world of nutrition for their known cancer-fighting properties. Cauliflower, for example, contains the two powerful anti-cancer "phytonutrients sulforaphane and indol-3-carbinol, or I3C."[49] (See the information earlier in this chapter on D.I.M!)

Sulforaphane apparently helps by assisting the body to form "enzymes" capable of flushing dangerous free radicals from the system before they can cause cellular harm. IC3, on the other hand, can cause the excretion of toxic estrogens from the body, thus protecting against hormone sensitive cancers of the breast and prostate.[50]

Pound for pound, cauliflower contains more vitamin C than tangerines or white grapefruits, but it is best to eat it raw, as cooking destroys much of the vitamin C and indole content. Cauliflower is also high in "purines," meaning those suffering with "gout" might enjoy other members of the cruciferous family for their anti-cancer properties, rather than cauliflower.[51] The high sulfur content of garlic also inhibits the growth of cancer cells, as do rutabaga, turnips, and watercress.[52]

How A Popular Mushroom Cured Breast Cancer!

The Maitake Mushroom AND D-Fraction, a book by Shari Lieberman, Ph.D., and Ken Babal, C.N., documents the story of a "45-year-old" woman who was cured of breast cancer taking maitake D-fraction. The patient opted for breast removal in 1992, "then received chemotherapy including 5-FU and ADM until February 1994." However, in spite of the surgery and the chemo, her **cancer returned** two months later! "She refused to take surgery this time and started taking 100 mg (about 100 drops) D-fraction and 5 g maitake tablets every day." After taking this amount for "six months, the dose of D-fraction…was reduced to 50 mg a day. In May 1995, complete regression of the recurred tumor was confirmed by her physician."[53]

You can find maitake supplements (including the maitake D-fraction) at some natural health food stores. Those with "multiple sclerosis" should not take maitake. There is "one form of interferon stimulated by maitake, gamma-interferon," that can cause "nerve tissue" to be destroyed, thus it is not recommended for those with MS, until more studies have been done.[53a]

Beta Glucan – The Yeast & Shiitake Mushroom Extract That Fights Breast Cancer

Website *www.newhope.com* describes "beta-glucan" as an extract of "baker's yeast." They further describe a "human study" from 1975 in "the *Journal of the National Cancer Institut,*" [sic] on the "anti-cancer effects of beta-glucan on nine cancer patients." These patients had either "skin, breast or lung cancer." When "beta-glucan" was "injected into their tumors," the tumors shrank "within five days," and this occurred "in all cases."[54] **These were amazing results, yet appar-**

ently, they did not catch the attention of the media or mainstream medicine!

According to C. Borek, Ph.D, at *www.newhope.com,* "Lentinan" is a "beta…glucan derived from the shiitake mushroom." It is used in Japan "for the treatment of advanced-cancer patients." When patients were given the extract intravenously, it "prolonged survival, sometimes five or more years."[55]

Lutein & Lycopene Fight Breast Cancer

Scientific research has shown that lycopene not only helps to inhibit the formation of breast malignancies, but it keeps the cancerous cells from multiplying![56] Lutein prevents this type cancer as well. Two of the best sources of lycopene are tomatoes and guavas. It is also found in watermelon, berries, red grapefruit, red peppers, carrots, and several other foods.[57] Good sources of lutein are dark green leafy vegetables such as spinach, collards, and turnip greens as well as egg yolks, but if using eggs, be sure they are organic! Avocados are also very high in lutein! Lycopene and lutein can also be purchased in supplement form in most health food stores, however, getting them from natural, organic food sources is always best, when possible. (Lutein is also a critical nutrient for maintaining eye health.)

Those who have a tendency to develop kidney or gallbladder stones should not consume large amounts of raw spinach due to its high "oxalate" content. Also, if you are taking "calcium supplements," wait "2-3 hours before or after" ingesting fresh spinach, since oxalates can inhibit calcium's assimilation by the body.[57a] Cooking destroys much of the oxalates. (See page 46 to prevent oxalate stones!)

VI. Soy Products & Breast Cancer

Soy contains "protease inhibitors," which, according to Don Colbert, M.D., in his book, *Walking In Divine Health,* are actually the soybeans' "defense against destruction. Birds can swallow the seed, but can't digest this substance. It is excreted. What is unique about a protease inhibitor is that it cannot be broken down," thus giving it the capacity to "block" cancer cell formation and growth.[58] Studies document that these substances can cause cancerous cells to actually revert "back to their original precancerous state."[59] (Weak phytoestrogens, such as those found in fermented soy products, like Haelan, can help remove harmful estrogens from the body in estrogen-positive cancers.) There is also a lot of information circulating regarding impurities in soy. (Fermented soy is fine!) For those who do choose to use soy products (such as with the Budwig flax oil diet), I would recommend using organic soy only.

Breast Cancer Cured With Haelan!

According to an article by Donna Sage, M.S.S.A., at website: *www.wellbeing journal.com/haelan.htm*, Haelan is nothing more than "a fermented soy beverage," but cancer patients are crediting this drink to curing their disease! The Chinese produced the drink over two decades ago for "a hospital nutritional supplement." It has high amounts of "the two main isoflavones" in soy, "genistein and daidzein," as well as "protease inhibitors," discussed earlier. Fermented soy contains many important vitamins and minerals.[60] (Note that genistein can also lower blood pressure.)

Many case studies are available of Haelan curing cancer, and Ms. Sage tells of one in particular involving Nina P. from Russia, who was told "in the late summer [of] 1996" that she had metastasizing "breast cancer" that had already spread "to her left arm, clavicle, hips, and spine." When her physician recommended surgery, she refused, and she was given "six months" to live. Nina changed her diet, "eliminating refined sugars." She consumed large amounts of "fresh vegetables, fish, and fruit," and began taking "vitamin supplements." She also started taking daily walks. Her son, Alexander, began looking for alternative treatments that might help his ailing mother, and he ran across Haelan.[61]

"Nina began to drink a bottle of Haelan per day in January 1997," along with her other lifestyle changes which had already helped her to survive five more months. At a follow-up visit with her physician in "March" of "1997," she had already outlived her six month life expectancy, so of course, her oncologist was quite shocked when she walked into their office! No trace of cancer could be found "in her bones or breasts," and "mammograms performed in April and November, 1997" were completely normal! She continued to take "four tablespoons of Haelan per day as a wellness dose to maintain optimum health."[62]

A report available (2000), noted that Nina was still cancer free at age 82. (It is interesting to note that Alexander's father "began taking two tablespoons of Haelan per day" for his "severe Parkinson's disease." He reported "a 90% reduction in tremors.")[63]

As of April 2005, Donna Sage informed me that Nina recently passed away, but not from cancer, from old age! Her cancer never recurred!

Another case history described by Ms. Sage is that of Patty Soccoman who was told she had "ductile carcinoma." After a biopsy (which confirmed the malignancy), her physician recommended "either a total mastectomy or a lumpectomy with removal of the lymph nodes under her arm followed by aggressive radiation...She chose a lumpectomy," but argued that she did not want to lose her "lymph nodes..." When she told her doctor, he wanted nothing to do with a mere lump removal. He insisted on breast removal. She was referred to an oncologist of whom she said:

> My doctor tried to scare me into surgery....I was anxious after my visit, because my doctor was so aggressive....He said that if he was my husband, he would duct tape my mouth shut and force me to have the radical surgery....That was the last time I went to that doctor![64]

In early November 1997, Ms. Sage says that Patty started to ingest "a bottle per day of Haelan." During this same time, she also "supplemented with flax oil, CoQ10, and fresh vegetable and fruit juices...chelation treatments...vitamin C," and an "80% raw, organic foods" diet.[65]

Six weeks went by and diagnostics showed that the breast tumor had decreased remarkably. Subsequent mammograms revealed that the tumor was progressively shrinking in size. When a mammogram in "August" of "1999" showed a mere "shadow" where the tumor was once located, "no evidence of metastases," and no other signs of cancer, Patty's "radiologist…Dr. Robert L. Turk" said that "in his 32 years of experience…'This doesn't occur; I have not seen these kinds of improvements.'"[66]

Dr. Turk also admitted that he "is skeptical about chemotherapy," and believed that just because a "cancer" protocol is given "FDA" approval is no indication that it is "safe." When asked if he recommends Haelan, "Dr. Turk said, 'My wife is on it, if that is any indication! Mrs. Turk is surviving colon and liver cancer.'"[67]

According to an update from Patty in 2000, at age 65, she was still cancer free. She also stated that since starting Haelan, her cataracts had disappeared. During her illness, she drank Haelan every day for "seven months" (one bottle). She said that she now takes about "2 oz every day" for "maintenance." Patty credits her dietary changes, renting comedy movies to boost her immune system, and her "strong faith in God," to helping her overcome cancer.[68]

I just recently learned from Donna Sage that, as of April, 2005, Patty Soccoman is still doing fine at age 70 with no recurrence of cancer! I also spoke to Patty in June of 2005 and she is doing wonderfully and still drinks Haelan as a preventative. She never had the radical surgery her physician recommended (just a lumpectomy), no radiation and no chemo! (Note that Haelan is usually taken on an empty stomach for maximum absorption.)

Fermented soy drinks are available at some health food stores. You can also purchase Haelan at website: *www.haelanproducts.com.*

VII. How The Right Fats Work To Prevent & Cure Breast Cancer

Flax – The Miracle Oil for Cancer Prevention

See Chapter 17 for the amazing curative properties of flax oil for all cancers! Borage oil and primrose oil are also discussed in that chapter.

CLA – Conjugated Linoleic Acid Prevents Metastasis

CLA, a "trace fatty acid," effectively prevents the formation of tumors as well as their spread throughout other areas of the body. It also promotes the self-destruction of tumor cells! Particularly impressive was a report published in *Anticancer Research* that in vitro and animal testing showed CLA blocked not only the growth, but the spread of human breast cancer. As explained on *Life Extension* website: "CLA alone increased lymphocyte numbers and their cell killing ability...[and] completely abolished the spread of breast cancer cells to the lungs, blood, and bone marrow." From the studies done, this fatty acid worked even better when combined with beta-carotene![69] (CLA supplements can be found at most natural health food stores.) Not to be confused with the harmful form of linoleic acid.

VIII. Herbs For Breast Health

Andrographis

According to website *www.herbs2000.com, "Andrographis paniculata"* is not a widely known herb, but it has "an extensive history in Asia" where the leaves and stems are highly cultivated. It is a medicinal herb used for "upper respiratory infections, fever, herpes, sore throat, and a variety of chronic and infectious diseases," as well as "cancer...headache," liver infections, "HIV" and "gallstone formation."[70] Recent studies show favorable outcomes with this herb against breast cancer cells. *"Androtech* (produced by BioTherapies)" combines this herb "with enchinacea."[71] *Herbs2000.com* also reports that andrographis can contribute toward infertility in both sexes. Do not use it "during pregnancy and nursing." Toxicity is rare and may include "dizziness and heart palpitations" in some persons. As with any herb, there is always the potential for "allergic" reactions, from "mild rash to more serious anaphylaxis."[72]

Cat's Claw Against Cancer

Cat's claw, also known as *Uno de Gato* can be found growing in the forests of the Amazon. It is known for its ability to enhance the body's immunity.

This herb is popular in Europe for treating a variety of ailments, and it is being investigated there "as a potential treatment for various cancers."[73] As described in Rita Elkins' book, *Cat's Claw (Uno de Gato),* one physician in particular had great success using this herb and others "in treating 14 types of accurately diagnosed cancer in 700 patients between 1984 and 1988." (The herb is also a "source of proanthocyanidin (pycnogenol)"[74]

Herbs2000.com explains that Uno de Gato should not be used with "hormonal drugs, insulin, or vaccines..." It should not be used for children, during pregnancy or lactation, without consulting a physician, nor if you have an "autoimmune illness, multiple sclerosis, or tuberculosis."[75]

Dandelion for Breast Cancer

According to *www.cancertutor.com,* the people of China "have used dandelion for breast cancer for over a thousand years." There are "7000 units of vitamin A per ounce" of "dandelion greens....In 1979, Japanese researchers found a dandelion extract...which inhibits Ehrlich ascites cancer cells."[76]

Dandelions are richer in "carotene than carrots," important for patients fighting cancer, because many cancer patients suffer from abnormally low levels of vitamin A. Dandelion greens are also rich in vitamins and minerals such as iron.[77] However, since dandelion can also have diuretic properties, be sure that if you drink dandelion tea or eat dandelion greens, you are getting extra potassium in your diet, even though dandelions do contain some potassium. You can some-times find organically grown dandelion greens at local health food stores reasonably priced. If you yank the greens from your front yard or some country roadside, first be sure that they haven't been sprayed with chemicals! You should not use dandelion if you have any type of biliary disease (or ulcers) since the herb can stimulate bile flow and increase gastric acid. Do not consume any herb high in iron if you suffer from a rare genetic disorder known as hemochromatosis. (Before beginning any herbal regimen, consult with your physician.)

Garlic for Cancer Prevention

Though considered more of a *spice* than an herb, garlic has proven effective in the prevention of many types of cancer, and apparently it does not take much. Less than one clove per day can boost the immune system. According to Optimal Diet Healthy Eating website (at *http://homodiet.netfirms.com)*, "Some researchers say that one medium-sized garlic clove has as much antibacterial power as 100,000 units of penicillin."[78]

Garlic can lower blood pressure and increase clotting (coagulation) time, so consult with your physician if you are on blood-thinners or blood pressure medications before taking large amounts of fresh garlic or garlic supplements, or if you are contemplating surgery, or just recovering from a surgical procedure.

Garlic is able to inhibit substances that promote cancer development, and has demonstrated the ability to significantly reduce tumor growth. It was found that mashing the bulbs releases the compounds that fight cancerous cells.

In her book, *The Food Pharmacy*, Jean Carper explains that in one animal test using garlic, scientists discovered that "fresh garlic completely wiped out breast cancers in the mice." They gave the credit to "garlic's allicin."[79]

Green Tea

Green tea is such a potent antioxidant it is discussed in detail in several other chapters of this book. I would recommend drinking several cups per day of decaffeinated organic green tea for anyone with cancer, auto-immune disorders, or simply for health maintenance.

Milk Thistle Inhibits Breast Cancer

According to *herbs2000.com*, this herb "binds to estrogen receptor sites on cancer cells," blocking harmful estrogen from entering the cells.[80] If milk thistle causes diarrhea, either cut down on how much you are taking, or "stop taking it" altogether.[81] (The loose stools "usually cease within two or three days," and occur because the herb promotes "liver and gallbladder activity.")[82]

In his book: *Natural Strategies for Cancer Patients,* Dr. Russell Blaylock says that an extract from milk thistle, *"silymarin,"* was shown to be "effective against...breast cancer, skin cancers, and other carcinomas."[83] (Milk thistle is also discussed in chapter eight of this book on liver cancer because of its amazing ability to rejuvenate and heal the liver. See the case history in that chapter of a terminal liver cancer patient who was totally cured using milk thistle! It is also being used to help fight colon and skin cancer!)

Be aware that if you have a chronic disorder such as hemochromatosis (the body absorbs too much iron – this is a genetic disorder that you would have been born with), you need to be sure that your physician approves your using milk thistle and other herbs. You want to be sure that if you are approved to take it, the herb you use is a standardized extract that is not high in iron! Also, if you are awaiting a transplant, or have already had one, you should never take any herbal preparations without consulting your physician, because they may interfere with your anti-rejection medications.

Pau d' Arco

Pau d' Arco (also known as *taheebo*) demonstrated in scientific studies in **humans,** the ability to prevent breast malignances from spreading.[84] (This tea is also known as *lapacho.* Be aware that lapacho was just one of the compounds extracted from pau d'arco tea and lapacho has blood-thinning properties.) Most health food stores have pau d'arco tea.

Red Clover & Rosemary

Rosemary, because of an ingredient that it contains known as "carnosol," may help cut the risk for malignancies of the breast.[85]

James Duke, Ph.D., in *The Green Pharmacy* says of "Red clover *(Trifolium pratense),*" that it contains a compound called "genistein," which prevents the formation of new "blood vessels," thus "starving tumors."[86] Note that this effect of blocking blood vessel formation is exactly how shark cartilage also works! Do not use red clover in excessive amounts without consulting your licensed health care practitioner. It can affect clotting (coagulation) time. Genistein can also lower blood pressure. Rosemary can raise blood pressure.

Rhodiola Rosea

Rhodiola is "a member of the family Crassulaceae," according to website *www.planetherbs.com,* and is "native to the arctic regions of Eastern Siberia," growing at very high altitudes! The old saying in "Siberia" is that "those who drink rhodiola tea regularly will live more than 100 years." It is a "potent antioxidant...able to combat all the diseases associated with aging."[87]

In Russia, "researchers have found that the oral administration of rhodiola inhibited tumor growth in rats 39 percent and decreased metastasis by 50 percent," and "in other experiments with various types of cancer, including...(cancer of glandular tissue such as breast cancer) and lung carcinoma," this herb "increased survival rate." It can be found at "Planetary Formulas Online Store."[88] See website: *www.planetherbs.com.* for the full article.

Schisandra

Schisandra "*(Schisandra chinensis)*" inhibits cancers of the breast, probably because it has a high amount of "lignans."[89] Schisandra seeds have numerous antioxidant ingredients that help prevent liver damage. It is also used by the Chinese to treat liver disease and inflammation.[90]

St. John's Wort

St. John's Wort, according to *www.herbs2000.com,* has demonstrated the ability to keep cancer from metastasizing to the "chest wall and lungs." It should not be used "if you are on prescription antidepressants or any medication that interacts with MAO inhibitors. Use it with caution during pregnancy." This herb also causes sun sensitivity, so be sure to avoid prolonged sun exposure when using it.[91] (MAO inhibitors are anti-depressant medications. Not all anti-depressants are considered MAO inhibitors. If you are taking any type of anti-depressant medication, your physician or pharmacist can tell you whether or not it is a MAO inhibitor and what foods and/or medications can be deadly if mixed with MAO inhibitors.)

Turmeric

Turmeric, rich in curcumin, can "activate" gene "p53" for combating cancer. This gene is important because it has the ability to suppress the genes that are responsible for causing cancer.[92] Turmeric is safe when used as a spice, however, if you are taking turmeric in supplement form, do not use if pregnant, nor if you have gallstones, since it stimulates the gallbladder. Like garlic, turmeric can slow clotting time, so it should be used in caution by anyone taking anti-coagulant medications,[92a] with blood disorders, or for anyone recovering from or contemplating surgery, or in those with ulcers.

Wormwood Used in Fighting Breast Cancer

According to website *www.cancertutor.com:* an herb known as *sweet wormwood* (containing the active ingredient artemisinin), has been tested for its effectiveness against breast cancer cells. One of the studies was "published in the *Journal of Life Sciences.*" The article "described how the compound killed virtually all human breast cancer cells exposed to it within sixteen hours…. Dr. Henry Lai…of the University of Washington," said that "…it's very selective…it's highly toxic to the cancer cells, but has a marginal impact on normal breast cells."[93]

Wormwood has long been a popular remedy for killing parasites and worms, and it is a cure for malaria, however, says Cancer Tutor™, "The UN and UNICEF refused to allow sweet wormwood to treat malaria…until it could be combined with a profitable pharmaceutical drug."[94] The website also points out the fact that malaria is caused by a parasite, and since wormwood kills cancer cells, perhaps the herb "could give credibility to the theory of some that cancer is caused by a parasite."[95] (Before beginning any herbal regimen, discuss with your physician.)

IX. Miscellaneous Supplements

Calcium D–Glucarate™ For Breast Cancer

D-glucarate is a normal component of many foods, especially "apples, grapefruits, broccoli and alfalfa sprouts."[96] As explained by Rita Elkins, M.H., in her book *D-Glucarate, Powerful Protector Against Breast and Prostate Cancers*, this substance was isolated by "Walaszek and his co-workers" and patented in "1986." It can rid the body of unneeded estrogen, and it "may not only work to prevent breast cancer, but has also reversed it in some animal test cases."[97]

Ms. Elkins says that there have been no reports of toxicity in "human trials" with D-Glucarate, "even at very high doses." However, since this nutrient works by detoxifying "hormones and chemicals" in the body, it may lower serum amounts of "prescription drugs" that you are taking, so be sure to clear usage with your physician.[98]

Cartilage For Breast Cancer Remission

Shark cartilage contains proteins that prevent tumors from forming new blood vessels, and, as noted by website *http://www.nutrition-farm.com/GLOSSARY/REPORTS/sharkrept.htm,* it works exceptionally well at shrinking tumors:

[T]he tumor can no longer receive nutrients necessary to sustain growth, form new tumors, and spread to other areas by way of these blood vessels...when all nutrient supply is stopped, the tumor will begin to turn upon itself, starve, die, and be consumed as dead cells.[99]

The compounds that inhibit this blood vessel growth are about "1000 times more concentrated in shark cartilage than in bovine cartilage," says *nutritionfarm.com*, thus you would have to ingest "enormous quantities" of bovine cartilage to get the same dosage as provided by shark cartilage.[100] "All forms of cancer can be treated with shark cartilage; however, the ideal types are tumor-forming cancers. It appears to be particularly successful in the treatment of breast cancer."[101]

See your natural health physician for specific dosing for your own particular condition. Do not use shark cartilage or bovine cartilage without consulting with your physician, especially if you are on prescription medications, have high blood pressure, a recent history of heart attack, surgery, transplant, or pending surgery or are pregnant, nor if you are taking chemo or radiation. It is not recommended for children. It is not for those with pheochromocytoma (adrenal tumor which can cause excessively high blood pressure), seafood allergies, ulcers or circulatory diseases. It is not for those with liver disease, except that it has been used successfully against liver cancer. For more information on dosing, see chapter six in this book.

Clodronate Prevents Breast Cancer Metastasis to the Bone

According to *www.cancertutor.com*, "Clodronate [a] biophosphonate," is said to prevent "breast cancer from spreading to the bones," however, it is "not available" in America due to "suppression" by the FDA, in spite of an article in the *"New England Journal of Medicine...Aug. 6, 1998,"* which said of clodronate that it had the ability to limit the spread of "breast cancer [in] high-risk breast cancer patients by 50%."[102]

Coley's Toxins Fight Breast Cancer

According to Dr. Ralph Moss, in his book *Cancer Therapy,* William B. Coley, M.D., was responsible for the development of "Coley's Toxins" in the late 19th century. They were actually developed from "two common bacteria." The results of treatment with Coley's toxins were "impressive" not only with breast cancer, but Hodgkin's, ovarian cancer, and melanoma malignancies as well. In studies done involving breast cancer patients, Dr. Moss says that "Thirteen of 20 of the inoperable (65 percent)...patients had five-year-survival." Coley's toxins are still being used today, predominantly in European countries and China.[103]

I believe it is best to use "natural" treatments for cancer prevention and treatment whenever possible. Coley's toxins are not "natural," but are being included here for informational purposes, and because of their reported success at prolonging the lives of cancer patients.

Hydrazine Sulfate & Breast Cancer

When Sharon W. was diagnosed with Stage IV cancer of the breast, it had already spread to nearly every vital organ of her body, as well as her lymph and skeletal system. She was told that she had less than two months to live. She refused chemo and any other conventional treatments and contacted Dr. Joseph Gold for hydrazine sulfate treatments. In less than three months, her pain had completely disappeared, and a new CT scan revealed that the only thing left of her massive cancer was three small hepatic growths. Two years have passed since she was given less than two months to live. She is still very much alive and doing quite well!

Be aware that hydrazine sulfate is a MAO inhibitor. As noted earlier in this chapter, there are certain foods and drugs that you can never combine with MAO inhibitors or the results can be deadly. Your physician can give you a complete list of foods and drugs that should never be combined with MAO inhibitors. See chapter 15 for more information on Dr. Joseph Gold and hydrazine sulfate.

Ukrain – Effective Non-Toxic Cure For Breast Cancer!

Ukrain is a combination of the plant "greater celandine" and a common drug "thiotepa," which are both toxic when used alone, but when combined, they are only toxic to cancer cells![104]

The main Ukrain website, *www.ukrin.com*, describes a human trial involving "363 cancer patients with 47 different types of tumour" that were all "treated with UKRAIN between September 1997 and January 2003 at the Villa Medica Clinic (Edenkoben, Germany) under the medical direction of Dr. Aschoff." Every patient, without exception had already "exhausted conventional means of therapy without success," and were either progressing in their cancer or had relapsed.[105] (In other words, all of them were terminal; conventional medicine had nothing left to offer them!) The website says that "the following rates of full remission were achieved":

> [B]reast cancer 31%, colorectal cancer 16.7%, bronchial adenocarcinoma 7.7%, small-cell bronchial carcinoma 21%, astrocytoma (brain tumor) 66.6%, neuroblastoma 60%, seminoma (testicular cancer) 75%, bladder carcinoma 50%.[106]

Ukrain is only available through alternative health clinics in the U.S., Canada and Europe. See the Ukrain website above for more information.

X. Low Fat Diet Inhibits Breast Cancer

Maureen Kennedy Salaman emphasizes the importance of a low fat diet in the prevention of breast cancer in her book, *Nutrition: The Cancer Answer II*: "One study shows women who reduce their fat intake from an average of 40-45 percent of total calories to 20 percent or less can reduce their chances of developing breast cancer."[107]

XI. Other Important Lifestyle Changes

Eydie Mae Hunsberger, Dee Simmons, Rita Myers, Johanna Brandt and others did not cure their cancers merely with a raw foods diet. (For one of the best websites on raw foods and a great recipe book, LIVING ON LIVE FOOD, see *AlissaCohen.com*.) Their diet plan incorporated a total way of living that involved many other aspects of health, besides dietary changes. Several of these are discussed later in this book. For example – proper rest, exercise, oxygen, fresh air, adequate water, prayer, a positive attitude, unselfishness, stress reduction, and faith in God – are all critically important in helping the body get well.

Though diet itself is the main focus of this chapter, it is not intended that the rest of these ingredients, so important for optimal health, be minimized. (Neither is this chapter, or this book, an exhaustive reference for vitamins, herbs and other nutritional remedies in fighting breast cancer and other cancers.)

The Importance of Water

According to the late Dr. F. Batmanghelidj, M.D., in his book, *Your Body's Many Cries For Water*, cancer patients are dehydrated. It is important that you get adequate amounts of water on a daily basis. This quantity of water requires extra salt. He recommended that "For every 10 glasses of water (about two quarts)" you drink, you need an extra "half teaspoon of salt per day."[108] Follow unless your physician has you on a special water-restricted or salt-restricted diet. See chapter 22 in this book *(Water, The Desperate Thirst)* for detailed information on the importance of water drinking for cancer prevention and health maintenance and amounts recommended, depending on your body weight.

CHAPTER 4

PAINLESS CURES & PREVENTIONS FOR PROSTATE CANCER

"More than one hundred thousand admissions to hospitals in the U.S. per year and more than sixteen thousand deaths each year are the result of upper-GI bleeding caused by the use of NSAIDS."
(Ray D. Strand, M.D., et al. from the book: *What Your Doctor Doesn't Know About Nutritional Medicine May Be Killing You.*)[1]

The Prostate Cancer That Vanished! Case #1

An herb from the Rainforest, known as *Graviola,* is showing great promise in the fight against several forms of cancer. Many documented cases of complete cures are being reported as a result of using this herb!

There are many case stories of cancer remissions from Graviola, including one from the Health Sciences Institute newsletter that tells of "an executive at a high-tech company in Texas." His name is "Daryl S.," and he discovered Raintree while he was "exploring alternative treatments to cure his prostate cancer." A "biopsy had confirmed...more than 20 tumors in his prostate!" His physician recommended surgery, but Daryl refused, knowing that surgery might mean a lifetime of "impotence and incontinence." As explained by Health Sciences Institute at website *http://www.hsibaltimore.com,* Daryl opted for something besides surgery for his cancer:

> Instead, he agreed to a far less invasive round of hormonal therapy to shrink the size of his prostate and began a rigorous supplement regimen that centered around the Graviola-rich supplement *N-Tense.* Within two months, Daryl's PSA level had dropped from 4.1 to 0.00. A sonogram and several other gamma-ray tests later confirmed that all **the malig-**

nant tumors inside his prostate had disappeared.[2] [Emphasis, mine.]

Case #2 – Another Prostate Cancer Disappears!

Dr. Abram Hoffer was able to bring about a complete prostate cancer cure in a patient who was told by his conventional medicine physicians that he was "untreatable." He was diagnosed with "sarcoma of the prostate" that had metastasized to his "pelvic bone." When the patient came to seek treatment from Dr. Abram Hoffer, he was only able to tolerate 10 grams of vitamin C daily by mouth, so Dr. Hoffer suggested injections of "10 grams of vitamin C twice weekly," as well as the oral doses. "After six months...the tumor was gone." He no longer needed the injections and he survived his ordeal living "another 9 years." He "died at age 80, but not from his cancer."[3] See the complete story at Dr. Abram Hoffer's webpage: *http://www.island-net.com/ ~hoffer.*

Avoid Milk – Cut Your Risk of Prostate Cancer

Another way to be sure to cut your risk of getting prostate cancer is to avoid milk and milk products entirely! See chapter 25 in this book for all the reasons why you should avoid cow's milk!

Life Extension's website at *www.lef.org*, has this to say about prostate cancer and milk:

> Plant foods are cancer protective, while animal foods tend to be cancer promoters....A study published in the journal *Cancer* shows that consuming three or more glasses of milk a day more than **doubles** the risk of prostate cancer...In European countries such as France and Switzerland where cattle hormone implants are banned, the incidence of prostate cancer is 50% less than in the U.S.; in Italy and Greece, it is about 75% below the U.S. rate.[4]

This study proves that the high amounts of hormones being injected into cattle in the U.S. are increasing our cancer statistics! Why are these harmful hormones allowed? If you insist on drinking cow's milk, buy organic, or better yet, use organic SOY milk products instead! Even though there is some controversy about soy products, if used in moderation, I believe they are safer than cow's milk! Chapter 25 will tell you exactly why! (Fermented soy products, such as Haelan, can help remove harmful estrogens from the body in estrogen-receptor positive cancers.)

Bee Pollen Extract Protects the Prostate

A common extract of bee pollen, *"Cernitin,"* prevents hyperplasia of the prostate and helps neutralize toxins. Animal research revealed that cernitin prevented poisonous cadmium from being absorbed in the body and it also reduced harmful blood lipids.[5]

Beta-Carotene Protects Against Prostate Cancer

Beta-carotene (as well as lycopene) has been shown to reduce the risk of prostate cancer. As described by Jack Challem in his book *All About Carotenoids Beta-carotene, Lutein & Lycopene,* in one research group involving thousands of "Harvard Medical School" physicians over a period of "twelve years," an analysis was made depending on the dietary levels of "beta-carotene" consumed. Some physicians supplemented with "50 mg. every other day," while others took varying amounts of the nutrient.[6]

Results showed that low dietary consumption of beta-carotene increased the risk of "prostate cancer" by "one-third," however Mr. Challem reports that dieters deficient in "fruits and vegetables" could still slash their risk of "prostate cancer…"36-percent" simply by supplementing with this critical nutrient.[7] Please note that Mr. Challem has a new book out: *Feed Your Genes Right: Eat to Turn Off Disease-Causing Genes and Slow Down Aging,* and it is described in detail at website *www.feedyourgenesright.com.*

Beta-Sitosterol Decreases Prostate Tumor Growth

In her book, *D-Glucarate, Powerful Protector Against Breast and Prostate Cancers,* Rita Elkins, M.H., reports that "beta-sitosterol" could reduce the "growth" of "cancerous tumors in the prostate" within just one week of treatment by "twenty-four percent."[8] See chapter five of this book for more information about instances when this supplement should not be taken.

You will find that many health food stores have combination herbal blends for prostate health. One example is *Zyflamend* from "New Chapter, Inc., Brattleboro, Vermont." This compound contains "rosemary, turmeric, ginger, holy basil and green tea," as well as derivatives of "hu zhang, Chinese goldthread, barberry, oregano and Scutellaria baicalensis." As reported by "the Society of Urologic Oncology," and noted by Karla Gale in *Reuters Health,* laboratory testing with Zyflamend against prostate cancer cells "led to a 78% reduction in cell number after 72 hours." It appeared even more potent than "curcumin alone."[9] This compound has blood-thinning effects. Always consult with your physician before beginning any new herbal regimen such as Zyflamend.

Boron Can Help Prevent Prostate Cancer

Reuters Health Information also reports that adequate amounts of boron in your diet can prevent prostate cancer! "Men who consume diets high in boron [found in fruits and nuts] have a reduced risk of developing prostate cancer."[10] When "the diets of 76 men diagnosed with prostate cancer [were compared] with those of 7651 healthy males...Dr. Zuo-Fen Zhang, from the University of California at Los Angeles School of public health...said that when the men were divided into quartiles based on their consumption of boron..." those with the highest boron consumption "had 'a 64% lower risk of developing prostate cancer.'" Apparently, according to the results "...the more boron-rich foods and beverages consumed, the greater the risk reduction."[11] Charlene Rainey, "president of Food Research, Inc., Costa Mesa, California," who "developed a boron nutrition database for the

World Health Organization," said that, "It looks like 3.5 servings of boron-rich fruits and one serving of nuts [a day] would put men in the top quartile…Good boron sources include grapes, dried fruits, avocados, red wine and grape juice, she said." See the full article at *www.OncoLink.com.*[12]

Burzynski's Antineoplastons

See chapter 13 of this book for amazing cases of cancer patients completely cured of "terminal" cancers, people who were basically sent home to die, then chose non-toxic antineoplastons from the Burzynski Clinic in Houston Texas. Also see many of the patient's own stories about their success in fighting cancer with antineoplastons at website: *http://burzynskipatientgroup.org/stories.html.* Many of these cases were prostate cancer patients. Many were "hopeless," very aggressive brain tumors. The main Burzynski Clinic website is at *www.cancermed.com.*

Calcium D-Glucarate™ For Prostate Cancer

D-glucarate can be found as a natural ingredient in many foods. Rita Elkins gives some of the best sources in her book, *D-Glucarate, Powerful Protector Against Breast and Prostate Cancers:* "apples, grapefruits, broccoli and alfalfa sprouts."[13] She says that it has the ability to decrease harmful estrogen (estradiol) and testosterone in the body, and in 1990, it was revealed that the compound had the capacity to stunt the growth of tumors, thereby preventing their spread.[14] In fact, D-glucarate is so efficient at removing harmful compounds from the body that Japanese researchers discovered when they dosed rats with "kanamycin" along with the D-glucarate, that the nutrient prevented the kidney toxicity that kanamycin usually causes.[15] D-glucarate has shown no adverse effects in human testing, not even when "very high doses" were given.[16]

Cherries Stop the Growth of Prostate Cancer Cells

Studies conducted at the "University of Iowa" by "Raymond Hohl, M.D," revealed that the "perillyl alcohol (POH)" in cherries is "extremely powerful in reducing the incidence of all types of cancer."[17] This remarkable study is described at *www.flavonoidsciences.com.* "Perillyl alcohol 'shuts down the growth of cancer cells by depriving them of the proteins they need to grow,' explains Dr. Hohl. 'It works on every kind of cancer we've tested it against.'"[18] This nutrient "performed favorably in the treatment of advanced carcinomas of the breast, prostate, and ovary." It was reported to be "up to five times more potent than the other known cancer-reducing compounds at inducing tumor regression."[19] The website further explains that the ingredients in tart cherries that fight cancer are the perillyl alcohol as well as "the presence of…melatonin," and "important flavonoids – isoqueritrin and queritrin, [and] ellagic acid." They also describe research (from "the Hollings Cancer Institute at the Medical University of South Carolina (MUSC"), which revealed that "ellagic acid may be the most potent way to prevent cancer. It also may inhibit the growth of cancer cells, and arrest the growth of cancer in subjects with a genetic predisposition for the disease."[20]

Raspberries are very high in this nutrient (as are pomegranates). See more information later in this chapter on ellagic acid. (You can get some very potent cherry and blueberry supplements at Flavonoid Sciences website: *http://www.flavonoidsciences.com/research/c3.htm.)*

DHEA & Prostate Cancer

Website *www.yourhealthbase.com* reports that DHEA prevents "prostate cancer." They state that "We do not usually report information based on animal experiments; however, the finding that DHEA can prevent or even reverse prostate cancer in laboratory rats seemed important enough to make an exception."[20a] Be sure to consult with your physician before taking DHEA. He or she will want to draw blood first to be sure that your levels of DHEA are low before recommending supplementation.

Deanna K. Loftis, R.N., B.B.A.

Diet & Life Style Change Cures Prostate Cancer

When Eric Gardiner was diagnosed with prostate cancer, he began a search for a natural alternative. He had no desire to go the cut, poison and burn route! He credited the cancer to a lifetime filled with stress, improper diet, and inadequate exercise, which damaged his immune system. When his physician recommended the conventional treatment that involved "cut, burn and poison," he was less than enthusiastic and describes why in his book, *How I Conquered Cancer – A Naturopathic Alternative:*

> This type of medicine always has a downside where some-thing bad always happens. It's called "consequences" or "side-effects." You have no doubt heard of people losing their hair or throwing up or the biggie – death. John Wayne did death. Millions and millions of people do death. *After* the chemo, after the radiation, after the surgery, they do death...[21]

Mr. Gardiner met with the same resistance that Eydie Mae Hunsberger experienced when she butted heads with the current health system. He found himself questioning the wisdom of orthodox treatment when statistics show that currently accepted methods of cancer treatment produce a dismal survival rate:

> Medical school is expensive. Inventing new medicines is expensive, and you out there with your prostate are going to pay. The American Cancer Society and its related and asso-ciated organizations take in money, hundreds of millions of dollars. They have thousands of employees and they want your prostate...For years insurance companies said "These are the good guys. Use them, we'll pay for it"...[22]

Eric also knew full well that, "[I]f you don't cure the source that caused the cancer in the first place, it will come back."[23] If you are diagnosed with cancer, cutting the cancer out may not solve your problem, because you are continuing to live the same lifestyle that caused the cancer in the first place, and it often returns. When Rita Myers, Eric Gardiner, Dee Simmons, Eydie Mae, and others were diagnosed with cancer, they did not return to the same lifestyle. They did not take up where they left off and resume their old habits. They completely changed their diet and lifestyle!

Eric Gardiner changed his diet and his lifestyle and conquered his cancer. He began a regular exercise program, cut down his fat intake, increased his intake of fresh fruits, vegetables, and water, and cut the junk food out of his diet. He used a bowel cleansing program and began using nutritional supplements. He also used Dr. Hulga Clark's herbal program to kill parasites in his system. He saw immediate results. Eric also recommends buying organic produce. For those who feel buying organic isn't worth the extra cost, he explains why it makes a difference:

> At first, you may find organic foods to be higher priced. If you factor in even a small part of the stomach remedies and other cures that you don't have to buy, and perhaps even a small part of the doctor bills you don't have to pay, you will find organic foods to be a real bargain.[24]

Dr. Clark's program of killing parasites in the body is discussed in chapter 27, later in this book.

Ellagic Acid Prevents Cancer Cells From Dividing

Ellagic acid (discussed earlier in this chapter) occurs naturally "in red raspberries, strawberries, blueberries, and certain nuts." According to *mnwelldir.org*, the richest source of "ellagic acid" is "raspberries…and it doesn't matter if the fruit is boiled, baked, canned, sugared, dehydrated, or fresh, the ellagic acid is still potent." The website points out that: **Eating just "one cup [of raspberries] per week stops prostate cancers (all prostate cancers) from growing for one week."** [Emphasis, mine.][25] A recent laboratory study from the "Hollings Cancer Institute," reported that this compound:

Stops cancer cells from dividing in 48 hours...causes normal cell death...**within 72 hours** in cases of breast, pancreas, esophageal, skin, colon and prostate cancers...prevents the destruction of the p53 gene...caused apoptosis (normal cell death) in HPV (human papilloma virus) exposed to it...one cup (150 grams) per day of red raspberries **prevents the development of cancer cells.**[26] [Emphasis, mine.]

Note – if you eat **raspberries** for their ellagic acid content, *mnwelldir.org* says "eat them on an empty stomach, before you eat anything else...If your fruit sits in your stomach too long, because you've eaten something prior, stomach acid will destroy its healthful properties." Apparently, ellagic acid is also powerful enough to "destroy the H. pylori bacteria responsible for stomach ulcers."[27] (Another natural source of ellagic acid is pomegranates. See the article later in this chapter on using pomegranate juice for recurring prostate cancer!) If raspberries are not in season, you can usually find them in the frozen section of your store. Many health food stores carry organic frozen berries.

Flaxseed for Treating Prostate Cancer

Preventing cancer and maintaining health of the prostate gland is very dependent on balancing EFAs (essential fatty acids) and the body's hormone level. Flaxseed, high in essential omega-3 oils for healthy prostate functioning, is an important dietary addition for men with prostate problems, or just those wishing to prevent them! It not only prevents cancer, but it should be considered a necessary adjunctive with any prostate cancer treatment program, as well as a colon cancer prevention.[28] (See chapters 13 and 17 of this book for details on the Budwig flax oil diet that has cured many *incurable* cancer cases, including *inoperable* brain tumors!)

Garlic Prevents Prostate Cancer

Multiple laboratory studies as well as animal and human research have shown that garlic prevents cancer. Just eating a small amount of garlic every day will drastically cut the risk for prostate cancer!

Ginger & Prostate Cancer

According to *Life Extension's* webpage, in their "Cancer Adjuvant Therapy" article under "Ginger (*Zingiber officinalis*)," the herb, ginger, not only has anti-inflammatory properties, but it stimulates the destruction of human prostate cancer cells, regardless of whether or not they are "hormone responsive." The dosage they suggest for this herb is "2 grams of ginger per day."[29] (Be sure to check with your physician before beginning an herbal regimen. Ginger has blood-thinning properties and it may interefere with other medications that you may be taking.)

Ginseng & Prostate Cancer

Studies done by "physiologist…Laura Murphy" showed that "a water extract of American ginseng slowed down the growth of human breast and prostate cancer cells in culture."[30] In an article by K. C. Jaehning at *http://news.siu.edu*, "Ms. Murphy calls ginseng a 'drugstore with 20 to 30 different compounds – I've never worked with anything that complex,' says the scientist from 'Southern Illinois University Cardondale's School of Medicine, who has studied' the herb 'since the early '90s.'"[31] Dr. Murphy, also an endocrinologist, "had access to a supply of human breast cancer cells grown for researchers," and as described at the above website:

> When she and her students began treating some of these cells with a ginseng extract, they found that the higher the "dose" of ginseng, the more slowly the cancer grew. In fact, with a high enough dose, they could actually stop the cells from growing at all. "Ms. Murphy said that 'it was consistent and repetitive – a very clean result….'"[31a]

When Dr. Murphy started to test ginseng in mice, she discovered that "tumors in mice injected with breast cancer cells treated with ginseng grew only half as big as they did in the mice that went without the herb." She does not promote ginseng used alone, because "it just slows the rate of growth [of the tumor], and if you take the animal off ginseng, the tumor will come back." She does explain that "if you can slow the growth maybe you can use something else that will kill that tumor." She also emphasizes that "ginseng's powerful effects come not from a single compound…but from the whole shebang working together…you have to use the whole root." It also isn't "recommended for those with estrogen-dependent cancers," because "ginseng can have estrogen-like effects." However (and this is very interesting) Dr. Murphy "and her associates found those estrogen-like effects in alcohol-based ginseng extracts but not in water-based extracts."[31b] Though it was American ginseng that they worked with, in an email to me on 2005, May 10, Dr. Murphy states that "all ginseng types have now been shown to elicit anti-cancer properties." The reason that she worked with American ginseng was "because Asian and Korean ginsengs had already been well-studied and not much was known about the American variety."[32]

(Though some herbal websites, such as *herbs2000.com*, recommend that you avoid certain ginsengs, including American and Brazilian if you have prostate cancer, see Dr. Murphy's information regarding the water-based ginseng as opposed to alcohol-based extracts above.)

Green Tea & Black Tea Slow Prostate Cancers

According to *www.nutraingredients.com*, recent studies have shown that men who drink green tea and black tea can "slow the growth of prostate cancer cells." The "polyphenols" in the tea are "quickly absorbed in human prostate tissue," and researchers from "the University of California, Los Angeles" have found the tea protective against prostate cancers.[33]

Lycopene Cuts Prostate Cancer Risk

The Reader's Digest book, *Foods That Harm, Foods That Heal*, points out that lycopene can reduce the risk for prostatic malignancies. When nearly 50,000 participating healthcare workers, many of them physicians, were followed in a research program conducted at Harvard, it was revealed that eating foods high in lycopene several times a week could cut their chances for prostate cancer in half.[34]

One of the best (and most popular) sources of lycopene can be found in tomatoes! Guavas are also rich in lycopene, and so are many other fruits and vegetables. Though most vegetables are more nutritious in their raw state (the way nature intended), cooked tomatoes may be the exception when it comes to preventing cancer. It has been demonstrated that cooking tomatoes brings out more of the lycopene than raw. Eating them cooked "reduces the risk of prostate cancer by 50%."[35] Another study showed that "those who ate two or more servings of cooked tomato products a week had one-third less risk of developing prostate cancer than those who rarely ate cooked tomato products..."[36]

Dr. James Balch, in his book *The Super Anti-Oxidants*, says that inhabitants of "Greece" and "Italy...where tomatoes and tomato-based foods" are a common staple, have very low rates for this type cancer.[37] In fact, this discovery about tomatoes and lycopene has been taken so seriously that researchers in Israel have actually come up with a hybrid tomato with quadruple the lycopene found in standard varieties![38]

According to "Dr. John W. Erdman" of the "University of Illinois in Chicago," to get the maximum dose of lycopene, you need to combine it with fat. This increases the absorption of lycopene in the colon.[39] (Good examples would be cooked or stewed tomatoes dressed with olive oil, a tomato salad with an olive oil dressing, flax oil with your tomato dish, or fresh avocado mixed with tomatoes or salsa.)

Dr. James Balch says that it isn't just prostate cancer that lycopene prevents, because scientists from the "University of Illinois" have discovered that women who eat foods rich in lycopene are **five times less likely** to develop "cervical cancer." [Emphasis, mine.][40]

According to Jean Carper, in her book, *The Food Pharmacy – Dramatic New Evidence That Food Is Your Best Medicine*, it is revealed that Hawaiians eat large amounts of tomatoes and they have fewer incidences of abdominal cancer. Americans and Norwegians who eat large amounts of tomatoes "(or carrots or cabbage)…" have slashed their risks of "lung cancer." She says that another study showed that "elderly" people who were avid tomato consumers were 50% less apt to succumb to cancers as their counterparts who ate fewer tomatoes, and studies in Wales revealed that tomatoes may inhibit "acute appendicitis."[41]

Taking vitamin E supplements with lycopene enhances its power, because vitamin E appears to trigger "the cancer fighting properties of lycopene."[42]

A news release recently stated that high levels of vitamin E could be harmful, contributing to overall mortality rates, however, what you were not told in this release was that most of the people involved in the study already had several other co-morbities or illnesses affecting them, so of course they had higher death rates.

Website *http://www.newstarget.com/001391.html,* recommends eating your tomatoes with broccoli to conquer prostate cancer, even stating that studies show this combo outperforms pharmaceutical drugs in preventing the disease![43]

Melatonin, Other Extracts, Herbs & Teas for Prostate Health

Several other natural herbs for prostate health are recommended by Dr. Ray Sahelian, M.D., (besides saw palmetto, discussed later) in his book, *Saw Palmetto Nature's Prostate Healer:*

> Pygeum africanum…Stinging Nettle…Rye Pollen Extract…Epilobium…Green tea…Beta-sitosterol…South African Star Grass…Pumpkin Seed…Zinc…Plant Estrogens, Flavonoids…Carotenoids…[and] Melatonin…[44]

Dr. Sahelian calls Melatonin **"Nature's Prostate-Shrinking Sleeping Pill."**[45] See his website at *www.raysahelian.com*, for more information, as well as his book! (Also see chapter nine in this book for more information on when you should, or shouldn't take melatonin!)

Milk Thistle Slows Growth of Prostate Cancer

Milk thistle, long known for its protective effects against liver damage, is discussed in great detail in chapter eight of this book because of its power to heal the liver. It is also important for prostate health because, as noted at *herbs2000.com*, it has the potential to "slow [the] growth of cancers that do not respond to hormone treatment."[46] Be sure to read other notes in this book (especially chapter eight) for those times when you should (and should not) take herbal preparations, even those as "safe" as milk thistle.

Mushrooms That Kill Prostate Cancer Cells

According to Shari Lieberman, Ph.D., and Ken Babal, C.N., in their book, *Maitake Mushroom AND D-Fraction*, researchers found that maitake D-fraction has the ability to cause cancer cells to self destruct, with a sort of "suicide gene."[47] Scientists conducting laboratory studies noted that D-fraction killed "prostate cancer cells" within "twenty-four hours."[48] Website, *Herbs2000.com,* recommends that you **do not** take maitake if you have "mutliple sclerosis....One form of interferon stimulated by maitake, gamma-interferon, can promote the destruction of nerve tissue, so people with MS should avoid maitake until this remedy has been more thoroughly tested."[49] This same website says that reishi mushroom extract proved effective as well, but it "induced a greater than 50 percent cancer-cell death...much less potent compared to the greater than 95 percent cancer-cell death achieved by Maitake D-fraction,"[50] and it was also discovered that when Maitake D extract is "combined with vitamin C, there was a synergistic effect. As little as 1/16 to 1/8 of the original maitake dose combined with vitamin C was found to be nearly as effective as the maitake dose alone."[51]

Pomegranate Juice for Recurring Prostate Cancer

According to an article from *Reuters Health Information*, drinking pomegranate juice may end up as a "treatment for recurrent prostate cancer."[51a] It has been found that "drinking 8 ounces per day of pomegranate juice increases the PSA doubling time* in men with recurrent prostate cancer, according to the results of a phase II study presented...at the annual meeting of the American Urological Association in San Antonio."[51b] As explained by "lead author" of the study, "Dr. Allen J. Pantuck, from the University of California at Los Angeles... 'The average doubling time before men began using pomegranate juice was 15 months, [and]...after treatment was 37 months. So, there was almost a 2-year increase in the doubling time.'" Not only is the juice very high in "antioxidants...the juice contains phytoestrogens [plant estrogens] that could be useful in combating prostate cancer, in particular." In this clinical trial, 48 men with prostate malignancies participated. There were "no serious adverse effects" and "none of the men developed metastatic disease." Some of the men had been through surgery, some through radiotherapy.[51c] (*Note that the longer the doubling time, the better! A shorter doubling time for PSA (such as 6 months) would mean a higher possibility of cancer metastasis, even after having a radical prostatectomy.)

Pumpkin Seeds for Prostate Health

It appears that eating pumpkin seeds may promote prostate health. Rita Elkins, in her book *D Glucarate*, says that this was demonstrated by "a randomized, double-blind study" conducted in "Stockholm" recently on more than four dozen participants with enlarged prostates, who were given the seeds, then followed for a 90 day period. All patients receiving pumpkin seeds experienced remarkable improvements without any adverse reactions.[52]

Reduce Fat Intake – Cut Your Risk of Prostate Cancer

As described by Maureen Kennedy Salaman author of *Nutrition: The Cancer Answer II,* a definite "link has been established between" high "dietary fat and prostate cancer." A vegetarian diet dramatically reduces the risk of prostate cancer. This is because fats in the diet raise testosterone levels and testosterone feeds prostate cancer. It has been proven that lowering male hormone levels of "testosterone," can inhibit these cancerous growths, and research has revealed that the higher the fat in the diet, the higher the death rate from prostate cancer.[53]

According to Ms. Salaman, "Peter Hill, Ph.D.," from New York City's "American Health Foundation," conducted a study on the effects of fat on hormone levels in men. This study showed that a group of men once considered "high-risk" for prostate cancer, could be "switched to a low-risk" group simply by changing their diet from "meats and fats," to a "low-fat diet."[54]

One really **big question** we should be asking ourselves is this: how in the world did we end up with such a deadly mixture of hormones in our meats and dairy products? It is because the FDA allows cancer-causing additives to be put into our food supply!

The FDA's primary drive since its creation has been to protect the elite, billion dollar drug industries rather than being concerned about the safety of American citizens![55] We've seen evidence just recently of drug companies being dishonest about testing and research with their products, covering up the truth about harmful side effects in their reports to the FDA. Much of this we have learned in news reports documenting fatalities among patients who were taking prescription medications.[56] (Remember Vioxx? Propulsid? Baycol? Rezulin?) The lure of wealth from the sale of millions in these drugs has warped the morals of many of the drug conglomerates. After all, why should they be worried about paying fines? A $300,000 fine is pennies for someone raking in billions of dollars in drug sales every year! It's a slap on the wrist!

While the FDA continues to approve many of the deadly drugs produced by the big drug conglomerates, they spend a great deal of time trying to ostracize and eliminate those producing and promoting natural health products, as Ms. Salaman further explains in *Nutrition: The Cancer Answer II*:

The message the FDA is sending to the public is very clear: The FDA will turn a blind eye if an Upjohn, an Eli Lilly or a Johnson and Johnson manufactures drugs that kill thousands – but be warned, the FDA will get you if you try selling food supplements or promote alternative medicine.[57]

Resveratrol Halts Prostate Cancer Cells

Recall *The Grape Cure* diet in chapter two? In an article at *Life Extension* website, *www.lef.org,* Terri Mitchell lauds the powerful anti-cancer properties of resveratrol (the antioxidant discussed in chapter two of this book):

> Good news for men concerned about prostate cancer. Resveratrol is a supplement that **blocks it at every stage, from beginning to end.** A polyphenol found in grapes and other plants, resveratrol was first identified as a multistage protector in 1997, and now is considered a leading agent against prostate cancer by researchers at Houston's M.D. Anderson Cancer Center and other institutions…this single supplement…has several mechanisms that stop cancer cells from multiplying, and even has the ability to destroy cancer cells.[58] [Emphasis, mine.]

Most amazing about "resveratrol," says *Life Extension*, "is that it can be very toxic to cancer cells but does not harm healthy cells; in fact, a person taking resveratrol for protection against prostate cancer may receive cardiovascular benefits as a side effect."[59] Resveratrol has proven itself "a 'chemopreventive' supplement that prevents DNA damage and destroys cancer cells from the earliest to the latest stages in both **human** and animal experimental models."[60]

Yet another study looking at prostate cancer cells, described at *Life Extension*, emphasizes that resveratrol:

> [H]alts the growth of hormone-positive and - negative cancers; works through multiple mechanisms to stop cancer cells from multiplying, is effective from the earliest to the latest stages of cancer, protects DNA from damage; and may inhibit cancer metastasis.[61]

My only question in all this is: **WHY ISN'T THIS BEING SHOUTED FROM THE ROOFTOPS?** How many men have been advised by their physicians during their yearly physicals to start eating **grapes, tomatoes (along with a fat source such as olive oil) broccoli, vitamin E, and raspberries** to drastically cut their chances of developing prostate cancer? (Especially since the studies are showing that resveratrol and raspberries could be useful in **halting prostate cancer once it has already been diagnosed!**)

Though resveratrol and lycopene are now available in supplement form at most natural health food stores, whenever possible, it is best to obtain the nutrients from fresh, natural food sources.

Saw Palmetto Inhibits Prostate Cancer Cells

Saw Palmetto is a popular herb for prostate protection. According to Ray Sahelian, M.D., in his book: *Saw Palmetto Nature's Prostate Healer,* a "1997 study done at Purdue University…" resulted in the identification of substances from the berries that inhibited "kidney and pancreatic cancer cells, [with] borderline activity against certain prostatic cancer cells."[62] (This information is also available at Dr. Sahelian's website at *www.raysahelian.com/saw.html*) Saw Palmetto has been used by many health care practitioners to treat problems with prostate inflammation and enlargement.

As described by Jean Carper in her book, *Miracle Cures*, saw palmetto is a best selling prostate treatment in Europe! Nearly two dozen scientific "studies" attribute the herb with the successful treatment of "enlarged prostate…90 percent" of the time! This is a much greater "cure power than pharmaceutical drugs and surgery can boast."[63] In "seven…studies (double-blind placebo)" using this herb, six of them revealed that saw palmetto is "superior to a dummy pill after one to three months of use."[64]

St. John's Wort

Italian scientists have very recently discovered that this herb, in animal testing, has the ability to inhibit malignancies in prostate cancer as well as suppress the spread of the disease. They concluded from the study that St. John's Wort may prove beneficial in fighting this type cancer.[64a] This herb should not be taken if you are on anti-depressants, especially if they are MAO inhibitors.

Sunshine Prevents Prostate Cancer

According to website *www.yourhealthbase.com*, adequate exposure to sunlight can significantly prevent prostate cancer. Studies in Great Britain involving more than 200 "men diagnosed with prostate cancer and 155 men with an enlarged prostate…" revealed that those participants who had "the lowest exposure were found to have a three times greater incidence of prostate cancer than did men with a high lifetime exposure…" to sunlight.[64b] If you have a hereditary tendency for melanoma, or other skin disorders, be sure to check with your physician before you attempt unprotected sunlight exposure.

Turmeric & Prostate Cancer

As described by "researchers at the 2002 annual meeting of the American Association for Cancer Research," the active ingredient in turmeric "*curcumin*," is effective at destroying cancer cells. This is explained at website *www.discount-vitamins-herbs.net/health:*

> An in vitro experiment with human prostate cancer cells revealed that curcumin works together with a naturally occurring molecule called TRAIL (tumor necrosis factor-related apoptosis-inducing lignan), which helps kill cancer cells. When curcumin was combined with TRAIL, the two agents killed two to three times more cancer cells than either treatment by itself. The combination killed up to 80% of the cancer cells.[65]

Turmeric "activates p53, a cancer control gene important in 50 percent of cases," and it also inhibits bone metastasis.[66] (Also note that the above website has many nutrient supplements available, including turmeric.) Turmeric is safe when used as a spice, however, if you are taking turmeric in supplement form, do not use if pregnant, nor if you have gallstones, since it stimulates the gallbladder. Like garlic, turmeric can slow clotting time, so it should be used in caution by anyone taking anti-coagulant medications,[66a] with blood disorders, or for anyone recovering from or contemplating surgery, or with ulcers.

Vitamin E & Selenium Protect Against Prostate Cancer

Website *www.infoaging.org* reports that when "scientists at the Stanford University Medical Center" compared "52 men with prostate cancer" to "96 men of the same age with no known prostate disease," those men with the "lowest levels of selenium" had a "four to five times" greater risk for "prostate cancer." It was interesting that "as the men aged," their "blood levels of selenium were also noted to drop," denoting a connection between aging, selenium deficiencies and increased risk for prostate cancer.[67]

Apparently, keeping high levels of vitamin E in the body can protect against not just "prostate cancer," but "bladder cancer" as well. According to *foodnavigator.com*, research, shows that high levels of vitamin E, from "both alpha- and gamma-tocopherol" sources were found to lower "the risk of prostate cancer, by as much as 53 per cent and 39 per cent, respectively."[68] They list some good **natural sources** of vitamin E ("alpha-tocopherol") as: "nuts and seeds, wholegrain products...beans and other vegetables...Spinach, green and red peppers and sunflower seeds..."[69] (Fresh sprouts are also a good natural source of vitamin E.)

Red Clover Destroys Prostate Cancer Cells

In a remarkable case described at *www.cancertutor.com*, "A 66-year-old physician with [a] PSA [of] 13.1...in March of 1996" underwent a "needle biopsy" that "confirmed the presence of a low grade adenocarcinoma." He then consumed a popular phyto-estrogen from red clover "for the seven days preceding his operation...(Promensil tabs – 4 x 40 mg/day)" at "a daily dose of 160 mg." Regardless, he still opted to have the prostate surgery.[70] Following the surgery, a comparison was made with "the biopsy tissue and the tumor tissue...." The website explains that the results showed a great number of cellular deaths in the tumor much like that obtained with "high-dose estrogen therapy and consistent with tumor regression." There were no undesirable reactions to the treatment.[71] (Be aware that red clover may affect blood coagulation time, so check with your physician before using this or any other herb.)

Soy Isoflavones & PSK Slow the Growth of Prostate Cancer Cells

A report at *www.herbs2000.com*, says that "soy isoflavone concentrate tablets" may halt "tumor growth," and decrease the possibility that it will "spread to [the] lungs." (Fermented soy products, such as Haelan, can help remove harmful estrogens from the body in estrogen-receptor positive cancers.) The addition to the diet of "Polysaccharide kureha (PSK) tablets," may be beneficial in slowing down the rate of tumor growth and metastasis.[72] They further explain that PSK, "also known as *krestin*," is a derivative "from the *kawaratake* mushroom...a powerful antioxidant and immune stimulant" that has been the focus of more than "200 scientific studies..." No toxicity has been reported when it is taken by mouth.[73]

Ukrain – A Non-Toxic Cure for Prostate Cancer

Ukrain is a combination of two ingredients: "alkaloids from the plant *Chelidonium majus L.* (greater celandine) and the pharmaceutical Thiotepa..." which are toxic when used individually, however, once combined they are only toxic to cancer cells![74] This from *www.ukrin.com*. The website also describes a remarkable human clinical trial that was conducted in a controlled study at the "Villa Medica Clinic (Edenkoben, Germany)," involving "74 patients with prostatic carcinomas," all of them having already received "conventional therapy protocols" for their cancer. Because of "relapse and/or progression of the disease [they] had no further conventional options available." (In other words, they were all terminal!) They were treated with

UKRAIN, "and partially at the same time with local hyperthermia." As a result, 73% of the men went into "complete remission" and 22% "partial remission," with "only 5% of patients showing no effect on the progress of the disease."[75] (See other cancer specific chapters in this book for amazing cancer cures using Ukrain, including the successful reversal of *terminal brain cancers* in chapter 13!)

Since Ukrain is considered alternative therapy, you can not obtain it from your local cancer clinic. You will need to seek an alternative health physician in the United States for Ukrain therapy, or travel to Europe or Canada where it is very popular. Their main website is *www.ukrin.com.*

Water Prevents Cancer

The late Dr. F. Batmanghelidj, M.D., in his book *Your Body's Many Cries For Water*, said that cancer patients are dehydrated. It is important that you take sufficient water on a daily basis (depending on your body weight). Extra water also requires extra salt. "For every 10 glasses of water (about two quarts)" you need a "half teaspoon of salt per day,"[76] unless your physician has you on a special water or salt-restricted diet. Many people who go on long fasts drink large amounts of water, forgetting that they also need to increase their salt intake. Do not use tap water. If you do not have a water filtering system, you may want to try steam-distilled water or a reliable purified water drink from your health food store. Avoid all chlorinated water and water with fluoride. See chapter 22 in this book for more information on the importance of water and how much your body needs.

Poly–MVA (Palladium Lipoic Complex)

See chapters 9 and 13 for information on Poly-MVA, an amazing nutrient that many cancer patients are crediting with healing their cancers completely, including prostate cancers.

CHAPTER 5

PAINLESS CURES & PREVENTIONS FOR COLON CANCER & ABDOMINAL CANCER

"Physicians want to help their patients, and most often they feel the only way to accomplish this task is by finding a disease process and beginning treatment with a prescription."
(Ray D. Strand, M.D., from his book: *What Your Doctor Doesn't Know About Nutritional Medicine May Be Killing You.*)[1]

I. Colon Cancer & Abdominal Cancer Vanish!

Case #1

George Malkmus had been a Baptist pastor for twenty years when he was diagnosed with colon cancer. He was 42-years-old and he refused to go the conventional medicine: cut, poison and burn routine. He asked:

> What was I to do…? As a pastor of 20 years, I had sat at the bedside of so many people and watched the devastating effects of chemotherapy, radiation and surgery experienced by others in the treatment of their cancers, I had also conducted the funerals for many of them.[2]

Reverend Malkmus cured himself completely of colon cancer, the same cancer that had killed his mother, who had been treated with conventional cancer therapy. He began a diet of raw fruits and vegetables that included large amounts of freshly-extracted juices. His diet is very similar to the one advocated by Eydie Mae Hunsberger and Ann Wigmore. His website at *www.hacres.com* gives details about his *Hallelujah Acres* diet:

> Emphasizing the wisdom of the Genesis 1:29 diet of raw fruits and vegetables handed down to mankind in the Garden

of Eden, Rev. George Malkmus delivers a powerful message of health through natural foods from a biblical perspective. Rev. Malkmus…combines the personal testimonial of his own recovery from colon cancer along with his research into nutrition and biblical teachings to develop a strong case for a vegetarian diet composed primarily of raw foods. He teaches that God created our bodies to be self-healing, and that this healing works best when we give our bodies nutrition in the form of raw foods as God intended.[3]

Rev. Malkmus believes that disease is caused when "mankind strays from the original Genesis 1:29 diet of raw fruits and vegetables [and], God intends us to earn this food by 'the sweat of thy face' (exercise)."[4]

The *Hallelujah Acres* "diet and lifestyle not only cured his colon cancer," but Rev. Malkmus said it also "gave him relief from a variety of other ailments…high blood pressure, hemorrhoids, hypoglycemia, and severe sinus and allergy problems," and he insists that "He has not been to a doctor, or even taken an aspirin, for over twenty years, and is now in his mid-sixties with more energy than he had as a teenager."[5] There are also several health products available at Hallelujah Acres website *http://www.hacres.com/products/products.asp.*

Case #2

When a physician had part of his stomach removed due to cancer, and it returned less than two years later, chemo was recommended. Few patients survive a year with this type cancer recurrence. Dr. E. refused chemo and opted instead to go on the Budwig diet, which "he religiously followed." The diet cured him, and that was 15 years ago. Today, he is still cancer free, and doing well "in his late seventies."[5a]

Johanna Budwig, at a "South German" radio station "September 11, 1967," described her success [using the Budwig diet] with a colon cancer patient:

It is amazing how quickly the tumor, for instance with colon cancer is being eliminated. Even with an old patient of 84 years who was scheduled for an operation because of his colon threatening to become blocked, I was able to achieve the complete elimination of the tumor and the patient's restoration to health within a few days. **These are not isolated cases.**[5b] [Emphasis, mine.]

The Budwig flax oil formula is given below. Please note, however, that the entire Budwig diet regimen includes many other specifics (for example restrictions on eating sugar and hydrogenated fats, etc.), which can be found in chapters 13 and 17 of this book as well as website: *www.healingcancernaturally.com/budwig_protocol.html*:

For each tablespoon of flaxseed oil, add 2 tablespoons of low-fat cottage cheese (or quark) or 6 tablespoons of yogurt. The flaxoil/cottage cheese or flaxoil/yogurt mixture should be fully blended until no traces of oil remain visible, proving that the highly unsaturated fatty acids have become water soluble (a hand-held mixer or a blender works well).[6]

This simple formula is eaten 3 – 4 times each day. See chapter 13 of this book for more details on the Budwig flax oil diet that has also cured many cases of inoperable brain cancer! Chapter 13 and chapter 25 of this book will also tell you why you may wish to substitute organic soy yogurt for the dairy cottage cheese. (Fermented soy products, such as Haelan, can help remove harmful estrogens from the body in estrogen-receptor positive cancers.)

Recently, *AntiCancer Research* reported in one of their articles, that flaxseed can help slow the expansion of breast malignancies, and intestinal growths that do not depend on estrogen. Flaxseed also reduces harmful cholesterol, elevates good cholesterol, and helps the body dump toxic estrogens.[6a]

Flax oil can be found in natural health food stores and even some popular grocery chains. If you purchase flax oil, it should always be refrigerated and **never heated**! One of the best ways to take fresh flax is to purchase the flax seeds whole, grind them in a coffee grinder and mix in water, juice, or oatmeal. You need to drink it quickly though, because flax thickens very fast! See chapter 35 in this book, *What To Do If You Are Already Ill*, for more information on using flax, and chapter seventeen for more details about the amazing anticancer properties of flax!

Abdominal Liposarcoma

Dr. Abram Hoffer, well known for his use of Orthomolecular Medicine (megadose vitamin and/or mineral treatments) as well as Complementary Medicine (combination of orthodox and Orthomolecular Medicine), was able to extend the life of a patient with abdominal liposarcoma for six years with Complementary Medicine. The details can be found at his webpage: *http://www. islandnet.com/~hoffer/*.[6b]

"The Maker's Diet"

Jordan S. Rubin, N.M.D., Ph.D., in his book, *The Maker's Diet*, documents a similar struggle of trying to regain his health when he rapidly deteriorated and almost died, not from cancer, but from Crohn's disease. He wasn't sure whether the MMR (measles, mumps, rubella) vaccine he received at age 15 (which has been implicated in causing digestive disorders like Crohn's and autism) may or may not have been a factor leading to his disease, but he realized that his unhealthy diet and lifestyle certainly contributed to his illness. Near death, he finally met a nutritionist who recommended a biblical diet to him that he followed and regained his health.[7]

Dr. Rubin began consuming organic *"kefir"* (a product of "naturally fermented milk from raw goat's and cow's milk; organically raised," biblically approved meats only, "ocean-caught wild fish and natural sprouted or sourdough breads made from yeast-free whole grains, as well as raw nuts and seeds, organic fruits and vegetables, raw sauerkraut, and carrot and other vegetable juices."[7a] He experienced the usual problem of feeling worse initially (the "Herxheimer reaction"), as is quite common when people are going through detoxification after years of eating processed food, junk diets. This is the time when your body is throwing off poisons that have accumulated in the system for years, and often causes indigestion and nausea. He also stated that: "Crohn's disease is supposedly incurable. Because of my experience, I can confirm that no disease is incurable."[8]

Dr. Rubin believes that since we are no longer in the Garden of Eden, we need protein from meats, but only meats as given in Deuteronomy 14 and Leviticus 11 of the Bible. The Israelites in the Old Testament were forbidden to eat scavengers such as swine, seafood without fins and scales, as well as those animals without cloven or split hooves that chew the cud.[9] (Further details of the dietary restrictions from the Old Testament of the Bible can be found in Deuteronomy 14 and Leviticus 11, as noted above.)

The Maker's Diet details the 40-day diet plan developed by Dr. Rubin (including a list of foods to avoid), which he says attacks "the three I's – insulin, infection, and inflammation."[10]

Dr. Rubin recovered from Crohn's disease using this biblically-based diet that he says many others with bowel problems are also finding successful. As far as the admonition regarding clean and unclean animals, much later in the Bible in the New Testament, the apostle Peter was given a vision from heaven revealing a change in dietary restrictions in Acts chapter 10, allowing many of the animals previously banned from the kosher diet. However, in spite of all this, our meat supply has become polluted with hormones, herbicides and pesticides. As for fish and seafood, our oceans are becoming toxic waste dumps, and it is widely known that mercury poisoning and other health issues with fish and seafood have existed for years.

If you include dairy products and meats in your diet, that is your decision, and if you are going to do so, at least **use only those as described by Dr. Rubin in his plan.** Buy certified ORGANIC only, so that you are assured you will not be consuming hormones and other toxins that will make you sick! Regardless of all this, I believe the evidence is overwhelmingly in favor of a raw foods vegan diet for cancer treatment, prevention and wellness, as opposed to one that allows meats and dairy. (I do make an exception when it comes to hard-boiled eggs, but they must be certified ORGANIC! Eggs contain many nutrients! However, if you are someone battling cancer, you may want to stick with the raw food vegan diet that so many have had success with! Consider the cases of Rev. Malkmus, Dr. Nolfi, Eydie Mae, and Ann Wigmore, described herein!)

See chapter 25 on milk, later in this book, before you decide to keep dairy products in your diet, organic or not! (Dr. Rubin said that a vegan diet did not work for him, but he was battling Crohn's, not cancer, and he does not give any specifics about the vegan diet he followed, as to whether or not he was including wheatgrass juices, etc.)

II. How Resveratrol Cured Abdominal Cancer

Resveratrol has proven so potent against cancer that an entire chapter in this book has been devoted to it. Please see chapter two for more information on this amazing ingredient found in common table grapes! Chapter two also tells the story of Johanna Brandt, author of *The Grape Cure*, who completely **cured her own abdominal cancer without surgery, chemo, or radiation!**

III. Herbs Effective Against Colon & Stomach Cancers

Artemisinin

Artemisinin (also called "wormwood") has been very popular in killing parasites, however, in a "series of successful experiments [it was] effective against a wide variety of cancers," most notably, "leukemia and colon cancer," and is described at *www.drlam.com*. They explain that this herb is capable of crossing "the blood brain barrier…and may be particularly suitable for curing brain tumors, together with Poly-MVA."[11] (See chapter 13 on brain cancer for more information on poly-MVA.) Do not use wormwood without consulting with your physician. Excessive dosing can be harmful.

Astragalus

Astragalus is an herb which boosts the immune system by enhacing the body's natural immunity in fighting cancer. This herb should not be used in the presence of a "fever or skin infection."[11a]

Graviola

According to website *www.mnwelldir.org,* a little known herb found in "the deep rainforest jungles along the Amazon" has "been used for centuries by…natives of South America to treat asthma, liver problems, arthritis and heart disease."[12] It is called *Graviola,* and some remarkable cancer cures are being credited to this herb. For example, a popular Christian television talk show host, who had surgery for colon cancer (then refused chemo and radiation afterwards), credits her complete healing from cancer to Graviola and her faith in God. (Graviola can be purchased at local health food stores and some internet sites such as *www.rain-tree.com.*)

Lab research that was apparently never published, indicated that Graviola may be "more powerful than Adriamycin, a commonly used chemotherapy" drug, however, Graviola has **none** of the toxic "side effects" associated with Adriamycin![13]

According to the *Wellness Directory of Minnesota's*™ website *(www.mnwelldir.org):*

> In laboratory studies, Graviola selectively hunts down and kills 12 different types of cancer cells (without harming healthy cells) including breast, prostate, lung, colon, and pancreatic cancer. Additionally, it actually boosts your immune system making the patient feel healthier and stronger and improves overall energy and outlook on life. The first rule of medicine: Do No Harm. This is one cancer fighter that follows that rule and Americans almost never heard of this because it was a Pharmaceutical company that did the studies, and when, after seven years of trying to synthesize the active agents in Graviola proved fruitless, THEY TRIED TO BURY THEIR RESEARCH.[14]

Apparently, the only reason the lid was blown off Graviola was because "an employee of the pharmaceutical company" performing the tests, leaked the entire story.[15]

Over a decade ago, "behind lock and key, this well-known drug giant began searching for a cure for cancer – while preciously guarding their opportunity to patent it and, therefore, profit from it." However, the drug company ran into "a big problem" when their attempt to "isolate and create man-made duplicates of two of the tree's most powerful chemicals" failed. When they tried to duplicate the original, the formula no longer worked, and according to "federal law...natural substances can't be patented." The result was that "the company couldn't protect its profits [and] the project it had poured millions of dollars and nearly seven years of research into." As a result of watching the prospect of big profits go down the drain, "testing on Graviola came to a screeching halt." They "shelved the project" and "refused to publish its findings in an independent journal."[16]

There was however, "one researcher, who...contacted Raintree Nutrition, a company dedicated to harvesting plants from the Amazon."[17]

Raintree began digging into everything they could find on the herb. Further studies came back that "supported the drug company's secret findings; Graviola had been shown to kill cancer cells"[18]

Health Sciences Institute website in a story at *http://www.hsibaltimore.com,* shares a very disturbing report about how information on this cancer-fighting herb was known by the National Cancer Institute as far back as 1976, but was never made public:

> One of the first scientific references to it [Graviola] in the United States was by the National Cancer Institute (NCI). In 1976, the NCI included Graviola in a plant-screening program that showed its leaves and stems were effective in **attacking and destroying malignant cells.** But the results were part of an internal NCI report and were, for some reason, **never released to the public.**[19] *[Imagine that! Can you guess why?]*

By now, you have probably realized that information regarding new discoveries in natural cancer prevention and cures are often purposely **suppressed** by the cancer industry! This little **oversight** by the National Cancer Institute is just one small example out of thousands!

H.S.I. also describes another very "recent study, conducted at the Catholic University of South Korea this year, which revealed that two chemicals extracted from Graviola seeds showed 'selective cytoxicity comparable with Adriamycin' for breast and colon cancer cells." The extracts not only "targeted and killed malignant breast and colon cells" in vitro, but they were "comparable" in efficacy to the "chemotherapy drug Adriamycin!"[20]

This was further confirmed by data publicized in the "*Journal of Natural Products,*" stating:

> Graviola is not only comparable to Adriamycin – but dramatically outperformed it in laboratory tests....***Graviola selectively targets cancer cells leaving healthy cells untouched. Chemotherapy indiscriminately seeks and destroys all actively reproducing cells – even normal, healthy ones.***[21]

Not only has it been shown effective against colon cancer cells, but lab studies also proved Graviola effective against lung cancer, pancreatic cancer, and prostate cancer cells. Though comprehensive clinical trials on humans have not yet been done, obviously some humans are already using the herb and having good results with it.

One astounding report of Graviola's curing abilities was documented by Daryl S., "an executive at a high-tech company in Texas," who had been diagnosed by "sonogram and biopsy" with "more than **20 tumors in his prostate.**"[22] When searching for alternative treatments (because he did not want to have surgery), Daryl found *Raintree.* His physician had already recommended surgery, but Daryl refused, believing that a "cure using this common conventional treatment would come at too great a cost."[23] See Daryl's full story in chapter four of this book, and how he used Graviola to completely **cure** his prostate cancer!

Raintree puts Graviola in their herbal formula known as *N-Tense*, which is available at their website *www.rain-tree.com*. The company says that there are "no side effects, apart from possible mild gastrointestinal upset at high dosages (in excess of 5 grams) if taken on an empty stomach."[24] *N-Tense* is composed of 50% Graviola along with other Rainforest cancer-fighting botanicals.

Essiac Tea – The Nurse Who Cured Hundreds (perhaps thousands) of Cancer Patients with Four Herbs

In 1924, Rene Caisse's aunt was diagnosed with advanced cancer of the stomach and liver. She was given "6 months to live." Rene, a Canadian nurse, asked her aunt's physician about using an herbal formula that she had obtained from another patient who had used the tea to cure her breast cancer! The story is described in Reese Dubin's book *Miracle Food Cures From the Bible*. The patient told Rene that she had been given the tea recipe by an "Ojibway (Chippewa) medicine man," a friend of her husbands. The physician approved for Rene's aunt to try the same herbal tea. It contained "sheep sorrel, burdock root, slippery-elm bark…[and] Turkish rhubarb…"[25] Rene's aunt used the herbal remedy for only 60 days. She was completely cured and outlived her ordeal by "another 21 years."[26]

Mr. Dubin describes the physician's reaction to the amazing cure: "The doctor, R.O. Fisher, M.D. of Toronto, was so fascinated by this miraculous recovery that together they began experimenting on mice inoculated with human cancer cells." Mr. Dubin says that "The results were so impressive that Dr. Fisher decided to try this herbal mixture on some of his advanced cancer patients. These patients too, showed definite improvement."[27]

The tea was called "*Essiac*" (Rene's last "name spelled backwards"). The news could not be contained. Other physicians began referring their terminally ill cancer patients to Rene. A short while later, a physician asked Rene to use her herbal tea remedy on a diabetic colon cancer patient. To their astonishment, not only did the tea and the injections made from the tea cure the bowel cancer, but the diabetes as well! Only three of the herbs were used in the injections, however, the exact **injectable** formula that was developed has been lost. It has since been available only as a tea.[28]

Mr. Dubin recounts that in 1926, physicians were so amazed at the results of Essiac tea, eight of them petitioned "the Department of National Health and Welfare of Ottawa, asking that Rene [be allowed] to test her remedy large scale," and to be "given facilities" to do so. Instead Ottawa's "Department of Health and Welfare sent two doctors with warrants for her arrest." However, when it was discovered that Rene was working under the supervision of "nine of the most eminent doctors in Toronto," the "Department of Health..." backed down.[29]

Over several decades, Dubin says that Rene ultimately went on to treat multiple hundreds of terminally ill cancer patients with her herbal tea remedy, many of which recovered completely. She did not charge for her services and always worked with prominent physicians. She accepted countless Canadian and American patients. Her own mother, now 72 "was diagnosed with cancer of the liver, inoperable because of a weak heart." After several days of treatment with Essiac tea and Essiac injections, her mother was completely cured, surviving her ordeal by "18 years," before dying at the age of 90 with heart problems.[30]

Cynthia Olsen, in her book, *Essiac A Native Herbal Cancer Remedy*, says that In "1932" a "headline" appeared "in the *Toronto Star*," which said, "Bracebridge Girl Makes Notable Discovery Against Cancer," but because of this article, Rene Caisse was again threatened with legal action, including "imprisonment for practicing medicine without a license."[31] Ms. Olson further explains that in 1938, Rene's supporters, including many physicians, petitioned the government of Ontario to pass a bill giving Rene permission to use her formula for cancer patients "without the constant threat of arrest." More than "55,000" people signed the petition! It fell three votes short of being passed, mostly due to "collusion by the Canadian Medical Association and the newly formed Cancer Commission."[32]

A short while later, in "1939...a public hearing was held by the Cancer Commission at the Royal York Hotel in Toronto," and says Ms. Olsen, "Caisse brought 387 patients to testify [however] the Commission only heard 49" of them. One patient in particular, "Herbert Rawson," was pushing fifty when two physicians told him, (in "1935") that he had rectal cancer, a diagnosis that was supported by x-ray exams. He declined surgery and came to Rene Caisse with a "written diagnosis and permission to treat with Essiac." He started Essiac "in April 1935" and received the "last of 30" treatments slightly more than a year later. Examinations shortly thereafter revealed no cancer whatsoever, and he outlived his ordeal another 25 years, dying "of a stroke at age 73."[33]

What was the verdict of the Royal Cancer Commission to all the records and testimonies made available to them? Reese Dubin in *Miracle Food Cures From The Bible*, says that they refused to acknowledge that Essiac was helping anyone with cancer. Their excuse was that they were not privy to the formula. Rene agreed to disclose the recipe, providing they would come clean and admit that cancer patients were receiving positive results with the herbal tea, but they would not do so.[34]

Because of continual threats of arrest and incarceration, Rene finally shut her clinic doors, but covertly continued to see patients over the next three decades.[35] However, Dubin says that she was constantly being observed "by officers of the Canadian Health Department," and faced years of imprisonment "if caught giving anything to help a cancer patient."[36]

Rene's fame came to the attention of "Fawcett" Publishing and one of their Editors, "Ralph Daigh" (who was suspicious of the medical establishment), as described by Cynthia Olsen in her above book:

> He believed he had concrete evidence that the medical establishment had suppressed information about the efficacy of Essiac. Through Daigh's efforts, Caisse worked with Dr. Charles Brusch, John F. Kennedy's personal physician....He regretted that John F. Kennedy did not live long enough to help influence the medical establishment in using Essiac throughout the medical organization.[37]

Dr. Brusch, never stopped endorsing Essiac, and stated:

> "The results we obtained with thousands of patients of various races, sexes and ages with all types of cancer definitely prove Essiac to be a cure for cancer. Studies done in four laboratories in the United States and one or more in Canada also fortify this claim." Later in life, Brusch developed cancer and cured it with Essiac.[38]

Of Essiac tea, *www.whale.to/m/quotes6.html* quotes Dr. Brusch as saying: "For I have in fact cured my own cancer, the original site of which was the lower bowels, through Essiac alone."[38a]

Cynthia Olsen says that it was with Dr. Brusch's help, that Rene tried to work with "Sloan-Kettering" a well known Cancer Institute, in the testing of her herbal tea. One of their physicians invited her to submit "some herbs for testing," which she was happy to do, along with "instructions on how to inject the herb." After testing, Rene received a reply telling her that there was "regression of sarcoma in 180 mice treated with Essiac."[38b] But then, Ms. Olsen says something rather curious happened. Rene found out "that Sloan-Kettering," against her specific instructions, had "frozen the herb," then later told her that "test results were negative." What happened to the report of the "180 mice" that had experienced "regression" of their tumors? Apparently, it wasn't publicized. "Cassie…in disgust…broke all ties with Sloan-Kettering."[39] In Ms. Olsen's words: "Rene Caisse…spent a frustrating life trying to save people's lives with a simple herbal tea, only to have that effort thwarted by the politics and greed of the medical establishment. Not much has changed since."[40]

Rene wanted nothing more than to help cancer patients with her herbal tea remedy, yet she endured years of incessant and needless harassment from the Canadian Ministry of Health.

According to Reese Dubin's account, Cassie finally sold her tea recipe for $1 right before her death. She died from problems related to hip surgery when she was 90-years-old. She had credited her own excellent health and lack of illness to the fact that she had taken Essiac tea "twice a week for nearly 50 years."[41]

Reese Dubin wrote that the best way to brew the Essiac formula is to purchase the four herbs organically from a natural health food store, rather than trying to gather them in the wild. He then recommends brewing your own herbal Essiac tea. (Note that burdock root "is a uterine stimulant," so should not be taken if you are pregnant.)[42]

Be sure that you always consult your physician about taking herbal preparations and do not give them to children without first consulting their health care practitioner.

The genuine Essiac formula can be found both in Reese Dubin's book, *Miracle Food Cures From the Bible,* and Cynthia Olsen's book,

Essiac A Native herbal Cancer Remedy, as well as many websites, including: *www.thebearbyte.com/Herbal/essiac.html.* (See below for obtaining this tea in a prepared formula ready to drink!)

If Buying Essiac Herbs in Bulk

The only herb in Essiac tea that is NOT powdered is the burdock root, which is cut, instead of powdered, according to Reese Dubin. He suggests that when purchasing slippery elm bark, ask for the "pure powdered...beige" colored herb. There are diluted formulas out there, which have been mixed with other ingredients and these are not acceptable. The "Turkish rhubarb" root "is yellowish-brown in color."[43]

Where to Find Ready-to-Drink Essiac Tea

If you do not wish to purchase the individual herbs and brew Essiac yourself, there are several commercial preparations of this tea. One very popular brand is called *Flor-Essence®,* found in most health food stores. It not only has the four Essiac herbs, but also watercress, kelp, blessed thistle, and red clover blossom. You can find *Flor-Essence®* in the dry tea form where you add water, boil it and follow the directions to prepare it at home, or you can buy it already bottled and ready to drink, another option albeit more expensive. There are other Essiac brands, one in particular, Resperin Essiac®, which can be purchased at *http://www.grand-strand.com/suebest/boywho.htm.* It is also available in many natural health food stores. Those who use Resperin Essiac® believe that it is so far superior to any other commercial Essiac tea on the market, it is incomparable. See Chapter 15 of this book for the story of a young boy cured of Hodgkins Disease using dietary changes, Resperin Essiac® tea and 714X injections. His parents were so impressed with the tea that they became distributors!

There are many other commercially prepared Essiac teas available. Reese Dubin gives several references in his book where you can purchase loose herbs in bulk. Several internet sites sell the herbs in bulk as do some local health food stores. Just be sure if you decide to make your own, you are not using tap water contaminated with chlorine and fluoride!

Garlic Against Abdominal Cancer

Garlic is also important in cancer prevention. A study was done in China testing the potency of garlic in cancer prevention. At the conclusion of the study, data showed that people who did not eat garlic had a much higher risk for developing cancer! The garlic eaters showed a drastically lower rate of abdominal cancers in comparison to the county where garlic was not eaten. It was found that those who had the lower cancer rates ate "more than half an ounce of garlic, onions, leeks, and similar vegetables every day." Scientists were surprised to find that if the garlic eaters also ate "fruits and dark green and yellow vegetables," they did not get "throat cancer."[44]

One does not necessarily need to consume large quantities of garlic to benefit from its protective action. Apparently, it takes a very small amount of garlic every day to decrease your risks of prostate cancer drastically! (Garlic has blood-thinning properties, so be sure to consult with your licensed health care practitioner before consuming excessive quantities.) Note that it won't do you much good to eat garlic every day to prevent cancer, if on the other hand, you are also eating large quantities of cancer-causing substances in meats and dairy products, or smoking cigarettes!

Goldenseal (Berberine) Suppresses Colon Cancer

According to *Life Extension's* website at *www.lef.org,* an ingredient in goldenseal known as *"berberine,"* can suppress the formation of colon cancer. It inhibits "bladder cancer," caused cellular death "in human leukemia cells…inhibited the development of skin tumors, [and] has potent antitumor activity against human and rat malignant brain tumors."[45] If taking this herb, the preparation should be "standardized to provide 5% hydrastine." *Life Extension* also says that there are some herbalists who recommend rotating goldenseal "with other herbals," rather than giving it continuously.[46]

Herbs2000.com recommends that you do **not** take goldenseal or other herbs that have berberine ("Barberry or coptis…or Oregon grape…) for more than two weeks, [or] if you are pregnant or have gallbladder disease. Do not take these herbs with supplemental vitamin B6 or with protein supplements containing the amino acid histidine, or if you have cardiovascular disease or glaucoma."[47] Goldenseal may raise blood pressure in some individuals.

Green Tea Protects Against Esophageal & Stomach Cancer

Researchers have known for many years of the anti-cancer properties of green tea. Studies show that when humans ingested "7 cups or more a day," stomach cancer rates dropped dramatically![47a] Scientists in China found that regularly drinking green tea cuts "gastric cancer" risk by as much as 50%! For cancer prevention, *Life Extension* website, *www.lef.org/protocols* suggests "5-10 cups a day (or five 350 mg capsules three times a day of a 95% polyphenol extract" of green tea.[48]

Milk Thistle Fights Colon Cancer

Though milk thistle (not to be confused with *blessed thistle*, a different herb), is most popular for its effectiveness at rejuvenating the liver, one of its components, "silymarin," was discovered by researchers to be "a powerful killer of colon and skin cancer." They also determined from "laboratory and animal studies," that silymarin fights "breast and prostate cancers, as well." This is described at *www.hsibaltimore.com*.[49] Based on this research, those with a strong family history of colorectal cancer and polyps may be able to prevent these cancers by supplementing with milk thistle.

As noted elsewhere in this book, do not take herbal preparations, even seemingly "safe" ones such as this if you are a transplant patient, or have any other type of chronic disorder or debility without consulting your doctor. See chapter eight later in this book, for more information on milk thistle, and instances when it should not be used.

Snow Rose Inhibits Colon Cancer

Longevity of life is not uncommon in what was once "part of the Soviet Union...the Republic of Georgia." **The population at last count was 3.2 million people and "almost 23,000" of them are "over the age of 100!"**[50] (Emphasis, mine.) These people have been the subject of much research due to their longevity, and according to an article by Nina Anderson, at *www.manyhands.com*, it has been surmised that their long and healthy life spans are due to their diets. They consume large amounts of Alpine Tea with "grain kefir containing eleven different probiotics. In addition, the water they drink is full of glacial minerals..." They also consume honey and wine. Alpine Tea's main ingredient is "Rhododendron caucasian," an herb harvested "at 10,000 - to 30,000-foot elevations in the Caucasian Mountains...(also known as 'snow rose')." Studies show that snow rose "inhibits or abolishes the activity of the enzyme hyaluronidase, known to be an initiator of colon cancer."[51]

The website further reports that snow rose has been studied for its effectiveness in treating coronary artery disease, "arthritis, gout, high cholesterol, blood pressure problems, depression, neuroses...psychoses, and concentration problems," and it was able to completely kill "12,000 staphylococcus aureus bacteria" in test tube experiments, outperforming both pine bark and grape seed.[52]

Rhododendron caucasicum is often combined with other herbs for increased potency. It can be found in some health food stores and internet sites. (Be aware that you can **not** harvest the rhododendron in your flower bed thinking it is the same herb. They are not the same.)

There are other herbal websites that sell snow rose or Alpine Tea. If you are purchasing Alpine Tea, be sure that it is the tea with *Rhododendron caucasicum.*

Suma ("Pfaffia") for Abdominal Cancer

According to *www.rain-tree.com,* "Suma *(Pfaffia paniculata)"* is often called "Brazilian ginseng," though it isn't "a true gingseng from the Panax plant family." Animal studies have shown that it may be important in fighting "abdominal cancer." *Raintree* explains that suma has more than a dozen "amino acids…" as well as multiple vitamins and minerals and many phytochemicals and nutrients. It has been referred to as "the Russian secret," since their athletes often take it for "muscle-building and endurance without the side effects associated with steroids."[53]

Raintree warns that the powdered root can cause "asthmatic allergic reactions if inhaled," and consuming excessive amounts of the tea may cause "mild gastric disturbances including nausea and stomach cramping." No known drug reactions have been reported with this herb.[54] For more information on suma, contact *www.raintree.com*.

Tian Xian for Gastrointestinal Cancer

When a patient was diagnosed with colon cancer and he failed to respond to chemo or surgery, he was given less than 60 days to live. A family member bought some Tian Xian for him. He began taking the herb and survived his ordeal, living on for several years.

Tian Xian is a Chinese herb ("pronounced *Dianne Sean*") that has been used in China to control, inhibit, and destroy cancer cells. Testimonials of people from all over the world who have been cured with this herb can be found at *tianxian.com*.

Turmeric: The Cancer-Fighting Herb

Turmeric contains curcumin, a potent antioxidant, shown to activate gene p53. This particular gene "stops defective cells from multiplying," thus inhibiting the growth and spread of cancer.[55] Note that turmeric is also being studied for its potential ability to help in the treatment of cystic fibrosis, and research has shown that it may help prevent diseases like Crohn's and colitis.

Turmeric is safe when used as a spice, however, if you are taking turmeric in supplement form, do not use if pregnant, nor if you have gallstones, since it stimulates the gallbladder. Like garlic, turmeric can slow clotting time, so it should be used in caution by anyone taking anti-coagulant medications,[56] with blood disorders, or for anyone recovering from or contemplating surgery, or those with ulcers.

Other Herbs Effective Against Colon Cancer

Bill Gottlieb recommends FOUR herbs for fighting colon cancer in his book, *Alternative Cures*, "Echinacea…Ginkgo…Astragalus…[and] Cat's Claw…" Cat's claw has long been important in colon cancer prevention. It helps promote the proliferation of "friendly, anti-cancer bacteria" in the intestines.[57] (This herb is also an excellent source of pycnogenols. You can find it in tea bags and in supplements.)

Website *herbs2000.com* recommends that you do not combine "cat's claw with hormonal drugs, insulin, or vaccines…" it should not be used for children without their doctor's knowledge, nor taken during pregnancy or lactation. It should not be used for those with "autoimmune illness, multiple sclerosis, and tuberculosis."[57a] Check with your physician first. Besides the herbs found in Essiac Tea and herbs such as garlic (already discussed in this book); see Chapter 18 for other anti-cancer herbs.

IV. Minerals And Nutrients For Colon & Abdominal Cancers

Calcium Prevents Colon Cancer

Research has shown that calcium can "reduce the risk" of some cancers (such as colon cancer) by as much as "75 percent." This is because calcium accelerates the removal of toxins from the digestive tract. If you decide on calcium supplements, you should find one that is combined with magnesium. Magnesium enables calcium to be utilized properly by the body.[58] (See the note on boron and vitamin D below.)

Calcium and magnesium are also important in the prevention of osteoporosis. In taking calcium and magnesium supplements for bone health, be sure that boron is included, and be sure that you are getting your vitamin D from natural sunlight. If you have a history of melanoma, consult with your physician beforehand. (See chapter 23!)

Quercetin Prevents Colon Cancer

One of the newest "superstars" in the anti-cancer nutrient arsenal is a potent bioflavonoid known as *quercetin.* It is described by Maureen Kennedy Salaman in her book, *All Your Health Questions Answered Naturally*:

> It is one of the strongest anti-cancer agents known. Various lab studies reveal that quercetin unleashes a one-two punch against cancer. It blocks cell changes that invite cancer and, if a tumor has already started, stops the spread of malignant cells. Red and yellow onions contain an incredible amount of quercetin – 10 percent or more of their dry weight. Not so white onions or, for that matter, garlic...[59]

In animal studies, quercetin inhibits the formation of intestinal cancers.[60] It is a powerful antioxidant, able to neutralize enzymes known to accelerate and initiate "tumor" expansion. Taking bromelain tablets will increase the body's ability to assimilate this powerful antioxidant. Bromelain is an extract from pineapples, so if you are allergic to pineapples, this substance is not for you! Also, this supplement is not recommended for those who may be taking certain immunosuppressant drugs and/or calcium channel blockers.[61] (Always check with your physician about supplements, especially if you are already on prescription medications.)

According to website, *www.news.cornell.edu/releases,* scientists at "Cornell University," have confirmed that "...Western Yellow, pungent yellow and Northern Red onions are higher in anti-cancer chemicals than other varieties tested."[61a] As noted by "Rui Hai Liu, M.D., Ph.D.," these chemicals can effectively inhibit "liver and colon cancer cell growth." Those varieties with the best anticancer effects for the colon were "pungent yellow and Western Yellow."[61b]

CoQ10: A Curative & Preventative

You may want to consider adding CoQ10 supplements to your daily diet if you are fighting cancer. As described by Dr. Stephen T. Sinatra, M.D., in his book, *The Coenzyme Q10 Phenomenon,* "anecdotal reports have demonstrated that high dose CoQ10 supplementation (i.e. 390 mg per day) has been associated with **complete remission**, even for patients with metastatic breast cancer." (Emphasis, mine.)[62] CoQ10 is also known as *ubiquinone.*

Dr. Sinatra also discussed studies by the late "Dr Karl Folkers," a primary researcher of CoQ10 who believed that insufficient amounts of CoQ10 and B6 could induce cancer in humans.[63]

Dr. Folkers tested 83 "patients in the United States...who had cancer of the breast, lung, prostate, pancreas, colon, stomach, rectum and other sites." They were ALL deficient in CoQ10![64] In another study, Dr. Sinatra found an alarming rise in breast cancer cases in women taking cholesterol lowering drugs. Apparently, they lowered cholesterol, but increased their risk of breast cancer![65]

CoQ10 & Multiple Sclerosis

There are other reasons that you may want to supplement with CoQ10 besides its cancer-fighting properties. Dr. Ray D. Strand, M.D., gives an amazing account of his experience treating a patient who came to him with **multiple sclerosis** in his book, *What Your Doctor Doesn't Know About Nutritional Medicine May Be Killing You.* When a young cowboy suddenly developed unexplainable weakness and numbness in his extremities, and was subsequently diagnosed with multiple sclerosis, he was fortunate enough to hear a lecture by Dr. Strand, and receive treatment that eventually resulted in complete remission. Dr. Strand explains what happened:

> It was about this time that Ross began looking into additional therapies for his MS. He heard me speak at a local meeting, and soon after began the nutritional supplement program I recommended to my patients with MS. Within

months he began to feel better. The numbness and weakness in his legs began to improve. Today, about three years later, Ross believes that he has fully recovered. The strength in his legs is back to normal, and he has absolutely no numbness in his legs, feet, or lower back. He is back to roping and again feels safe in the saddle.[66]

Dr. Strand also describes current MS treatment and how he used nutritional supplementation in Ross' case:

[P]hysicians are now using Betaserone and Avonex (which is actually interferon), drugs known to improve the immune response. Nutritional supplementation with potent antioxidants, minerals, CoQ10, grape seed extract, and essential fats do basically the same thing; however, they don't have all the adverse side effects. Again, I always encourage patients to continue taking all their prescription medications along with their supplements. Some MS patients do improve so much that they discuss going off their medication with their physicians.[66a]

It is noteworthy that vegetarian diets and low fat diets significantly reduce the risks for M.S. Research has also shown that curcumin may be beneficial in fighting M.S. because it appears to have a protective effect on nerve cells. Curcumin does have a blood-thinning effect and may increase bile and gastric acid output, something to consider if you have gallbladder disease or ulcers.

Grape Seed Extracts

See chapter two for more information about the powerful ingredient in grapes (Resveratrol) that has demonstrated amazing curative properties for nearly all cancers!

Dr. Ralph W. Moss says that "Pycnogenol® is the proprietary name of a product derived from the bark of the French maritime pine tree...," rich in "bioflavonoids," in his book *Antioxidants against Cancer*.[67] These bioflavonoids, reports Dr. Moss, are also found in the seeds of grapes and are sold as supplements. They are super antioxidants, important in preventing disease and boosting the immune system. These extracts are said to be "20 times as potent…as vitamin C and 50 times more potent than vitamin E." Apparently, nothing outperforms pycnogenol's ability to neutralize "free radicals" except for "green tea extract."[68]

Folic Acid & Colo-Rectal Cancers

Folic acid is critically important in the prevention of colon cancer. At his website *www.newmediaexplorer.org*, Chris Gupta discusses the fact that it was three decades before the FDA finally admitted that this vitamin had the capacity to "prevent neural tube birth defects." In the meantime, many countless birth defects occurred because the FDA refused to allow vitamin manufacturers to recommend the vitamin during pregnancy.[69] Chris also describes the results from the "famous Nurses' Health Study," which was done at "Harvard Medical School," revealing that those nurses who had taken the vitamin over a long period of time ("400 micrograms of folic acid a day for 15 years") reduced their chances of intestinal cancers by "75%." Apparently, this is one time that "supplements" worked better and proved more "protective" than ingestion of the vitamin via dietary means.[70] It is also important to note that the "90,000 women" who took part in this study had greater protection the longer they used folic acid. Those using the vitamin briefly experienced only "marginal protection."[71]

Zinc Combo Stops Abdominal & Esophageal Cancers

Though we need only small amounts of the mineral, zinc, a deficiency has been connected to many cancers, especially those of the esophagus and upper abdomen.[72]

Remarkable evidence of the link between cancer and zinc was revealed in data from a research study conducted in Linxian, China in the 1990s. This province holds an infamous reputation for "being the 'world capital' of cancer of the esophagus and upper stomach." It was theorized that the area lacked adequate amounts of "zinc and selenium" in the soil.[73] Chinese researchers collaborated with those in the U.S. to try to determine the exact cause. Zinc, selenium, and beta-carotene studies were done "between 1982 and 1991" that used "30,000" Chinese participants given "various food supplements," as described by Dr. Ralph Moss in *Antioxidants against Cancer:*

> The dosages were from two to three times the Recommended Daily Allowances. What they discovered was nothing less than astounding. Stomach cancer among those who received the zinc and vitamin A combination was decreased...62 percent compared to those who did not receive these supplements....[A] combination of beta-carotene, vitamin E, and selenium caused a 42 percent reduction in esophageal cancer.[74]

Dr. Moss said of the Chinese study, "I can only guess at what these scientists said privately about their ability to reduce esophageal cancer by 42% with a simple vitamin-mineral pill. Publicly they merely called this study 'a hopeful sign' which should encourage additional studies...in larger numbers of subjects.'"[75] He was disappointed that the results of this study generated very little media coverage. These were two dreadful cancers and small amounts of supplements were proven to prevent them, yet how many people who lived in or near the province not involved in the study were given this information? How many people succumbed to these two cancers years after this study because the findings were merely labeled "a hopeful sign," and never given the publicity they deserved?[76]

V. Vegetables for Healing

Fiber, Cruciferous Sulfur Veggies, & Colon Cancers

Many prestigious medical journals have touted the importance of fiber in preventing colon and other cancers. Perhaps no other source of fiber has become more prominent lately than cruciferous vegetables. As pointed out by John Heinerman in *Heinerman's New*

Encyclopedia of Fruits & Vegetables: "...the sulfur and histidine in broccoli, brussel sprouts, cabbage, cauliflower, kale, kohlrabi, and mustard greens inhibit the growth of tumors, prevent cancer of the colon and rectum, detoxify the system of harmful chemical additives and increase our body's cancer-fighting compounds."[77]

Other vital nutrients found in cruciferous vegetables such as cabbage, broccoli, and brussel sprouts are called *indoles*. Recent studies have shown that they are critically important in preventing and treating colon and abdominal cancers.

It is best to eat cruciferous vegetables raw as cooking destroys much of their vitamin and enzyme content. Consuming them with **"cloves"** and an "indian spice" known as ***"jambul"*** has been associated with decreasing the risk of stomach cancer.[78]

Lutein Inhibits Colon Cancer

Lutein is a carotenoid found in many fruits and vegetables. Research has documented that people who regularly eat dark leafy greens and other foods high in lutein could dramatically reduce their risk for cancer of the colon. In fact, statistics have proven that lutein-rich diets are colon-healthy! (Lutein is also critical for healthy eyes!) Avocados are lutein-rich!

Mushrooms That Inhibit Colo-Rectal Cancers & Prevent Their Spread

Maitake mushroom is an important stimulant for the immune system. According to *www.herbs2000.com*, an extract from this mushroom, *Maitake-D,* has shown impressive anticancer properties, including the ability to slow the "growth of new tumors."[79]

The "most potent" form of this mushroom is the "*Grifola frondosa.*" Taking "vitamin C" along with this mushroom makes absorption more efficient.[80]

According to website *herbs2000.com*, PSK or "*Polysaccharide kureha,*" also commonly "known as *krestin,* is an extract from the kawaratake mushroom." It can be found growing wild in several countries, and it has been the subject of over "200 scientific studies." Apparently, it prevents metastasis of tumors by neutralizing the "enzymes" that allow tumors to proliferate.[81]

Outside of the United States, PSK is considered the most popular anti-cancer drug in the world. It is also given as an adjunctive with other cancer treatments.[82] For colorectal cancers, **Reishi mushroom** tablets are also recommended for their ability to boost the immune system.[83]

Lentinan is an extract of the **Shiitake** *("Lentinus edodes")* mushroom. Deanne Tenney, in her book, *Medicinal Mushrooms*, reports that this extract has demonstrated the ability to trigger the body's manufacture of immune cells that destroy mutations, such as cancer cells.[84] It also "enhances the production of Interlukin," a compound well known to halt the formation of "cancer cells and viruses."[85] Lentinan "intramuscular injections or powder," known for their successful treatment of "stomach cancer," are considered *alternative therapy*, so you will have to seek an alternative practitioner to administer them![86]

Research revealed that shiitake can increase survival time for terminal cancer patients, without major adverse reactions. Also, if you have already had surgery to remove cancer, it is believed that this mushroom may help keep it from returning.[87]

VI. Fruits That Can Save Your Life!

Cherries Prevent & Treat Stomach Cancer

An ingredient found in cherries, a "monoterpene" known as *"perillyl alcohol"* is effective at preventing "cancers of the breast, lung, stomach, liver, and skin," according to "animal" testing conducted at "Indiana University School of Medicine in Indianapolis."[88] This is described in Selene Yeager's *Doctors Book of FOOD REMEDIES*, from a report by "Charles Elson, Ph.D…professor of nutritional sciences at the University of Wisconsin, Madison…" Dr. Elson states: "We're not just showing that this compound fights cancer, meaning that it neutralizes cancer-causing toxins. We're also showing that it is effective in animals with existing tumors."[89]

Papaya – A Healing Fruit for Colon Cancer

See Chapter 20 for examples of papaya extract's ability to shrink colon cancer and even put metastatic cancer into remission!

VII. Other Supplements & Treatments For Abdominal & Colon Cancers

Beta-Sitosterol Inhibits the Spread of Colon Cancer

Beta-Sitosterol is a naturally occurring plant nutrient "found in…rice bran, wheat germ, corn oils, and soybeans."[90] At his website *(www.drlam.com),* Dr. Lam reports that most diets have deficient levels of this nutrient. It has been found to inhibit the growth of colon cancer cells, being one of the main nutriceuticals from soy that inhibits cancer formation. It also has the ability to "heal ulcers," as well as keep "blood sugar" stable and boost the immune system, and is effective against prostate cancer and "lymphocytic leukemia."[91] (Fermented soy products, such as Haelan, can help remove harmful estrogens from the body in estrogen-receptor positive cancers.)

Of course, you should not take this supplement without first consulting your physician. It should not be taken by anyone with any type of atypical health problems or disorders that interfere with their ability to properly assimilate fats. Some examples are beta sitosterolemia (see website: *http://rarediseases.info.nih.gov/html/reports/fy2003/nhlbi.html*[92]) or "cerebrotendinous xanthamosis" (see website: *http://www.ninds.nih.gov/disorders/leukodystrophy/leukodystrophy.html*[93]) This supplement is available at natural health food stores in tablet or capsule form, and you may find it combined with herbs or other nutrients.

Burzynski's Antineoplastons

See chapter 13 of this book for amazing cases of cancer patients completely cured of "terminal" cancers, people who were basically sent home to die, then chose non-toxic antineoplastons from the Burzynski Clinic in Houston, Texas. Also see many of the patient's own stories about their success in fighting cancer with antineoplastons at website: *http://burzynskipatientgroup.org/stories.html.* The main Burzynski Clinic website is at *www.cancermed.com.*

Vitamin Supplements

A good balanced vitamin-mineral supplement is recommended for anyone fighting cancer or any other serious illness. Many foods that you juice will have natural forms of vitamins and minerals (such as beta-carotene and calcium in carrot juice). All vitamins and minerals are important in cancer prevention and treatment.

For example, in the body, **vitamin D** is turned into a hormone that can cling to and neutralize colon cancer cells. Adequate vitamin D can cut your threat of colon cancer in half![94]

One of the best ways to get adequate amounts of vitamin D is 10-20 minutes a day of full sun exposure without using sunscreen. According to an article from *www.herbs2000.com*, studies have shown that "even modest amounts of vitamin D can hasten recovery from Stage I colon tumors…[and] 500-1000 mg of vitamin D" are necessary every day.[94a] Avoid taking iron supplements, [unless ordered by your physician for anemia or other blood disorders], because "iron supplements and iron-rich foods, such as organ meats," appear to cause "colon damage."[94b] Check with your physician about sun exposure if you have a prior history of skin cancer or are taking medications that may cause sun sensitivity.

Shark Cartilage Halts Abdominal Tumor

When scientists discovered that sharks rarely get cancer, regardless of how contaminated their environment, investigations began into the secret of their resistance to this disease. As described by Maureen Kennedy Salaman in her book, *Nutrition: The Cancer Answer II*, this disease resistance found in sharks has been researched and documented by "Dr. William Lane, Ph.D.," who wrote in "*Sharks Don't Get Cancer*" that it is the "cartilage" that shields "them from cancer," because cartilage prevents the growth of "new blood vessels."[95] Cancer cells must be fed to survive. Within two weeks of growth, cancer cells "develop a system of arteries. Shark cartilage blocks this tumor-survival effort," and this essentially "starves" the tumor to death, explains Ms. Salaman.[95a] She also describes a case where a physician from Central America successfully used shark cartilage to treat one of his patients "who had an inoperable, grapefruit-sized abdominal tumor." Within 30 days, "the tumor stopped growing...and after six months shrank to the size of a walnut."[96] (This extract has also been successful against ovarian, cervical, and uterine cancers, and is discussed further in chapter six.)

Shark cartilage is not for use with children, nor during pregnancy, or if you have recently had a heart attack, transplant, surgery, chemo or radiation. It is not for those with high blood pressure, pheochromocytoma (adrenal tumor which can cause excessively high blood pressure), ulcers, allergies to seafood, or circulatory diseases. It is not for those with liver disease, except it has been used successfully against liver cancer itself. Dosing information can be found in chapter six of this book. Be aware that you should always consult with your naturopathic health physician for specific dosing for your own individual needs before using this supplement.

Soy Supplements

Soy is the source of potent antioxidants. One of them, known as *daidzein,* has been shown to inhibit the growth of colon cancer cells. Another soy product, *Haelan,* has been responsible for the remission of several different types of cancers. There is some controversy about soy products, but fermented soy is fine.

Haelan is nothing more than a "fermented soy beverage," however, according to Donna Sage, M.S.S.A., it has been used successfully against cancer, though it was originally "developed in China in the early 1980s as a hospital nutrition supplement."[97] Haelan has high amounts of "the two main [soy] isoflavones genistein and diadzein," reports Ms. Sage, as well as "protease inhibitors," which are known to "prevent the mutation of healthy cells into cancerous cells." Fermented soy is also very high in many vitamins and minerals.[97a] See chapter three in this book for more detailed information about Haelan's cancer-fighting properties. (Fermented soy products, such as Haelan, can help remove harmful estrogens from the body in estrogen-receptor positive cancers.)

How Wheat Grass Juice Cured Colon Cancer!

According to Steve Meyerowitz in his book, *Wheatgrass Nature's Finest Medicine,* "Gary Garrett" of "Gainesville, Florida" was given a poor prognosis when a baseball-sized colon cancer was found growing though the "wall" of his "colon." It had already metastasized to "six lymph nodes" and his "liver." Physicians told him that chemotherapy and radiation would buy him **six months of life**. He had surgery, but refused both chemo and radiation and began a wheat grass regimen. He lived another three years, then died while hospitalized for a liver infection during a time he did not have access to fresh wheat grass juice! His wife felt that had he been able to drink fresh wheat grass juice during that time, he would still be alive.[98]

See more information about the amazing healing properties of wheat grass juice and other green juices later in chapter 16 of this book, *God's Great Grasses.*

Ukrain Effective Against Colo-Rectal Cancer Without Toxic Side Effects

Ukrain, discussed in previous chapters, was named after the country of the physician who developed it (without the "e"). It is a merger of two compounds, a plant called *"greater celandine"* and the drug "thiotepa," both highly toxic. However, it was found that when these two ingredients are combined, they are only toxic to cancer cells! Ukrain has proven effective against many different cancers in laboratory studies and clinical trials with **hundreds of cancer patients! (These are HUMAN studies, not animals!)**[99]

At the main Ukrain website, *www.ukrin.com*, they report that "96 patients with colorectal carcinomas" were part of "a randomised [sic] study carried out by Prof. Zemskov (National Medical University Kiev, Ukraine)...(15 of them with metastasising [sic] and 33 with non-metastasising [sic] colorectal tumors)."[100] 48 of the 96 patients received Ukrain and the other 48 received radiation and the common chemo drug 5-FU. 21 months later, **75% of those "treated with Ukrain" were still alive, while only 33% of the patients on the conventional chemo and radiation were still alive!**[101]

Another randomized study was done involving "48 patients with rectal carcinoma. Dr. Bondar (Regional Cancer Centre, Donetsk)," headed up the study. As *ukrin.com* further reports, Dr. Bondar treated 24 of the patients before they had surgery with "5-FU" and "high dose radiotherapy" and the other 24 had "one series" only of "Ukrain therapy" before having surgery ("10 mg every second day, to a total of 60 mg) and one series after the operation (to a total of 40 mg)."[102] Within a period of "14 months," one fourth of those on the chemo and radiation relapsed, "but only 8.3% of patients who had received UKRAIN" relapsed. When the patients were checked "two years later...33.3% of patients who had received" chemo and radiation "had relapses but only 16.7% of the patients who had been treated with UKRAIN."[103] The Ukrain repeatedly outperformed both chemo drugs and radiation therapy!

In spite of all this, if you are diagnosed with cancer, don't expect your physician to know a thing about Ukrain, unless he or she is an alternative medicine doctor. You will have to seek an alternative health physician in the United States, Europe, Canada, or the Ukraine where it is popular therapy. You can find out more about ukrain therapy at *http://www.ukrin.com*.

Water Can Prevent Cancer

So important to our survival (it isn't actually considered a supplement), water, in recent studies, has been shown to decrease the risk of developing cancer! To benefit from water, be sure that you drink it chlorine-free and fluoride-free!

According to website *www.herbs2000.com,* research "in Taiwan" found that men drinking "more than 8 glasses of water" on a daily basis experienced a "92 percent lower risk of developing colon cancer than men who drink fewer than 8 glasses of water a day, even when all other factors are taken into account." The men in this study were between "thirty-three and eighty" years of age.[104]

Cancer patients are usually dehydrated. This according to the late Dr. F. Batmanghelidg, M.D., in *Your Body's Many Cries For Water.* Lack of sufficient water has been linked to the cause of asthma, lupus, Crohn's Disease, diabetes, irritable bowel syndrome, degenerative disc disease, arthritis, migraines, cancer, and all autoimmune disorders! Remember when drinking water, you need to increase your salt intake. Dr. Batmanghelidg recommended that "for every 10 glasses of water (about two quarts)" you need a "half teaspoon of salt per day."[105] See website *www.watercure2.org.* Always check with your physician if you are on a water-restricted or salt-restricted diet, and be sure to read chapter 22 later in this book for more information on using water for optimal health.

Poly–MVA (Palladium Lipoic Complex)

See chapters 9 and 13 for more information on the amazing nutritional formula known as Poly-MVA that many "terminal" cancer patients have credited to bringing their cancers into total remission! The main Poly-MVA website is located at *www.polymva.net.*

CHAPTER 6

PAINLESS CURES & PREVENTIONS FOR CERVICAL, UTERINE & OVARIAN CANCERS

"Biologists have been telling medical doctors for thirty years that it is possible to destroy cancerous tumors by just giving the patient drugs that interfere with the development of new blood vessels. Why hasn't organized medicine listened to them?"
(Dr. Burt Berkson, from his book: *The Alpha Lipoic Acid Breakthrough)*[1]

I. Natural Foods That Prevent & Kill Cervical, Ovarian, & Uterine Cancer Cells

Berry Extract Kills Cervical Cancer Cells

Researchers have discovered that compounds taken from blueberries and strawberries actively inhibited the growth of both cervical and breast cancer cells.

Beta-Carotene Fights Cervical & Endometrial Cancer

The most important indicator (among nearly a dozen that were tested), for the risk of cervical cancer, is insufficient amounts of "beta-carotene..." This, according to Jack Challem in his book, *All About Carotenoids Beta-carotene, Lutein & Lycopene.* Mr. Challem explains that this was true not only for "cervical dysplasia," but "cancer of the cervix," as well. It was also discovered that the "synthetic form" of beta-carotene did not offer the same protection as that supplied by nature![2] One of the best ways to get beta-carotene naturally is to juice raw carrots and other foods rich in beta-carotene. The body converts beta-carotene to vitamin A.

In *Earl Mindell's Food as Medicine*, Dr. Mindell suggests the following dietary regimen for the prevention of cervical cancer: "...foods rich in beta-carotene (sweet potato, carrots, kale), lycopene (ruby red grapefruit, red pepper, tomato), folic acid (asparagus, spinach, wheat germ), and vitamin C (cantaloupe, cauliflower, berries)."[3] These same foods fight other cancers (e.g. oral and pancreatic) as well!

When Swiss and Italian researchers checked the dietary trends of hundreds of their citizens, they discovered that it did not take much to protect against endometrial cancer.[4] They found that women eating very small quantities of "beta-carotene…[daily] the amount in one cup of baked winter squash," slashed their "risk of endometrial cancer" in half![5]

Broccoli Prevents Cervical Cancer

Scientists conducting a research study discovered that women could dramatically reduce their risks of developing cervical cancer by increasing their dietary intake of broccoli![6]

Cherries Inhibit Ovarian Cancer

Dr. Raymond Hohl, M.D., from "the University of Iowa," revealed that the "perillyl alcohol (POH)…" in cherries "…is extremely powerful in reducing the incidence of all types of cancer. As described at *www.flavonoidsciences.com,* "perillyl alcohol 'shuts down the growth of cancer cells by depriving them of the proteins they need to grow…'" Dr. Hohl explains that "it works on every kind of cancer we've tested it against."[7] This nutrient, says *flavonoidsciences.com*, "performed favorably in the treatment of advanced carcinomas of the breast, prostate, and ovary." In animal testing, it was reported to be "up to five times more potent than the other known cancer-reducing compounds at inducing tumor regression."[8] (You can find some very potent cherry and blueberry supplements at website: *http://www.flavonoid sciences.com/research/c3.htm.)*

Citrus Pectin Prevents Cancer Metastasis

Modified citrus pectin is found in all plants. In animal studies, it has been shown to inhibit the metastasis or spread of cancer cells.[9]

According to Russell Blaylock, M.D., in his book, *Natural Strategies For Cancer Patients,* the compound was tested against many forms "of human cancers – prostate cancer, two breast cancer types, melanoma, and laryngeal epidermoid carcinoma..." and successfully prevented "metastasis" in all of them![10] (It also lowers unhealthy cholesterol.)

Website *http://www.breadbeckers.com/bulkuponfiber.htm* describes some very good NATURAL sources of pectin including: "apples, bananas, cabbage, citrus fruits, dried peas and okra."[10a] Of course anything containing these ingredients, such as jams and jellies (e.g. apple jam and marmalade), would also be high in pectin.

Ellagic Acid Fights Cervical & Other Cancers

Dr. Daniel Nixon from "MUSC...began studying ellagic acid in 1993." As described at *www.cancer-prevention.net*, "his recently published results" revealed that "cervical cancer cells [and] HPV (human papilloma virus) exposed to ellagic acid" were destroyed.[10b] The antioxidant also prevented "cancer cell division," as well as "destruction of the P53 gene by cancer cells," a gene that prevents normal cells from mutating. There were "similar results for breast, pancreas, esophageal, skin, colon and prostate cancer cells."[10c] One of the richest natural sources of ellagic acid is raspberries. Cherries, berries and pomegranates also contain this nutrient.

Flaxseed Reduces Uterine & Cervical Cancers

A research study involving flaxseed revealed that women who consume flaxseed supplements can reduce their risk for several types of cancers. The main gist of this research emphasized that using flaxseed may prevent and "treat" many ominous types of cancer, including "breast, uterus, and cervix..."[11]

An excellent way to incorporate flax oil into the diet is to use fresh organic whole flaxseed (either the golden or the brown). Put 2 tablespoons in a coffee grinder. Grind until powdery (about 5 seconds), mix in 8 ounces of water (shake well) and drink. Just be sure to drink it immediately. If you let it sit, even for a few seconds it will thicken too much. Drink additional water or juice if needed. It can be used as a breakfast drink, then again later in the day, up to 2 - 3 times per day. (Each tablespoon of flax gives you about one teaspoon of flax oil). Or add one tablespoon of flax oil to a baked potato or your favorite salad dressing, fruit smoothie or juice. (Most of us need 2 - 3 tablespoons of flaxseed oil per day.)

Lycopene & Endometrial Cancers

Lycopene, discussed earlier, is a potent anti-oxidant and, in laboratory studies, was effective against endometrial cancer. As noted by Dr. R.W. Moss in his book, *Antioxidants against Cancer,* lycopene was found to be "four times stronger than alpha-carotene, and ten times stronger than beta-carotene at inhibiting tumor growth" when tested against cultures of "human endometrial, breast, and lung cancer cells."[12] High levels of lycopene were also linked to dramatic reductions in cancers of the head and neck, "stomach...colon," and "rectum...."[13] Look for this nutrient in veggies and fruits such as watermelon, guavas, carrots, and red tomatoes.

Mushrooms that Inhibit Cancer

Mushrooms (reishi, maitake, shiitake, and several others) have been shown to inhibit cancers. According to the *Wellness Directory of Minnesota's™* website, *http://www.mnwelldir.org,* one mushroom in particular that is effective against ovarian cancer is the agaricus mushroom "(Agaricus Blazei Murill or ABM)."[13a] You can use this mushroom much like any other mushroom. It contains a polysaccharide that was found "effective against Ehrlich's ascites carcinoma, sigmoid colonic cancer, ovarian cancer, breast cancer, lung cancer, and liver cancer as well as against solid cancers."[13b] *Mnwelldir.org* explains that in Japan, when "mice were fed ABM as a preventative and then injected with a very powerful cancer causing agent (sarcoma 180), 99.4% of them showed no tumor growth. Conventional medicine has **nothing as powerful as this**," and "...studies in Japan showed ABM to be 80% more effective than the world's [outside the U.S.] number one cancer drug, PSK."[14] (Emphasis, mine.) PSK is discussed below.

These mushrooms can be ordered at "*www.agaricus.net*," one of the "largest suppliers in the world." They can also be purchased at "*www.mitobi.com.*" They are available from "*http://www.hplus.com/a36.html*" in "freeze dried extract" capsules. You can also "order mushrooms in bulk, wholesale from China," at "*http://www.abmcn.com.*"[15] (See chapter 24 of this book for more information about the amazing healing and curative powers of mushrooms and their extracts.)

Polysaccharide Kureha (PSK)

PSK is an important supplement for preventing the spread of tumors. "Also known as *krestin*…[it]…is an extract from the kawaratake mushroom." *Herbs2000.com*, explains that it is a potent antioxidant that boosts the immune system, and the Japanese have been using the complex polysaccharides in this mushroom for more than 20 years.[16] "It is virtually nontoxic and readily bioavailable when taken orally," and is often used in conjunction with other cancer therapies. It can also be found in tablet form. You should consult your physician if you intend to use it.[16a]

Wellness Directory of Minnesota's™ website notes that PSK is "the world's number one cancer drug," but this is excluding the U.S. Most Americans don't even know this supplement exists! This is because when you are diagnosed with cancer in Japan (for example), they start using the **least toxic** medications **first** then progress to the most toxic.[17]

We do things **backwards** in America. Cancer patients are given the deadliest treatments first, and if the cancer is still there, they are either zapped with more chemo until it sucks out what little life they have left in them, or else they are told they are *terminal*, and nothing else can be done for them! Conventional physicians rarely tell them about the safer, alternative treatments available. (Mostly, because many conventional physicians don't know what is available in alternative treatments.) Patients only hear about them from a relative or a friend who has researched them, or from reading a book such as this one! Often, their immune system has already been irreversibly **obliterated** by toxic chemo and radiation! However, remember this, as long as you are still alive, it is NEVER too late, regardless of what your diagnosis is! There are many cases in this book of *terminally ill* cancer patients, completely cured of cancer using natural therapies! See chapter 13. Also, see chapter 35, *What To Do If You Are Already Ill,* for more information.

II. Hormones Against Cancer

Being Estrogen Dominant Increases Your Risk For Ovarian Cancer

See chapter 21 in this book *(Prescription HRT, The Great Tragedy Of the 20th Century)* on hormone replacement therapy for information on the dangers of estrogen dominance and how it contributes to uterine cancer, breast cancer, ovarian cancer, excess weight, mood swings, infertility, cystic breasts, uterine fibroids, and a host of other maladies!

In *What Your Doctor May Not Tell You About Menopause,* Virginia Hopkins and the late Dr. John Lee discuss how correct levels of "ovarian hormones using saliva," can be determined. Dr. Lee and Ms. Hopkins wrote that the high "estrogen levels" found "in the West" are abnormal, and may be the reason for our "current epidemic of breast and ovarian cancer." Lack of exercise and excessive calories were also contributing factors.[18]

The reason that our calorie intake in the West is so much higher than in less industrialized nations is because of the high "fat content of our diet. Some 40 per cent of our calories come from dietary fat... Excess calories = excess fats = higher estrogen levels = greater incidence of breast and uterine cancer."[19]

Besides controlling high estrogen levels by eating less and exercising more, see chapter 21 on how natural progesterone cream can play a part in the prevention (and reversal) of estrogen dominance, cancer, and all of the health issues noted above.

III. Vitamins & Minerals That Fight Cancer

Cervical Cancer, Vitamin C & Poly–MVA

Apparently, even in small amounts, vitamin C can prevent cancer. In the book *Healing With Vitamins*, by the editors of *Prevention* Health Books, it was noted that researchers were looking for an explanation as to why "cervical cancer" rates are so high in "Latin America," as compared to the rest of the world. They discovered that if women there would supplement with even small amounts of vitamin C on a daily basis, they could slash their risk of this cancer by greater than one-third, and it did not require much – slightly more than 300 milligrams daily![20] (See chapters 9 and 13 for info on Poly-MVA.)

Folate & Vitamin C Prevent Cervical Cancer

The amount of vitamin concentration in our tissues varies greatly. Dr. Blaylock in *Natural Strategies for Cancer Patients*, says that a woman's body actually contains greater amounts of "vitamin C and folate" in her cervix than is found in her "gallbladder." It should therefore, be no surprise that insufficient amounts of either of these nutrients can increase a woman's chances tenfold of getting "cervical cancer...."[21]

Some good natural sources of folic acid are: "Asparagus, Avocados, Bananas, Beans, Beets...Cabbage...Cantaloupe, Citrus Fruits/juices, Endive...Green, leafy vegetables, Lentils, [and] sprouts."[22] Natural sources of vitamin C are cherries, oranges, currants, papaya, cantaloupe, peppers, leafy green vegetables, watermelon, berries, and many other fruits and vegetables.

Vitamin E & Glutathione Prevent Cervical Cancers

The risk of invasive cancers can be decreased "threefold" simply by supplementing with "200 to 400 international units of vitamin E per day..." Also, as noted by *herbs2000.com*, insufficient levels of "the amino acid glutathione" are associated with an increased incidence of cervical cancers.[23] Having a pap test with "atypical" cells, however, does not necessarily mean a cancerous condition. Lesions that are "cancerous or pre-cancerous" in the cervix will "turn white when exposed to vinegar. In most cases, this change can be observed visually by a physician or trained nurse-midwife."[24] An excellent natural source of glutathione is asparagus. (See chapter nine for a list of many natural glutathione-rich foods.)

Selenium Fights Cervical & Ovarian Cancer

Selenium, discussed earlier in this book, is gaining much attention for its ability to fight cancer. In the Reader's Digest Book, *The Healing Power of Vitamins, Minerals, and Herbs,* it is explained that selenium combined with vitamin E has anti-inflammatory properties. When two different universities conducted "a five year study" on this mineral, they discovered that "200 mcg [micrograms] of selenium daily" slashed all incidences of "prostate...colorectal...lung malignancies," and "overall...cancer deaths."[25] The statistics were remarkable. It has also been shown to prevent just about every other cancer imaginable, and insufficient blood "levels" of this mineral increased the risks for malignancies, metastasis, and reduced "survival rate..."[25a]

IV. Herbs That Prevent & Treat Ovarian, Cervical & Uterine Cancer

Andiroba Inhibits Cervical Cancers

According to *www.rain-tree.com*, andiroba *"(Carapa guianensis)"* is a very tall tree found in the "Amazon Rainforest" as well as other areas. Oil from the tree has been used for a multitude of purposes, including pain relief.[25b] Recently, scientists have discovered that this tree has anti-cancerous effects. As recently as 2002 scientists noted that "the seed oil could prevent and even reverse cervical dysplasia." Also, "the leaf, bark, seeds, and flowers have shown some activity against sarcoma cancer cells in vitro..."[25c] The oil is used to treat skin disorders, says raintree, including skin cancers, parasites, rashes, and fungi. Though there are no known drug interactions or toxicity reported from andiroba, it is always possible for some individuals to be allergic to certain herbs.[26] For more information on this herb, contact *www.rain-tree.com*.

Astragalus Tincture or Capsules

Astragalus is important in slowing the progression of malignancies and triggering the body's immunity. This herb is not recommended for those with an active infectious process.[27]

Cat's Claw

Cat's claw raises levels of white blood cells that kill cancer cells. Do not use it however, if you are breast feeding or pregnant. Do not combine it with hormones or diabetic medications, including insulin.[28] This herb, according to *herbs2000.com*, is not recommended for those with "autoimmune illness, multiple sclerosis, and tuberculosis."[29]

Chinese Skullcap

Chinese Skullcap "(Scutellaria baicalensis)" is described by website *www. compassionateacupuncture.com,* as having the ability to inhibit "many viruses including tumor viruses and the HIV virus....It is also anti-inflammatory and induces cell death in a number of cancer cell lines including two sarcomas and cervical cancer. (Yance, 1999)" [30]

Emodin & Cervical Cancer

Emodin has been an herb of choice in Chinese medicine for years. It has anticancer properties against many types of cancers, including those of the cervix in human cells. In laboratory testing, it has the ability to cause cancer cells to undergo a type of suicidal death.[30a]

Essiac Tea & Advanced Ovarian Cancer

Chapter five of this book has more details on the herbal remedy, Essiac tea, and the story of the Canadian nurse who used the tea to cure many of her cancer patients. In an article at *www.1001herbs.com,* a case history is given of Myrna, a patient diagnosed with an aggressive metastasizing cancer of her ovaries that was already in her lungs and lymphatic system. Physicians told her that surgery to remove all of her cancer was not possible due to the large amount of tumors. They did however, perform a hysterectomy, gave her "six months," and she was basically sent home to die.[31]

When Myrna asked her doctors if anything could be done from an alternative approach, such as using nutrition to extend her life and retard the disease, she was told that nothing could be done. She was however, given "a new hormonal therapy," and she also obtained the herbs for Essiac tea, which her grandmother brewed for her.[32] She went to her physician on a weekly basis and x-rays showed that the tumors were slowly shrinking! Not only were the tumors disappearing, but "her blood count returned to normal." Shortly over "a year after beginning Essiac, the doctor called to tell Myrna she was an official miracle. Her charts showed no indication of cancer in any systems…" That was three years ago and there has been no recurrence.[33] (The "hormonal therapy" was not identified.)

Espinheira Santa Inhibits Ovarian Cancer

Espinheira santa is an herb often referred to as "South American holly." According to *herbs2000.com*, it is used medicinally for many ailments and has been found to have notable antitumor properties. Laboratory studies show that this herb may be effective against "some forms of lung cancer," and that "it slows [the] growth of ovarian tumors."[34]

The herb can be purchased in tincture form and is also sold in bulk-tea format. If interested in purchasing the herb, contact *www.rain-tree.com.* There are many websites and natural health food stores that offer herbal remedies.

German Chamomile

Chamomile is commonly prepared in tea bags. It contains compounds that suppress the ability of malignant cells to attach themselves to "new sites," thus preventing their spread.[35] Be sure to discuss this herb with your physician before supplementing.

Graviola

See Chapter four and five for more information on how a common herb, *Graviola,* from the Amazon Rainforest was used to bring about total remission in two types of cancer.

Green Tea

Green tea is an excellent source of very powerful antioxidants that inhibit the ability of estrogen to be absorbed by tumor cells. It is best to wait at least 60 minutes after drinking green tea before you take any "other medications."[36]

Resveratrol

See Chapter two in this book for information on cases of ovarian and cervical cancers that were completely healed using resveratrol (in grape juice).

Snow Fungus Inhibits Cervical Cancer

Snow fungus *"(Tremella fuciformis),"* also called "white jelly leaf...white tree-ear," and other common names, grows on trees and "decaying logs."[36a] *Herbs2000.com* says that this herb has been used for many centuries in China and Japan for medicinal purposes. The fungus has been identified as an important stimulant for the immune system having "antitumor activity," cholesterol lowering abilities, anti-inflammatory properties, and it "protects the liver."[37] The website also notes that there are polysaccharides in snow fungus that "fit like keys into receptor sites on certain immune cells." This causes an increase in immune boosting chemicals. Snow fungus can slow down the "rate at which cancers spread." In laboratory studies, extracts from this fungus have been able to "kill cervical cancer cells, as well as those taken from other types of tumors."[38]

Turmeric Fights Cervical Cancer

Turmeric is a popular spice used throughout the world. It contains a very impressive antioxidant known as *curcumin* that triggers genetic activity to suppress the multiplication of malignant cells.[38a] Excessive levels of harmful estrogen inhibit this gene from doing its job adequately, as do toxins. It is the curcumin in turmeric that motivates this gene and enables it to work efficiently, thus inhibiting cervical dysplasia. Turmeric can be purchased at your local grocery store as a spice or in supplements at natural health food stores.[39] Be aware that turmeric has blood thinning effects. It can be consumed in large amounts by most people without problems, however turmeric intake is not recommended if you have gallbladder disease, such as gallstones.[39a]

Inflammation & the Cancer Process – Ovarian Cancer

There appears to be a close connection between an underlying infection and the subsequent development of cancer. This is probably the reason that the media recently publicized that following an aspirin regimen reduced the incidence of "lung cancer" in "women" by 50% over those not on the regimen. They claimed the same protection against other cancers, such as "breast cancer and colon cancer."[40]

Aspirin usage, however, has some very unpopular side effects. Many people are hospitalized yearly with fatal complications (i.e. bleeding ulcers) from using aspirin and NSAIDS. Rather than using aspirin, there are natural plant flavonoids that can block the enzymes responsible for inflammation. Several of these substances are given in Dr. Russell Blaylock's book, *Natural Strategies For Cancer Patients*, and they can be found in "ginkgo biloba…celery, parsley…curcumin…kale, turnip greens, broccoli, black tea, strawberries…black currants, green tea…onions, apples, cranberries…green beans…[and] grapefruits."[41]

V. Other Anti-Cancer Supplements & Treatments

Burzynski's Antineoplastons

See chapter 13 of this book for amazing cases of cancer patients completely cured of "terminal" cancers, people who were basically sent home to die, then chose non-toxic antineoplastons from the Burzynski Clinic in Houston Texas. Antineoplastons are also used to treat ovarian, uterine and cervical cancers and nearly every other cancer imaginable. Also, see many of the patient's own stories about their success in fighting cancer with antineoplastons at website: *http://burzynskipatientgroup.org/stories.html.* Many of these cancers were "hopeless" very aggressive tumors. The main Burzynski Clinic website is at *www.cancermed.com.*

Hydrazine Sulfate Inhibits Cervical Cancer

See Chapter 15 for details on hydrazine sulfate, a product promoted by Joseph Gold, M.D., for treating many forms of cancer, including cervical cancer.

Painless Treatments that Cured Uterine, Cervical, and Peritoneal Cancers

When a biochemical researcher began experimenting on sharks to find out why they rarely develop cancer – regardless of how polluted their environment – Reese Dubin in his book, *Miracle Cures From The Bible*, says that the next step was human testing. Three physicians: "Dr. Ernesto Contreras, Sr., M.D. and his two sons," treated ten cancer victims without charge, all of them having advanced cancer with less than "6 months" to live.[42] One patient left the study and one died, leaving eight to participate, explains Mr. Dubin. Though these were considered "hopeless cases," in "seven" patients tumors decreased and some were considered "miracle cures," and Mr. Dubin describes three of them:

(1.) "A 48-year-old woman" who was diagnosed "with a Stage III inoperable…uterine and cervix cancer with invasion to the bladder." She had received radiation treatment earlier, but it had not halted the progression of her cancer. After trying "shark-cartilage therapy" for 49 days, her pain had nearly disappeared and the cancerous mass had shrunk by "80 percent…After eleven weeks, there was a complete (100 percent) reduction in tumor size."[43]

(2.) "A 62-year-old female" with "previously treated cervical and uterine…cancer" that had metastasized "to the right sacroiliac." This metastasis was found "in an area that had been previously radiated." The patient underwent "9 weeks of shark cartilage therapy" after which the tumor shrank by "80 percent…" **Nearly three months into the treatment, the tumor had completely disappeared. She "was considered cured."**[44] (Emphasis, mine.)

(3.) "A 36-year-old" woman "with a stage IV peritoneal carcinoma from a colon primary cancer." She was basically cut open, sewed back up and told she was terminal. For nearly two months, she was given "shark cartilage treatment." She then underwent a surgical procedure "to remove an abscess," and it was discovered that her tumor had shriveled by "80 percent…**At eleven weeks, the patient was tumor-free and was considered by the doctors to be a 'miracle cure.'"**[45] (Emphasis, mine.)

It is remarkable that one of the first benefits of shark cartilage was its ability to reduce pain, and in all of the clinical trials done, there were some patients who did not "respond" at all, some who "improved," then relapsed, but, as explained by Mr. Dubin, there was *"absolutely no toxicity…noted at any dosage level."*[46] He says that the "shark cartilage…used [was] 100 percent pure…" Patients having advanced tumors ("Stage III and Stage IV") were given "1 gram of shark cartilage per 2 pounds of body weight" daily as a "retention enema" or "orally if necessary."[47]

It appears that giving shark cartilage has not only benefited several cancer patients, but those suffering from arthritis, psoriasis, and enteritis as well, explains Reese Dubin. One particular case involved a patient bedridden with "rheumatoid arthritis."[48] The patient opted for shark cartilage treatment as he had suffered for more than two decades with severe pain, misshapen joints, and everything conventional medicine could offer, which had not helped. He was placed on capsules of shark cartilage: "one capsule per 11 pounds of body weight for 21 days, then four capsules per day for the next 21 days." In another "three weeks," he was completely pain-free and "his spinal column [had] straightened."[49]

Since shark cartilage works by preventing new blood vessels from growing (which tumors depend on to survive) it is not recommended during pregnancy, for children, or for patients recovering from surgical procedures, heart attacks, transplants, taking chemo or radiation, or contemplating surgery. It is not for those with high blood pressure, pheochromocytoma (adrenal tumor which can cause excessively high blood pressure), seafood allergies, liver disease (though it has been used successfully in treating liver cancer itself), ulcers or circulatory diseases. See above for more information on dosing. Also you should be consulting with your natural health physician for specific dosing for your own individual needs before taking this supplement.

According to "Harvard Medical School," the spread of blood vessel networking is called *angiogenesis*," a process where "a network of blood vessels grows to nourish the tumors. These researchers recommend 2,000 mg. a day." Shark cartilage is available at most health food stores.[50]

Conventional medicine has never recognized shark cartilage as a remedy for cancer, in spite of its anti-angiogenesis factors. But you will never guess what a pharmaceutical company began pushing last year to target tumors! It is a new chemo drug described as having the ability to inhibit the formation of new arteries and veins to prevent tumors from being supplied with the nutrients they need to survive, something that shark cartilage also does.

This ability to cut off circulation to tumors is not really new. This is what shark cartilage does. The only catch is this: the new chemo drug has some very toxic side effects, some of them even fatal, such as ruptured intestines with hemorrhage! That is only one of about thirty toxic side effects! Others include kidney disease, congestive heart failure, blood clots and potentially fatal blood disorders!

Are you getting a picture of how the drug *system* works? Do you know how many potentially toxic side effects shark cartilage has? Thus far there have been no serious side effects associated with the use of shark cartilage. Shark cartilage, a natural product **can not be patented**. Better to CREATE a synthetic drug (with two dozen or more potentially deadly side effects) that can be patented and sold for millions of dollars, than to tell the public that a NATURAL substance that inhibits new blood vessel formation (without **TOXIC side effects)** is already available! (See notes earlier about when you should not take shark cartilage)

Shark cartilage has repeatedly demonstrated its anti-angiogenesis properties. As described at website *http://www.enerex.ca/articles/shark_cartilage.htm*:

> Dr. Judith Folkman and her research team at Children's Hospital in Boston several years ago showed that without access to a constantly expanded and replaced supply of blood, cancerous tissues stop growing as soon as the tumors have reached a size of 1 to 2 cubic millimeters....no toxicity has been reported in any of the studies conducted using shark cartilage.[51]

Also, see the story in chapter 16 of this book of an 89-year-old woman diagnosed with "Stage IIIA, Grade 3, papillary serous carcinoma...in the left ovary and omentum" who underwent surgery to remove the cancer, but refused the "traditional 6-round chemotherapy with paclitaxel and cisplatin" that her oncologist prescribed. Instead, she opted for a nutritional, alternative cancer program which included the use of wheat grass juice, even though her "oncologist... family physician...gynecologist, and a referred John Hopkins oncologist tried to convince her to "accept chemotherapy." She went into remission and has had no recurrences or cancer metastasis since. The diet she followed is given in more detail in chapter 16.[51a]

Soy Isoflavones & Endometrial Cancer

Soy contains a powerful antioxidant, *genistein*, which has been shown to inhibit the "growth of estrogen-dependent cancers."[52] Website *herbs2000.com,* recommends that those with endometrial cancer avoid the herbs "cordyceps, dan shen, fennel seed, licorice, [and] peony."[53] There is some controversy about soy. When choosing soy products, choose organic, and use in moderation, however, fermented soy products are fine. (Fermented soy products, such as Haelan, can help remove harmful estrogens from the body in estrogen-receptor positive cancers.) Genistein can also lower blood pressure.

Ukrain

See other cancer specific chapters in this book for information on Ukrain and its amazing history of curing many hopeless cancer cases!

VI. Other Risk Factors

Low Fat Diet Reduces Risk of Ovarian Cancer

Reducing the amount of dietary fat in your diet will improve your overall health and prevent chronic diseases. It also slashes the risk of many cancers. Scientists revealed that the incidence of ovarian cancer could be decreased one-fifth merely by having women limit their fat intake by "just 10 fewer grams…a day."[54]

Fiber Lowers Risk of Endometrial Cancers

Research also shows that women can reduce their risk of endometrial cancer by almost half, simply by increasing their fiber intake. The more fiber, the lower their incidence of endometrial cancer.[55]

Milk & Dairy Products Increase Risk
of Ovarian Cancer

In her book, *All Your Health Questions Answered Naturally*, Maureen Kennedy Salaman explains that consuming dairy products may have ominous consequences. For example, the type of sugar found naturally in milk ("galactose"), has been linked with an above average occurrence for "ovarian cancer." This was determined from a "1989" study conducted by "Harvard… gynecologist Daniel W. Kramer…"[56] See chapter 25 of this book for more information on the ominous link between cancer and dairy products!

Vaccinations & Cancer

According to Robert Morse, M.D., in his book, *The Detox Miracle Sourcebook*, think carefully before you choose vaccinations:

> Vaccinations have been linked to many cancers, and the sharp rise in diabetes (especially juvenile), multiple sclerosis, Bell's Palsy, vascular disorders, arthritis, and other conditions. The American Academy of Pediatrics knows of the toxic and horrific side effects of vaccinations and *still* recommends their prolific use.[57]

(They have also been implicated in autoimmune disorders and digestive disorders, as well as SIDS.)

Water

See chapter 22 for more information on how adequate water intake can dramatically reduce the risk of all cancers and chronic diseases.

CHAPTER 7

PAINLESS CURES & PREVENTIONS FOR LEUKEMIA & MULTIPLE MYELOMA

"Hundreds of cancer survivors each year develop leukemia as a result of previous therapy...these malignancies tend to be chemotherapy resistant or difficult to treat. Conventional medicine calls them secondary leukemias, and they are being identified with increasing frequency."
(Maureen Kennedy Salaman, from her book,
All Your Health Questions Answered Naturally.)[1]

Types of Leukemia

Leukemia is sometimes referred to as *blood cancer*. When a person is diagnosed with leukemia, usually what occurs is a dramatic elevation in their white blood cell count, because immature, cancerous white blood cells (called *blasts*) are multiplying so rapidly that they crowd out normal blood cells, causing hemorrhage. (There may not be enough platelets for proper clotting.) Infections occur since there may not be enough normal, mature white blood cells to fight viruses and bacteria, etc.), and severe weakness and anemia (and many other symptoms) because normal red blood cells may be crowded out. (The cells in *hairy cell* leukemia actually develop tiny hairy-looking little outgrowths from the cellular wall that are obvious under a microscope, hence its name.)

Every year, many thousands of people in the U.S. are diagnosed with various leukemias. In acute leukemia (as opposed to chronic leukemia) the cancerous blood cells that develop are immature and unable to function and they multiply rapidly, crowding out normal, healthier cells. The disease progresses quickly. In chronic leukemia, the cells are more mature, thus slightly more efficient (than the more immature cells of acute leukemia), and they divide and multiply much more slowly, thus, the progression of the disease is less rapid.

Leukemia is named for the cells in which it is found, and there are many subclasses of leukemia. Most of our blood cells form in the body's bone marrow, though some do form in the spleen. We depend on red blood cells for vital functions, such as carrying oxygen and other nutrients to and from the cells, while white blood cells are the body's immune system policemen, protecting us from outside invaders and inside mutants! When the immune system becomes compromised (such as during times of acute and chronic stress; through exposure and ingestion of harmful chemicals, toxins, radiation, medications; lack of proper rest, diet, exercise, and fluids), the result can be the malignant proliferation of cancerous blood cells. These malignancies then crowd out the healthy cells causing serious complications, hemorrhage, nutritional starvation, and eventually results in death if left untreated.

There are also some circumstances where people may be genetically predisposed to developing certain types of leukemia, and it is a well known fact that radiation, toxins, and nuclear fallout can cause leukemia. Unfortunately, many people who undergo radiation or chemotherapy treatment for one type of cancer often develop leukemia later as a result of the radiation (or chemo) they received for the prior cancer! This is a well-known (but often not discussed) *side effect* of radiation (and chemotherapy) treatment!

Just as other cancers can be prevented and often cured by immunotherapy (boosting the immune system by natural means to help the body heal itself), the same can be said of some leukemias.

Myelomas

Myelomas are tumors that have their origin in "bone marrow" cells. When these cancerous cells multiply and invade the bone and bone marrow forming multiple tumors, the disease is known as *"multiple myeloma."* This causes an "inadequate production of normal antibodies" making "patients susceptible to infection."[2]

As for multiple myeloma, many oncologists believe that this disease can not be cured, though there are treatments available. They also say that one can not prevent the disease and usually by the time a person is symptomatic, their cancer has severely progressed.

Is it true though that multiple myeloma cannot be prevented? Cancers, including myeloma and leukemias are the result of an immune system gone berserk. If we can prevent illnesses such as the common cold and flu by boosting the immune system, (i.e. juicing and proper nutrition, exercise, getting plenty of rest, fresh air, prayer, positive mental attitude, etc.), is it not reasonable to assume that we can also prevent diseases like leukemia and myeloma by strengthening the immune system?

Bone Marrow Transplants (BMT)

Conventional medicine attempts to treat some forms of leukemia and myeloma with chemotherapy drugs in a procedure known as a bone marrow (or stem cell) transplant. Acute lymphocytic and non-lymphocytic leukemias, brain tumors, Ewing's sarcoma, breast cancer, Hodgkins and non-Hodgkins lymphoma, neuroblastoma, ovarian cancer, and small cell lung cancers are some of the cancer types that conventional medicine treats with BMT.

There are three different kinds of bone marrow transplants, depending where the cells are taken from: "*Allogeneic* transplants," where a donor (other than an identical twin) provides the cells, "*Autologous* transplants involve cells being taken from the patient, stored, then reinfused following high-dose therapy; and *Syngeneic* transplants are where the donor is an identical twin."[3] (Note that some bone marrow transplants may involve the use of stem cells taken from cord blood.)

Part of the bone marrow transplant may involve what is known as TBI or *total body irradiation.* The goal during this time is the *total destruction of your own bone marrow and the complete disablement of your immune system!* Make no mistake – this is a DELIBERATE and total **destruction of your immune system** – there is nothing accidental about it!

During many of the actual phases of the bone marrow transplant, you are subjected to multiple rounds of chemotherapy. Right before the transplant, you will usually be given very high dose chemotherapy, all insults to the immune system. During much of the time, you will be very susceptible to infection, disease, and excess bleeding, hence the reason for *reverse isolation.* You will receive large doses of antibiotics, which in themselves often cause toxic side effects such as massive yeast infections, allergic reactions or kidney damage. You will also be taking blood products to help you fend off infections. (Keep in mind that after destroying your entire immune system, your oncologist will now try everything possible to *fix* **the damage** that he or she has done to you!)

The newly implanted bone marrow cells begin growing and dividing in a process known as *engraftment,* usually around the 14th day or so after the BMT. Nurses working with bone marrow transplant patients know that engraftment is a critical stage. If all goes as planned, you should eventually start producing your own white blood cells, platelets, and red blood cells, and you will be sent home from the hospital. (You may spend up to two months in the hospital during this process!) It may take another six months to a year before your life will ever resume a semblance of normalcy!

If you receive your own cells, you are generally at a lower risk for complications and may return to your usual routine quicker than patients receiving allogeneic transplants.

Patients who undergo bone marrow transplant from a donor often experience a serious problem known as GVHD or *graft-versus-host disease.* Their body actually begins to reject the transplanted blood cells (much like someone getting a kidney transplant will reject a donor kidney). If the rejection is mild, prognosis is good. If GVHD is severe, death may be imminent.

As described at *cancerbacup.org,* sometimes, a purging of "the donor's bone marrow" is done, using "antibodies to remove a type of white blood cell (T-lymphoycyte) which is thought to cause the graft-versus-host disease," especially "if a severe graft-versus-host reaction is possible – for example, if bone marrow from an unrelated donor is used."[4]

It is a sad irony that one of the many possible adverse side effects of getting a bone marrow transplant for multiple myeloma and other cancers is *leukemia!* Patients may survive the BMT, return to their normal routines, then a year or two later be diagnosed with leukemia – a result of all the chemotherapy and total body irradiation! It is not at all unusual to come down with secondary cancers after taking chemotherapy or radiation.

Chemo and radiation patients can be lulled into a false sense of security (believing they have beaten their cancer odds), because they go along for a year or two living out their normal routine, only to end up with a worse cancer than the one they started with from all the chemo and radiation received! I saw this happen over and over again in my own experience while following bone marrow transplant cases.

According to *Taber's Cyclopedic Medical Dictionary*, "patients who have received immunosuppressive agents [such as chemo drugs and radiation, for example] have **a more than 100 times** greater chance of developing NHL [Non-Hodgkin's Lymphoma], probably owing to the immunosuppressive agents activating tumor viruses."[5] (Emphasis, mine.) Do you realize what they are SAYING here? They are telling you that if you take chemo or radiation, your chances of getting this OTHER cancer (NHL) is "100 times" greater as opposed to those NOT taking chemo and radiation. How do you like THOSE odds!? When your physician tries to push chemo and radiation onto you or your loved ones, ask them about THESE ODDS!

During the time that I worked as a Transplant Coordinator R.N. for an insurance company, I followed telephonically, the cases of hundreds of transplant patients from beginning to end. I recall that the BMT patients were some of the most miserable of people. In anguish, they would tearfully cry to me about all the horrible side effects they were experiencing from the toxic chemo drugs or radiation they had been given. I could understand their terrible desperation, and though I would try to reassure them that they were doing well and stood a good chance of recovery, in my innermost being, I knew that many of them were dying. I knew that the BMT process had inflicted upon their immune system a fatal blow from which they might never recover. It was a depressing job and one of the many reasons that burdened me to begin investigating alternative cancer therapies, which led to this book! **The remainder of this chapter deals with natural ways to prevent and fight leukemia and multiple myeloma, many of which have even cured those already with the active disease!**

I. How Vitamins, Minerals, & Nutrients Have Prevented & Cured Cancer

High Dose Vitamin C Cures a Teenager's Cancer!

Have you or someone you love been diagnosed with leukemia? Be sure that what you (or they) have really **is** leukemia and not a vitamin C deficiency, or even a folic acid or B12 deficiency! Those words of warning from Maureen Kennedy Salaman in her book, *Nutrition: The Cancer Answer II!* Though the story she describes below with Dr. Rimland involves Hodgkins disease, she explains that a vitamin C deficiency (scurvy) can resemble leukemia, as can folic acid and B12 deficiencies.

When "Bernard Rimland, Ph.D.," world reknown for using nutrition for emotional and psychiatric disorders, was told that his teenage daughter had cancer ("a terminal type [of] Hodgkins disease, stage 4B"), he began her on a high dose vitamin C regimen. The cancer had aggressively attacked the teenager's "liver and kidneys." Doctors told him that she had the worse case of "kidney" impairment they had ever seen, and she was given "six to eight months to live." Her father immediately started her on high doses of vitamin C every day – large doses – "40 grams" per day! He also gave her "a gram of niacinamide [1000 mg.], 50 mg of the other B vitamins, 800 I.U. of vitamin E and 75,000 I.U. of vitamin A, as well as calcium, magnesium and other minerals in normal amounts."[6]

The oncologists in his daughter's cancer ward had absolutely no faith in Dr. Rimland's nutritional supplement program! In Dr. Rimland's words as told to Maureen Kennedy Salaman (from her book, *Nutrition: The Cancer Answer II)*:

> Although the oncologists were giving her chemotherapy – those horrible chemicals – and she lost all of her hair, they assured me their efforts wouldn't help a case this far gone. (Despite their contentions), she began to improve at a spectacular rate.[7]

Dr. Rimland explained how he persistently gave the oncologists taking care of his daughter hard copy documentation of the "efficacy of vitamin C." They completely ignored him and never read the material. Though his own daughter improved and completely recovered after receiving the high dose vitamin C regimen, he sadly commented that the oncologists refused to treat other children in the ward with vitamin C as he had done for his daughter, despite her remarkable recovery:

> [T]he (other) kids – in my daughter's words – most of them with leukemia – were dying like flies. I remembered Irwin Stone's writing which noted that the symptoms of leukemia are identical to those off scurvy. Stone used to say, "If you run a vitamin C blood test, someone with leukemia would have almost zero vitamin C. If you gave that person a lot of vitamin C, the blood level would still measure zero. So you have to give them massive amounts to get the blood level anywhere near normal."[8]

Dr. Rimland said that if you gave leukemia patients large doses of vitamin C, "the symptoms of leukemia would go away," and he added that "Irwin Stone" documented and "published case histories of people who recovered and did very well, just as my daughter did. She's perfectly normal today." Dr. Rimland's high dose nutritional program saved his daughter's life and he feels might have spared other children in the same "ward" with her. The problem was that he could not convince the oncologists. He said, "It has to be their way or no way…"[9]

(What were they afraid of? Afraid that maybe a natural substance (a vitamin) could cure a deadly disease that their toxic drugs were powerless against? Afraid of repercussions from the manufacturers of those same toxic drugs? Afraid of the FDA which exists to promote the drug tzars? Fearful of having their judgment questioned? ALL of the above?)

As further described by Ms. Salaman, the amounts of nutritional supplements that Bernard Rimland gave his daughter during this time and he and his family continue to take (what he calls his "anti-cancer formula") on a daily basis are as follows:

> 10-12 grams of vitamin C in water or juice, 200 micrograms of selenium; 400-800 I.U. of vitamin E; and 25,000 to 80,000 I.U. of vitamin A....of course we eat a lot of fresh vegetables, adding about 1000 mg of calcium, which is very important to prevent colon cancer...[10]

(Note: Since vitamin A can be toxic in large doses and natural beta-carotene is not, I would recommend taking the vitamin A as described by Dr. Rimland above, in beta-carotene form by juicing fresh carrot juice daily! The body converts natural beta-carotene into vitamin A!)

Dr. Rimland split the large dosage of vitamin C into several divided doses throughout the day.[11] For those who experience stomach upset from high dose (oral) vitamin C, you can obtain buffered C powder or crystals in health food stores. High dose vitamin C is also given intravenously by many alternative health physicians.

More Evidence for Vitamin C

Linus Pauling was an early advocate for high dose vitamin C therapy. He won the Nobel Prize twice, once in 1954 for chemistry, and again in 1962 the Nobel peace prize. He authored several books on chemistry, quantum mechanics, vitamin C, and cancer. He has been followed by others who have taken up the banner in favor of megadosing with vitamin C, including Dr. Abram Hoffer, and Dr. Robert Cathcart.

Dr. Cathcart's website at *www.orthomed.com* gives startling revelations about diseases such as "Ebola...and West Nile," as well as many others that he says could possibly be "cured or ameliorated by massive doses of vitamin C."[12] I spoke at length with Dr. Cathcart by phone on 07/05/05 regarding many of these issues.

If you look at a table of the U.S. RDA (Recommended Daily Allowance or sometimes referred to as the Recommended Dietary

Allowance) for vitamin C, it is very low at only 60 milligrams. (Most people could probably burn this much up during 2 minutes of stress!)

Did you know that scientists are very concerned about the health of their laboratory monkeys? They have to keep them on healthy diets so that they stay well! Dr. Abram Hoffer explains how this is accomplished, and the answer will surprise you!

> Because of the importance of keeping laboratory monkeys in good health, careful studies have been made of the health of monkeys in relation to their daily intake of vitamin C. As a result of these studies, the chow for monkeys provides a far larger amount of this vitamin than the RDA for humans, roughly 50 times as much. This fact suggests that the optimum daily intake for humans might well be a megavitamin amount of this vitamin, perhaps 2,500 milligrams, instead of the RDA of 60 milligrams.[13]

Did you note that lab monkeys get **"50 times"** as much vitamin C to keep them healthy than what the U.S. Food and Nutrition Board recommends for adult humans? What does that tell you? If it takes this megavitamin dosage of C to keep a monkey healthy, why would anyone in their right mind assume that humans can maintain wellness on a puny 60 milligrams a day? Dr. Hoffer suggests a more sensible intake – the *"Optimum Intake"*:

> It is now clear that there are two important daily intakes for each vitamin. One is the RDA, the intake recommended by the Food and Nutrition Board of the U.S. National Academy of Sciences, the amount considered to be enough to prevent obvious signs of the corresponding deficiency disease for most people. The other intake, which we consider to be the most important one, is the optimum intake, the one that leads to the best of health. For most vitamins this intake is much larger than the FDA and may be said to be in the megavitamin range.[14]

If you still have doubts about the way that natural cancer cures are being suppressed, consider the findings on vitamin C and what happened when it was discovered that vitamin C was "highly toxic" to certain **cancer cells**. Dr. Abram Hoffer explains:

> L. Benade, T. Howard and D. Burke, working in the laboratories of the National Cancer Institute, found that ascorbate [vitamin C] was highly toxic to Ehrlich's ascites carcinoma and caused profound structural changes in the cancer cells; the institute ignored this work, however.[15]

Dr. Hoffer also says that "There is clearly good evidence that the regular ingestion of mega amounts of vitamin C (1 to 20 grams per day) and of other vitamins increase the state of health and well-being, increase the length of life, and decrease the incidence of cancer, heart disease, and other diseases."[16]

Vitamin E & Leukemia

Vitamin E substances known as "Tocotrienols" are found "in palm oil, rice bran oil…wheat, grape seed oil…barley…and a few other foods," and according to Ralph Moss, Ph.D., in his book, *Antioxidants against Cancer*, these compounds reduce harmful fats that circulate in the blood, act as anti-inflammatory agents, decompose unwanted "proteins," and are potent "anti-oxidants…." They also inhibit "breast cancer, melanoma, and leukemia cells."[17]

Treating Leukemia with Vitamin A & Zinc

In *All Your Health Questions Answered Naturally*, Maureen Kennedy Salaman describes research presented by "Dr. Frank L. Meyskens" at a cancer conference in "1993," where he explained that minimal supplementation with "vitamin A helps increase the survival rate of patients with CML" (chronic myeloid leukemia). It appears that Vitamin A also plays an important role in tumor prevention.[18]

Ms. Salaman also describes a report where "79 patients with acute promyelocytic leukemia" were given a form of synthetic vitamin A by "Raymond Warrell, M.D...[and] 86 percent" went into "complete remission."[19] She adds that another study from "Acona, Italy" involving "91 young patients affected by acute lymphoblastic leukemia..." revealed a close connection between relapse and low blood levels of **zinc and thymulin**.[20] *Yourhealthbase.com* reports that researchers in "Houston, Texas" have found that "Vitamin A (retinol) and its biologically active metabolite, retinoic acid, are known to be useful in the prevention and treatment of certain cancers such as acute promyelocyte leukemia," as well as "prostate cancer."[21]

Dr. Abram Hoffer, M.D., F.R.C.P(C), in his book *Healing Cancer – Complementary Vitamin & Drug Treatments*, describes in his experience, that it is very common for cancer patients to have excessive levels of copper in their body, possibly caused by a lack of zinc:

> There is an inverse relationship between copper and zinc. A deficiency of one will cause an increase in the amount of the other. The easiest way to bring down copper levels is to increase the intake of zinc. Fortunately zinc is a very safe trace mineral and can be given in useful dosages for long periods of time with hardly any side effects. In summary, patients with cancer have elevated serum copper levels, elevated ratios of copper/zinc, and may have low zinc levels. The higher the ratios are, the more malignant is the disease and the poorer the prognosis.[22]

Vitamins & Selenium

Vitamin A and selenium have been shown to destroy bone cancer cells during in vitro testing. Vitamin E and selenium work together. As noted at *herbs2000.com*, about "150 **micrograms** of selenium" are needed on a daily basis, as well as "200 to 400 international units of vitamin E daily."[23] Vitamin A blood levels can be maintained by juicing fresh fruits and vegetables, such as carrots.

Vitamin D helps to normalize the manufacture of bone cells "slowing the rate at which cancer cells multiply..." however, taking synthetic vitamin D as a supplement is not recommended as it may cause the release of calcium from bones that are already deficient from the cancer.[24] Vitamin D is manufactured in the skin when direct sunlight strikes the skin. It takes about 20 minutes of full spectrum direct sunlight each day for sufficient vitamin D synthesis in most people. (You should consult your physician about sun exposure, especially if you have a history or genetic tendency toward melanoma.)

Beat Leukemia With Beets

A simple garden vegetable may be one of the most potent detox agents for the human body and blood known to man. It is none other than beets! Beet juice is very potent and concentrated as an antioxidant (much like wheat grass juice in potency), so much so, that it is always best to combine it with another juice such as carrots or apples or a green juice like broccoli or spinach. Never start out drinking several ounces at a time! Begin with two ounces a day, then four, and work up to six to eight ounces at a time, added to another juice. (You can also obtain powdered beet root in health food stores.) It is interesting that a vegetable juice that so closely resembles blood (in appearance) is actually GOOD for your blood! Beet juice has proven useful for treating leukemia and other cancers. Beets can be kept fresh for weeks in the refrigerator.

Website *herbsfirst.com* (now linked with *http://herballegacy.com/id118.htm*) recommends consuming "a couple of pounds of raw, mashed beets daily [as a] therapy for leukemia and tumors."[25]

I prefer to juice beets. Fresh beets are hard as rock. They are difficult enough to slice up for juicing and even harder to mash when raw, (unless you are using a food processor to shred them!)

Barley Grass Halts Leukemia Cells

In an article for *sproutnet.com*, Steve Meyerowitz's website, International Specialty Supply, says the following of Dr. Y. Hagiwara and **barley grass juice:**

As a doctor, Hagiwara facilitated a large body of university level research on dried barley grass juice. He found that it contains 11 times the calcium of cow's milk, 5 times the iron of spinach, 4 times the B1 of whole wheat flour, 7 times the vitamin C in oranges and an abundance of vitamin B12, 80 mcg per hundred grams....Barley grass is especially rich in...anti-oxidants...[26]

One of the antioxidants identified by Steve Meyerowitz in his article above was "vitamin E succinate (VES) [which] stopped the proliferation of prostate, breast, and leukemia cancer cells."[27]

CoQ10 Deficiencies & Multiple Myelomas

Studies by Dr. Folkers and colleagues revealed that patients with "breast cancer and multiple myeloma" often had CoQ10 deficiencies as compared to the rest of the "population."[28] This was reported by Dr. R. W. Moss in his book, *Antioxidants against Cancer*. As a matter of fact, evidence over a period of "35 years" revealed that taking CoQ10 increased "survival [for] cancer patients" by as much as "5 to 15 years, says Dr. Moss."[29]

Folic Acid & Adult Leukemia

You may want to be sure that you are not deficient in folic acid (vitamin B-9 or folate), first found within "spinach leaves in 1941," if you wish to prevent adult leukemia. Dr. Moss explained that a genetic mutation that affects 1/3 of the population has been found to inhibit some cancers, so this is one mutation that is actually good for you! It causes "folic acid" to be easily assimilated for the job of repairing damaged "DNA..."[30]

Scientists discovered that if men having this defective gene did not consume alcohol, their chances of having "colon cancer" were greatly lessened. However, if they began consuming alcohol, their nutritional advantage evaporated.[31] Dr. Moss further points out that those having the genetic aberration, have a 2/3 less risk for "acute lymphocytic leukemia" (ALL). Because of this, scientists are convinced that a lack of folic acid in the diet dramatically increases the chances of colo-rectal cancers, and may also lead to the "development of ALL..."[32]

As seen from the words of Maureen Kennedy Salaman at the front of this chapter, many of today's cases of leukemia are being diagnosed in patients who had prior chemo and radiation for other cancers. She describes research from one study which found that taking chemo can elevate your chances of getting "leukemia by as much as 12 times compared to surgery. Radiotherapy increased the risk ten times," however, there is some "good news....Folic acid can protect against this effect." According to Ms. Salaman, another study revealed that women having insufficient amounts of "folic acid" in their blood (who had received chemotherapy for breast cancer), also experienced "a high frequency of mutant cells following chemotherapy...," indicating that adequate amounts of folic acid can protect against this threat![32a]

Some excellent natural sources of folic acid given by Dr. H. Winter Griffith in *Vitamins, Herbs, Minerals & Supplements*, are: "Asparagus, Avocados, Bananas...Beets...Green leafy vegetables... Lentils...[and] Sprouts..."[33]

Is it Leukemia Or is it a Folic Acid or B-12 Deficiency?

If you are diagnosed with leukemia, be sure to get more than one opinion! Maureen Kennedy Salaman warns in her book, *All Your Health Questions Answered Naturally,* that "two out of every three patients diagnosed as having leukemia actually had a severe deficiency of folic acid and vitamin B12 – pernicious anemia." A month or two on vitamin therapy and their blood counts were completely normal![34] And just how widespread is this problem? No one really knows.

Have you or a loved one been diagnosed with leukemia recently? Be sure first of all, as stated earlier, that you get a second opinion, and next, be sure that what you have is indeed leukemia and not a lack of B12, folic acid, or even a vitamin C deficiency! (Vitamin B12 and folic acid are also available in sublingual tablets that you simply place under your tongue and dissolve; however the best way to be sure you are getting adequate B12, is with B12 injections from your physician. You can also check out Dr. Andrew W. Saul's website at *http://www.doctoryourself.com/nasal.html* for his recipe on the use of nasal B12!)

GLA (Gamma Linolenic Acid) & Leukemia

GLA, already discussed in a previous chapter, is commonly found in borage oil and evening primrose oil, but according to Russell L. Blaylock, M.D., in *Natural Strategies For Cancer Patients*, the best source is borage oil. GLA can kill cancer cells and has shown its ability to do so in a variety of cancers. In laboratory tests, when leukemia cells were treated with GLA, nearly half of them died. In the absence of the GLA, only one fifth "of the cancer cells died."[34a] Dr. Blaylock says that the leukemia cells were taken from patients "with alpha-cell chronic lymphocytic leukemia." Apparently, the addition of cortisone increased the effectiveness of GLA, killing a much greater percentage of the unwanted cells.[35] Note that the **NORMAL cells were not affected!** When GLA was injected "directly into a [human] brain tumor (glioma,)" it went into regression![36]

More isn't necessarily better in the case of GLA! Larger doses can cause "inflammatory reactions," which may increase tumors rather than inhibit them! Because of this "narrow window of effectiveness," Dr. Blaylock does not "recommend taking more than 2,000 milligrams of GLA a day as a supplement."[37]

Some providers of organic flax oil also add borage oil and/or evening primrose oil as a combination oil supplement in their flax products. Flax itself has been shown to prevent the growth of new cancer cells. See chapter 17 for further information on flax for cancer prevention and treatment, and chapter 13 for the famous Budwig flax oil diet that has cured many cancers!

Flavonoids & Cell Protection

Protecting blood cells from mutation means ensuring that cellular DNA does not mutate! Once cells begin to mutate, and the immune system is sick, the end result is often a debilitating cancer such as leukemia, sarcoma, or multiple myeloma.

The protective ability of phytochemicals (plant chemicals, such as those found in green and black tea) was shown in a recent report where three flavonoids outperformed the rest in protecting DNA. These three, according to Dr. Blaylock, were "luteolin...(celery), myricetin...(black currants), and quercetin...(teas, apples, and onions)."[37a] Parsley, silymarin, and ginkgo biloba (high in quercetin) also have ingredients that inhibit the growth of cancer cells. In the fruits that were tested, those with the greatest ability at protecting DNA were found in "blackberries, sweet and sour cherries, black currants, pineapples, and watermelon."[38]

Grapes (Resveratrol) Block Leukemia Cells

The amazing nutrient in purple grapes called *resveratrol,* was discussed in chapter two, yet it is again coming up as being important in fighting leukemia. Researchers have also noted that this compound inhibits many types of malignant cancers, including leukemia!

Grapes are one of the best sources of reveratrol! According to website *herbs2000.com,* resveratrol also works to inhibit the process of cancer by the promotion of cellular "differentiation, a process by which the unrestrained multiplication of cancer cells is stopped and white blood cells are returned to their normal life cycle. Since this announcement, nearly 100 scientific studies have attributed other cancer-fighting effects to resveratrol."[39] Reservatrol also has the ability to mobilize "a gene named p53, which acts as a kind of 'molecular patrolman' to destroy cells with damaged DNA."[40] The website also reports that researchers have found "resveratrol" can halt the manufacture "of a chemical called *NFkB*, which inflames the tissues surrounding a tumor and is essential for leukemia viruses to activate leukemia." In other words – resveratrol stops the chemicals responsible for the development of leukemia dead in their tracks! Not only that, but scientists have discovered that "reservatrol acts" very similar to a popular chemo drug known as "tamoxifen...in laboratory tests..."[41] However, resveratrol does not have the toxic side effects found in tamoxifen!

With all the cancer fighting properties that resveratrol has, is it any wonder that Johanna Brandt witnessed so many amazing cures with her grape diet? (See chapter two!)

Mangosteen for Leukemia

Mangosteen fruit contains more than two dozen "xanthones," a good source of antioxidants. The ORAC test ("Oxygen Radical Absorbance Capacity") is a measurement of an antioxidants ability to "absorb free radicals," and of course, the foods you want to eat are the ones with the highest ORAC rating! Mangosteen is very high on the ORAC list.[42] Website *cancertutor.com* reports that one "ounce of mangosteen juice has 20 to 30 times the ability to absorb free radicals than one ounce of most fruits and vegetables."[42a] (See chapter 19 for a sample ORAC list!)

According to website *members.aol.com/jonbio/nutrition.htm,* the ORAC score for carrots is "200, Pomegranates [is] 3,037...[and] Mangosteen...[is] 17,000." This same website offers a product known as XanGo™, a "whole fruit puree of the mangosteen."[43]

Six different nutrient compounds from this fruit were tested on leukemic cells in laboratory tests. All six successfully inhibited the cancers. (Note that **mangosteen is not the same** as the mango fruit.)

A Mushroom Extract Cures Leukemia!

Writers Sheri Lieberman, Ph.D. and Ken Babal, C.N., describe Dr. Peter D'Adamo, N.D.," of "Greenwich, Connecticut," as a long term user of maitake mushroom for health in their book *Maitake Mushroom And D-Fraction.* In *"Eat Right For Your Type,"* Dr. D'Adamo recounts the details of a case where he had used *maitake D-fraction* supplement against terminal leukemia. This particular patient had already taken chemo, but the tumor invaded "her spleen" within a "year after the treatment."[44] (Not surprisingly, another chemo failure!)

The tumor was aggressive and grew rapidly. When the patient came to Dr. D'Adamo she had an enlarged spleen. He "gave her D-fraction" and instructed her to "take a half teaspoon twice a day." The tumor eventually "completely disappeared," and according to Dr. D'Adamo, "this was not a particularly rare case."[45] He has successfully treated many types of cancer and "HIV-positive patients" with "maitake mushroom" combined "with a few other natural remedies." He has also had very good results treating "prostate cancer patients" when chemotherapy failed to help them, as well as cancers "of the liver, breast and colon," and he believes that taking "maitake" enhances the effectiveness of "shark cartilage."[46]

Maitake is not recommended for anyone with "multiple sclerosis…" This, according to website *herbs2000.com*. The precaution is because there is "one form of interferon stimulated by maitake, gamma-interferon, [which] can promote the destruction of nerve tissue, so people with MS should avoid maitake until this remedy has been more thoroughly tested."[47]

Shiitake mushrooms have been the focus of much research. Oriental populations have used them for thousands of years. They support immunity and are useful against "cancer, leukemia, lymphosarcoma, and Hodgkins Disease," as well as HIV. According to *http://www.stoneycreekmushrooms.com:*

> One shiitake mushroom, eaten with a tablespoon of butter, actually reduces serum cholesterol. In Japan it is taken to prevent heart disease because it regulates both high and low blood pressure. As an anti-inflammatory, it improves stomach and duodenal ulcers, neuralgia, gout, constipation and hemorrhoids. Shiitake also counteracts fatigue, generates stamina and improves the complexion.[48]

A note of caution: if you are taking medications that thin the blood, check with your physician, because shiitake affects clotting time. It can also cause rashes in some people.[48a] A supplement containing not only shiitake but the mycelia of several other mushrooms that is said to enhance the body's natural immunity is AHCC. AHCC is available at *discount-vitamins-herbs.net*. Some health food stores also carry the supplement. (Fresh shiitake is best if cooked. Always buy organic when possible!)

Quercetin for Leukemia

Quercetin, discussed earlier, is a very potent flavonoid protective against cancer. As described in *All Your Health Questions Answered Naturally*, by Maureen Kennedy Salaman, its effects are increased when combined with ascorbic acid, it has been useful "in the treatment of acute leukemia...[and] it works with rutin, a related flavonoid" (also known as *"vitamin P"*). Research has shown that the combination of these three powerful flavonoids, "quercetin, rutin and vitamin C together may contribute toward a reduction in leukemia cells."[49]

A few good natural sources of quercetin are "onions, cayenne pepper, garlic and green tea."[49a] Rutin can be found in berries, prunes, paprika, chervil, cherries, grapes and the skins of citrus fruit as well as many other foods.

Ms. Salaman believes that in choosing onions for quercetin, that it is best to choose either "red" or "yellow...onions" not "white." Red and yellow onions are much higher in this nutrient than are white onions.[49b]

Royal Jelly Inhibits Leukemia

According to website *www.cancertutor.com*, in a Canadian study, one group of mice with "leukemia" were fed "royal jelly," while the "control" group with "leukemia" were not given the nutrient. Those not receiving the royal jelly succumbed to "ascitic tumors in less than 14 days," while "mice receiving appropriate mixtures of cells and royal jelly all failed to develop tumors," showing the protective effects of royal jelly against leukemia.[50]

Soy Isoflavones & Leukemia

Two powerful soy isoflavones known as "genistein and diadzein," may protect against some forms of cancer, including "prostate cancer, breast cancer, leukemia, glioblastoma multiforme, and bladder cancer."[51] Soy should be taken in moderation. Instead of consuming high amounts of soy, you may want to try genistein and diadzein supplements, which you can find at most health food stores. (Fermented soy products, such as Haelan, can help remove harmful estrogens from the body in estrogen-receptor positive cancers.) Note that genistein can also lower blood pressure.

Strawberries & Cherries Inhibit Cancer Cells

In a revealing note by Jean Carper in her book, *The Food Pharmacy*, researchers placed strawberries at the top of a list of foods that they felt were responsible for decreased rates of fatalities from cancer among "a group of 1271 elderly Americans in New Jersey."[51a] Those eating larger amounts of strawberries decreased their risks for getting cancer three-fold over "those eating few or no strawberries." It was also found that strawberries effectively destroyed "the poliovirus, echnovirus, reovirus coxsackievirus, and herpes simplex virus."[52] (Raspberries, cranberries, cherries, and blueberries have similar cancer-fighting compounds!)

An ingredient in cherries, *"perillyl alcohol,"* was shown (in animal testing) to suppress leukemic cells.[52a] (This ingredient is also described in earlier chapters of this book.) Cherries, especially sour cherries, have long been used as a popular treatment for gout.

II. Herbs, Plants, & Teas That Inhibit Leukemia

Algae

In recent years, different types of algae are proving to be deadly to cancer cells. According to Dr. R. W. Moss in *Cancer Therapy*, it was discovered that a "beta-carotene-rich algae named Dunaliella bardawil…'markedly inhibited' spontaneous breast cancers in mice."[53] Chlorella, a "one-celled algae," has been the subject of intense study, revealing that it too has impressive tumor fighting abilities! When researchers in Japan fed mice "chlorella *(pyrenoidosa)*…every other day for ten days," then followed this with injections of three types of cancer, "breast, leukemia or Ehrlich ascites," the amazing results were described by Dr. Moss:

> All of the untreated mice died within 20 days. But over 70 percent of the treated animals survived over 60 days. Since chlorella does not directly kill cancer cells, the scientists concluded that its effects were caused by boosting the immune response.[54]

You can purchase chlorella at your local health food store, but be sure to choose an organic brand that is **broken cell wall** chlorella such as *Sun Chlorella* or *Kyoto Chlorella*. If the cell wall is not broken, it is not easily absorbed by the body. Also, be sure to purchase algaes and seaweeds from reputable sources! (Chlorella also contains essential omega-3, omega-6 and ALA fatty acids.)

Aloe's Anti-Leukemic Factor

Japanese scientists looked into the effect of aloe on various kinds of cancer in mice, isolating a chemical by the name of *"aloe emodin,"* (also discussed in chapter six). It was this chemical that was responsible for fighting leukemia in animal studies. Not only that, but in their studies of the effect of aloe on other cancers, they noted that the compound decreased the rapid proliferation of some types of tumors in the test animals and even cured a particular type of malignancy. Initial results revealed that it works by stimulating immunity.[55]

Aloe emodin has also been isolated from the herb sheep sorrel, one of the ingredients that is found in Essiac Tea. According to website, *DrLam.com,* "aloe emodin, isolated from sorrel," does show "significant anti-leukemic activity…." Dr. Lam also reports that Dr. Chester Stock at Sloan-Kettering tested aloe emodin and found that it is "responsible for the destruction of cancer cells in the body."[56]

Oriental researchers found that aloe-emodin halts a specific type of leukemia cell by preventing its metastasis. Be sure to consult your physician before beginning an aloe regimen.

Artemisinin

Artemisinin, also known as *"wormwood,"* has been a popular remedy for centuries for treating parasites, with the ability to cross the "blood brain barrier," meaning it "may be particularly suitable for curing brain tumors, together with Poly-MVA."[57] This according to Wellness Directory of Minnesota™ website: *www.mnwelldir.org* and *drlam.com*. It is "effective against a wide variety of cancers as shown in a series of successful experiments," especially against "leukemia and colon cancer." Some cancer activity was also shown against "melanoma, breast, ovarian, prostate, CNS [central nervous system] and renal cancer." Note that not all wormwood contains artemisinin![58] (See chapter 13 for more information on Poly-MVA.)

A word of caution: do not take excessively high doses of this herb. "Therapeutic levels (dosages) for those with active cancers can be 1,000 mgs per day, divided into 4 parts, while some physicians recommend 1,600 mg per day based upon a 100 pound female."[58a]

Astragalus

This herb is important in restoring depleted immune cells. (Do not use it if you have "a fever or a skin infection.")[59]

Autumn Crocus

Autumn Crocus *"(Colchicum autumnale),"* long used as a successful remedy for the pain associated with "gout," has also been used "with some success" for treating leukemia and "Behcet's syndrome, a chronic disease marked by recurring ulcers and leukemia." Do not use this herb without first consulting with your physician, because even in low doses, it can be associated with severe adverse effects.[59a]

Butcher's Broom

This is an herb with known vasoconstrictive "(blood vessel narrowing)" effects. Twelve "steroidal saponins" were recently isolated from butcher's broom by "Japanese researchers," and two of them killed leukemia cells.[60] (Butcher's broom can be found in tea form as well as supplements.) Cattle ranchers once used it as a snake-bite remedy.

Cat's Claw Fights Leukemia

Also known as *Uno de Gato,* cat's claw is popular in tea form. According to Rita Elkins, M.H., in her book *Cat's Claw Uno de Gato*, it has proven antioxidant properties and the ability to scavenge for and destroy cancer-causing substances. Research has also revealed that this herb can hone in on aberrant cells. "...scientific studies have shown that it can specifically target cellular mutations such as leukemic cells and inhibit their development."[61] Ms. Elkins explains that the herb demonstrated its ability to fight leukemia without harming "normal bone marrow cells...." Its uncanny "ability...to differentiate between leukemic cells and normal cells..." could make it a valuable alternative "treatment for people with acute leukemia."[62]

Cat's claw can be found in supplements as well as tea bags. *Herbs2000.com* explains that it is not recommended "in autoimmune illness, multiple sclerosis, and tuberculosis," or for women who are "pregnant or lactating....European practitioners avoid combining it with hormonal drugs, insulin, or vaccines."[62a]

Chaparral & Leukemia

Chaparral "*(Larrea tridentate)*" which is often consumed as a popular tea, is believed to have the ability to inhibit tumors and "leukemia...."[63] (This herb is discussed in more detail in chapter 31 on teas.)

Essiac Tea

See chapter five of this book for details on the cancer-fighting properties of Essiac tea and the nurse who healed hundreds (perhaps even thousands) of her cancer patients using this herbal formula.

Garlic Inhibits Promyelocytic Leukemia

Laboratory research studies have recently demonstrated that compounds in garlic can arrest the activity of this type leukemia.

Green Tea Prevents Leukemia

Certain ingredients in green tea known as "catechins….(*epigallocatechin gallate)"* EGCG, have the ability to prevent DNA damage. During testing, this tea was successful at suppressing the "growth" of "leukemia" cells.[64] As a matter-of-fact, mixing black and green teas together greatly enhanced their protective power. There is not a great deal of difference between green and black teas. When black tea is "raw," it is called "green tea."[65] (It is best to use decaffeinated tea because caffeine acts as a diuretic, dehydrating the body, and most cancer patients are already dehydrated. Removing the caffeine does not affect the antioxidant potency.)

Another study reported at *foodnavigator.com* "from patients with B-cell chronic lymphocytic leukemia (CLL)" (common in people in their sixties, and for which there is no known cure), revealed that green tea interrupted the "communication signals needed by cancer cells to survive, prompting them to die in eight of 10 patient samples tested in the laboratory."[66]

Goldenseal & Berberine Fight Leukemia

An ingredient isolated in the popular herb, goldenseal (known as *berberine),* was able to **cause leukemia cells to self-destruct**.[67] As described earlier, *herbs2000.com* recommends that herbs containing berberine ("barberry…coptis… goldenseal or Oregon grape…")

should not be taken during pregnancy or in suspected "gallbladder disease," nor with "supplemental vitamin B6 or protein supplements containing the amino acid histidine. Do not use goldenseal if you have cardiovascular disease or glaucoma"[68] (This herb may also increase blood pressure in some individuals.)

"Other anticancer herbs" given in *The Complete Encyclopedia of Natural Healing* by Gary Null, Ph.D., are: "African cayenne, bilberry, bloodroot, comfrey, dandelion root, goldenseal, pau d'arco, and suma..."[69] (Do NOT use comfrey root **internally**. Consult with your physician before using comfrey.) Also, remember that any herb has the capacity to cause allergies in some individuals.

Lapacho Used for Leukemia

Lapacho "*(Tabebuia avellandedae, and T. impetiginosa),* also commonly known as pau d'arco" and taheebo tea, is described in detail at website *www.rain-tree.com.* It is very popular "for many ailments, including cancer (esp. leukemia), candida" and many other disorders. "It is considered one of the world's great tonic herbs."[70]

Be aware that lapacho is actually just an extract from the main tea, pau d'arco, but the names get intertwined. When using the herb, you need to be sure that you are using pau d'arco – the entire tea.

According to *holistic-online.com*, supporters of this tea say that "it is one of the most important anti-tumor agents in the entire world...especially useful in the treatment of leukemia."[71] It is believed that it works by stimulating "the production of red blood cells in bone marrow." Lapacho is the main ingredient in this herb, and when used alone, it had "severe side effects," however, "when the whole herb was given it produced clinical anticancer effects without the toxic side effect."[71a] It is also important to be aware that sometimes when teas such as this are tested, an extract of one of the teas main ingredients will be used in the test, rather than the entire tea. Of course, in using teas such as this, one needs to use the whole tea, not one or two extracts isolated from the main tea!

Holistic-online.com further explains that "Lapacho [pau d'arco] is highly toxic to many kinds of cancer cells..." It was given a "clean bill of health in 1981," by the FDA.[72]

Genuine pau d'arco tea should come from the tree's bark (the"inner lining.") It has been used for many years, especially in South America, as an effective way to manage "cancer and other dread diseases."[73]

This tea is often very effective for some people, when others do not respond to it. Possibly because some sources are not using the "inner bark" of the tree, the most potent and healthful. Website *www.oralchelation.com,* says do not purchase it except from reliable sources. It should be manufactured only from the "inner lining (or phloem)" of the tree.[74]

Saffron Destroys Cancer Cells

Some spices appear to be able to destroy cancer cells on contact! Saffron is one of them. As noted by Selene Yeager in the *Doctors Book of FOOD REMEDIES:*

> In laboratory studies, for example, compounds from saffron were placed on human cancer cells, including cells that cause leukemia. Not only did the dangerous cells stop growing, but the compounds appear to have no effect on normal, healthy cells...[75]

Seaweeds, Viva Natural, & PTZ Fight Leukemia & Other Cancers

Viva Natural is a nutritional compound taken from seaweed. This extract was effective in animal studies against leukemia and lung cancer cells and was even considered more effective "against lung cancer than the standard drug *Isoprinosine.*"[76] In his book, *Cancer Therapy: The Independent Consumer's Guide to Non-Toxic Treatment and Prevention,* Dr. Ralph Moss says of Viva Natural and PTZ: [pretazettine hydrochloride]

> Viva Natural...showed progress against leukemia, as did another natural substance PTZ, an alkaloid from the narcis-

sus plant....Mice with cancer that were given PTZ showed a 90 percent increase in survival while methrotrexate-treated mice had only a 71 percent increase....PTZ was even able to **cause a complete remission of advanced leukemia...**[77] [Emphasis added.]

Dr. Moss describes a "brown kelp" known as "*Laminaria,*" which may be responsible for Japan's "low breast cancer rates....Another extract of brown sea algae called *Sargassum kjellmaniaum* also has anticancer effects." It was effective at stopping "the growth of sarcoma cells...," and when it was combined "with sulphur" in a compound known as "*sulfated SKCF...*it was effective against leukemia."[78] (Kelp should only be taken in very small amounts and not by those with thyroid disorders, unless cleared with their physician, because it is high in iodine!) Other types of seaweed have been discussed earlier in this book.

Turmuric Stops the Spread of Multiple Myeloma

According to an article from *www.discount-vitamins-herbs.net*, scientists in 2003 at the "University of Texas M.D. Anderson Cancer Center" revealed that "curcumin," found in the common "spice turmeric, can stop the spread of multiple myeloma..." Not only that, but the curcumin also caused the "cancer cells" to undergo "apoptosis – a process where cells program themselves to die." At a conclusion to the study, it was "suggested that patients suffering from multiple myelomas be treated with this 'pharmacologically safe agent.'"[79] Yet how many physicians treating their cancer patients tell them this, do you think? Do you or someone you know have multiple myeloma? If so, has anyone ever told you (or them) that turmeric was shown to halt the spread of this type cancer? This herb is said to be "extremely safe," and "has been used in large quantities as a food with no adverse reactions." Consult with your physician before taking large quantities as it may interfere with blood clotting time, making you more susceptible to bleeding. (Do not use the herb if you have gallbladder disease.)[80]

Selene Yeager in *Doctors Book of FOOD REMEDIES,* reports that "India's National Cancer Institute" is so impressed with the power of turmeric in cancer prevention, it is highly promoted in that country. In animal testing, she says, it has been shown to "reduce the risk of colon cancer by 58 percent," and may inhibit melanoma as well.[81] Turmeric has anti-inflammatory properties that assist in wound healing, and may be important in preventing Alzheimer's, as found in animal studies.[82] Note that if you are interested in turmeric and other herbal supplements, as well as many vitamins and other nutrients at reasonable prices, see *www.discount-vitamins-herbs.net.*

III. Other Supplements & Treatments For Leukemia

Alpha Lipoic Acid Inhibits Leukemia

See other chapters in this book (e.g. chapter 19) for more information on alpha lipoic acid. It not only protects the liver, but inhibits leukemia as well. Potatoes, broccoli, brewer's yeast, and spinach are excellent sources of alpha lipoic acid. This is one nutrient you will need to supplement with to get adequate amounts.

Those who have a tendency to develop kidney or gallbladder stones should not consume large amounts of raw spinach due to its high "oxalate" content. Also, if you are taking "calcium supplements," wait "2-3 hours before or after" ingesting fresh spinach, since oxalates can inhibit calcium's assimilation by the body.[82a] (Cooking destroys much of the oxalates. See page 46.)

Beta-Sitosterol – Works Against Lymphocytic Leukemia

Beta-sitosterol, as described at www.*drlam.com*, is a naturally occurring nutrient that can be "found in rice bran, wheat germ, corn oils, and soybeans," but most diets are deficient.[83] It fights "lymphocytic leukemia…[and] normalizes blood sugar" in "type II diabetics…" and can also "relieve inflammation, heal ulcers, [and] enhance uterine tone…"[84] Beta-sitosterol should not be taken during lactation or pregnancy, nor by those with atypical hereditary diseases which may interefere with the body's correct assimilation of fats (see chapter five for examples and more information.)

Burzynski's Antineoplastons: Nox-Toxic Help for "Hopeless" Cancer Cases

Though not discussed at length in this chapter, see chapter 13 for more information on Burzynski's antineoplastons and his very successful treatment of **leukemia, lymphomas, bone and breast cancer, as well as "terminal" cases of inoperable brain cancers** and many other cancers! The Burzynski Clinic is located in Houston, Texas, the only state in which the FDA permits him to practice antineoplaston therapy. Their main website is *www.cancermed.com*. Also, read the remarkable stories of many people who have been <u>cured</u> using non-toxic antineoplastons: *http://burzynskipatientgroup.org/stories.html.* You will find many email addresses and mailing addresses from some of these survivors, should you wish to contact them about their amazing recoveries using antineoplastons.

DHEA & Leukemia

DHEA "(*Dehydroepiandrosterone*)" is a naturally occurring hormone produced by the adrenals that may play an important role against leukemia. As explained by Dr. James F. Balch, M.D. in his book, *The Super Anti-Oxidants*: "rats with virus-induced leukemia" were given DHEA and the results were impressive. The DHEA was effective against harmful free radicals and stimulated the animals' immune systems.[85]

A word of caution though before you decide to supplement with DHEA – consult your physician for a blood test to see if you have low blood levels of DHEA and related hormones. Dr. Balch explains that this hormone is not for women with insufficient "estrogen levels," who are "postmenopausal."[86] He also recommends the following for anyone thinking of taking DHEA supplements: avoid extremes – either physicians who are completely ignorant about this subject – or those who overly prescribe it. Be sure that you do not indiscriminately begin using the hormone without lab work to "determine your current blood levels of DHEA." Don't supplement if you are under 30, or if you have a prior "history of breast, ovary, or prostate cancer."[87] DHEA is a stimulant-type hormone that may be helpful in preventing muscle loss and "the onset of diabetes," in reducing body fat, and it may even "reverse Type II diabetes." It can also raise glutathione levels, increase the speed of healing, and may prevent osteoporosis.[88]

Mullaca: Toxic to Leukemia Cells

Mullaca *"(Physalis angulata)"* also known as *"cape goose, wild tomato, winter cherry,"* and other common names, is a Rainforest herb that fights leukemia cells.[89] Website *www.rain-tree.com* describes the herb in detail and says that the extracts of mullaca that are anti-leukemic are plant steroids known as *"physalins."* They have been shown to work against several kinds of malignancies such as "lung, colon...liver, cervix, melanoma and glioma (brain) cancer cells..."[90] In Taiwan, scientists revealed that this herb could halt the advancement of "five different types of acute leukemia, including lymphoid (T & B), promyelocytic, myeloid and monocytic."[90a]

Again, during 2001, Houston scientists discovered a compound in mullaca that was toxic to "nasopharynx cancer cells, lung (adenocarcinoma) cancer cells as well as leukemia in mice," says Raintree. The scientists believed that the herb may function by damaging the DNA of cancer cells so that they are not capable of reproducing![91]

Though no drug interactions have been reported, mullaca may lower blood pressure and affect blood clotting time, and may have a mild hypoglycemic effect. Mullaca is also used as an "analgesic...antiviral...sedative, [and] vermifuge (expels worms)."[92] For more information on mullaca, contact Raintree Nutrition at *www.rain-tree.com.*

Simarouba, Anamu, & Amargo Against Leukemia

Simarouba *"(Simarouba amara, glauca)"* is an herb that has been well known in some cultures for many years, but in vitro testing did not begin until 1976. At that time it was found to contain potent phytochemical anti-leukemia inhibitors called "quassinoids," and three of them were active "against lymphocytic leukemia..."[92a] In spite of this, no testing has been done on humans.[93] (Raintree says that excessive doses of this herb may cause "increased perspiration and urination, nausea and/or vomiting.") They also point out the anti-viral properties of the herb and ponder its potential use one day against the "West Nile Virus."[94]

Anamu *"(Petiveria alliacea),"* kills cancer cells directly and boosts the immune system by triggering the activity of white blood cells. Raintree Nutrition reports that laboratory research in 1990 showed that "extracts of anamu retarded the growth of leukemia cells and several other strains of cancerous tumor cells." After three years, the scientists did a follow-up study showing that these same compounds were destroying cancer cells, not just stunting them! The conclusion of the study was that "the whole herb water extracts of anamu were **toxic to leukemia and lymphoma cancer cells** but only **inhibited** the growth of breast cancer cells."[95] (Emphasis, mine.) Further lab studies done in 2001 and 2002 showed anamu to be toxic to cancerous liver cells and it "retarded the growth of brain cancer cells."[96] This herb does contain coumarin, so use with caution if taking blood-thinning medications, if you have a blood disorder, or are contemplating or recovering from surgery. Do not use it without first consulting with your physician. Since extracts of the herb can "cause uterine contractions," it should never be used during pregnancy. It can also lower blood sugar.[97] Both Anamu and Simarouba are in Raintree's *N-Tense-2*, available at their website *http://www.raintree.com/anamu.htm*. Another little known herb found in Raintree Nutrition's *N-Tense-2* that has shown activity against leukemia is **amargo**.[97a]

Vassourinha's Anti-Leukemic Extracts

Vassourinha "(*Scoparia dulcis*)" is an herb found abundantly not only within the Rainforest, but the U.S. as well. Some of the extracts of this herb have been very impressive against leukemia, cancer, and viruses such as HIV, and it has also demonstrated the ability to work against "malignant brain tumors, bone cancer and melanomas (without harming healthy cells)." Be sure to let your physician know if you are taking herbals such as this one, because vassourinha may lower blood pressure.[98] When Raintree Nutrition found that leukemia was not responding to Graviola in their product *N-Tense*, they developed *N-Tense-2* with mullaca, cat's claw, and vassourinha, as well as other cancer-fighting herbs specifically for aiding in the fight against leukemia. They are both available at *www.rain-tree.com.* You can also find dosage information there.[99]

Note that **Raintree Nutrition does not make *curative* claims for their herbs.** They report the results of tests conducted on various herbs, and they suggest that herbs be part of an overall comprehensive health treatment plan. Many of the plants discussed at their website can be purchased by the pound in cut leaves or in powdered form.

IV. Miscellaneous Herbs & Supplements

Andrographis Inhibits Leukemia

Andrographis "(*Andrographis paniculata)*" is an herb found in Asia with an ancient history of medicinal usage. Research of its use against cancer is very promising as well as against many pathogens. Studies show that andrographis can cause "leukemia cells" to "differentiate."[100] This is important, because as described earlier, if cells differentiate (like they are supposed to) they do not mutate and become cancerous! Getting them to revert back to a differentiated state means healthy cells! Extracts taken from andrographis leaves, in some tests, were able to halt the replication of abdominal "cancer cells," and they have shown success with other cancers as well, such as melanoma, "prostate cancer, breast cancer cells, and non-Hodgkins's lymphoma."[101]

Andrographis has very low toxicity. In rare cases, as reported by *herbs2000.com*, it can cause "dizziness and heart palpitations" or "mild to severe" allergic reactions.[102] The herb is available in a brand known as *"Androtech"* produced by "BioTherapies," and it is "standardized" and combined with "Enchinacea and zinc."[103] If you are trying to get pregnant this is NOT the herb for you! It should not be used if you are breast feeding or pregnant.

Bitter Melon Fights Leukemia

This herb with the repulsive-sounding name has shown activity against multiple cancer cell lines in laboratory testing, including human leukemia, skin cancers, liver cancer, and sarcomas.[104] (Excessive amounts may lower blood sugar or cause diarrhea.) Do not use it without consulting your physician, especially if you are taking diabetic medications.[104a]

Buckthorn Bark Inhibits Lymphocytic Leukemia

Buckthorn bark is one of the ingredients in Harry Hoxsey's tea formula. A research study revealed that "certain buckthorn preparations showed significant inhibition of P-388 lymphocytic leukemia in mice."[105]

Dyer's Woad Root Extracts Inhibit CML

Dyers's Woad *"(Isatis Indigotica Fortune)"* has been part of "traditional medicine" in China for many years. According to *www.nutrition2000.com*, "Root extracts have been used to treat patients with solid tumors and leukemia...Review of several published trials from China found oral administration of 150-200 mg of purified Dyer's woad per day led to remission in **60 percent of patients** with **chronic myelocytic leukemia**." [These were **HUMAN patients**, not lab animals!] This herb has also been shown to kill various bacteria, parasites, and viruses.[105a] (Emphasis, mine.)

Scutellaria

Another herb popular in Asian countries, scutellaria has been in use medicinally for hundreds of years. It is rich in plant flavonoids and effectively destroys pathogens ("bacteria and viruses") in patients "with multiple myeloma…" Do not use the herb if you have bowel problems such as "diarrhea."[106]

Shark Liver Oil Inhibits Leukemia

Though shark **cartilage** has been shown to be helpful in attacking other cancers, for leukemia, shark liver **oil** is more commonly used. In one particular case reported by Reese Dubin in his book, *Miracle Food Cures From the Bible*, an elderly woman who had been fighting "chronic lymphatic leukemia for 15 years," had good results when her physician placed her on "eight 500 mg. capsules of shark-liver oil daily." Within "6 months," her white blood counts, which previously had been extremely elevated, dropped to normal levels![107] Though no serious problems have been associated with using this supplement in normal dosages, it can cause atypical epigastric discomfort in some people. See your licensed natural health physician for individual dosing to fit your needs.

Tian Xian & Multiple Myeloma

Tian Xian is a Chinese herb that has been credited with many cancer recoveries, including multiple myelomas! You can read case histories of many cancer survivors, some given only two to six months to live, who went into complete remission using Tian Xian at *www.tianxian.com*. Many are still alive today, years after their ordeal!

Ukrain Fights Leukemia

Ukrain, discussed in prior chapters, is given by injection, so it is not exactly painless, however, it is included here due to its success rate with several types of cancer, and the fact that it is non-toxic! It is described by Dr. Ralph Moss at his website *www.ralph-moss.com/ukrain* (as well as the main ukrain website, *ukrin.com)*. It was discovered in "1978" by "Dr. Wassyl J. Nowicky…Director of the Ukrain Anti-Cancer Institute of Vienna, Austria."[107a] It is a combination of an herb "greater celandine" and the drug "thiotepa," a chemo drug. These two ingredients when used alone were very toxic, but once merged were found to be completely non-toxic except to cancer cells![107b]

A study that involved 70 "terminal" cancer patients discovered that Ukrain was toxic "to **human leukemias,** non small and small cell lung cancers, colon cancers, central nervous system cancer, melanomas, ovarian cancer and renal cancer."[108] (Emphasis, mine.)

You won't be able to find Ukrain at your local conventional medicine practitioner. It can only be found at alternative medicine clinics in the U.S. or in Canada, the Ukraine, or another country in Europe, where it is commonly used. It is discussed in several other cancer-specific chapters in this book. The main website for Ukrain therapy is at *www.ukrin.com.*

Xi Shu

Xi Shu "*(Camptotheca acuminata)*" is an herb that has been used by the Chinese for several millennia. They have used it for treating leukemia, and for this reason, it is often referred to as the "cancer tree."[109]

V. Other Issues Involving Leukemia

Childhood Leukemia Statistics & Hot Dogs

In her book, *All Your Health Questions Answered Naturally*, Maureen Kennedy Salaman discusses the newspaper headline (from the *Los Angeles Times,* June 3, 1994) that linked hot dog consumption to the development of childhood leukemia:

John Peters, a University of Southern California epidemiologist reported in the scientific journal Cancer Causes and Control, that **children who eat more than 12 hot dogs a month** have nine times the normal risk of developing childhood leukemia. Two other reports in the journal suggest children born to mothers who eat at least one hot dog a week during pregnancy have double the normal risk of developing brain tumors, as do children whose fathers ate hot dogs before conception.[110] [Emphasis, mine.]

Avoid Cow's Milk, Avoid Leukemia

Of great concern, is the use of cow's milk, especially in children. Dr. Russell Blaylock, M.D. in *Natural Strategies For Cancer Patients*, explains that eliminating cow's milk from your diet may protect you from getting leukemia because "...two of the most common diseases in cattle...[are] leukemia and lymphoma..." Note that pasteurization does **not** always kill all of these viruses![111] (Avoiding cow's milk may also protect your children from juvenile or Type I diabetes! See chapter 25 in this book for more information on why you are better off permanently getting cow's milk out of your diet!)

Flax Oil & The Budwig Diet

See chapters 13 and 17 of this book for information on the famous Budwig flax oil diet that many have credited to complete cancer cures!

Poly–MVA for Leukemia

See chapters 9 and 13 for more information on this amazing nutritional supplement that many cancer survivors have credited to bringing them into total remission, even from leukemia. Their main website is *www.polymva.net.*

CHAPTER 8

PAINLESS CURES & PREVENTIONS FOR LIVER CANCER

"I now believe, in many cases of cancer diagnosis, we often have a case of uninformed doctors leading uninformed, trusting, patients."
(Burt Berkson, M.D., Ph.D., from his book:
The Alpha Lipoic Acid Breakthrough)[1]

The Liver Cancer That Vanished!

As described by Jean Carper in her book, *Miracle Cures,* when a CAT scan diagnosed a "52-year-old carpenter" with liver cancer, a follow-up biopsy confirmed the diagnosis, as well as the presence of a "4.5 cm" tumor "on the right lobe of his liver [that] had already spread to the left lobe." He had been "a heavy drinker and smoker" for more than 20 years, and physicians at the "University of Maryland" determined that surgery was hopeless, due to the late stage of the cancer. They sent the patient home, assuming a rapid death. (Terminal "liver cancer...patients" generally are given a life expectancy of only a few months!)[2]

Imagine the surprise of these physicians when their patient showed up nearly 12 months "later," in "June 1991," not only alive and well, but much improved! As further noted by Ms. Carper, he told them that he had quit smoking and drinking since being diagnosed with liver cancer, and that he felt very well and had even gained weight. They were astonished when subsequent ultrasound and CAT scan showed no signs of the tumors, and several biopsies done at the prior location "where the previous massive tumor was located," were negative.[2a] Doctors noted that this was highly unusual. So unusual in fact, that it occurred "only once in 60,000 to 100,000 patients," and "only eight cases of complete regression of liver cancer have ever been published in the entire world medical literature, the doctors noted."[2b] Though they surmised that giving up cigarettes and alcohol contributed to the patient's healing, they had no real answers to the total regression of the deadly cancer. It turns out that the patient himself had the answer, as Ms. Carper explains: immediately upon leaving the "hospital with his incurable liver cancer in 1990, he started taking a dose of 450 milligrams of silymarin, or milk thistle, daily, prescribed by his local physician. He had downed it religiously, he said, every day for eleven months."[3]

Though the physicians would not admit that it was the milk thistle that cured the liver cancer, Ms. Carper says that they were in favor of using the herb, seeing that there were no toxic side effects, "and the herb is known to neutralize free radicals and regenerate liver cells."[4]

Why were these physicians so reluctant to **admit** that the only thing that this patient did differently to **cure** his liver cancer was using milk thistle? It does not take a rocket scientist to figure out exactly what cured his inoperable liver cancer! Let's face it, many people quit smoking and drinking immediately when they are diagnosed with liver cancer, (or lung cancer) but that does NOT CURE them! This is simply another case of conventional medicine refusing to admit that something besides a toxic chemo drug CURED a deadly cancer!

Milk thistle can be found at any natural health food store as a supplement and in tea bags. It is also sold in bulk.

Be aware that if you have a chronic disorder such as hemochromatosis, diabetes, hepatitis, are taking prescription medications, or you are a transplant patient, you should never begin a new herbal regimen without consulting with your physician. If you have hemochromatosis, you need to be sure that the milk thistle supplement you purchase does not have iron. (Also, be aware that if you are diabetic, milk thistle can lower blood sugar.)

The Mushroom Poisoning Cure

Is milk thistle the miracle herb many believe? YES! There is no doubt that it helps **protect** and *regenerate* the liver.

In *Miracle Cures*, Jean Carper describes the case of a scientist from Germany, "Dr. G. Vogel of the University of Munich," who found in the early 80's that milk thistle saved the lives of dozens of victims in Europe who had ingested the lethal "amanita mushroom, also called the ***death cap***."[5] While amanita usually kills nearly half of those who ingest it (even with medical treatment), no one given milk thistle experienced a fatality, even though they were not treated until **48 to 72 hours after they ate the mushrooms!** Dr. Vogel believed the herb competes for poison receptor sites within the liver, shielding "liver cells from further damage and healing those already damaged."[6]

As far as dosing, Ms. Carper further explains that some physicians will suggest a dosage of "280 milligrams" of silymarin (milk thistle) per day as a preventative, however, for those already having liver dysfunction, a higher dosage of "420 milligrams of silymarin taken in three divided doses every day may be needed." [e.g. you would be taking 140 milligrams morning, noon and evening.] Once serum levels show an improvement, the amount is "cut back to a daily dose of 280."[7] (Remember that the liver cancer patient described in the earlier story (above) was ingesting 450 milligrams of silymarin per day for 11 months!)

James A. Duke, Ph.D., (with Michael Castleman) documented a similar study on the power of milk thistle in preventing death from the amanita mushroom in their book, *The Green Pharmacy, Anti-Aging Prescriptions:*

> In one study, 60 people were given silymarin for Amanita poisoning. None died. In another study 189 people received standard medical care for Amanita poisoning, while another 16 were given silymarin. Among those receiving standard medical care, 46 died. Among those taking silymarin, **none died**...In one laboratory study using animals, silymarin prevented liver damage from large doses of acetaminophen...[8]

The use of "standard medical treatment," says Dr. Duke, normally means "activated charcoal."[9] In a *nutshell*, the patient is given a vile-looking black liquid charcoal to drink. The charcoal is supposed to soak up all the toxins and excrete them from the body, preventing damage to vital organs such as the liver, however, it sometimes doesn't work, especially if too much time has passed since the "toxic" substance has been ingested! Activated charcoal can also be given through gastric lavage if the patient is not conscious, for example, during cases of drug overdose. The charcoal really works best if given within a half hour of the time the toxin is ingested.

Believe it or not, the U.S. is so far behind Europe in medical technology that silymarin is not even available in emergency rooms for treating mushroom poisoning, yet it is commonly used in European countries! Some U.S. hospitals are finally getting in alpha lipoic acid, but I am sure it is probably **only because** of the unselfish and heroic efforts of doctors like Burt Berkson, M.D. (See his book, *The Alpha Lipoic Acid Breakthrough.*)

Milk Thistle & Other Cancers

Not only has milk thistle proven to protect the liver, but research has shown that the herb may be "effective against breast cancer, skin cancers, and other carcinomas."[10] See chapters four and five of this book for information on how this herb is being used against prostate and colon cancer as well!

Milk thistle has been used for over 2000 years. It is actually the seeds of the plant that are therapeutic, containing several flavonoids "collectively known as silymarin."[11] This, according to Dr. Mark Stengler in his book, *Natural Strategies for Cancer Patients.* He points out that milk thistle is "ten times more potent" in its antioxidant power than vitamin E. It works by actually prompting liver cells to regenerate, and it keeps the liver from absorbing "toxic substances."[12]

Milk Thistle, Glutathione, Skin Disorders & Endometriosis

Glutathione is another major antioxidant found throughout the human body, and there are few substances you can take that will increase its production. Milk thistle is one of them! Milk thistle also helps raise the body's amount of "superoxide dismutase, (SOD)," another potent antioxidant. Dr. Stengler points out that the ability of milk thistle to rejuvenate the liver is vitally important for people suffering with "hepatitis, fatty liver, and cirrhosis of the liver." It also prompts the regeneration of kidney cells and stimulates "bile" secretion, improving the digestion of fats.[13] Of course you will need to check with your doctor before using this herb if you have problems with "large gallstones"[14] or any other sort of biliary disease.

Though vitamin C aids the body in making more glutathione, according to Dr. James F. Balch in *The Super Anti-Oxidants,* milk thistle actually keeps glutathione reserves from being exhausted in the liver, and it appears to be "more potent than either vitamin E or C…"[15] Other nutrients that increase the body's production of glutathione (besides vitamin C), explains Dr. Balch, are the amino acids that can be found in "asparagus, avocado, Brussel sprouts, cabbage, [and] walnuts."[16] Foods rich in sulfur (e.g. onions, broccoli, garlic, and red cabbage) are also very protective to liver function.[17] (See chapter nine for a list of glutathione-rich foods.)

Milk thistle also acts as an anti-inflammatory for skin disorders such as "psoriasis." It may help relieve the painful symptoms of endometriosis since it assists liver cells in estrogen metabolism.[18] Scientists have discovered that (in animal testing), if the skin suffers dangerous sun exposure, then silymarin used topically, it could reduce the incidence of melanomas by two-thirds![19]

No side effects have been reported from the use of milk thistle. Though it has a reputation for being exceptionally safe, some users of the herb experience diarrhea on initial use (for about the first 24 to 48 hours).[20] It is recommended that the herb be ingested on an empty stomach. There have been no reports of adverse effects when milk thistle was taken with other routine medications.[21] (Of course, as with any herb, there is always the possibility of allergic reactions in some individuals.)

Milk Thistle & Chemo

Website *http://content.nhiondemand.com,* notes that one of the flavonoids in silymarin, "silibin," may lessen the cellular injury that chemo drugs such as "paracetamol, cisplatin, and vincristin" cause.[22]

In another study, when rats were fed poison and silymarin both, **the herb prevented them from getting liver damage!**[23]

Milk Thistle & Hepatitis

James A. Duke, Ph.D. in his book, *The Green Pharmacy Anti-Aging Prescriptions*, recounts the story of a lady with **hepatitis A**, whose "liver was functioning at just 40 percent of its normal capacity." She "received an injection of vitamin K," then began taking milk thistle. After taking milk thistle for 3 weeks, Dr. Duke says that "a second test showed liver function had improved to 82 percent."[24]

When Lloyd Wright contracted **hepatitis C** from blood transfusions, he healed himself naturally with milk thistle and wrote a book called *Triumph Over Hepatitis C*. At his website: *www.hepatitisCfree.com*, he describes how he uses milk thistle:

> I use the organic seeds, simmering them for two hours and then drink the tea iced. It is also important to take at least 1000 mg. of milk thistle per day in addition to the tea, as silymarin is not water-soluble. There are other active ingredients in milk thistle that are important but, unfortunately, most of them are eliminated from the processed capsule form. This is why I recommend taking both the tea and the capsules. I've reviewed many articles and studies on milk thistle and hope that some of them will find their way to all those liver doctors who told me there was nothing I could take to help my liver regenerate.[24a]

Mr. Wright also has information on new products containing milk thistle and other important liver healing herbs at his website above.

There are cases of **"chronic persistent hepatitis"** actually going into remission within "six months to a year" of using milk thistle! Jean Carper, in *Miracle Cures*, says that this herb is "considered so safe in Germany that there are no government warnings against using it even during pregnancy and lactation." (Emphasis, mine.)[24b]

Standardized Milk Thistle

As recommended by Maureen Kennedy Salaman from her book, *All Your Health Questions Answered Naturally,* when purchasing milk thistle supplements, check that the brand you are purchasing has "standardized extract" of "80% silymarin."[25] If you purchase the herb in loose bulk format, follow the directions given at the herbal store where it is purchased. Most health food stores where you buy loose herbs should provide you with directions on brewing them.

Aloe Emodin Effective Against Liver Cancer

Aloe emodin, an ingredient taken from "aloe vera leaves" has been researched for its anti-cancer properties in fighting liver cancer, with amazing results. *Life Extension's* website (*www.lef.org)* contains a published report of studies conducted using aloe-emodin to treat cancer. It was useful against liver and lung tumors in animal studies. Also, aloe-emodin was able to suppress "the growth of neuroectodermal tumors...in mice" (even though their immune systems were severely compromised), "without any appreciable toxic effects on the animals."[26] (When cells that are supposed to eventually develop into **nerve tissue** turn into cancerous cells instead, they are called *neuroectodermal tumors.* This is an example of what happens when cells do NOT differentiate as they are supposed to.)

Other studies reveal that aloe-emodin could be an important preventative for liver malignancies by causing liver cancer cells to undergo a type of self-destruction ensuring their demise. (Aloe-emodin was also found in sheep sorrel, one of the herbs used in making Essiac tea.)

Alpha Lipoic Acid Heals Liver Damage, Prevents Cancer, & May Eliminate The Need For A Liver Transplant!

Alpha lipoic acid is a natural ingredient that our bodies make, but "as we grow older...we manufacture less and less of it," however we "must maintain a high ALA level to stay healthy." Dr. Burt Berkson, M.D., Ph.D., in his book, *The Alpha Lipoic Acid Breakthrough,* lists just a few of the amazing health benefits of alpha lipoic acid (ALA):

> ALA can inhibit the production of the AIDS virus...may prevent cataracts of the eye...protects the kidneys...possibly prevents diabetes...enhances your immune system...helps fight many disease processes, including cancer...prevents leukemia...can be used for treating diabetes...and serious liver disease...protects the heart and brain from the necrosis (cell death) that follows a heart attack or stroke.[27]

Dr. Berkson has also treated several of his **hepatitis C patients with ALA,** patients who were told that they would die without a **"liver transplant."** (Emphasis, mine.) After treatment with ALA therapy, "all of the patients (except one)" had returned to their jobs or school and reported higher "energy levels." The alpha lipoic acid was part of a structured nutritional program that included "stress reduction...and exercise..." All of the participants received not only ALA, but milk thistle and several vitamins as well. Dr. Berkson believes that before anyone even contemplates "liver transplant surgery, a doctor should prescribe a course of alpha lipoic acid."[28]

Have you been diagnosed with liver cancer, hepatitis, or liver failure? Has your physician considered prescribing milk thistle or alpha lipoic acid supplements for you? Has he or she explained the importance of lycopene in liver health? (Note that Dr. Berkson also cured four mushroom-poisoned patients with alpha lipoic acid. See chaper 33 later in this book for that incredible story!) Though potatoes, broccoli, brewer's yeast, and spinach are food sources of alpha lipoic acid, you can not get sufficient daily amounts without supplementing with this nutrient.

Those who have a tendency to develop kidney or gallbladder stones should not consume large amounts of raw spinach due to its high "oxalate" content. Also, if you are taking "calcium supplements," wait "2-3 hours before or after" ingesting fresh spinach, since oxalates can inhibit calcium's assimilation by the body.[28a] (Cooking destroys much of the oxalates. See page 46.)

Apples for Liver Health

Is it possible that simple ingredients in apples may be powerful enough to prevent cancer and slow its growth? Researchers have discovered through laboratory testing that compounds in these fruits can suppress both hepatic and intestinal cancers and since both the pulp and peelings contain the cancer fighters, wash your apples thoroughly, but don't peel before eating!

Astragalus – Herbal Power for the Liver

Astragalus in capsule form boosts the immune system, activating immune cells to fight tumors. Astragalus should not be used if you are running a temperature or during the presence of an infectious process.[29] This herb is very popular as a tea. You can find astragalus tea bags in natural health food stores as well as in supplements.

Beets for Liver Health

An excellent liver cleansing drink to boost liver health is beet root juice. As noted by John Heinerman in *Heinerman's Encyclopedia of Healing Juices,* Hungarian physician, "Dr. Alexander Ferenczi" discovered that "beet root juice and its powdered form arrested the further development of many different kinds of cancer." When given to test animals with "malignant tumors," not only did their cancer disappear, but they survived an average of "20 percent longer" than those animals not given the beet juice.[30]

Always start ingesting beet juice slowly to build tolerance. It is very potent, and consuming too much at once can detoxify too rapidly and make you feel worse! Always mix beet juice with another vegetable juice such as carrot, celery, or green juices, rather than drinking it alone.

Cherries Prevent Liver Cancer

According to Selene Yeager in the *Doctors Book of FOOD REMEDIES:* "A monoterpene that is found in cherries...*perillyl alcohol*...[inhibits] cancers of the breast, lung, stomach, liver, and skin." This was demonstrated by animal testing at the "Indiana University School of Medicine in Indianapolis." Researcher, "Charles Elson, Ph.D.," said this ingredient not only "fights cancer" by neutralizing "cancer-causing toxins," it is also "effective in animals with **existing tumors**."[31] (Emphasis, mine.) You can find some very potent cherry and blueberry supplements at website*: http://www.flavonoid-sciences.com/research/c3.htm.*

Cinnamon for the Liver

Just one teaspoon per day of grated cinnamon can work wonders for your liver because it "deactivates plasmin, a substance that allows cancer cells to invade healthy tissue."[32] This is described at website *herbs2000.com.*

I purchase cinnamon at a local health food store sold in bulk and use 1-2 teaspoons at a time, usually when I make fresh apple juice. (Cinnamon can also help stabilize blood sugar, and it may help prevent food poisoning.) See chapter 30!

The 390 mg. Daily Regimen of CoQ10 That Cured Liver & Breast Cancer

Research has shown that high doses of Coenyme Q10 given to cancer patients may help them win the fight against several different types of cancer. In a 1994 study, two women having breast cancer experienced complete remission during a clinical trial where they were given either 300 mg. or 390 mg. of CoQ10 daily. In the patient receiving 390 milligrams, the tumor completely vanished withn a 60 day period of taking the supplements.[32a] A year later, another human study was conducted. A middle-aged patient experienced total remission of a liver cancer that had previously been marked by multiple tumors. All the tumors totally vanished! Another middle-aged lung cancer patient on CoEnzyme Q10 enjoyed complete remission after a period of several months. An elderly patient with breast cancer, experienced no further cancer after she had a lump removal and was on the CoQ10 treatment.[33]

CoQ10 supplements are available in health food stores, pharmacies, popular grocery chains and internet sites such as *www.discountvitamins-herbs.com.*

A popular chemo drug, Adriamycin, causes CoQ10 to be depleted from cardiac muscle, resulting in cardiac injury, one of the adverse complications of the drug. However, patients who receive CoQ10 supplementation when they are given this drug do not experience this problem! "(Yance, 1999)"[33a]

Essiac Tea & Other Herbs

See chapter five of this book for information on Rene Cassie and the many patients she treated and cured of various cancers with Essiac tea, **including her own mother.** If you do not wish to buy your own herbs for this tea and brew it from scratch, there are preparations on the market that contain the herbs already pre-mixed. One example is known as *Flor-Essence®*, which not only has the Essiac herbs, but kelp, blessed thistle, and red clover for boosting the immune system. *Flor-Essence®* comes already made into a tea, or in a dry mix that you can brew to make the tea yourself. It is available at most health food stores.

Another brand of Essiac tea known as *Resperin Essiac®* was partly responsible for curing a young boy of Hodgkins disease, as described in chapter 15 of this book. You can get more details of his personal story in that chapter, as well as online at: *http://www.grandstrand.com/suebest/boywho.htm.* His parents were so impressed with the tea, they became distributors, and you can order it from their website, above. (If you wish to start from scratch and make your own Essiac, websites with the original Essiac recipe are given in chapter five of this book.)

Some herbalists don't recommend buying a ready made dry mix of the Essiac herbs, believing that the four herbs should be kept separate until the tea is made. Marie Nadine Antol in her book, *Healing Teas,* recommends the following herbs for their benefit in promoting liver health: "Alfalfa, cascara sagrada, chamomile, dandelion, feverfew, garlic, goldenseal, gotu kola, horehound, licorice, milk thistle, pau d-arco, propolis, sarsaparilla, [and] uva ursi."[34] (Note that some of these herbs have blood-thinning effects, may increase bile secretion or gastric acids, or elevate your blood pressure. Do not use them without first consulting with your licensed health practitioner.)

Graviola

Refer to chapters four and five for more information on how this herb has been used to bring about cancer cures.

Goldenseal Halts the Multiplication of Liver Cancer Cells

According to website, *www.herbs2000.com,* goldenseal contains berberine, an ingredient that "stops multiplication of liver cancer cells." Other herbs that contain berberine are "barberry...coptis... [and] Oregon grape."[35] It is also noted that "herbs that contain berberine" should not be used in those who are "pregnant...lactating," or may have "gallbladder disease...Do not take these herbs with supplemental vitamin B6 or protein supplements containing the amino acid histidine." It is not for those with "cardiovascular disease or glaucoma."[36] (Berberine or goldenseal may increase blood pressure in some individuals.)

Grapes (Resveratrol) Inhibit Liver Cancer

Research recently credits resveratrol (a super antioxidant) to the prevention of liver cancer. It works by preventing malignant cells from invading the body, and halts the formation of a compound identified with malignant breast cells as well. See Chapter two of this book for more information on the amazing curative powers of this nutrient, which is found in common table grapes!

Green Tea for Liver Health

Green tea is rich in polyphenols, bioflavonoids that are also "super antioxidants." In his book, *Dr. Earl Mindell's What You Should Know About The Super Antioxidant Miracle,* Dr. Mindell says that these bioflavonoids (known as "catechins") have been known to eliminate dangerous lipids, reduce "cholesterol and blood pressure," inhibit processes that trigger cancer, stop the growth of pathogens, assist in "digestion," protect "against ulcers and strokes,"[37] and it also "protects the brain and the liver," works as an "antibacterial... [and] cures gum disease..."[38]

Green tea is much higher in catechins than black tea. (As discussed earlier, for some cancers, combining both teas is more effective.) Green tea catechins are available at health food stores in supplement form if you do not wish to drink the tea. Note that cancer patients should stick to **caffeine-free** tea, because caffeine is very dehydrating.

Studies have shown that the ability of green tea to inhibit all types of cancer is very impressive. Dr. Mindell describes one such example:

In one [study], the lung cancer rate in mice fed green tea was reduced by 45 percent. Other animal studies suggest that green tea can cut the rate of stomach and liver cancer and slow the progress of skin cancer...but green tea doesn't just stop the cancer from ever getting started, it can also stop tumor growth in its tracks...[39]

According to an article at *herbs2000.com*, green tea can help prevent the development of liver cancer if a person is not already infected with "viral hepatitis – if soy lecithin is also taken."[40] In order to reduce the chances of having hepatitis advance to a cancerous liver, "licorice and scutellaria [herbs] can be used together in tea form. Take 1 cup of each (from bags) daily."[41] Note that licorice, unless it is deglycyrrhizinated (DGL), can raise the blood pressure. *Herbs2000.com* further explains that you should not use undeglycyrrhizinated licorice if you have "glaucoma, high blood pressure, or disorders affected by estrogen." Always consult with your physician first. When taking this herb, also "take a potassium supplement daily…[and] avoid scutellaria during diarrhea."[42] (You can purchase DGL licorice in health food stores. If you get the chewable wafers, they taste somewhat like coffee beans!)

Green Foods & Liver Health

Chlorella is an algae "found in fresh water" that is even richer in chlorophyll than wheatgrass, alfalfa, and all other green foods, including other algae. It has higher levels of chlorophyll than any other plant, including spirulina. C. M. Hawken in *Green Foods "Phyto Foods" for Super Health,* says that chlorella stimulates the immune system by producing extra white blood cells and increasing the levels of interferon in the body. It has been shown to "slow down and even reverse the progression of certain tumors."[43]

Chlorella has magnesium, beta-carotene, calcium, zinc, protein, many other vitamins and minerals, and several carotenoids, which are heart protective and cancer inhibitory.[44]

Be sure in purchasing chlorella that you obtain a brand that has broken-cell-wall. Without the cell wall of this one-celled organism being broken, it is not easily absorbed by the body.

If you are wondering about chlorella dosages for those with cancer, Dr. Joseph Mercola of *www.mercola.com* states:

> It is not uncommon for people who have cancer to take as much as 30 grams of chlorella per day. One person with bone cancer showed tremendous results after 6 months of

taking 20 grams of Chlorella per day....The specific dose and application of chlorella ideally should be monitored by a nutritionally oriented physician or a certified clinical nutritionist.[45]

In Ann Wigmore's *The Wheatgrass Book*, chlorophyll is described as being so similar in structure to hemoglobin that physicians have even used it "to treat anemia." It can be important for delivering "oxygen throughout the entire body, including the brain."[46]

Wheat grass (though not as high in chlorophyll as chlorella) is another green food that greatly enhances the immune system! Ms. Wigmore said that there are three important compounds in wheatgrass that benefit the liver: "choline, [which] works to prevent the deposition of fat," "magnesium," important in pulling out "excess fats," and "potassium," which rejuvenates.[47]

Hormones & Liver Cancer

Recent studies have shown that using birth control pills increases a woman's risk of liver cancer three times over those who do not use them. Maureen Kennedy Salaman in her book, *All Your Health Questions Answered Naturally,* warns that for those using the pill "five or more years," their risk was "5.5 times" greater than women never using the pill. Tests showed that the ingredient in the pills causing liver cancer was the "synthetic estrogen!"[48]

See chapter 21 in this book entitled, *Prescription HRT – The Great Tragedy of the 20th Century,* for more information on how pharmaceutical companies knowingly promoted their synthetic estrogen and progesterone prescriptions to the public, when they knew full well that natural estrogen and natural progesterone (found in nature) were already available, and without toxic side effects!

IP-6 for Cancer Prevention

According to Dr. Michael T. Murray at website *www.doctormurray. com*, IP-6 is a naturally occurring ingredient extracted from "whole grains and beans," but it "is absorbed much better when it is taken on its own in pill form." Though not tested on humans, this natural substance is "inexpensive," and "poses absolutely no health risk, yet holds the promise of being a real answer to one of the most deadly diseases on this planet – cancer." Being an antioxidant, it enhances the immune system. Thus far, "in animal experiments, IP-6 has demonstrated impressive effects in preventing and reversing cancer." Dr. Shamsuddin, "world-renowned expert on IP-6," suggests "a total daily amount of 1 - 2 g of IP6… [however] for individuals with a high risk of cancer or cardiovascular disease, kidney stone, fatty liver, etc., this amount should be doubled. And finally for treatment of existing cancer, Dr. Shamsuddin suggests even high[er] dosages." Dr. Murray said that he recommends this supplement to all his cancer patients.[49]

Lycopene Power & Liver Health

If you are interested in a drink that will rapidly improve the health of your liver, try tomato juice. For "hypoglycemia, chronic fatigue syndrome, yeast infection, and mononucleosis," John Heinerman in *Heinerman's Encyclopedia of Healing Juices*, recommends drinking "tomato juice" with "a pinch of cayenne pepper and dash of hot sauce" to rejuvenate "the liver and adrenal glands within" 30 minutes.[50]

Lycopene was proven to inhibit the formation of cancers of the liver. Research on **humans** demonstrated that lycopene can cut the risk for cancer of the liver in half! (Also, see my liver tonic recipe at the end of this chapter.) Other good food sources of lycopene (besides tomatoes) are watermelon and red peppers.

Limonene Halts the Growth of Tumor Cells

Laboratory research shows that an ingredient in citrus fruits known as "limonene" has anti-cancer properties.[51] "Professor of human oncology at the University of Wisconsin Medical School in Madison…Michael Gould, Ph.D," said that limonene causes "cancer cells to self-destruct. It assists them in their own suicides…"[52] This is detailed by Selene Yeager in *Doctors Book of FOOD REMEDIES*. She further reveals that giving laboratory animals "a diet consisting of 10 percent limonene" shrank tumors by "70 percent…"[53] (These studies involved mostly lung and breast cancers.) When scientists fed laboratory animals "with early stages of liver cancer…" an "extract of orange juice," the "pre-cancerous lesions dropped 40 percent." (They had first removed the "vitamin C" from the juice.[54])

Mushrooms That Prevent Liver Cancer & Metastasis

Animal studies proved that feeding mice a diet of "20 percent maitake powder" and maitake "D-fraction" (from maitake mushrooms), reduced the occurrence of liver cancers after the mice had been fed a carcinogen. Of the group receiving no mushroom at all – every single one of them developed liver tumors![55] It was also found that maitake prevented the metastasis of cancers in the lab mice to whom it was given![56]

Maitake should not be taken by those with "multiple sclerosis," cautions *herbs2000.com*. This is because maitake increases the formation of "gamma-interferon, [which] can promote the destruction of nerve tissue, so people with MS should avoid maitake until this remedy has been more thoroughly tested."[57]

Lentinan injections from the shiitake mushroom have been shown to stop the progression of cancerous liver growths.[58] However, since they are considered *alternative therapy*, you will have to seek an alternative medicine practitioner for this treatment.

Reishi mushroom extract may also help suppress the advancement of malignances in the liver.[59] (It is available in tablet form.)

As described at website, *mnwelldir.org,* another mushroom that helps in the fight against liver cancer is the agaricus mushroom *("Agaricus Blazei Murill").* This mushroom "can be used in cooking" just as any other mushroom, explains Wellness Directory of Minnesota™. It has a polysaccharide that was found "effective against Ehrlich's ascites carcinoma, sigmoid colonic cancer, ovarian cancer, breast cancer, lung cancer, and liver cancer as well as against solid cancers." These mushrooms can be ordered at *"www.agaricus.net*...one of the largest suppliers in the world."[60]

(See chapter 24 in this book for more information about the marvelous curative and disease prevention power of mushrooms!)

Onions Prevent Liver Cancer

Researchers at "Cornell University" in "Ithaca, N.Y.," believe that it is very possible that an "Onion a day keeps [the] doctor away."[61] Details on this study can be found at *www.news.cornell.edu/releases/Oct04/onions.cancer.ssl.html.* It also appears that the variety of onion you eat makes a big difference! In the article, scientist "Rui Hai Liu, M.D., Ph.D...associate professor of food science," says that "shallots, Western Yellow, pungent yellow and Northern Red onions are higher in anti-cancer chemicals than other varieties tested." According to him, "onions are one of the richest sources of flavonoids in the human diet." They also kill viruses, inhibit allergies and are "anti-inflammatory." The best onions to fight liver cancer are "Western Yellow, shallot and pungent yellow." Apparently the "more pungent" the onion and the "more bitter," the greater the anti-cancer potency. They reported that "Western Yellow onions had 11 times more flavonoids than Western Whites, the onions with fewest flavonoids."[61a]

Other Liver Nutrients

As described by Maureen Kennedy Salaman in her book, *All Your Health Questions Answered Naturally,* it has been discovered, in animal testing, that deficiencies in "choline and lecithin...may cause" enough harm to your liver to "eventually" give you cancer! "[T]ake lecithin, [and] you'll be getting your choline." Your body can make choline, says Ms. Salaman, but only if you take a combination of "folic acid, B12 and the amino acid methionine," at the same time.[62] She further explains that borage oil," rich in "linolenic acid," can keep toxins from harming your liver. It is often used to treat cases "of mushroom poisoning" that might "otherwise be fatal."[63] (Two more substances used for this purpose are milk thistle, and alpha lipoic acid, as discussed earlier in this chapter.)

Other ingredients to fortify your liver, as described by Ms. Salaman are: aged "liquid garlic extract," the B vitamins, "vitamin E, beta carotene...selenium [and] beets and beet tops...." Even patients fighting hepatitis have been helped by drinking beet root juice, says Ms. Salaman, but only if they consume "a quart or more a day," regardless of whether it was chemically or virally induced.[64]

From what I have researched on garlic, I believe that next to eating fresh organic garlic, the best garlic extract is Kyolic®. They received an award from the National Nutrition Foods Association, and use a stringent manufacturing and aging process. When cooking, it is best to use fresh, organic garlic. Chicory, a close relative of milk thistle, also has liver-protective abilities.

Do not suddenly start drinking large amounts of beet juice as it detoxifies the body so rapidly, it may make you worse initially! Start by drinking small amounts (two ounces at a time) and always mix it with a few ounces of another vegetable juice such as carrot or celery.

Phyllanthus for the Liver

This herb ("Phyllanthus niruri"), also known as the "kidney stone tree...is not related to gooseberry." It "inhibits liver cancer," and is the source of a "vaccine" used against "Hepatitis B..."[64a] It should not be used without your physician's advice since it may lower blood pressure. It may also have some "diuretic" and "hypoglycemic"properties. For more information on this herb, see *www.herbs2000.com*.[64b]

Selenium Prevents Liver Cancer

Selenium is so important for liver cancer prevention that "a clinical trial in China involving 100,000 people," revealed that selenium could reduce liver cancer deaths by more than one-third! The study lasted eight years. This mineral is particularly important for anyone fighting "hepatitis B."[65]

Too much selenium can be toxic, however, most people don't get enough of this mineral on a daily basis. According to Dr. James F. Balch, in his book: *The Super Anti-Oxidants: Why They Will Change The Face of Healthcare in the 21st Century,* "unless you are eating a couple of acres of parsley each day," you may be deficient in this vital mineral! He recommends about "200 micrograms" per day, though "doses of as much as 700 micrograms daily have proven safe, even for extended periods."[66] Some good natural sources listed in Dr. H. Winter Griffith's *Vitamins Herbs, Minerals & Supplements* are: "Bran, Broccoli, Brown rice, Cabbage...Mushrooms...Oatmeal, Onions, Seafood, Tuna [and] whole-grain products."[66a] (Brazil nuts and kelp are also very rich in selenium, however, kelp should be used sparingly because of its iodine content.)

Help From the Sea for Curing Liver Cancer

Shark cartilage is discussed in Chapter six in more detail for its treatment of cervical, ovarian, and uterine cancers, however, it has also been effective against other cancers. In her book, *Nutrition: The Cancer Answer II*, Maureen Kennedy Salaman discusses "Dr. Ernesto Contrearas, Jr." of Panama, who placed "eight terminal cancer patients" on the supplement for 60 days. Seven of the "eight showed a reduction in tumor size of 30 to 100 percent," and one "patient with an advanced liver tumor experienced complete remission after eight weeks of shark cartilage therapy."[67] Shark cartilage is not for use with children, nor during pregnancy, or if you have recently had a heart attack, transplant, surgery, chemo or radiation. It is not for those with seafood allergies, liver disease (though it was used successfully in the case above for liver cancer), high blood pressure, pheochromocytoma (adrenal tumor which can cause excessively high blood pressure), ulcers or circulatory diseases. See chapter six for more information on dosing. You should also consult with your natural health physician for specific individual dosing to fit your own situation before taking this supplement.

Soy Lecithin, Arginine, & Jerusalem Artichokes – Nutrition to Prevent Liver Cancer from Progressing

Soy lecithin works against free radicals to inhibit cancer development. "Arginine" is an "amino acid" found in foods "such as chocolate, coconut, hazelnuts, [and] sunflower seeds."[68] It helps suppress the advancement of malignancies of the liver, but does so in such a way that the body does not suffer protein-starvation. On the other hand, "Jerusalem artichokes…contain inulin," an ingredient discovered (in lab studies) to suppress the growth of liver malignancies.[68a] (This is INULIN, **not insulin**.) Do not use arginine if you have genital herpes, or the herpes virus that causes fever blisters and shingles. Be sure to get organic artichokes, because most artichokes are heavily sprayed!

Tian Xian Effective Against Liver Cancer

Tian Xian, a Chinese herb, is said to be effective in fighting several forms of cancer, including liver cancer. As reported at *www.tianxian.com*, in November of 1992, 83-year-old Mr. "N. Zentaro" of Japan, was diagnosed with liver cancer as well as stomach cancer. His physician felt that due to his age and the fact that the cancer was in two sites, surgery would not be feasible. Not only that, but even if he had opted for surgery, he was told he would "only have a few months to a year to live."[69] His daughter told him about Tian Xian and he began taking it. Not only was he cured, but six years later, alive and well, he reported in a testimonial that he is still taking the herb and all of his checkups "are normal…even [his] doctors were surprised."[69a]

This supplement is available at some health food stores and on several websites including: *www.tianxian.com*.

Vitamin K for Cancer Prevention

Vitamin K may be important in preventing liver cancer. According to the consumer health news service *HealthDay.com,* in an article by reporter Serena Gordon, a study published "in the July 21 issue of the *Journal of the American Medical Association...*" revealed that participants supplementing with vitamin K experienced much "lower rates of liver cancer."[70] The study was done from 1996 to 1998 and involved "40 women with viral cirrhosis...most of the women enrolled in the study had hepatitis C. The average age of the study participants was around 60..." The participants were given "45 milligrams of vitamin K2 daily." Researchers discovered that the women taking "vitamin K supplements were nearly 90 percent less likely to develop liver cancer."[70a] (Note that leafy greens such as spinach and broccoli are rich in vitamin K.)

Those who have a tendency to develop kidney or gallbladder stones should not consume large amounts of raw spinach due to its high "oxalate" content. Also, if you are taking "calcium supplements," wait "2-3 hours before or after" ingesting fresh spinch, since oxalates can inhibit calcium's assimilation by the body.[70b] (Though raw is better for you, cooking destroys much of the oxalate content.)

Miscellaneous Herbs for Liver Health

Actinidia is a root popular in China for medicinal uses. When test animals were "injected" with this herb, according to Dr. Ralph Moss in his book, *Cancer Therapy*, they experienced a remarkable percentage of tumor suppression and inhibition of their "liver cancers..."[71] (Note that **Kiwi fruit** is a type of actinidia!)

Bitter orange has large amounts of "monoterpenes," which help suppress malignancies of the liver.[72]

Bupleurum has something in common with an herb that **is used to fight liver cancer** – milk thistle! Bupleurum rejuvenates a sluggish liver. It has a reputation as an anti-inflammatory and, according to *herbs2000.com*, it is used in Japan to successfully treat "hepatitis and other chronic liver problems."[72a] It has also been used for bone cancer.[73] Be aware that excessive dosing of this herb can cause epigastric problems and swelling. It should not be taken if you are running a temperature or taking other medications.

If bupleurum causes epigastric problems such as "stomach upset," your herbalist or natural health practitioner may need to lower the amount that you are taking.[74] For more information on this herb, see website *www.herbs2000.com/herbs/herbs_bupleurum.html.*

Chinese peony in "various species" demonstrated the ability (in animal studies) to prevent liver damage caused by chemicals, as noted by Dr. James Duke with Michael Castleman in their book: *The Green Pharmacy Anti-aging Prescriptions.* It is recommended by WHO, "the World Health Organization" for liver health. Medical practitioners in China generally give "between 3 and 20 grams of peony root a day."[74a] Do not take this herb without consulting your physician.

Dandelion has been used for hundreds of years in rural areas for treating "jaundice."[75] According to Marie Nadine Antol's *Healing Teas*, this herb is a powerhouse of "nutrients…vitamins, minerals and trace elements" necessary for liver health. Though it has many medicinal uses, she says that dandelion tea is "free of any toxic side effects."[76] See other chapters of this book for more information on dandelion and vitamin A.

Be aware that dandelion can increase hydrocholoric acid and bile secretion, something to consider if you have ulcers, gallstones, biliary disease or other stomach disorders. Excessive amounts of dandelion could cause dehydration since it is a natural diuretic.

Indian Almond *("Terminalia Catappa")* extract can protect the liver against chemical damage as discovered "in animal studies." This herb can be found growing wild in some states.[77]

Kudzu *("Pueraria Montana")* is another herb containing liver protecting "saponins."[78]

Macela *"(Achyrocline satureoides)"* is a potent herb from the Rainforest of the Amazon. As described at website: *www.rain-tree.com,* laboratory research has shown that a compound taken from these flowers can suppress the proliferation "of cancer cells by 67% in vitro."[79]

Rain-tree.com further explains that in "2002" studies from "Argentina" (laboratory testing) reported that the herb is "toxic to liver cancer" cells. It was also effective against "HIV" and "Pseudorabies (a type of animal herpes virus)."[79a] Animal studies have shown no reports of toxicity with the herb. It is used in Brazil as a tea and has been used in herbal medicine for years, either "the entire plant or just its flowers..." It has a blood sugar lowering effect as well.[80] For more information on this herb, contact Raintree Nutrition at *www.rain-tree.com.*

Picrorrhiza *("Picrorrhiza kurroa")* is an herb from which the extract "picroliv" comes. This extract is currently undergoing testing "in human trials in India," where it is popular for treating hepatitis.[81]

Schisandra has a high lignan content, making it important as a "breast cancer" inhibitor.[82] There are over two dozen substances that are "liver-protective" in schisandra "seeds....The herb is used in China for treating hepatitis, the usual dose being 1 to 7 teaspoons of the berries a day."[83]

An article at www.*NewHope.com* website discussed the use of schisandra berries in treating many ailments, including diabetes and "liver cancer." When human studies were done in China on patients with liver disease, "lignans" in schisandra increased levels of "glutathione" and were "reported to be beneficial in treating viral– and chemical-induced hepatitis and liver cancer."[84] Most health food stores have schisandra supplements, and tea bags.

Scutellaria and Licorice - While scutellaria has been shown to kill "liver cancer cells," *herbs2000.com* says that it can be combined with "licorice [in] tea form to help prevent hepatitis from progressing to liver cancer."[84a] Licorice should not be taken by anyone with "glaucoma, high blood pressure, or disorders affected by estrogen..." If you decide to use this herbal combo, the website recommends that you "use for 6 weeks then take a two-week break."[85] When taking it, eat foods that are high in "potassium…or take potassium supplements daily…[and] avoid scutellaria during diarrhea."[86] (One way to prevent the problems associated with licorice use is to obtain DGL or *de-glycyrrhizinated* licorice, available in health food stores.)

Tamarind juice, and Bottle gourd protect the liver from damage. Dr. James Duke in *The Green Pharmacy Anti-aging Prescriptions*, describes "Bottle gourd…(Lagenaria Siceraria)" as one of the richest sources of "choline, [a] B vitamin" important for liver protection. "Eat it like butternut or acorn squash." He says that you can find liver protective "Tamarind juice…*(Tamarindus Indica)*…in Latin American markets."[87]

Turmeric is a popular spice which contains curcumin, a protective ingredient for liver cells. It has performed impressively in studies inhibiting cancer growths and has already been discussed in several other chapters in this book. Turmeric is safe when used as a spice, however, if you are taking turmeric in supplement form, do not use if pregnant, nor if you have gallstones, since it stimulates the gallbladder. Like garlic, turmeric can slow clotting time, so it should be used with caution by anyone taking anti-coagulant medications,[88] with blood disorders, or for anyone recovering from or contemplating surgery, or those with ulcers.

Keeping the Liver Healthy

It is important to realize that prevention of liver damage in the first place is your priority for liver health! The liver is important for the metabolism of amino acids, carbohydrates, and fats. It is so important in detoxifying harmful chemicals that we can not survive long without it! Chemicals, including prescription drugs and excessive use of over-the-counter medicines such as Acetaminophen, are toxic to liver cells. The liver must work overtime to flush what it considers to be poisons, from the system, as well as harmful food additives that the body does not recognize. Also, be aware that certain vitamins such as vitamin A and D are not water soluble and are stored in the liver. Excess amounts of these vitamins can be harmful. This is why your best source of vitamin D is sunshine, and your best source of vitamin A is NATURAL beta-carotene (not the synthetic form found in pills)! The body turns beta-carotene into vitamin A.

Many patients are on the transplant waiting list because of adverse drug reactions to medications they have taken! Some are there because they thought it was safe to consume RAW seafood, which contained viruses capable of destroying liver cells! Stay away from raw clams, oysters, other raw seafoods and any type of under-cooked meats! Other substances like hormones, pesticides, and herbicides used recklessly in commercial farming are harmful to the liver. Alcohol consumption is very damaging to the liver. The thousands of people who succumb to cirrhosis and other diseases brought about by excess alcohol consumption are a sad testimony to this fact every single day!

Note that you should always check with your physician before beginning any herbal regimen, including relatively "safe" herbs such as milk thistle. If you have already received a transplant, certain herbs (even milk thistle) may interfere with the anti-rejection medications that you must take. If your liver damage was caused by excess iron (a genetic disorder known as *hemochromatosis*) for example, you must be sure that if taking milk thistle, you use a standardized preparation that is **not** high in iron, or it could do you more harm than good! This is another reason you should discuss herbs with your physician before self-medicating.

There are many herbs that, if consumed in large amounts, or taken over long periods of time, can cause liver damage. A few of these are "comfrey, germander...and pennyroyal," and of course, be sure to purchase your mushrooms in your local grocery store or natural health food store (preferably organic). Don't take chances gathering them in the wild if you are not familiar with varieties that can be deadly if ingested.[89] You may want to keep a bottle of milk thistle (silymarin) in your first aid kit for emergencies! (e.g. you go on vacation and your pet decides to eat half-a-dozen deadly mushrooms at the campground site, or a chemical spill near your home exposes you to toxic chemicals that can cause liver damage.) Also, see the information in this chapter about the benefits of alpha lipoic acid for liver health!

Other Non-Toxic Treatments for Liver Cancer

Though these treatments are not exactly what I would consider *pain-less* or *natural*, they do not involve the use of toxic chemotherapy and are being included here for informational purposes for that reason. They are considered an alternative to surgery.

Bland Embolization & Ablation

Bland embolization and ablation are both procedures that researchers believe may prolong the lives of some liver cancer patients. In radiofrequency ablation, heat is used in an attempt to destroy malignant cells, an alternative to surgery which may be much riskier for some debilitated patients!

In Embolization, a procedure is done that cuts off blood supplies to the tumor, thus starving the tumor to death. These procedures are also being used for other forms of cancer. (Shark cartilage also works by preventing the growth of blood vessels that feed tumors, thus starving them!)

LITT – Laser-Induced Thermotherapy

There is a great deal of information on the internet and in medical journals on a laser procedure that is apparently increasing survival time (over surgery) for some patients with primary tumors that have metastasized to other organs, such as the liver or bone. It is called LITT – laser-induced thermotherapy, and is also used for some cancers which, for one reason or another, have been deemed inoperable. The treatment uses a laser to eradicate cancerous growths. Thousands of patients have already been treated successfully with this procedure. Most have a primary cancer that has metastasized to other organs.

Liver Flush

The following is my liver tonic recipe that I use occasionally for its detoxification and antioxidant value. It is also included in chapter 35.

Juice the following organic items in your juicer:

- 2 medium carrots
- 3 medium tomatoes
- Small bunch of parsley
- ¼ sweet green or red pepper (also add the seeds to the juicer)
- 1 medium beet
- 2-3 kale or collard leaves
- 6-12 spinach leaves
- 1 large celery stalk
- 1/2 small red or yellow onion
- Small bunch of cilantro
- ¼ tspn grated ginger (optional)
- ¼ tspn grated lemon peel

To the finished juice add 1 tbspn lemon juice, ½ tspn of turmeric (do not use turmeric if you have "gallstones," biliary disorders, or[90] ulcers), 1 tbspn flax oil, ¼ tspn cayenne pepper (optional, as tolerated), 1 crushed garlic clove, and one serving of a green powder such as Green Miracle, chlorella, barley, or kamut (or 1 oz. fresh wheat grass juice if available). Add 3-4 oz. of water to dilute, only if desired. Mix well with the juice and drink. This drink is very nutritious, and detoxifying. (Be aware that some of the ingredients in this flush have blood-thinning properties.)

Poly–MVA for Liver Cancer

See chapters 9 and 13 for information on an amazing nutritional supplement known as Poly-MVA, a palladium lipoic complex, that contains several vitamins, alpha lipoic acid, and amino acids that many cancer survivors are crediting to bringing them into total remission.

CHAPTER 9

PAINLESS CURES & PREVENTIONS
FOR LUNG CANCER

"The natural treatments for cancer that work best take about two years to reverse the cancer. It takes about 3-6 months for the tumor to regress, to disappear, but the detoxification that needs to happen takes longer, because cancer is the end stage of a body toxicity and just because the tumor is gone doesn't mean that the toxicity is gone."

(Sandra Goodman Ph.D. and Mike Howell, from
"An Interview with Udo Erasmus" *Positive Health* Magazine)[1]

Types of Lung Cancer

Lung cancer and the type of diagnosis given is sometimes "non-small cell" or "small cell lung cancer," depending on "how the cells look under a microscope," and as noted at website *www.cancer-healing.com,* "non-small cell lung cancer can be further divided into various types named for the type of cells in which the cancer develops, typically: squamous cell carcinoma, adenocarcinoma, and large cell carcinoma."[2]

I. Nutrients To Prevent & Halt Lung Cancer

Apples Cut Lung Cancer Risk by 50%

A study showed that eating apples appears to reduce the risk of getting "lung cancer by over 50 percent."[2a] Juicing fresh apple juice and adding cinnamon is doubly nutritious, but remember not to discard the vitamin-rich peelings!

The Lung Tumor That Disappeared!

Heinerman's Encyclopedia of Healing Juices, by John Heinerman, tells of a physician in a "Budapest hospital" who treated a "50-year-old" man with a "lung tumor" with beets [raw]. "After 6 weeks of treatment the tumor had disappeared…after 4 months of treatment he gained 10 kg (22 lbs.) in weight."[3]

Vegetables containing sulfuric compounds, "cabbage, kale, kohlrabi, Brussel sprouts, cauliflower, mustard greens, watercress, radish…garlic, [and] onion," are effective at "preventing as well as treating tumors."[4]

According to Dr. Ralph W. Moss, in his book, *Cancer Therapy: The Independent Consumer's Guide to Non-Toxic Treatment & Prevention*: a substance isolated from "broccoli," known as "*sulphoraphane*," was theorized by a prominent medical college to be possibly "the most powerful anti-cancer compound ever detected."[5] (This cancer fighting compound is not just in broccoli. It is also found in all the foods listed above, and apparently, it is not diminished by "microwaving or steaming.")[6]

Beta-Carotene

Beta-Carotene is effective at lung cancer prevention, however, it has also been discovered that natural beta-carotene (rather than the synthetic supplemental form) is much more effective! When a popular study was conducted on the effects of beta-carotene on smokers, it was reported that taking the vitamin in supplement form "actually increased the risk of lung cancer." However, there is one very **big fact** that was left out of the media reports on this study! They neglected to tell you that the beta-carotene used in the study was SYNTHETIC beta-carotene supplements, NOT natural beta-carotene.[7] The media also failed to report that "the risk was only among those who smoked more than a pack of cigarettes a day and/or drank a daily drink (or more) of alcohol." As further described at *jrussellshealth.com*, those men with "adequate levels of beta-carotene or vitamin E were intentionally excluded from this Finnish study, which meant that only men with very high risk factors for developing lung cancer (poor diets and heavy smoking) were allowed to participate."[8] (The government disbanded the research when the participants taking **SYNTHETIC** forms of beta-carotene had increased risks for cancer development!)

As noted by Dr. Ralph Moss in his book, *Antioxidants against Cancer,* studies point to the need for NATURAL forms of beta-carotene and vitamin A for health, rather than the synthetic forms. Dr. Moss also reports that scientists in China have determined from their studies that "synthetic beta-carotene could actually be harmful to the genes while natural beta-carotene 'could be of practical value in tumor prevention and supplementary treatment.'" When scientists from Israel emphasized that one should be very aware of what type of beta-carotene was being used (natural as opposed to synthetic), **they were ignored.**[9]

Is it possible that the body does not distinguish synthetic beta-carotene and vitamin A as it does when the natural forms are provided by nature, as given to us by our Creator, God?

As a matter of fact, according to Dr. Moss, there is a huge difference in the natural and the synthetic form of this vitamin, as reported in a scientific article revealing that "cancerous changes in stomach cancer cells," could be "reversed" by "natural beta-carotene," but not by the "synthetic" form of the vitamin![10] Is it any wonder that something man-made is so far inferior to what God intended for us in nature?

Another study known as the "Physicians' Health Study...[of] over 22,000 male physicians...found no adverse health effects" in taking beta-carotene. The study was described at *http://ods.od.nih.gov*, and it was further noted that "'only those men who consumed more than 11 g per day of alcohol (approximately one drink per day) showed an adverse response to B-carotene supplementation' in the lung cancer trial.'"[11] (This study used synthetic beta-carotene supplements!)

The physician conducting the study determined that eating foods rich in beta-carotene could help "prevent from 15,000 to 20,000 lung cancer deaths a year," and it wouldn't take much – just "the amount [of beta-carotene] found in ONE carrot!"[12] (Have you had YOUR carrot today?)

Once people quit smoking, they are at risk for "laryngeal cancer" until the larynx heals. It has been found that adequate amounts of beta-carotene are vital in the healing process to prevent this type of cancer.[13] Even in those who are non-smokers, consuming "carrots" is probably their best cancer insurance, as revealed by a study from Sweden.[14]

Beta-carotene can be taken in large doses, as long as it is the NATURAL form [e.g. from foods like carrot juice and yams], because the body excretes excess amounts once the "body stores are full." This "limits further increases in storage levels," and even though consuming high levels of "carotenoids" may color the skin a slight yellowish-orange, this is temporary and not harmful.[15] Though carrots, cantaloupe and yams are high in beta-carotene, one of the highest sources of this nutrient is the blue-green algae, spirulina. Just be aware that if you have any type of chronic disease, liver disorder or biliary problems, you should be checking with your physician before consuming large amounts of herbs, minerals or vitamins, including vitamin A and beta-carotene.

Spriulina is anti-viral to the extent that it has shown the ability to "completely stop the viral replication," of the "HIV-1" virus.[15a] This according to C.M. Hawken in *Green Foods – "Phyto-Foods" for Super Health.*

Cherries Inhibit Lung Cancer

As described in other cancer specific chapters of this book, a "monoterpene that is found in cherries, called *perillyl alcohol,*" in animal tests, was shown to prevent "cancers of the breast, lung, stomach, liver, and skin..."[16] As explained by Selene Yeager in the *Doctors Book of FOOD REMEDIES:*

> Charles Elson, Ph.D., professor of nutritional sciences at the University of Wisconsin Madison, [states] "We're not just showing that this compound fights cancer, meaning that it neutralizes cancer-causing toxins. We're also showing that it is effective in animals with existing tumors."[16a]

More evidence for the health-promoting benefits of fresh fruit! Cherries and their juices are also popular natural remedies for treating gout! Tart cherries are especially effective. You can find some very potent cherry and blueberry supplements at website: *http://www.flavonoidsciences.com/research/c3.htm.*

CoQ10 – The Super Antioxidant

CoQ10 (also known as *"ubiquinone"*) is one of the greatest antioxidants of the new millennium, and the human body can not function without it. It is a naturally occurring ingredient in all cells, much like a vitamin, though it is not classified as one. Some amounts are produced by our body, but levels decrease as we age.[16b] Low blood levels of this nutrient have been linked to many diseases and disorders. A complete lack of CoQ10 in your body results in death. The amount of food that has CoQ10 that would have to be eaten in order to give you adequate daily amounts would be impossible for most people to consume.[17]

CoQ10 has proven so critical that there are actually cases of patients who have been able to get off the **heart transplant waiting list** after taking CoQ10 supplements, and there are no toxic side effects with this nutrient! However, it takes considerably large doses. See Dr. Andrew Saul's website at *http://www.doctoryourself.com/congestive.html.*[17a]

In humans, research has demonstrated that "high dose CoQ10 supplementation (i.e. 390 mg per day) has been associated with complete remission, even for patients with metastatic breast cancer."[17b] This per Dr. Stephen T. Sinatra, cardiologist, in his book *The Coenzyme Q10 Phenomenon.* As a matter-of-fact, explains Dr. Sinatra, one of the primary scientists involved in research on this nutrient, "Dr. Karl Folkers," believed that "the exceptional fatality of pancreatic cancer" is due to "extremely high deficiencies of CoQ10."[18] Dr. Sinatra calls CoQ10 a "Miracle in our midst." He tells of one case study in particular when a man asked him to take over the care of his "79-year-old mother," who was suffering with heart failure and pneumonia. The patient had been ventilator-dependent for 3.5 weeks and was not expected to live, yet when her son, a "Ph.D...biochemist" and expert on "CoQ10," asked her physicians to put her on the supplement, they refused because it was not on the hospital "formulary" and it was unconventional![18a] The patient, already semi-comatose, was transferred to another hospital and Dr Sinatra took over her care. He immediately began giving her CoQ10 ("450 mg…through her feeding tube daily"). She was also given "one gram of magnesium intravenously" daily and "a multi-mineral/vitamin preparation" that Dr. Sinatra had developed.[19]

Dr. Sinatra noted that the CCU doctors and nurses were all skeptical of his alternative therapy, however on "the 3rd day" after starting the CoQ10, the patient began to rouse from her comatose state. Ten days later, "she was weaned from the ventilator…. Four days" after coming off the vent, she was "sitting up in a wheelchair and using only supplemental oxygen" and went to an "extended care facility." Since that time, Dr Sinatra said that he has seen the patient in his office several times. He said that she stays on "360 mg" of CoQ10 every day, along with some "conventional medical therapy," and when he "last spoke with her family, she was reorganizing a vast library of about 3000 books."[20]

Dr. Sinatra has used CoQ10 to treat many of his cardiac patients, only to discover that it has also helped those with "cancer, arthritis, impaired immunity, peridontal disease, diabetes and neurodegenerative diseases."[21] He believes that the indifference of modern medicine toward this nutrient is costing lives, and can not understand the reluctance of the medical profession to use it. As he explains in his book, *Coenzyme Q10 and the Heart:*

> The rejection of Coenzyme Q10 as a potent nonpharmacological treatment defies the imagination. It is apparently difficult for highly trained medical personnel…to believe that anything so simple and so natural can be as effective as the highly engineered drugs modern medicine has to offer.[22]

Research has shown that Parkinson's disease, peridontal disease, and accelerated aging may all be linked to deficiencies in CoQ10, and that this supplement may be valuable in preventing "memory loss, stroke, or cancer," due to its tremendous ability at fighting free radicals.[23]

Are you struggling with cancer, such as pancreatic cancer or breast cancer, an auto-immune disorder, heart disease, or a lung disorder? Does your physician have you on CoQ10? <u>If not, ask them, **WHY**</u>? If you have a chronic disorder or disease, small doses of CoQ10 will not be effective, however, you should begin with a small dose, such as 30 mg, then gradually increase the dosage until you are taking 300-400 mg daily in DIVIDED dosages, not all at once. Check with your physician as he or she can instruct you on gradually progressing your dosage of this nutrient. There is so much overwhelming evidence in favor of using CoQ10, that it is difficult to understand why any physician would be reluctant in recommending this very valuable, safe, non-toxic supplement to their patients!

Ellagic Acid

Nuts and berries contain a "phenol" known as "ellagic acid," an important cancer fighter. When two researchers in Ohio fed test animals a diet rich in this nutrient, then injected them with cancer 14 days later, the group of animals receiving the ellagic acid had a "60 percent" reduction in cancerous tumors.[24] One of the richest sources of ellagic acid is raspberries. Other sources are strawberries, nuts, pomegranates, and grapes.

Grape Seed Extract – Pycnogenol®

"Pycnogenol®" is a product extracted from "pine tree" bark, rich in bioflavonoids. These "bioflavonoids" are also found in the seeds of grapes and are popular supplements. As explained by Dr. Moss in *Antioxidants against Cancer,* they are super antioxidants, important in preventing disease and boosting the immune system.[24a] They are "20 times as potent an antioxidant as vitamin C and 50 times more potent than vitamin E," says Dr. Moss, and, according to one researcher, the only thing better at zapping free radicals is "green tea extract."[25] (If you are fighting cancer, **grape seed extract and CoQ10** should be in your nutritional arsenal for healing your immune system!)

Limonene Prevents Lung Cancer

Lemon (citrus limon) has a potent antioxidant protection in it's peeling, fruit and juice in the form of *limonene,* a proven cancer preventative. Dr. James Duke and Michael Castleman in *The Green Pharmacy Anti-Aging Prescriptions*, explain that test animals "injected" with "lung cancer...were also given a single 25-milligram dose of limonene." The group receiving limonene "developed 78 percent fewer tumors."[26]

The "best source of limonene" isn't actually lemons, says Dr. Duke. It's "caraway seed." Limonene can also be found in "cardamon, celery, fennel, lime, orange, spearmint, tangerine, and thyme."[27] (Rye bread is great for lowering blood pressure and if you bake your own, be sure to add plenty of caraway seeds!)

Lentinan: A Mushroom Extract for Lung Cancer

Lentinan comes "...from the...**shiitake mushroom** *(lentinus edodes)."* It boosts the immune system, with few adverse "effects." Dr. Moss in *Cancer Therapy*, reports that in animal testing, it reduced malignancies and increased their lives by nearly 50%. In one particular study, if test animals having "lung cancer" received "early treatment" with lentinan, they experienced a cure rate of "25 to 75 percent..." He explains further:

> Scientists reported in *Cancer Research* that even if lentinan therapy was begun after tumors were allowed to grow large, the results were dramatic: "complete tumor regression and cure" of 29 to 63 percent of the mice in three separate experiments...[28]

You can find shiitake mushroom in tea form by *Alvita®.* (There are some alternative health care providers who give lentinan injections.)

Lycopene

Lycopene is a potent antioxidant found in fruits and vegetables such as tomatoes, and guavas. It is "four times stronger than alpha-carotene, and ten times stronger than beta-carotene at inhibiting tumor growth."[29]

Lycopene should always be taken with a fat source for absorption.[30] A good example would be tomatoes and olive oil, tomatoes with flax oil, tomato sauce mixed with olive oil, or fresh avocados mixed with tomatoes or salsa.

Niacin, Vitamin C, & Lung Cancer

Dr. Abram Hoffer, Ph.D., M.D., FRCP(C), has been a pioneer in Orthomolecular Medicine (using megadose vitamins and minerals to heal the body). When a patient with lung cancer and psychiatric problems was referred to him, he prescribed high dose vitamin therapy, which included 1000 mg of niacin and 1000 mg of vitamin C after meals. The patient fully recovered, not only physically, but mentally.[30a]

According to Dr. Hoffer, "Very rarely niacin will cause obstructive jaundice, which clears when the niacin is stopped."[30b]

Resveratrol

Resveratrol, an ingredient in **grapes** has proven so potent against cancer cells, that an entire chapter in this book has been devoted to it. Please see chapter two for more information on resveratrol.

II. Minerals, Vitamins, & Nutrients For Lung Cancer Prevention

Alpha Lipoic Acid

Alpha lipoic acid is an important amino acid considered by some to be "the universal antioxidant" with a great deal of documentation supporting its ability to prevent malignancies. It can also bond with and "neutralize" poisonous metals in the body.[31] ALA can be purchased in supplement form. As we grow older, our bodies produce less and less of this vital nutrient, making it next to impossible to get the amount we need from diet alone. (e.g. if you want the amount of ALA, in "a hundred milligram capsule," Dr. Burt Berskon in *The Alpha Lipoic Acid Breakthrough,* says you should be prepared to "eat about 100 pounds of spinach.")[32] Other food sources of this nutrient (besides spinach) are potatoes and brewer's yeast.

If you are looking for a place to find herbs, vitamins and supplements that are reasonably priced, check internet site *www.discount-vitamins-herbs.net.* Not only do they provide a tremendous variety of supplements, but they also have a wealth of information from scientific studies that have been done on several different nutrients. They market timed-released supplements such as alpha lipoic acid which are not always easy to find.

Vitamin C

Vitamin C appears to have a "protective" or shielding effect on cells, and apparently it does not take much to do the job. Research revealed that participants ingesting less than 200 milligrams per day (or the equivalent of eating "about two oranges"), were 50% "less likely to develop lung cancer as those getting less than 90 milligrams a day."[33]

Dr. Gladys Block, who is affiliated "with the Division of Cancer Prevention and Control at the National Cancer Institute" (NCI), confirmed that Vitamin C plays an important role in the prevention of cancer.[34]

See Chapter seven in this book for the story of a Ph.D. biochemist who cured his teenage daughter's Hodgkins disease using high dose vitamin C (also known as Orthomolecular Medicine.)

Vitamin E & Lung Cancer Growths

There is a definite proven link between vitamin E deficiencies and several different cancers. Research studies have linked high levels of vitamin E to a decrease in the risk for getting either stomach or lung cancer. In one particular animal study, described in *Dr. Earl Mindell's What You Should Know About The Super Antioxidant Miracle*, "two groups of hamsters" were "exposed" to a known cancer causing agent. None of the animals receiving vitamin E developed cancer. Every single one of those not receiving the vitamin, developed cancer.[35]

Be sure in buying vitamin E to purchase the natural form ("**d-alpha**-tocopherol" and other "mixed tocopherols"). Dr. Mindell cautions that you should not purchase the "synthetic" form ("**dl-alpha** tocopheryl," which is more difficult for the body to absorb). Natural vitamin E in a dry form is more easily absorbed by the body. Food sources of this vitamin are: "dark green leafy vegetables such as broccoli and kale...soybeans, eggs, wheat germ...unrefined vegetable oils. Most vitamin E is made from soybeans."[36] (Fresh sprouts also contain vitamin E.)

Glutathione Prevents Lung & Other Cancers

Glutathione is another amino acid important in cancer prevention. It is produced within our own cells "from three amino acids: cysteine...glutamic acid, and glycine."[37]

Dr. Allen H. Pressman, author of *The Glutathione Phenomenon*, states, "[g]lutathione helps in preventing and battling weight gain, hyperactivity, alcohol, sugar and caffeine addictions, allergies, arthritis, cataracts, lung and skin, and prostate and bladder cancers."[38]

It may not be wise to take glutathione in supplement form (orally) because of poor absorption. This is explained by Dr. James Balch in his book, *The Super Antioxidants.* Taking Vitamin C keeps "glutathione" elevated, but does not produce more of it. He says it is best to "take cysteine and let your body do the rest," or you can take a supplement known as NAC ("N-acetylcysteine") which will "temporarily, raise glutathione levels."[38a] Glutathione also helps the body maintain constant supplies of vitamins C and E by "recycling" these vitamins once the body has "oxidized" them.[39] (Cooking destroys much of the glutathione in foods.)

See the chart below for some excellent natural sources of glutathione:

Table 1. Comparison of Glutathione in Fresh vs. Cooked Foods (in milligrams per 3 1/2 oz (100 g) serving)	
Food	**Glutathione Content**
Apples	Uncooked: 21.0 mg Cooked: 0.0 mg
Carrots	Uncooked: 74.6 mg Cooked: 0.0 mg
Grapefruit	Uncooked: 70.6 mg Cooked: 0.0 mg
Spinach	Uncooked: 166 mg Cooked: 27.1 mg
Spinach (4)	Uncooked: 9.65 mg Cooked: N/A mg
Tomatoes	Uncooked: 169 mg Cooked: 0.0 mg
Asparagus (4)	Uncooked: 28.3 mg Cooked: N/A mg
Avacado (4)	Uncooked: 27.7 mg Cooked: N/A mg
Purslane (4)	Uncooked: 14.81 mg Cooked: N/A mg

(1). JONES DP, COATES RJ, FLAGG EW, et al. (1992) Glutathione in Foods listed in the National Cancer Institute's Health Habits and History Food Frequency Questionnaire. Nutr Cancer 17: 57-75

(2). BLOCK G, DRESSER CM, HARTMAN AM, CARROLL MD (1985) Nutrient sources in the American diet: Quantitative data from the NHANES II Survey. I. Vitamins and Minerals. Am J Epidemiol 122: 13-26

(3). BLOCK G, DRESSER CM, HARTMAN AM, CARROLL MD (1985) Nutrient sources in the American diet: Quantitative data from the NHANES II Survey. Macronutrients and Fats. Am J Epidemiol 122: 27-40

(4) SIMOPOULOS AP, NORMAN HA, GILLASPY JE (1995) Purslane in human nutrition and its potential for world agriculture. World Rev Nutr Diet 77: 47-74
(Reprinted with permission of website: *http://www.nutritionadvisor.com/glutathione_foods.php.*)[39a]

As you can see from the chart, the highest source of this nutrient is uncooked spinach and tomatoes![40]

According to Steven Petrosino, Ph.D., at website *www.nutrition advisor.com,* you can also increase your body's glutathione levels with "undenatured whey protein isolate," as well as with "the herb milk thistle...[and] curcumin...alpha lipoic acid...vitamin B6, riboflavin...selenium...asparagus, avocados, squash, okra, cauliflower, broccoli, potatoes, spinach, walnuts, garlic, and raw tomatoes...."[41] You can find undenatured whey protein isolate at their website above in a brand known as *Immunocal,* as well as more information on the scientific studies performed on this supplement. It is the only whey protein isolate listed in the *Physician's Desk Reference* (PDR), but you do not need a prescription to obtain it.

Selenium Prevents Lung Cancer

During 1973, in a scientific study known as "The Willett Study," blood was drawn from over four thousand healthy men, after which they were followed over a period of "5 years." Dr. Ralph Moss in *Antioxidants against Cancer*, says that during the duration of the study, "111 of the men developed cancer."[41a] Blood comparisons were made to the men who were still healthy. It was found that those men who developed cancer had very low amounts of the mineral selenium. As a matter-of-fact, those having the lowest levels of selenium were twice as likely to have cancer as the men with much higher amounts of the mineral. Apparently, says Dr. Moss, their greatest risk was for "cancers of the digestive tract and the prostate."[42]

The "Willett study" generated so much interest that the NCI (National Cancer Institute) sponsored yet another study on selenium that lasted for eight years, whose primary intention was to test the mineral's effects on skin cancer. They wanted to see if selenium was able to "prevent skin cancer." They were in for a surprise however, says Dr. Moss, because the mineral did not influence the incidence of melanoma, but the participants given selenium experienced **50% fewer fatalities from other cancers such as "lung, colon, rectum, and prostate than the placebo group."**[43]

Some good natural food sources of this mineral as given by Dr. H. Winter Griffith in *Vitamins Herbs, Minerals & Supplements*, are: "bran, broccoli, brown rice, cabbage...mushrooms, nutritional yeast, oatmeal, onions...whole-grain products," and "garlic (grown in selenium-rich soil)."[44] (Brazil nuts are also very rich in selenium.)

In taking selenium supplements, it is always good to do so in combination with "vitamin E." Too much selenium can be harmful.[45]

A physician by the name of *"Emanuel Revici"* developed a cancer therapy with "selenium" at its heart. For 40 years, he was very successful in treating cancer at his "New York" clinic, but he was eventually "driven out of practice by the New York Medical Board."[46] See website *www.cancertutor.com* for more information.

Melatonin – Antioxidant

Melatonin is described at *healthyroads.com* as "one of the new 'miracle' hormones." It is "produced by the pineal gland, which begins to shrink at about age twenty," meaning as we get older, our body makes less and less of this vital hormone, "about 1 percent a year" less.[47] Long popularized as "an aid for sleep, jet lag, and insomnia caused by working at night," the website explains that "it has also been claimed that melatonin is a powerful antioxidant that helps with aging and immunity, and reduces the risk of cancer and heart disease."[48]

In a **human study** described by *health-n-energy.com*, it has been demonstrated that melatonin possesses anti-cancer properties:

> An article in Cancer Research, 1998 Vol. 18 Iss. 2B, pp 1329-1332 confirms that melatonin activates the immune system in Cancer patients. In a study of 31 patients, who failed to respond to other therapies, melatonin administered at 10 mg per day showed significant results, with 12 patients (39%) achieving disease stabilization after 3 months. None had adverse reactions. This study concluded [that] melatonin plays a significant role in defending the body against the progression of cancer.[49]

Melatonin crosses the blood/brain barrier, something many other antioxidants are not capable of doing. Website *health-n-energy.com* explains why this is so important:

> Dr. Russel Reite, author of "*Your body's natural Wonder Drug – Melatonin*" describes it as one of the most powerful antioxidants, and advocates its use for this reason, for free radical damage to the brain is known to be the cause of a large number of serious diseases such as Alzheimer's, Parkinson's, Down syndrome and muscular dystrophy. Vitamin E, the universal antioxidant, does not cross the blood/brain barrier to prevent oxidation. **Melatonin does!**[50]

Melatonin has also proved useful in the prevention of "cachexia," a "wasting syndrome" experienced by many sufferers of terminal cancers, however, there are some restrictions to the use of the hormone. It is not recommended that patients with "leukemia, lymphoma and myeloma" take melatonin. There is a possibility that melatonin may accelerate the advancement of these type cancers.[51] In addition to this precaution for Melatonin, website *healthyroads.com* advises that "some studies suggest that melatonin can induce depression and exacerbate allergies," and since "Melatonin counteracts the effects of cortisone…patients taking cortisone should avoid it."[51a] It is also possible that the hormone "may cause constriction of blood vessels, may inhibit fertility, may suppress the male sexual drive, and may produce hypothermia and retinal damage. As with any powerful hormone, melatonin should not be taken by pregnant women."[52] Significant amounts of natural melatonin can be found simply in eating tart cherries![52a]

III. Herbs Effective Against Lung Cancer

Aloe Vera Juice for Smokers

Aloe juice may be important in preventing the progression of cancer in smokers. It halts the conversion of toxic compounds (found "in tobacco smoke") into cancer causing chemicals. If you have diarrhea, stomach cancer, or any type of chronic disease, discuss aloe with your physician before ingesting large amounts.[53]

Aspilia

Aspilia *("Aspilia mossambicenisis"),* also known as "Wild Sunflower," not only kills parasites, but acts much like an antibiotic. *Herbs2000.com* reports that the herb has demonstrated the ability to destroy malignant cells in "solid tumors," for example, those of the "lung and breast."[53a]

Astragalus

Astragalgus has a healing effect on the lungs, and is reported to enhance the body's natural immunity.[54]

When researchers took an alkaloid from a variety of this herb "(oxyphysus)," they found that it halted melanoma in animal testing. According to Dr. Ralph Moss in his book, *Cancer Therapy*, when they fed it to mice, it took only one day before it "inhibited over 80 percent of tumor colonies in their lungs."[55]

Do not take this herb if you are running a temperature or during an infectious process involving the skin.[56]

Cat's Claw

Cat's Claw (also known as *"Uno de Gato"*) is a known immune system stimulant. This herb has been able, in some cases to put "lung cancer" into remission. It should not be used during pregnancy or lactation or if you are taking "insulin for diabetes,[57] nor for those with "autoimmune illness, multiple sclerosis, and tuberculosis."[58]

Cayenne Powder

Cayenne pepper powder may be useful for smokers as it appears to be able to prevent one of the chemicals in tobacco smoke from becoming harmful.[59]

Espinheira Santa

This herb *("Limaosinho maytenus")* is widely used in South America for medicinal purposes. It has been popular in ulcer healing since it appears to balance the body's "production of hydrochloric acid," and lab studies have confirmed that it may work just as well as "the common prescription drug cimetidine (Tagamet)."[59a] This was reported at *herbs2000.com.* Also, researchers believe that compounds extracted "from the trunk bark..." are toxic to some types of lung cancer, ovarian cancer cells, and other cancers as well.[60]

Essiac Tea & Graviola

See Chapter five in this book for the story of a Canadian nurse who healed hundreds (perhaps thousands) of her cancer patients (many of them terminal), using an herbal tea remedy containing four herbs. Also see chapters four and five for information on the ability of an herb from the Amazon Rainforest to successfully bring about cancer cures without toxic side effects!

Green Tea Inhibits Lung Cancer

One of the main ingredients in green tea is "epigallocatechin gallate (EGCG)." In his book *Cancer Therapy*, Dr. Ralph Moss explains that green tea not only prevents skin and gastrointestinal tumors, but laboratory animals receiving EGCG grew far fewer cancers of the lung than those not fed the tea.[61] When mice were specifically "bred" so that they would be prone to get "liver cancer," Dr. Moss said that giv-ing them green tea prevented the development of any "tumors…"[61a] It was also found that if mice were given green tea as their only "source of liquid," they had 60-63% reductions in "stomach and lung cancer," however, "90 percent of the control mice" not receiving the tea all "developed cancer."[62] (Studies show that drinking black tea can also reduce lung cancer risk.)[63]

Parsley Inhibits Lung Tumors

Parsley is an overall cleanser. The seeds have an anti-inflammatory effect. The herb is often dried and used in teas. It contains a com-pound known as "myristicin," which inhibits the development of can-cerous growths in the lung.[64]

Do not use parsley if you are pregnant as it can cause premature labor. It should not be used during an infectious process especially involving the kidneys. (Parsley oil can cause skin irritations and is highly toxic.)[65] Fresh, organically grown parsley (in small amounts) is best! If you buy it in herb form, be aware that if the tea comes from the root, it is much more potent than tea made from the leaf.

Psoralea Seed Inhibits Lung Cancer

Psoralea seed is actually a "climbing bean" that grows throughout China. It is popular in traditional Japanese and Chinese herbal medi-cine for many different ailments. It is used for lung cancer because it contains compounds which prevent "osteosarcoma and lung cancer cells" from proliferating.[66] Since this herb can increase your sensitiv-ity to sunlight, if using it limit sun exposure, or avoid it altogether![67]

Rhodiola Rosea for Carcinoma

Rhodiola Rosea is a native herb from the "arctic regions of Eastern Siberia." The saying in Siberia, according to *planetherbs.com* is that "those who drink rhodiola tea regularly will live more than 100 years."[67a] It is very popular in middle Asia, and was named "rosea" because it smells like roses. It is a powerful "antioxidant" that has shown the ability to increase the "survival rate" of "lung carcinoma" patients as well as in those having other types of cancers.[68] See the website above for more information on rhodiola rosea.

Seaweed

Many sea vegetables (seaweed) are not only nutritious, but healing and curative as well. An extract taken from "seaweed" known as "Viva Natural" has shown promising anti-cancer activity. It proved effective in lab tests with mice "against lung cancer cells...as well as leukemia." It was even more effective than the common chemo drug, "isoprinosine."[69]

Viva-Natural, according to Jean Carper in her book, *The Food Pharmacy*, is merely "a dried version of wakame." In one animal study, it not only helped "prevent lung cancer," but it also **cured** lung cancer! Scientists participating in the study were amazed that this seaweed nutrient was so potent at boosting cellular immunity.[70]

Laminaria is another species of seaweed important in cancer prevention says Ms. Carper. Scientists in Japan discovered several species of the weed effective at preventing and suppressing "colon" and "intestinal cancers" in laboratory animals.[71]

(It is important to note that many seaweeds like kelp, are very high in iodine and should not be eaten more than once per week. Those with thyroid disorders should consult their physician before consuming herbs and seaweeds.)

Tian Xian – Herbal Treatment for Lung Cancer

Tian Xian ("pronounced 'Dianne Sean'") is an herbal supplement from China promoted for its ability to control, inhibit, and destroy cancer cells.[72] There are many testimonials at their website of cancer patients from all over the world who have experienced complete cancer cures using this herb, several of them having lung cancer.[73] It has also been used by survivors of nearly every other type of cancer imaginable. Their web address is www.tianxian.com.

Turmeric (Curcumin)

The *Cancer Tutor*™ webpage describes this herbal spice as a "natural substance so smart it can tell the difference between a cancer cell and a normal cell; so powerful it can stop chemicals in their tracks," and so potent, it has the ability to protect DNA "from lethal amounts of radiation."[74]

Turmeric is available as a spice that you can get at your local grocers or in higher, more concentrated forms at natural health food stores as a supplement.

There is a gene known as the "p53 gene" that has the ability to prevent "defective cells" such as cancer cells from replicating. Turmeric appears to have the ability to activate this gene to "fight small lung-cell cancer."[75] Turmeric is safe when used as a spice, however, if you are taking turmeric in supplement form, do not use if pregnant, nor if you have gallstones, since it stimulates the gallbladder. Like garlic, turmeric can slow clotting time, so it should be used in caution by anyone taking anti-coagulant medications,[75a] with blood disorders, or for anyone recovering from or contemplating surgery.

IV. Other Supplements & Treatments That Fight Lung Cancer

Beta Glucan

Beta glucan is an extract of "baker's yeast" and is available in supplement form at most health food stores. It is also extracted from mushrooms "such as shiitake...and maitake." As explained by C. Borek, Ph.D., in an article from *newhope.com,* research was published in "the *Journal of the National Cancer Institute"* in 1975 as a result "of a human study...on nine cancer patients." These patients had either "skin, breast, or lung cancer." When beta glucan was "injected into their tumors..." they shrank in less than a week! The beta glucan caused the body's "immune cells" to concentrate at the site of the cancer, thus destroying it![76]

Lentinan, discussed earlier, is a beta glucan extracted from "shitake" mushrooms. *Newhope.com* says that it is used in Japan to treat "advanced cancer patients" and when given "by intravenous injection," it has often extended the life of cancer patients by "five or more years."[77]

One website in particular *http://www.cancer-treatments.net/cancer.html,* promotes the use of "oat beta glucan," which they claim is superior to "yeast beta glucan," the form most popular in health food stores. According to them, "Recent research has demonstrated that oat beta glucan will cause a three times greater production of interleukin from the macrophage cell as compared to yeast beta glucan." However, the website tells me that there is now available an even more potent "whole cell beta glucan from baker's yeast."[77a] Contact them at: *http://www.cancer-prevention.net.*

Burzynski's Antineoplastons – Non-Toxic Cancer Cures

Antineoplastons are non-toxic cancer treatments provided by Dr. Stanislaw Burzynski at his clinic in Houston, Texas, which have <u>cured</u> many cancer patients. They are mentioned in several other cancer specific chapters of this book and in great detail in chapter 13 due to their remarkable success with terminal brain cancer patients. They are used for lung cancer patients and nearly every other cancer imaginable. (They are also used with mesothelioma cancers, discussed later in this chapter.) See their main website at *www.cancermed.com,* and read some of the many testimonials of patients who have successfully used antineoplastons to cure their cancers at *http://burzynskipatient-group.org/stories.html.*

Burzynski's Antineoplastons & Mesothelioma Cancers

Mesothelioma is a very rare cancer caused by asbestos exposure. It usually affects the thoracic cavity where the heart and lungs are located, but can affect other areas of the body. Non-toxic antineoplastons discussed above have been used at Burzynski's Clinic in Houston,

Texas for treating this disease. See their website at *www.cancermed.com.*

Calcium D-Glucarate™

D-glucarate™ *("D-glucaric acid calcium salt tetrahydrate")* is a naturally occurring ingredient in "fruits and vegetables" mainly in "apples, grapefruits, broccoli and alfalfa sprouts."[78] It is described in detail by Rita Elkins, M.H. in her book: *D-Glucarate™, Powerful Protector Against Breast and Prostate Cancers.*

D-glucarate™ was isolated and patented in "1986." It decreases levels of harmful estrogen (estradiol) and testosterone in the body, explains Ms. Elkins, and it assists the body in ridding itself of harmful toxins![79]

This nutrient is organ protective and it reduces serum cholesterol levels. It works by binding itself with toxic compounds facilitating their quick exit "from the body," and Ms. Elkins also notes that it is so efficient, researchers discovered when they gave "Kanamycin, a toxic antibiotic" to rats, it protected them from the kidney impairment that this drug usually causes.[80] A report published in *"Anticancer Research"* revealed that test animals given the nutrient had their risk of tumor formation decreased by half, as compared to those not receiving it.[81]

D-glucarate™ is an important supplement for "ex-smokers" because it effectively blocks carcinogens. Also, this compound has been shown in "animal testing" to prevent "breast cancer," even **reversing it** in some cases![82]

There has been no evidence of toxicity in using glucarate, however, you should still discuss taking it with your physician, especially if you have a chronic condition or are taking prescription medications.[83]

Noni Juice & Lung Cancer (Lewis Lung Carcinoma)

According to research studies, noni juice (*"Morinda citriolia"*) can inhibit malignancies of the lung. It is believed that it works by stimulating immune cells, possibly one reason why the juice is also said to fight infections. Noni can kill e-coli, "salmonella...shigella...and staphylococcus aureus" germs.[84] You can find noni juice in most health food stores.

Ukrain – An Effective Non-Toxic Cancer Treatment

Ukrain, as discussed earlier, is a combination of the plant "greater celandine" and a common drug "Thiotepa," which are both toxic when used alone, however, when combined they are only toxic to cancer cells.[85]

A **human trial** was done involving "363 cancer patients with 47 different types of tumor" that were all "treated with Ukrain between September 1997 and January 2003 at the Villa Medica Clinic (Edenkoben, Germany)." The results are described at *www.ukrin.com*. All patients, without exception, had already exhausted every means of "conventional" treatment available and were all worsening. They were either progressing in their cancer or had relapsed.[86] (In other words, **all of them were terminal**; conventional medicine had nothing left to offer them!) "The following rates of full remission were achieved" with Ukrain: "breast cancer 31%, colorectal cancer 16.7%, bronchial adenocarcinoma 7.7%, small-cell bronchial carcinoma 21%, astrocytoma (brain tumor) 66.6%, neuroblastoma 60%, seminoma (testicular cancer) 75%, bladder carcinoma 50%."[87]

The main website for ukrain is at *www.ukrin.com*. It is only available through some alternative medicine practitioners in the U.S, and is a very popular cancer treatment in Europe. Dr. Shantha's clinic in Atlanta, Georgia also provides this treatment, though there are others. See more information on his clinic in chapter ten.

V. Flax Oil & GLA

See chapter 17 for more information on the curative, healing properties of flax oil!

Gamma-linolenic acid (GLA) is found in "borage seed oil or evening primrose oil" and helps promote normal cellular "growth." It can help suppress malignancies of the lung. Do not use GLAs without consulting your physician, especially if you are taking chemo.[88]

VI. Water

The importance of adequate fluid intake cannot be over-emphasized for cancer patients and for prevention of all illnesses. Be sure to consult with your physician about salt and fluid intake if you are on a low salt, fluid restricted diet or any other type of special diet. Do not use water with chlorine and fluoride. If you do not have a filter system at home, you may want to resort to steam-distilled water for drinking and cooking purposes or a reputable purified water from your local health food store. See chapter 22 in this book for more information on the importance of water drinking in cancer prevention and treatment!

A Word About Smoking & Lung Cancer

Smoking is actually the main culprit most responsible for lung cancer. One simple reason is because the smoke that comes out of a cigarette actually creates toxic free radicals that have the capacity to change the DNA in your cells. Once this genetic material in your cells begins to change or mutate, the new defective cells begin multiplying rapidly, especially when "exposed" to additional carcinogens. You may not even be a smoker, but when you inhale secondhand smoke, the same toxic free radicals are entering your cells as those of the person who lit the cigarette! Every time a person "lights up a cigarette, more than two thousand chemicals are released in that smoke." (Toxic chemicals!)[89]

As suggested by Maureen Kennedy Salaman in her book, *Nutrition: The Cancer Answer II,* your best protection against "lung cancer" may be "Beta carotene."[90] Breathing in toxic air pollutants causes the body to use up excessive amounts "of vitamin A," prompting the liver to change beta-carotene into more vitamin A. Ms. Salaman further explains that "vitamin E and selenium" sacrifice themselves to prevent vitamin A from oxidizing on its way to the pulmonary system.[91]

It is always important to remember, especially for smokers, or ex-smokers, that you should be taking beta-carotene in its NATURAL form, rather than synthetic forms of the vitamin. For example, when you drink carrot juice, you are taking in a natural form of beta-carotene. **The body takes the natural beta-carotene that you ingest and converts it into natural vitamin A, which is a great deal healthier than synthetic vitamin A or synthetic beta-carotene!**

Poly–MVA for Lung Cancer & All Other Cancers

See chapter 13 for more information on Poly-MVA, a potent nutrient compound that many cancer patients are crediting with curing their cancers. Also, read the many testimonials of cancer survivors who describe using Poly-MVA to help cure their lung cancer as well as Stage IV adenocarcinoma, "hopeless" brain cancers, ovarian, uterine, endometrial and breast cancers, anaplastic carcinoma, bladder and prostate cancers, ALL leukemia, Hodgkins and non-Hodgkins lymphomas, multiple myelomas, osteosarcoma and pancreatic cancers at website: *http://www.S94567060.onlinehome.us/survivors/testimonials.html*. The main Poly-MVA website is located at *www.polymva.net*. Many of these patients refused chemo and radiation and opted only for alternative therapies, such as Poly-MVA. Some began with chemo and radiation, but their cancers returned much more aggressively. Others successfully used Poly-MVA against cancers CAUSED by the radiation and chemo that they received! Some used Poly-MVA in conjunction with other alternative or conventional treatments.

CHAPTER 10

PAINLESS CURES & PREVENTIONS FOR MOUTH, THROAT, NOSE, & THYROID CANCERS

"Today's flawed system of drug approval needs a major overhaul or Americans will continue to perish while effective therapies exist in other countries."

(Chris Gupta, *www.newmediaexplorer.org)*[1]

I. Mouth, Throat, & Nose Cancers

The Mouth Cancer That Disappeared!

Once again beta-carotene has shown evidence of curing yet another type of cancer – cancer of the mouth. As described by Jack Challem in his book: *All About Carotenoids Beta-Carotene, Lutein & Lycopene:* multiple "human studies conducted at the University of Arizona in Tucson, and other research centers" have shown that this nutrient has the ability to "reverse...oral leukoplakia, a precancerous lesion of the mouth or throat" that can ultimately result in "oral cancer if left untreated." This condition, which has been linked to alcohol and tobacco consumption, has also been reversed with "vitamin A and vitamin E."[2]

Halting mouth cancer does not necessarily even require natural vitamin A. Not according to Dr. Ralph Moss in *Antioxidants against Cancer.* When "Steve Otto" of "Washington, D.C." developed cancer of the mouth, he underwent several months of chemo and "radiation," which did absolutely nothing to stop the progression of his tumor! He jumped at the chance for something new when he was offered a synthetic "vitamin A" known as *"retinoic acid."* He only took "eight pills per day" for a few months, explains Dr. Moss, "before his tumor shrank and then" totally vanished.[3] This was not in vitro or animal testing. **This was a case of vitamin A CURING MOUTH CANCER, yet how much publicity did it receive from the medical com-**

munity? How much media attention was given to it? Most of mainstream America never heard of it!

It is worth noting that even though a synthetic form of vitamin A cured this patient's oral cancer, "natural beta-carotene" has been shown to "reverse cancerous changes in stomach cancer cells..." something the "synthetic" pill was unable to do. Dr. Moss explains further that taking the synthetic beta-carotene caused blood levels of "lycopene" to drop, another reason why natural beta-carotene is best![4] Fresh carrot juice is beta-carotene rich as are most of the green juices and seaweeds.

Increased consumption of fresh "fruits and vegetables," says Dr. Moss, is linked to lower rates of "head-and-neck cancers" and a reduced occurrence of "second primary tumors."[5]

Brazilian Peppertree Inhibits Throat Cancers

Brazilian peppertree is not only "antimicrobial," but Health Sciences Institute at *www.hsibaltimore.com,* says that laboratory testing proved that "it is effective against a specific type of cancer cell that can be found in cancers of the throat, esophagus, and other areas, in addition to exhibiting general anticancer activity."[6]

This herb may cause uterine stimulation and blood pressure drops. It is not for long term use.[7] For more information on the herb, contact *www.rain-tree.com.*

Burzynski's Antineoplastons for Head & Neck Cancers

Antineoplastons are non-toxic cancer treatments provided by Dr. Stanislaw Burzynski at his clinic in Houston, Texas which have cured many cancer patients. They are used for cancers of the head and neck as well as nearly all other cancers, and are discussed later in this chapter in more detail under the section on *thyroid cancer.* They are also discussed in great detail in chapter 13 of this book. Dr. Burzynski's webpage is at *www.cancermed.com.*

Chlorella, Folic Acid, Resveratrol, Limonene, Cherries & Essiac Tea

Other nutrients that fight the ravages of head-and-neck cancers include: wheat grass, algaes such as chlorella and spirulina, essiac tea, limonene, cherries, and grape juice (resveratrol). These nutrients and herbs are discussed in several other chapters of this book.

Ellagic Acid Prevents Esophageal Cancer

Commonly found in nuts, cherries, berries, grapes, tea and apples, ellagic acid inhibits esophageal cancers. Scientists in Ohio tested the nutrient's proficiency in stopping cancer of the throat in animals. Test results showed a "21 to 55 percent" drop in tumor formation in the test animals. "Precancerous growths" were also inhibited.[8]

One of the richest sources of ellagic acid is raspberries. When test animals were given the berries as part of their daily diet, there was a dramatic decrease in malignancies of the throat, in some cases, greater than 50%, and strangely enough, in this particular instance, more wasn't necessarily better, because smaller amounts worked best. When researchers doubled the amount of berries, results were not as remarkable. Berries used in the study were black raspberries.

This nutrient has also shown effectiveness at halting the growth of prostate cancer cells and promise against cervical cancer. (Other sources of ellagic acid are nuts and pomegranates.) See chapters four and six for more information on ellagic acid and these two cancers.

Essiac Tea & Graviola

Refer to Chapter five in this book for information on the herbal tea remedy used by a Canadian nurse to cure hundreds (perhaps even thousands) of her terminally ill cancer patients, and the herb from the Amazon Rainforest (Graviola) with cancer curing properties.

Garlic Inhibits Cancer of the Esophagus

Physicians from "M.D. Anderson" were shocked to discover that mice treated with a compound found in garlic ("diallyl sulfide") were two-thirds less likely to develop "tumors" when given a toxin that caused colon cancer. Dr. James F. Balch in *The Super Antioxidants,* explains that when they tried the same test against esophageal cancer, the results were even more dramatic![9] According to "Dr. Michael Wargovich," the animals receiving garlic were "exposed" to a very powerful cancer causing chemical, yet *"not one got cancer."* He believes that the garlic somehow activated processes in the liver that reduced the toxicity of the "carcinogens."[10] Garlic not only prevents cancer, but it can also help normalize blood pressure, kill bacteria, viruses and "parasites," reduce harmful lipids, fight "yeast infections...lower blood sugar," and boost the immune system, says Dr. Balch.[10a]

The same remarkable potency of garlic against other cancers is discussed in cancer specific chapters of this book.

Green Tea Protects Against Esophageal & Stomach Cancer

Life Extension's webpage at *www.lef.org* discusses the important anti-cancer properties of green tea. When humans ingested "seven cups" of this tea "or more a day," stomach cancer rates decreased dramatically![11] According to *Life Extension*, a study in "China" found that:

> [L]ong-term green tea drinkers had approximately 50% less risk of developing gastric cancer compared to individuals consuming little or no tea...Green tea reduces the damaging effects of nitrites in the acidic environment of the stomach with greater efficiency than vitamin C.[11a]

Researchers at "Harvard Medical School" reported that the main ingredient of green tea "(epigallocatechin gallate EGCG), has chemo-preventive effects on cancers affecting a number of organs in the digestive tract."[12] *Foodnavigator.com* explains that the research team also revealed that EGCG "inhibits the growth and reproduction of cancer cells…associated with Barrett's esophagus" (A type of cancer caused by continuous acid damage from the stomach backing up into the esophagus).[12a]

It is very alarming that "in the UK 7,200 people a year are diagnosed with cancer of the esophagus, up 65 per cent in the last 30 years," however, a study presented by *"Digestive Disease Week"* has blamed this alarming trend on the increased "consumption of fizzy drinks."[12b] (For more information, see *foodnavigator.com.*)

Lycopene Decreases Risk for Mouth & Throat Cancers

Lycopene intake, mentioned at length in earlier chapters, is also associated with decreased risk for cancers of the mouth, throat and pharynx, by more than one third![13] Good natural sources of lycopene are red tomatoes, guavas, watermelon, carrots, and red peppers, as well as many other vegetables and fruits.

Molybdenum Prevents Esophageal Cancers

According to Dr. Moss in his book *Cancer Therapy: The Independent Consumer's Guide to Non-Toxic Treatment and Prevention*, Lack of molybdenum, a common "trace mineral," may be responsible for the occurrence of some cancers.[13a] Part of the problem may be linked to its lack in the soil. When this mineral (along with "vitamin C") is added to the soil as well as the "food supply," cases of esophageal cancer are reduced, and apparently, says Dr. Moss, it does not take much. When added to the water supply at "just two parts per million," both stomach and throat cancer were dramatically reduced.[14]

Mullaca Effective Against Gliomas & Nasopharynx (Nose & Throat) Cancers

Mullaca is a Rainforest herb that is toxic to gliomas. (Gliomas are a type of brain tumor.) Clinical research is ongoing with this fascinating herb, and preliminary laboratory and animal studies have shown that it is "an effective immune stimulant," is deadly to many different "types of cancer and leukemia cells," and is an effective "antimicrobial."[15] In laboratory testing, says Raintree Nutrition (*rain-tree.com*), extracts of mullaca known as *"physalins"* have shown impressive anti-cancer effects toward multiple forms of "human and animal cancer cells including lung, colon, nasopharynx, liver, cervix, melanoma and glioma (brain) cancer cells."[16]

Because Mullaca may intensify or lessen the effects of some prescription medications, be sure to consult with your physician before using it.[17] (Also, see chapter 13 for more information on gliomas and other brain tumors.)

Onions Inhibit Oral Cancer

Harvard animal studies revealed that "putting onion extract on oral cancer cells" greatly reduced some of the cells, and even destroyed others. This according to Jean Carper in her book *The Food Pharmacy*. She says that onions can also lower blood sugar levels.[18]

Photodynamic Therapy for Oral Cancers

See chapter 11 for more information on the use of photodynamic therapy. Though it is discussed there in conjunction with pancreatic cancer, this procedure has also successfully treated other forms of cancer, including mouth and throat cancers.

Riboflavin (B-2), Chinese Herbs, Vitamin A, Selenium, & Zinc Prevent Mouth & Esophageal Cancer

Experiments done in China to see if vitamins could stop the high rate of esophageal cancers common in some parts of the country had remarkable results! In *Cancer Therapy*, Dr. Ralph Moss says that in one area, thousands of people aged "40 to 65 were examined." More than half of them already had signs of cancer of the esophagus with significant abnormal cell growth.[18a] Over two thousand had "mild dysplasia." Patients were given either "riboflavin or a placebo," or a specially prepared herbal mix called "antitumor B," vitamin A (retinamide), or a placebo, depending on how extensive the dysplasia was. When the participants were checked 36 months later, the group receiving the herbal formula had slightly over fifty-percent **fewer cancers** than the placebo group. Those receiving vitamin A and riboflavin had "33.7 and 19 percent" fewer esophageal cancers.[19] (The ingredients in the herbal mix "antitumor B," were not identified.)

The combined nutrients, "zinc, vitamin A...riboflavin, and selenium," can reduce the incidence of "mouth cancer."[20] Researchers from India discovered in 1995 that using a combo of these 4 nutraceuticals decreased the incidence of damaged DNA by "72 to 95 percent" in a group of volunteers receiving it.[21] Out of "300....heavy smokers" tested, Dr. Ralph Moss says that 150 were given the vitamin mineral combo and the other half, a placebo. Of those participants given the "supplements...57 percent" had "complete remissions," however, in those given "the placebo" there were remissions in "only 8 percent..."[22] Research has proven that oral doses of zinc, taken by those with increased susceptibility can decrease the incidence of mouth and throat cancer. In lab studies, scientists were able to reverse abnormal cell growth (potentially cancerous) in animals by merely feeding them zinc.

Spirulina Inhibits Oral Cancers

Spirulina-Dunaliella is a type of blue-green algae, high in beta-carotene and other anti-oxidants. Animal studies have shown that this alga is important in helping to prevent the formation and spread of mouth cancers.[22a]

Simarouba Inhibits Cancer of the Pharynx

Simarouba is another Rainforest herb that has shown inhibitory activity against "human epidermoid carcinoma of the pharynx."[23] Excessive dosages ("three times the traditional remedy") may result in "increased perspiration and urination, nausea, and/or vomiting." According to Raintree Nutrition, there have been no "drug interactions…reported" from the use of this herb.[24] For more information on simarouba, contact them at *www.rain-tree.com.* As with any herbal remedy, be sure to consult with your physician first. Do not give herbal preparations to children without first consulting their licensed health care practitioner.

Transfer Factor™

The initial development of "transfer factor" can be credited to Dr. H. Sherwood Lawrence in 1949. He was researching T.B. and discovered that he could take an "extract of leukocytes" [white blood cells] and transfer the immunity that those white blood cells contained from a donor to a recipient. This factor that contained the "immune response," he referred to as "transfer factor."[25] Website *cancertutor.com* reports that since that time, more than "3000 scientific papers documenting the benefits of transfer factors, [have been written, and] $40,000,000 has been spent on research." This immune enhancer has recently become available to the public in supplement form.[26]

As described at *realsuccess4life.com,* an "Independent Study by [the] Institute of Longevity Medicine" was done in 1999 on transfer factor, comparing it to "196 of the worlds' most popular nutrients."

The testing according to "Jeunesse, Inc." claims that "Transfer Factor™ is 500% more powerful than any other nutrient or substance found in any nutritional or medical literature." They say that it outperformed "Noni...Aloe Vera...Cordyceps Formula, Shiitake Mushroom, Echinacea...[and] IP6." This nutrient works by increasing natural killer (NK) cell activity within the immune system.[27] Transfer factor is available at website *www.realsuccess4life.com.*

4Life Research Company has recently developed a patented high antioxidant liquid blend containing not only Transfer Factor EF-X but juice from the popular Brazilian Rainforest berry, the acai berry, as well as pomegranate, purple grapes, elderberries and blueberries in a drink known as *RioVida.* You can read more about *RioVida* at *www.RioVida.com.* The antioxidant power of the acai berry is claimed to be ten times more potent than grapes and twice as potent as blueberries. For those interested in this product, *RioVida* can be ordered at *http://jbramlett.my4life.com.* Go to "shop" at the bottom of the webpage, then to the *4Life Transfer Factor* column and scroll down to *RioVida.*

Ukrain Effective Against Esophageal Cancer Without Toxic Side Effects

The plant "greater celandine" is very toxic to humans, so is the drug "Thiotepa," however, one physician discovered that when the two were combined, a new drug (they named *Ukrain)* was developed that was only toxic to **cancer cells!**[28]

Ukrain has been effective against cancer in clinical trials involving hundreds of patients, yet it is non-toxic to normal cells in humans. One patient in particular, who was diagnosed with "squamous cell esophageal carcinoma," was deemed "inoperable." He was treated with three rounds of standard chemotherapy as well as radiation. **The chemo and radiation failed and the patient worsened.** He was then started on Ukrain therapy ("46 ampoules"). After receiving Ukrain, all of his symptoms disappeared, x-rays showed "no residual cancer," and four years later he was still in complete remission from his throat cancer.[29]

Another patient, 32-year-old Mr. R.K.J., after "a three-month history of difficulty in swallowing," was diagnosed by "barium swallow...histology and endoscopy" with a "poorly differentiated squamous cell carcinoma about 23 cm in the distal third of the esophagus." After his physicians finished their exam, they informed him that he was inoperable. This was in 1990. He underwent "40 courses" of radiation treatment "with the maximum tolerable dose" beginning in November of 1990. He also underwent "three courses of chemotherapy...cisplatin, methotrexate and bleomycin." **His condition worsened after the conventional treatment and diagnostics showed that the cancer remained unaffected.**[30]

In March of 1991, the patient began Ukrain treatment. He received four ampoules ("5 mg each ampoule) on alternate days for two weeks, and then two ampoules every alternate day to a total of 46 ampoules (230 mg Ukrain)."[31]

After beginning his therapy with Ukrain, the patient was able to speak and eat without difficulty. He began a remarkable improvement. "Surprisingly, all medical tests, barium swallowing and scans were normal. No signs of cancer were seen." An x-ray exam done the following November 1991 (8 months since beginning Ukrain treatment) revealed no abnormalities of the esophagus, no "irregularities" whatsoever. One year later, x-rays were still completely normal, and "check-ups for the last three and a half years have shown no recurrences" of his cancer.[32] More details of remissions such as the ones above, brought about by Ukrain therapy can be found at their website: *www.ukrin.com.*

Ukrain is considered alternative therapy, so you will have to seek an alternative health care physician in the United States for Ukrain therapy, or travel to Canada or Europe, where Ukrain is widely used. You can find Ukrain therapy at Dr. T. R. Shantha's clinic in Atlanta, Georgia, discussed below in this chapter.

Vitamin C Inhibits Esophageal Cancer

The high rate of esophageal cancer in "Linxian County...China," was investigated and finally linked to not only mineral poor soils, but to a cancer-causing substance found "in pickled vegetables called RRME." In animal testing, this chemical was responsible for more than 60 percent of the cancers. When treated with "massive doses of vitamin C and a form of vitamin A," both nutrients inhibited the work of the carcinogen.[33]

II. Thyroid Cancers

There are four types of thyroid cancer, depending on the location and cellular origin, papillary, medullary, follicular, and anaplastic. Thyroid cancer is usually treated by surgically removing the cancer. This may involve a partial or total thyroidectomy, depending on the extent of the cancer. Afterwards, of course, thyroid hormone replacement therapy is prescribed. Other treatments involve the use of radioactive iodine therapy, CAAT or Controlled Amino Acid Therapy (an alternative therapy), as well as the usual chemo and radiation that orthodox medicine advocates.

One of the best ways to protect the thyroid is a highly nutritious diet, including the use of sea salt containing iodine, however you need to use any type of iodine supplement under medical supervision especially if you have a thyroid disorder, or if you are taking thyroid medication.

Note that Dr. T. R. Shantha, M.D., Ph.D., at *Integrated Medical Specialists* in Atlanta, Georgia, has successfully treated thyroid cancer using Ukrain and IPT therapy combined. (IPT, or Insulin Potentiation Therapy is described later in this book in chapter 15, as well as more detailed information on Ukrain therapy.) Also see chapter 13 for more information on Ukrain. You can contact Dr. Shantha's clinic, *Integrated Medical Specialists* at #1-866-353-5315. They are located in Atlanta, Georgia. Their website is located at: *http://weheal-cancer.org/contact.html*. There are many other alternative clinics that use Ukrain, but they may not use it in combination with IPT.

Some of the other alternative therapies mentioned in this book have been successful with thyroid cancers. For example: hydrazine sulfate, developed by Dr. Joseph Gold, details of which can be read in chapter 15 of this book. Dr. Gold's clinic does not take calls from patients, but you can have your health practitioner call them at #315-472-6616. They are located at Syracuse Cancer Research Institute, Inc., Presidential Plaza, 600 East Genesee St., Syracuse N.Y. 13202.

Thyroid Cancers & Burzynski's Antineoplastons

Antineoplastons are non-toxic cancer treatments provided by Dr. Stanislaw Burzynski at his clinic in Houston, Texas, which have cured many cancer patients. They are mentioned in several other cancer specific chapters of this book and in great detail in chapter 13 due to their remarkable success with "terminal" brain cancer patients. They are also used for thyroid cancer patients and nearly every other cancer imaginable. See their main website at *www.cancermed.com,* and read some of the many testimonials of patients who have successfully used antineoplastons to cure their cancers at *http://burzynskipatient-group.org/stories.html.* (Many of those who have been cured with antineoplastons at the above website have left their email addresses or phone numbers where they can be contacted if you wish to discuss with them their experience with the Burzynski Clinic.) Antineoplastons are not entirely *painless,* because they are given intravenously; however, they are sometimes given in capsule form.

Poly–MVA (Palladium Lipoic Complex)

See chapters 9 and 13 for more information on this amazing nutritional supplement that many cancer survivors credit with bringing their cancers into complete remission. The main website for this supplement is *www.polymva.net.*

CHAPTER II

PAINLESS CURES & PREVENTIONS FOR CANCER OF THE PANCREAS

"It is with pancreatic cancer that conventional medicine fails most miserably. The American Cancer Society reports that a mere three percent of patients live more than five years after diagnosis. They also report no progress in treatments or mortality rate since the early 70s claiming that 'very little is known about what causes it or how to prevent it...' Somebody hasn't been reading their medical journals."

(Maureen Kennedy Salaman, from her book,
All Your Health Questions Answered Naturally)[1]

The Pancreatic Cancer That Disappeared!

Case #1

The Complete Encyclopedia of Natural Healing by Gary Null, Ph.D., details the story of a patient with pancreatic cancer, who followed Gerson Therapy for a year and experienced a total cure. He had no chemo, no surgery and no radiation. In the patient's words, "That's 11 years ago, and I have had absolutely no problem since."[2]

Max Gerson was a "1907 graduate of the University of Freiburg Medical School." He moved to New York and practiced medicine there for many years, until his death. Afflicted with "migraines" that nearly disabled him, he ended up finding a cure for them with a restricted sodium, abundant "fresh fruits and vegetables" diet. He believed that cancer could be prevented and controlled by dietary means, much to the fury of the AMA, which was completely against him and what they considered his absurd ideas of preventing and halting cancer with dietary methods.[3] In no uncertain terms, they announced: "'There is no scientific evidence whatsoever to indicate that modification in the dietary intake of food or other nutritional essentials are of any specific value in the control of cancer...'"[4]

Even though we now understand how important nutrition is in cancer prevention, the cancer establishment really hasn't changed much! They have only recently admitted that certain foods may decrease your risk of cancer, but they still believe the answer to treating this dread disease is in toxic chemicals and radiation, rather than helping the body get well with the right nutrients as provided by our Creator God to heal and restore an immune system gone awry.

In his book *Cancer Therapy*, Dr. Ralph Moss said that one of Gerson's patients was none other than "Nobel laureate Albert Schweitzer, M.D.," who said of him: "'I see in him one of the most eminent medical geniuses in the history of medicine.'"[5]

It is interesting that one of the components of Gerson Therapy included over a dozen glasses a day of freshly squeezed fruit and vegetable juices, mainly carrot juice. Ann Wigmore and Eydie Mae Hunsberger also used several glasses of fresh juices daily for optimal health. However, there is an element of New Age Philosophy in Gerson Therapy, something that I do not advocate. I believe that those cancer patients who have done well on Gerson Therapy, have done so primarily because of the **13 glasses a day** of healthy fruit and vegetable juices the diet teaches! This sort of diet puts the body in a balanced state of alkalinity, enabling the immune system to heal.

At one time "*JAMA*...published an article of his," but later "attacked Gerson and called him a quack," says Dr. Gary Null in *The Complete Encyclopedia of Natural Healing*.[6] Gerson worked on ways to help "lupus" and "tuberculosis" patients. At that time, very little had been done in the medical field for either disease, however, Gerson successfully reversed "the disease process" in some of his patients by recommending a natural juicing diet of fresh "grasses and vegetables.... [and he] was something of a superstar in Europe until the 1930s."[7]

Dr Null further reports that about the time Gerson was in the prime of his career, "Senator Claude Pepper of Florida" was charged with "a special senate investigation" of Max Gerson's work. Gerson was invited to bring forth patients and their records substantiating his claims. He produced "50 patients" he had treated, who had once been diagnosed as "terminally ill," yet all were still "alive and well," after "five years." The senator and the entire committee were so overwhelmed with the amazing results of his work, that rather than con-demning him, "they actually commended him…" His work still prospers today, kept alive (in Mexico, of course!) by "his daughter, Charlotte Gerson Strauss."[8] You can contact them for more information at their website: *www.gerson.org.*

Case #2

Dr. Abram Hoffer, a long time advocate of Orthomolecular and Complementary Medicine, says of pancreatic cancer: "This kind of cancer is considered by oncologists to be untreatable by any conventional therapy, with survival time after diagnosis never as long as five years."[9] However, he goes on to describe a patient who, at 58-years-old, came to see him with terminal pancreatic cancer. She was seeking advice about high dose vitamin C regimen (she had been given "3 to 6 months to live"). Dr. Hoffer not only started her on vitamin C megadoses of 40 grams per day, but also prescribed other nutrients, including "vitamin B-3, selenium and zinc sulfate."[10] (Before she came to see him, she had been taking "10 grams" of vitamin C daily on her own.) Dr. Hoffer said that "six months later she called me at home in great excitement. She had just had a CT scan. No tumor was visible." Her physician was so disbelieving that he ordered the test a second time. The results were the same – the tumor was gone! She survived her ordeal, living a normal life for another "22 years after she was told she would die."[11]

Burzynski's Antineoplastons: Non-Toxic Cancer Cures

Antineoplastons are non-toxic cancer treatments provided by Dr. Stanislaw Burzynski at his clinic in Houston, Texas, which have cured many cancer patients. They are mentioned in several other cancer specific chapters of this book and in great detail in chapter 13 due to their remarkable success with terminal brain cancer patients. They are also used for pancreatic cancer patients and nearly every other cancer imaginable. See their main website at *www.cancermed.com,* and read some of the many testimonials of patients who have successfully used antineoplastons to cure their cancers at *http://burzynskipatient-group.org/stories.html.*

Cherries & Limonene Shrink Pancreatic Tumors

Perillyl alcohol, a naturally occurring ingredient of cherries, limes and lemons helps kill cancer cells, but is harmless to normal cells. It has been shown to prevent breast, liver and skin cancers. "D-limonene and perillyl alcohol" are "monoterpenes."[12] As described by *cancer-tutor.com,* "perillyl alcohol was shown to reduce the growth of pancreatic tumors injected into hamsters to less than half that of controls," [and] "16% of pancreatic tumors treated with perillyl alcohol completely regressed..." yet there was no shrinkage in any of the untreated tumors. Perillyl alcohol also prevents "colon...prostate and lung cancer."[13]

In *The Food Pharmacy* by author Jean Carper, she reveals that the Swedes studied groups of people "with and without pancreatic cancer" and discovered that the most important way to prevent the disease was the consumption of "citrus fruits (and carrots)..."[14] Not only that, but these foods all decrease the incidence of gastric cancers. In animal studies, Japanese scientists found that an extract taken from the rind of grapefruit, "when injected under the skin of mice...stopped their tumor growth and caused a partial or complete remission" of cancer.[15]

CoQ10 – Low Levels Linked to Pancreatic Cancer

This nutrient, also called "ubiquinone," has been the subject of many scientific double-blind **human studies**, and is so important in fighting cancer it is mentioned in several other cancer specific chapters in this book. It is found in all of our cells and in some foods, but amounts decrease as we age. Some natural food sources of this nutrient are "salmon, broccoli, spinach... [and] nuts..."[16]

The late Dr. Karl Folkers was a prominent scientist greatly interested in the effects of ubiquinone on cancers. In his studies, he found that cancer patients had drastically low levels of CoQ10! **Patients**

with pancreatic cancers had the lowest levels of CoQ10 than with any other cancers studied! He believed that the "exceptional fatality of pancreatic cancer" is linked to critically low levels of this nutrient. The same low blood levels of CoQ10 were discovered in children with "leukemia."[17]

Essiac Tea

See chapter five of this book for more information on this herbal tea blend using four herbs that a Canadian nurse used to cure hundreds (perhaps even thousands) of her cancer patients.

Figs That Fight Cancer

An anti-cancer chemical isolated from figs known as *"benzaldehyde,"* has shown remarkable ability to shrink tumors by more than one-third in mice injected with the compound. In her book *The Food Pharmacy*, Jean Carper explains that Japanese scientists began giving "oral doses" of this extract "to human cancer patients, with some success." However, when they used **injectables** containing the extract, results were much more remarkable! More than 50% of participants having "advanced cancer improved...seven...went into complete remission, [and] twenty-nine into partial remission," says Ms. Carper. The fig nutrient extended their life spans, and it **was amazingly more "effective on human malignant tumors** than on experimental tumors in mice..."[18] (Emphasis, mine.) Juice from figs also showed the ability to destroy parasites and bacteria.[19]

Geraniol Effective Against Pancreatic Cancer

Geraniol is a plant nutrient that can be found in "citrus fruit" peelings. Website *extoxnet.orst.edu* says that the compound is often used to flavor "ice cream, sweets, baked goods, gelatins, puddings [and] chewing gum."[20] This phytochemical is also capable of inhibiting tumor growth as demonstrated by scientific testing. Extensive testing on humans has not yet been done. Also found in ginger and rosemary.

GLA Increases Survival Rates in Pancreatic Cancer

In her book, All *Your Health Questions Answered Naturally*, Maureen Kennedy Salaman describes a study by a prominent researcher from Canada who gave "30 patients...with inoperable pancreatic cancer...gamma-linolenic acid (GLA)," and he discovered that the supplement tripled their "survival rates."[21] The nutrient also worked "in smaller numbers with terminal breast and colon cancer..." and without toxic "effects."[22] Ms. Salaman explains that though the best natural source of GLA is "borage oil" (which is over ¼ GLA), other good natural sources are "evening primrose oil, black currant oil...and spirulina."[23] GLA is available in natural health food stores.

Graviola & Resveratrol

See chapter two for an amazing ingredient in common table grapes credited to preventing and curing cancers, and chapter five for information on the herb *Graviola*, from the Amazon Rainforest. Both of these chapters describe case histories of people that have credited their total cure from cancer to these natural substances. (Some patients have credited Graviola with curing their pancreatic cancer.)

Lycopene & Beta-carotene Cut Pancreatic Cancer Risk

Already mentioned earlier, lycopene is an important nutrient in preventing pancreatic cancer. More than 28,000 people in the U.S. died from pancreatic cancer during 2000.[24] This deadly disease "has a mortality rate of more than 90 percent," however there is more than enough evidence to substantiate that its cause could be dietary.[25]

One research study revealed that those people who exclude vegetables from their diets are four times as likely to develop this deadly cancer "than those who ate five or more servings of vegetables [per day]." The type of vegetables eaten mattered as well. Most importantly, was the consumption of foods "high in beta-carotene and especially lycopene..."[26]

If you are still not convinced (as some in the scientific community) that food and the dietary choices we make greatly influence our chances of having pancreatic cancer, consider a report in the book, *All Your Health Questions Answered Naturally,* by Maureen Kennedy Salaman on the work done by George Comstock "of the Training Center for Public Health Research in Hagerstown, Maryland..."[27] After studying more than "25,000 volunteers," he discovered a definite link between lycopene deficiency and this type of cancer. Ms. Salaman gives some good natural sources of lycopene as "tomatoes...apricots...[and] watermelon..."[28] Several other fruits and vegetables contain lycopene including red peppers, guavas, carrots, pink grapefruit, and papaya.

Poly–MVA for Pancreatic Cancer

See chapter 13 for more information on this nutrient-rich formula, which may be helpful in reversing pancreatic cancers (as well as brain cancers).

Pancreatic Enzyme Therapy

According to Ms Salaman, pancreatic enzymes have been used to treat not only pancreatic cancer, but "degenerative and autoimmune diseases," as well. The enzyme therapy appears to work by doing away with the gummy "coating that allows cancer cells to stick to the body," halting the spread of the disease.[29] Physicians in Germany have been able to "dissolve" tumors with these enzyme injections, says Ms. Salaman, and apparently, "vitamin A" enhances the process and "is given in conjunction" with the enzymes.[30] She recommends the following vitamin A rich foods eaten "as fresh as possible: dandelion greens, carrots, yams, kale, parsley, turnip greens, collard greens, chard, watercress, red peppers, cantaloupe, persimmons, apricots, broccoli, mangoes, pumpkin and peaches." She also advises that the best way to heal your pancreas, and it "will heal itself if you let it," is to help it out by taking "digestive enzymes so it doesn't have to work so hard..."[31] Ms. Salaman has two excellent enzyme supplements, *Multi-Enzyme*, and *Enzyme Ease®* at her website, *www.mksalaman.com.* Just go to the product section at her website for the *Maximum Living Quality Supplements* for ordering either formula.

(And of course, don't forget that ounce-for-ounce chlorella and spirulina are highest of all in natural beta-carotene!)

Photodynamic Therapy for Pancreatic Cancer

Though I do not look at this treatment as *natural* or *painless* since it is an invasive procedure done in an operating room, it is being included in this section for informational purposes, and because it has been a successful alternative to toxic chemo drugs and radiation for many patients. According to the article, *Light Therapy Tackles Cancer,* from BBC News at *bbcnews.com* (used with their permission), "Beams of light could be the latest weapon for doctors fighting a tough-to-treat cancer which kills nine out of ten patients," and it is called "Photodynamic Therapy."[32] As explained at their website above:

> This therapy reportedly increased the expected lifespan of many of the 16 pancreatic cancer patients who underwent it. There are two stages to the treatment. Firstly, a drug is given which "sensitizes" cells to the effects of light. If these cells are exposed to strong light, they die. Then, a fibre-optic cable is placed near the target tumour, and light is precisely aimed through it. When the beam hits the tumour cells, it kills them, hopefully without damaging too many surrounding cells.[33]

This study was conducted by "University College London and detailed in the journal Gut," and it "involved patients with inoperable advanced cancer, who were not expected to live long. Surgery and radiotherapy are difficult in pancreatic cancer, because the gland is tucked away close to vital organs and blood vessels."[34] The website further details the procedure:

Doctors gave the patients a sensitising (sic) agent called Foscan, then three days later inserted six needles carrying the laser light fibres into their tumours. The tumours shrank in all the patients, and although the average prognosis was six to 10 months of life, almost half were alive a year later, two survived for two years, and one managed 30 months. Side-effects were also far lighter than alternative treatments, with patients eating and drinking within 48 hours and leaving [the] hospital 10 days after treatment. The authors of the study said they were encouraged by the results. The drugs used in the experiment are not without their own risks. Because they are not particularly "selective", being present in normal as well as tumour cells, there is a danger that too much "collateral damage" can occur to tissue surrounding the tumour.[35]

Not only that, but after the procedure, patients are told that they "must avoid skin exposure to bright light for some time after treatment, as this can cause significant damage." Even after the treatment, they were "kept in dimly-lit rooms." They are also told that they must completely avoid sunlight for an extended period of time. Other professionals working with the procedure are trying to develop "photosensitising (sic) chemicals which are far more selective."[36] This procedure appears to be gaining popularity. According to "Professor Stanley Brown, director of the Leeds Centre for Photobiology and Photodynamic Therapy: 'Photodynamic therapy allows a targeted approach – it can be far less traumatic than surgery. I think in the future it will be used far more to treat early cancer and pre-cancerous conditions, as better screening picks them up.'"[37] This treatment has also been successfully used for those with mouth and esophageal cancers.

R.N. Cures Her Own Pancreatic Cancer With Diet

See chapter 23 for the story of an R.N. who cured her pancreatic tumor with dietary changes and **topical** applications of hydrogen peroxide gel.

Saw Palmetto Inhibits Pancreatic Cancer

The herb, saw palmetto, long important for prostate health, was shown in a study from Purdue University to have "moderate activity against certain kidney and pancreatic cancer cells…" As described by Dr. Ray Sahelian in his book, *Saw Palmetto, Nature's Prostate Healer,* physicians conducting the study "isolated two compounds from SP berries, called mono-laurin and mono-myristin," responsible for the above results.[38]

Turmeric Inhibits Pancreatic Cancer

Curcumin, the ingredient in turmeric that gives it that golden glow, has been discussed in other chapters in this book for its cancer fighting properties. Research revealed recently that when scientists tested varying strengths of curcumin on cancerous cells of the pancreas they discovered that the curcumin inhibited the growth of tumors, and it may also offer some protection against Alzheimers. Turmeric is safe when used as a spice, however, if you are taking turmeric in supplement form, do not use if pregnant, nor if you have gallstones, since it stimulates the gallbladder. Like garlic, turmeric can slow clotting time, so it should be used in caution by anyone taking anti-coagulant medications,[38a] with blood disorders, or for anyone recovering from or contemplating surgery. It is not for those with ulcers.

Vitamin C Lowers Risk for Pancreatic Cancer

When researchers in Europe studied over one hundred "cases of pancreatic cancer," and compared "them to 195 patients without the disease," they discovered lower rates of this type cancer among people who consumed vitamin C rich foods and "unsaturated fats" in their diet.[39] This according to Maureen Kennedy Salaman in *All Your Health Questions Answered Naturally.*

There are also impressive success stories of people healing their pancreatic cancer with mega-doses of vitamin C given intravenously.

An email friend of mine was diagnosed with pancreatic cancer just this past December 2004. Ms. J. C. immediately started taking "megadoses of vitamin C (intravenously through an alternative health practitioner). **She is currently cancer free!** She started with "50g three days a week; went to four days a week, then 5 days a week." In her words, she said that she "felt wonderful the whole time and kept working without any side effects except the first few days when" she was "detoxing." She reports that "I continue to feel great and go once a week." (This is also known as Orthomolecular Medicine.) She was tested at the end of April 2005 and now her doctor claims that he must have "made a mistake." (Yeah, right! That's what they all say when someone is cured of cancer without chemo, radiation and surgery! They try to tell you that the original diagnosis must have been in error, or that you never had cancer to begin with!)

How Tian Xian Cured Pancreatic Cancer

Tian Xian is a Chinese herb that has been promoted for its usefulness in controlling, destroying and inhibiting cancer cells. When Maribel C. Lim (Philippines) was put through a battery of testing and diagnosed with pancreatic cancer, she was told that even if she opted for surgery, she would not survive longer than 6-12 months. Her physician insisted she have surgery, but she refused, opting instead on an herbal regimen of Tian Xian. She also changed her diet, eliminating "sugar, salt, fat, oil, [and] white flour." Two years later, she was still alive, still taking the herb and doing very well.[40]

Tian Xian is a Chinese herb that has been credited with many cancer recoveries, including pancreatic cancers! You can read case histories of many cancer survivors, some given only two to 6 months to live, who went into remission using Tian Xian at *www.tianxian.com*. Many are still alive today, years after their ordeal!

Ukrain Retards Growth of Pancreatic Cancer Cells

Ukrain, discussed in several cancer specific chapters of this book, was developed by combining two ingredients that when given individually are very toxic, but once combined, they are **no longer toxic**, except to **cancer cells**![41] (Author's note: Since this compound is generally given by injection, I wouldn't exactly classify it as *natural* or *painless,* but it is being included in this section because it is completely non-toxic, and because of its success against pancreatic cancer!)

Ukrain has very powerful anti-tumor effects. Many patients that have been treated outside the "hospital environment" with Ukrain have gone into complete remission lasting "19 years" beyond treatment.[42]

"[T]he National Cancer Institute (Bethesda, Maryland, USA)" conducted lab studies showing that Ukrain was deadly to "all solid cancer cell lines tested." This included "melanomas, for brain, ovarian, kidney and small cell and non-small cell lung carcinomas, and also for intestinal cancer cell lines for which no other medication has shown a malignotoxic effect..." It was effective against over "100 cancer cell lines," including those of pancreatic cells that "were resistant to the chemotherapy drug Cisplatin, as well as human tumor transplants." Healthy cells were not harmed! The dosage effective at killing cancer cells would have to be multiplied **100 times** before it would ever harm normal cells![43]

The most amazing thing about the study results to me was the lack of further testing and publicity the results were given! How many people are aware of the non-toxic effects of Ukrain at killing cancer cells? Most cancer patients are given three choices for treatment when diagnosed: chemo, radiation or surgery. WHY are they never told about Ukrain? (Or antineoplastons?) Since it is considered alternative therapy, if you desire to use Ukrain, you will have to seek an alternative health physician in the United States, Canada or Europe for Ukrain therapy. It is a sad fact that since it **isn't toxic to healthy cells**, it is not widely promoted in the U.S! See the Ukrain website at *www.ukrin.com* for more information. (See chapter ten for information on a clinic in Atlanta, Georgia that uses this therapy.)

CHAPTER 12

PAINLESS CURES & PREVENTIONS FOR BLADDER & KIDNEY CANCERS

"Nutritional science offers us the greatest hope in our fight against cancer and several other degenerative diseases."
(Ray D. Strand, M.D. from his book, *What Your Doctor Doesn't Know About Nutritional Medicine May Be Killing You.*)[1]

Astragalus Inhibits the Spread of Kidney Cancer

Astragalus is an herb that enhances the body's immunity. It may be important in preventing kidney cancer metastasis,[2] because it activates "gene p53," which prevents "defective cells" from replicating. Do not use astragalus if you are running a temperature or have an infectious process involving the skin.[3]

Berberine for Bladder Cancer

Herbs that contain "berberine...(Goldenseal, Barberry, Goldthread, and Oregon Grape)" have "anti-inflammatory properties," and have shown effectiveness "against bladder cancers."[4]

According to website *healingpeople.com*, since "berberine has been reported to cause uterine contractions and to increase levels of bilirubin," herbs with berberine are not recommended during pregnancy. They should not be used by "young children, nursing women, or those with severe liver or kidney disease."[5] They may also increase blood pressure.

Though goldenseal "appears to be safe when used as directed...[and] side effects of oral goldenseal are uncommon," says the website, there have been reports of gastrointestinal distress and increased nervousness in people who take very high doses."[6] *Herbs2000.com* recommends that you do not take herbs containing berberine "with supplemental vitamin B6 or...supplements containing the amino acid histidine. Do not use goldenseal if you have cardiovascular disease or glaucoma."[7]

Burzynski's Non-Toxic Antineoplastons Have Cured Bladder Cancers

Stanislaw R. Burzynski, M.D., Ph.D., working with peptides and amino acids, developed "peptide fractions" that he believed would treat cancer effectively. These came to be known as "antineoplastons." He manufactured the non-toxic substances in his own lab and eagerly shared his findings with other scientists.[8]

When he gave "19 bladder cancer patients [grades II to IV, without distant metastasis…"] his antineoplastons, the results were amazing. The patients were all treated then studied over the next decade. At the study's completion, the following results were reported: "thirteen" of the participants were in "total "remission…two [in] partial remission…one [had] stable disease [and] three" were advancing in the disease. **Antineoplastons have been found to be safe and nontoxic, even in large doses.**[9] (They are not the same as antineoplastics.)

Dr. Burzynski's story is an interesting one. He has had a great deal of success in treating cancer patients, many of them diagnosed as terminal, but he has spent a good portion of his life fighting constant harassment by the medical establishment in much the same way that Rene Cassie did. Apparently, their success rate against cancer made those who were promoting toxic treatments uncomfortable! Antineoplastons are non-toxic! Some insurance companies are finally covering antineoplastons, but not unless you have gone through their "accepted" treatment first, meaning chemo and radiation! If the chemo and radiation don't kill you, then they MIGHT approve antineoplastons for you! There are a few exceptions, such as terminal brain cancers, which are easier to get approved. If you wish to pursue this treatment in the U.S., the only place it has been approved is at the Burzynski Clinic in Houston, Texas. You can reach them at their website: *www.cancermed.com.*

Cat's Claw Fights Bladder Cancer

Cat's claw herb enhances the body's natural immunity against cancer cells. It should not be used during pregnancy or lactation, for children (unless under medical supervision),[10] or for those with "autoimmune illness, multiple sclerosis, and tuberculosis." Do not combine it with "hormonal drugs, insulin, or vaccines."[10a]

Chlorine Causes Bladder Cancer

Research has shown that drinking chlorinated water increases the risk of bladder cancer. As noted at website *www.wizardofeyez.com/chlorine.html,* in a study from 1992 (reported in the "July issue of the American Journal of Public Health"), researchers at "the Medical College of Wisconsin in Milwaukee" disclosed a very alarming trend:

> [P]eople who regularly drink tap water containing high levels of chlorine by-products have a greater risk of developing bladder and rectal cancers than people who drink unchlorinated water. The study estimates that about 9 percent of all bladder cancer and 18 percent of all rectal cancer cases are associated with long-term consumption of these by-products. This amounts to over 20,000 new cases each year.[11]

You can greatly add to your health risks by drinking water containing chlorine or fluoride. Some excellent filters are available that keep unwanted chemicals out of your drinking water, as well as the option of using spring water or distilled water. See chapter 22 of this book for more information on the importance of adequate water consumption.

EFA's (Essential Fatty Acids) & Bladder Cancer

When a group of "urologists" at Aberdeen Royal Infirmary drew "blood" from "96 bladder cancer patients…" and compared them to the general population, they found that those with bladder cancer were lacking in efficient levels of fatty acids, thus showing that lower amounts of these EFA's may greatly contribute to the incidence of bladder cancer in humans![12] According to Siegfried Gursche in his book, *Good Fats and Oils,* some natural sources of essential fatty acids are "unrefined pumpkinseed oil," unrefined "walnut oil...[and] flax seed oil," to name a few. Never heat "pumpkinseed...walnut [or] flax oil."[13] A few other essential fatty acid sources include fish oils, borage oil, perilla oil, evening primrose oil, and avocados.

Garlic Fights Bladder Cancer

Aged garlic extract was found in U.S. testing on animals to be superior to warding "off bladder cancers than a well known cancer 'vaccine' called BCG"[14] (Bacillus Calmette-Guerin.)

This is documented in Jean Carper's book, *The Food Pharmacy,* as well as the fact that multiple animal tests have proven that not only can "fresh garlic...immunize animals against tumor development," but it can "reverse it, once under way." Japanese researchers were able to cure breast cancers in mice with "fresh garlic," reports Ms. Carper and they were further amazed to find out that garlic out-performed vitamin E's antioxidant ability at reversing "liver damage." She explains that it is so potent that "Chinese physicians recently used it in high doses to cure cryptococcal meningitis, a fungal infection that is frequently fatal."[15] Also, scientists studying the spice recently reported that when taken by mouth, garlic can suppress a highly destructive type of malignant bladder growth.

Grapes (Resveratrol) & Bladder Cancer

Chicago researchers noted in the "journal *Science*" that "resveratrol stops not one but all three major stages of cancer development."[16] Resveratrol is found naturally in grape juice and is also available in supplemental tablet form.[17] See chapter two in this book for more information on resveratrol and how Johanna Brandt cured her own abdominal cancer without chemo, surgery, or radiation by using common table grapes and a raw food diet! Reservatrol supplements are now available in some health food stores.

Graviola & Essiac Tea

See Chapter five for more information on the herb from the Amazon Rainforest *(Graviola)* that fights cancer, as well as the herbal tea *(Essiac)* that a Canadian nurse used to cure hundreds (perhaps thousands) of her cancer patients!

Indoles – Vegetables That Can Save Your Life

Cruciferous vegetables, those containing indoles, such as "broccoli, Brussel sprouts, cabbage, collard greens, radishes, turnips and turnip greens" are important for keeping bladder cancer patients in remission. Recent studies involving nearly 48,000 male participants revealed that "eating broccoli and cabbage on a regular basis (five or more servings per week)" can significantly reduce the incidence of this type of cancer.[18] **(These were HUMAN, not animal studies!)**

Mushrooms That Fight Cancer

Shiitake mushrooms have been the focus of much research. Oriental populations have known about them for thousands of years. They have been used to fight "tumors and viruses...Cancer, hepatitis B, leukemia, lymphosarcoma, Hodgkin's disease and even HIV."[19] They are effective at boosting the immune system. The Japanese use shiitake for treating blood pressure, heart disease, fatigue, and complexion problems. However, a note of caution: if you are taking anti-coagulant medications, check with your physician, because shiitake has a blood-thinning effect. (It may cause "skin rashes" in some people.)[20]

Shiitake is popular in Japan for abdominal cancers. One of its extracts, lentinan, discussed elsewhere in this book, has shown significant anti-cancer properties in test animals. Lentinan is usually given as an injection by alternative health care providers, so it isn't exactly what I would consider *painless,* however it is being included here for its obvious benefits to the immune system. Its ability to fight viruses was demonstrated in one particular case, when an AIDS patient went into complete remission after receiving lentinan injections.

Maitake mushroom may reduce the incidence of bladder cancer return, after surgery.[20a]

pH & Bladder Cancer

See chapter 29 of this book for the story of a cancer patient who was completely cured of Stage III bladder cancer simply by changing his body's high acidity level to an alkaline pH!

Rhodiola Rosea – A Simple Herb for Bladder Cancer

Rhodiola Rosea is an herb with an odor much like that of "roses," says *planetherbs.com*, hence its name. It is very popular in Asia for treating many ailments, including stress-related issues and high cholesterol. It is also used for performance improvement in athletes, hearing improvement, blood sugar regulation, liver protection, and cancer prevention.[20b] The website also says that rhodiola is a very powerful antioxidant. Researchers in Russia discovered that oral ingestion could prevent the formation of tumors, as well as their spread (in animal testing). The herb not only enhanced the immunity of patients with malignancies of the bladder, but it also extended the lives of those with lung and breast cancer.[21]

Saw Palmetto Fights Kidney Cancer

Saw Palmetto, long popular for fighting prostate problems, was shown in a 1997 study to possess "moderate activity against certain kidney and pancreatic cancer cells…"[22] This was reported by Dr. Ray Sahelian in his book *Saw Palmetto Nature's Prostate Healer.*

Shark Cartilage

See other chapters in this book, including chapters six and thirteen for further information on how shark cartilage has been used to fight various cancers and their metastasis.

Skullcap Extract – Baicalein Against Bladder Cancer

According to website *www.nutrition2000.com,* the main "flavonoids in skullcap are baicalein and its glycoside baicalin….scutelliarin is only a minor component." Baicalein's performance in lab studies as an anti-cancer agent involving "human prostate and bladder cancer cell lines," was impressive. It also **killed** prostate cancer cells.[23]

Ukrain Effective Against Bladder Cancer

Ukrain (discussed in other cancer-specific chapters of this book) is a cancer treatment composed of two ingredients, both of which are toxic individually, but once combined, they are toxic only to cancer cells![24]

According to website *www.ukrin.com*, a research study was conducted using Ukrain on 28 patients having **carcinoma of the bladder**. They were split "into three groups for a…controlled clinical trial using either one, two or three cycles of UKRAIN therapy with a two-week interval between cycles. Each cycle consisted of 10 mg/day intravenously, over 10 days." The tumors were checked before this treatment "and two weeks after the end of treatment." Diagnostics used were "cystoscopy and ultrasound." Nine of the patients were given "one cycle" of UKRAIN, ten received "two cycles," and 9 were given "three cycles…. Four from nine patients receiving one cycle of Ukrain" enjoyed "either complete remission or partial remission" of their cancer; five out of the ten that received two cycles had "either complete remission or partial remission," and eight out of the nine that were given "three cycles" had either "complete remission or partial remission." There were no incidences where tumors grew in size, and it was "concluded that...longer treatment" with **ukrain** resulted in the best outcomes![25]

It is noteworthy that with most drugs, the dosage between what is therapeutic and what becomes toxic is a slim margin. This is not the case with Ukrain. Unlike toxic chemotherapy, **human testing has revealed no adverse side effects from Ukrain!**[26] This treatment is only available at alternative therapy clinics in the U.S., Canada, Europe, and Asian countries. Their main website is *www.ukrin.com.* Dr. T. R. Shantha's clinic in Atlanta, Georgia provides Ukrain treatment. They are located at website: *http://wehealcancer.org/contact.html.*

Vitamin C – For Bladder Cancer Prevention

In her book, *Foods That Heal*, Maureen Kennedy Salaman explains that bladder cancer occurs more commonly in smokers than in non-smokers. At the end of the sixties, "Tulane University scientists – Dr. Jorgen U. Schlegel...and George Pipkin," revealed that large doses of vitamin C can actually eliminate the carginogens "that precede bladder cancer in smokers."[27] Ms. Salaman says that for purposes of the study, "1500 mg. of vitamin C" in 3 divided doses were used. The results of the study prompted Schlegel to suggest such a regimen for those susceptible to bladder cancer (e.g. cigarette-smokers).[28] Ms. Salaman also lists some natural food sources of vitamin C: "rose hips...acerola cherries...guavas...black currants...spinach...cabbage...raspberries and romaine lettuce."[29]

When choosing your vitamin C, if you use supplements (rather than natural food sources), it is better to choose natural derivatives from acerola or rose hips rather than the sodium ascorbate form of vitamin C. The ascorbate may aggravate "symptoms."[30]

Vitamin D & Sunlight Inhibit Cancer Spread

There are so many warnings about sunlight causing skin cancer that many people are going overboard and avoiding any sun exposure whatsoever, forgetting that the sun is our most natural, important source of **vitamin D!** When sunlight hits the skin, a chemical process occurs that creates vitamin D in our bodies! We need about 10 - 20 minutes of sunlight (without sunscreen) every single day for vitamin D synthesis, an actual total of about 20 minutes because it also boosts the immune system and lowers blood pressure! This is why it is so easy to fall asleep when you are lying on a beach sunbathing! Sunshine lowers blood pressure, stimulates the immune system, and it relaxes you! (When getting your daily sunshine, avoid exposure during the hottest times of the day, and discuss with your physician, especially if you or a close family member has a prior history of melanoma, of if you are taking medications that increase sun sensitivity.)

Vitamin D may be important in preventing renal cancer from metastasizing to "the bones," as well as inhibiting tumor formation in the kidneys.[31]

Sadly, many parents are becoming so over anxious about bundling up their children against the sun, there is an alarming increase in this country of ricketts, a bone growth disorder caused by a lack of vitamin D in the diet, especially critical for children with their fast-growing bones!

Vitamin E Protects Against Bladder & Prostate Cancer

As described at *foodnavigator.com*, new research has found that vitamin E can inhibit "both prostate cancer and bladder cancer..." A controlled study showed that increasing dietary amounts of "alpha-tocopherol" could slash the "risk of bladder cancer by greater than 50%." Researchers also concluded that "both alpha-and gamma-tocopherol lowered the risk of prostate cancer, by as much as 53 percent and 39 percent respectively"[32]

Dr. H. Winter Griffith in *Vitamins Herbs, Minerals & Supplements,* gives some excellent sources of vitamin E: "Almonds, Asparagus...Brazil nuts, Broccoli...Fortified cereals...Peanuts...Spinach, Sunflower seeds...and Wheat germ."[33] (Fresh sprouts also contain vitamin E, especially wheat berry sprouts!)

Deanna K. Loftis, R.N., B.B.A.

Vitamin Combo Therapy for Bladder Cancers

When researchers gave "bladder cancer" patients…"high daily doses of vitamins A (40,000 IU), B6 (100 mg), C (2000 mg), and E (400 IU)," they experienced "40 percent fewer tumors than a control group" not taking the vitamins, plus their life span doubled! This study was reported in *Earl Mindell's What You Should Know About The SuperAntioxidant miracle.* As a result, it was concluded that "high dose" vitamin therapy may lower the "high recurrence rates" often found in these type cancers.[34]

It is important to note in this study (and the one discussed below), that we are talking about clinical trials **involving humans, not lab mice**!

In another "double-blind clinical trial" to determine the efficacy of using mega-dose vitamins for 65 bladder cancer patients (conducted by Dr. David L. Lamm "and colleagues [at the] West Virginia School of Medicine)" participants were treated "with a standard treatment called BCG."[35] (BCG is a weakened strain of the microbe that is administered in TB vaccinations.) They gave 30 of the patients "RDA" (recommended dietary allowance) amounts of antioxidants, and the other "thirty-five" were given the following "megadoses.…Vitamin C, 2000 milligrams; vitamin A, 40,000 international units; vitamin B6, 100 milligrams, vitamin E, 400 international units [and] zinc, 90 milligrams."[36]

Although the recurrence for bladder cancer is usually very high, less than a year later, the recurrence of bladder cancer "in the megadose group began to fall." Five years later, those who had received high dose vitamins had a 41 percent recurrence rate "compared with 91 percent in those" who had been given the lower dosages. By the completion of the study, eighty percent "of patients in the low-dose group" relapsed, "while" forty percent "in the high-dose group had new tumors."[37] This was startling evidence in a **human trial** that giving bladder cancer patients mega vitamin/mineral doses, slashed their cancer recurrence rate by over half! As explained by Dr. Ralph Moss in his book, *Antioxidants against Cancer*: "This is the kind of study that the medical establishment has demanded as proof of the benefits of megadose antioxidant therapy."[38]

270

(Yet, how many bladder cancer patients do you think are being placed on a megadose antioxidant therapy program like the one described above to keep their cancer from recurring?)

It is important to realize that if you take high doses of synthetic vitamin A and E, you should be monitored by a physician. These are "fat-soluble vitamins" and they can be stored in body tissues and organs and cause toxicity if excessive amounts are taken.[39] One way that you can avoid this problem (e.g. in the case of vitamin A) is to take natural sources of beta-carotene such as carrot juice, which the body then converts into NATURAL vitamin A!

What do you think happened when these very important studies came out? Absolutely nothing. Dr. Moss lamented the fact that, **"After these studies were done, it was business as usual in the world of conventional cancer treatment.** No follow-up studies were done and few cancer patients have ever heard about it."[40]

Why should we be surprised at this finding? There isn't much profit for the cancer industry if you turn to megavitamins and antioxidants to treat cancer and prevent its recurrence instead of turning to them for their immune-destructive radiation and toxic poisons! Many alternative physicians are providing vitamin megadosing for their cancer patients, otherwise known as *Orthomolecular Medicine.*

Water Prevents Bladder Cancer

So important to our survival, research has shown that drinking adequate water can decrease your risk of developing cancer! Studies have shown that men who drink at "least 11 glasses" of water per day can cut their "risk of bladder cancer" by 50%.[41]

Dehydration is common in cancer patients. Years of chronic dehydration have been linked to the cause of asthma, lupus, arthritis, degenerative disc disease, and all autoimmune disorders! Be sure that the water you are drinking does not contain chlorine and fluoride. If you do not have access to a good filtration system, you may want to try a reputable spring water from your local health food store, or more inexpensive steam-distilled water. (See Chapter 22 in this book for more details on the vital importance of water drinking for optimal health and disease recovery.)

Wheatgrass Juice Fights Bladder Cancer

Dorothy Naylor of "Naples, Florida" was diagnosed with multiple bladder tumors. Every time she had chemo or radiation, the tumors would return. She obtained a *Green Power* juicer and began juicing wheatgrass on a daily basis until she was tolerating "6 ounces per day." She finally cured herself completely of bladder tumors drinking wheatgrass juice.[42] See chapters three and sixteen for more information on other amazing cancer cures involving wheatgrass juice.

Poly–MVA for Bladder Cancers

See chapters 9 and 13 for more information on this palladium lipoic complex that contains vitamins, alpha lipoic acid and amino acids that many cancer survivors are crediting to bringing about total remission from their cancers, some even sent home to die, who recovered completely using this alternative treatment nutritional drink. Their main website is *www.polymva.net.*

CHAPTER 13

PAINLESS CURES & PREVENTIONS FOR BRAIN CANCER & NEUROBLASTOMA

"As a retired physician, I can honestly say that unless you are in a serious accident, your best chance of living to a ripe old age is to avoid doctors and hospitals and learn nutrition, herbal medicine and other forms of natural medicine unless you are fortunate enough to have a naturopathic physician available. Almost all drugs are toxic and are designed only to treat symptoms and not to cure anyone. Vaccines are highly dangerous, have never been adequately studied or proven to be effective, and have a poor risk/reward ratio...In short, our main stream medical system is hopelessly inept and/or corrupt. The treatment of cancer and degenerative diseases is a national scandal. The sooner you learn this, the better off you will be."

(Dr. Allan Greenberg 12/24/2002)[1]

Non-Toxic Cures for Inoperable "Terminal" Brain Cancers!

Have you or someone you know been told that they have an inoperable brain tumor or that they are terminal and the type tumor they have can not be cured? Do not let someone convince you of that – because there are many people who have been cured of "terminal" brain cancer without chemo and without radiation! This chapter will tell you about case histories of several of them, but they are not "unique" or "isolated" cases. They are routine "cures" for an alternative cancer therapy that most cancer patients are never told about. This is a blatant *coverup*, and make no mistake about it, it is very intentional. The modern cancer establishment would much rather have you spend your dollars taking useless radiation and chemotherapy than to tell you the truth, because their resources, funding and way of life would DRY UP if the truth were widely known! They are concerned about their wallets!

There is one website in particular where you can read about the individual case histories of more than two dozen people who were told that their brain cancer was incurable, many of them children! People who are in complete remission today, living normal, healthy lives without brain tumors! Some of the patients initially received chemo and/or radiation, but the tumors returned! See website *http://burzynskipatientgroup.org/stories.html.* Many of the people you will read about at this website have included their email addresses, or home addresses where you can feel free to write to them! A few of those cases are described briefly in this chapter.

Antineoplastons are not always painless since they are usually given intravenously, however they are also given in capsules. I have included them here because of their success rate against terminal brain cancers!

The Medulloblastoma that Disappeared!

This type brain cancer is quite rare, but deadly. When a three-year-old little boy, Dustin K. was diagnosed with medulloblastoma, his parents were given little hope. He initially had surgery; however doctors were not able to remove all of the tumor. They wanted to follow up with chemo and radiation, to which the parents objected. Instead, they sought treatment at the Burzynski Clinic in Houston, Texas for non-toxic antineoplastons.

Dustin was treated with antineoplastons and within months, his tumor had disappeared. When it returned a short while later, he was treated again with antineoplastons, and the tumor again disappeared and has not recurred. He is now totally cancer-free at 13-years-of-age and living a normal, healthy life! His uncle is a practicing physician, who had advised his parents not to treat with Burzynski initially. However, in reading the case history of this child, it is his uncle who had a change of heart, and tells part of the story! You can read it for yourself at *http://burzynskipatientgroup.org/dustink.htm.*[1a] What's more, this is NOT an isolated case!

A Malignant Rhabdoid Brain Tumor Cured!

This same webite describes the story of a four-year-old little girl who was diagnosed with a rhabdoid brain tumor, Crystin S. Her parents were advised that the tumor was incurable and all they could hope for was to possibly extend her life a short time by giving both chemo and radiation at the same time. The tumor initially shrank then returned. Her parents took her to Burzynski's Clinic in Houston, Texas for antineoplaston treatment, which ultimately resulted in a complete cure. For several months, the little girl seemed fine; however her parents were later to find out that something dreadful had happened to her. The oncologist, certain that Crystin was going to die anyway, had given her double the radiation dosage that she should have received. After being completely cured of brain cancer on Burzynski's antineoplastons, the little girl died several months later. Upon autopsy, her parents were told that her death was caused by the massive doses of chemo and radiotherapy she had been given, which had resulted in irreversible injury to her brain![1b] Had the child never received chemo and radiation to begin with, she would probably still be alive today!

Stage III Inoperable Anaplastic Astrocytoma Cured Without Chemo or Radiation!

See the amazing story of Jodi. G., who was completely cured of an inoperable, stage III Anaplastic Astrocytoma (brain tumor) using only Burzynski's antineoplastons. Jodi refused chemo and radiation because doctors never talked "cure," to her. All they discussed was possibly extending her life. Her story is posted at website: *http://burzynskipatientgroup.org/jodig.htm.* Four years have passed since Jodi was diagnosed. She remains cancer free![1c]

Inoperable Brain Tumors That Disappeared!

Antineoplaston treatment was devised by Stanislaw Burzynski, M.D., Ph.D., and is still being used at his Houston, Texas clinic, the only

place in the country that the FDA allows his treatment. (See his website below.)

Dr. Burzynski believed that second to the body's "immune system," there is a "biochemical defense system" that is programmed to
protect us "against defective cells." He developed a group of peptides
he called *antineoplastons,* that were found to be effective against a
variety of cancer cells in lab studies, yet they **were non-toxic to normal cells**.[2] It is believed that antineoplastons work by "reprogram-
ming defective cells," such as cancer cells, so that they revert back to
normal cells. The compounds do occur naturally in humans, but for
some unknown reason, at very **low levels in cancer patients**. Dr.
Burzynski's antineoplastons have been used successfully against
"breast cancer, lymphoma, leukemia, and bone cancer," and have
been especially effective against malignant brain cancer cells.[2a]

In 1988, he "treated twenty patients" diagnosed with "a fast-
growing type of brain tumor" known as "*astrocytoma.*" They were all
in an advanced stage of the disease. (This is a malignant type of brain
tumor with a dismal chance of survival! Very few patients live longer
than two years once they are diagnosed.) All the patients (several of
them children) received the antineoplastons administered (outpatient
intravenously) over a seven hour period during the night "while sleeping." As a result of the treatment, most of the patients "improved rapidly." Within "six weeks," all the children and most of the adults were
able to return to school or "part-time work….Nearly 80 percent of the
patients responded well." A checkup **four years later on all of them**
revealed that many were still in total remission carrying out their
"normal activities."[3] (This is remarkable when you consider that
every one of them had advanced, inoperable brain cancer, yet FOUR
YEARS LATER, they are all still very much alive!)

Dr. Burzynski "showed MRI slides [to] the 1990 World Research
Foundation Congress" of a "thirty-six-year-old" woman who had a
very "fast-growing astrocytoma." Within 60 days of antineoplaston
treatment, there was obvious "shrinkage" of the tumor, and "after six
months of treatment the tumor was entirely gone." Not only that, but
"Dr. Burzynski emphasized" the fact that the space where the tumor
had once been was **completely healed over with normal brain tissue** – there were no gaping holes or shadows showing scar tissue!

"Today, five years later, [in 1995, he explained in his report] the patient remains symptom free and is enjoying a normal life."[4]

Glioblastoma is another very deadly and "aggressive type of malignant brain tumor." Most people "don't live longer than nine months" from the time they are diagnosed. When "Dr. Burzynski found that his seven-hour nighttime IV drip" was not working with glioblastoma cancer, he created "a small pump" device that would attach "to the patient's clothing or belt." Thus, the antineoplastons could be given in continuous infusion over a 24-hour period.[4a] One of his first patients to try the pump was a "ten-year-old boy" with "a brain stem glioblastoma…" an inoperable location. He underwent radiation first and the tumor shrunk initially, but then began **growing again a short time later**.[5] (Another radiation failure!)

Dr. Burzynski started the child on the pump he developed. **The brain tumor disappeared completely within 4 weeks, replaced by "normal, brain tissue."** He revealed diagnostic pictures of this case in 1990 from the child's MRI results. A follow-up three years later showed the child still cancer-free. The new pump delivery system has had "favorable results in approximately 60 percent of the patients who have been treated with it."[6] (This is particularly remarkable when you realize that most of the patients receiving this treatment are **terminal cases of inoperable brain cancer!**)

It is noteworthy that Dr. Burzynski has had great success at curing some of the most aggressive, deadly cancers, especially terminal patients having malignant brain cancers. (I wonder how many patients in the U.S. diagnosed with "hopeless" inoperable brain tumors are ever told about antineoplastons by the physicians treating them? Do YOU know someone recently diagnosed with an inoperable brain tumor? Has their physician mentioned this alternative treatment?) Some insurance companies are **finally** beginning to cover antineoplastons. Be prepared, however, to butt heads with the FDA if YOU try to pursue antineoplastons. Only those with lymphomas or malignant brain tumors can use them. Any other type of cancer and the FDA will tell you that you must first use chemotherapy or radiation before trying antineoplastons, even though they are toxic treatments and **antineoplastons are NOT toxic!** (Isn't it amazing how a government agency like the FDA tries to play "God" with your life?!)

The FDA has vigorously attacked Burzynski from day one of his discovery. They charged that one of his patients died of "septicemia" (from an intravenous infusion), yet the report was very "vague" without giving any specifics, and not at any time, did Dr. Burzynski ever receive documentation of a patient of his "dying from septicemia." All studies ever done on these compounds have shown them to be safe. They are "natural products," accepted "by the body even in high doses, without any of the serious side effects" found in chemotherapy agents.[7] The trumped up attack by the FDA was just one more attempt to try to find something negative in a desperate attempt to discredit this very successful alternative cancer therapy! Their tactics over the years haven't changed in the least!

Dr. Burzynski's story has been mainly a "fight to survive" since he has had to spend a great deal of his time and finances fighting legal and political battles "brought against him by the FDA, the American Cancer Society, National Cancer Institute, large insurance companies, [and] the medical board and health department of Texas..." However, during this same period of time, he has gained global fame for his work. Clinical trials are still being conducted around the world with his discovery.[8] If you are interested in more information on antineoplastons, Burzynski's Clinic website is at *www.cancermed.com*. Additional information can also be found at *www.curezone.com*.

At Burzynski Patient Group website *http://burzynskipatient-group.org/stories.html,* you can also read the case histories of more than 38 cases of brain tumors, glioblastomas, astrocytoma, astrocytoma III, anaplastic astrocytoma, brain stem gliomas, ependymoma, pineoblastoma, and neuroblastoma brought into remission with antineoplastons. There are also case histories of remarkable remissions in many other cancers at this website, including multiple myeloma, lymphocytic lymphoma, non-Hodgkins lymphoma, prostate cancer, breast cancer, ovarian cancer, and esophageal cancer. There is even a case history of a patient who has had good results using antineoplastons with a rare type of cancer known as *Waldenstrom's* macroglobulinemia, and a patient whose lupus was brought into remission as well. Dr. Burzynski also treats other autoimmune disorders.

What I find most disturbing about so many of these cases, including those involving young children, is that when they were given a poor prognosis and asked their oncologist if there was anything available that could offer hope apart from devastating chemo and radiation, they were told NO! In one case in particular, a doctor KNEW the history of a patient who had been cured of an aggressive brain tumor at the Burzynski Clinic, and still never revealed this information to his brain cancer patient, pushing them instead to go through with chemo and radiation! In many cases, cancer patients were also told that the only thing chemo or radiation could do was *possibly* gain them a few more months of life at the most, yet they were not told about antineoplastons!

The Burzynski Clinic also treats many other cancers and disorders including: CLL and CML (leukemias), fibrous histiocytoma, mesothelioma, neuroendocrine tumors, Wilm's tumor, mantle zone lymphoma, Hodgkins & non-Hodgkins lymphoma, mycosis-fungoides-sezary syndrome, choroid plexus neoplasm, craniopharyngioma, mixed olioma, high-grade gliomas, visual pathway gliomas, and many others, too numerous to mention here. The main webpage for the Burzynski Clinic is *www.cancermed.com.*

See the section in this chapter under *Mullaca Inhibits Brain Cancer (Gliomas),* for more information on several types of brain tumors, including some very rare brain tumors.

Artemisinin

Artemisinin, also called *"wormwood"* has been popular in killing parasites, however in a "series of successful experiments," it was also "effective against a wide variety of cancers," most remarkably, "leukemia and colon cancer."[8a] Artemisinin is capable of crossing "the blood brain barrier…and may be particularly suitable for curing brain tumors, together with Poly-MVA."[8b] Excessive doses of artemisinin can be harmful. According to website *Wellness Directory of Minnesota*™, "long-term toxicity is not known at this time."[9] Do not take this herb without consulting your physician, especially if you are already taking radiation therapy. (Poly-MVA is discussed later in this chapter.)

Deanna K. Loftis, R.N., B.B.A.

How Cartilage Supplements & Dietary Changes Cured a Child's Neuroblastoma

Neuroblastoma is a very common type of virulent cancer that affects primarily children "from birth through age 14 years." As described in detail at website *www.chem-tox.com/neuroblastoma/default.htm*, the tumor is "solid...seen most often in the newborn period and the median age at diagnosis is 2 years."[9a] These type tumors are usually found "in the abdominal area either in the adrenal gland...or around the spinal cord in the neck, chest, or pelvis," and prognosis or outcome is not good. If the tumor is "localized," [meaning it has not yet spread] it "can be cured by surgery alone but those with bone metastases usually have a fatal outcome..."[10] A link between this disease and "exposure to the termite pesticide chlordane" has been found. Supposedly, it was no longer used after 1988, but it was so widely used before that, "it is still being found in the air of approximately 75% of homes built before 1988 and at dangerously high levels in approximately 7% of pre-1988 homes."[11] You may want to check out that next home you buy for chlordane levels (if it was built before 1988), especially if you have small children toddling around.

When eleven-year-old Kyle S. awoke one morning with unbearable "hip and groin" pain, he had no idea what was happening to him. "Within 24 hours Kyle couldn't walk," and a short time later, he was diagnosed with stage IV neuroblastoma. Trusting in the modern medical establishment, Kyle's parents promptly took him to "the prestigeous [sic] St. Judes' Hospital for whole body radiation and Autologous Bone Marrow Transplant (ABMT)."[11a] As noted by a writer at website *www.karlloren.com,* his father describes what happened next as a horror story of "Going to Hell and back again." Though his young son went through a year "of chemotherapy using different drugs and transfusions for neutropenia, and...weeks of solitary isolation, **there was no change in Kyle's tumor**." (Emphasis, mine.) His parents were told that the tumor was "chemo-resistant," nothing further could be done for the child. They were then advised to take him home and to "enjoy him while you can."[12]

Kyle's parents were not about to give up. During the next few months, Kyle was given "oxygen therapy, chelation therapy," and improvements in "his diet and nutrition with nutritional supplements." His parents also got in touch with "John Prudden MD, a Harvard graduate and former professor of medicine at Columbia College of Physicians and Surgeons. Prudden prescribed **Bovine Cartilage (VitaCart®) at 9 grams per day** as a non-toxic means of killing tumor cells." (Emphasis, mine.) Kyle's family also "contacted Dr. Jack Taylor at the Taylor Wellness Center for his Metabolic Assessment Program." (See their street address and their website below.) This nutritional program helped them with "diet, supplements and detoxification organized specifically to Kyle's body chemistry."[13] (Note that the VitaCarte® I have seen on the internet is spelled with an "e.")

Not only was Kyle taking VitaCarte® and other supplements as noted above, but his family was involved in a prayer support group. Kyle's father explains what happened:

> Now one year later we have totally reversed Kyle's prognosis...The tumors are gone and we continue to pray for the knowledge and resources to reverse the horrendous damage we allowed the doctors to inflict on Kyle's body.[14]

The type of cartilage Dr. Prudden used, "VitaCarte®," is made by "Phoenix Biologics, Inc.," and can be ordered by contacting #800-947-VITA. Their website is *www.vitacarte.com.*

Dr. Jack Taylor's Wellness Center website is located at *www.biotor.com.* Dr. Taylor's program is not promoted as a cancer program – it is a metabolic nutritional wellness program.

Cayenne – A Spice Cures Inoperable Brain Cancer

Cayenne pepper has been used to promote heart health for years. "Dr. Christopher...often called Dr. Cayenne," has given this natural remedy "to help cure almost every malady that appeared in his office." For "stomach ulcers, he recommended one teaspoon of cayenne pepper in a glass of water three times a day, and cured many a stomach ulcer." If you opt to take capsules, always take them with food! For heart attacks, he says that "the capsules will not work." As *described on the*

Wellness Directory of Minnesota™ and *Alternative Cancer Therapies'* website:

> Dr. Christopher witnessed time and time again that one cup of hot cayenne pepper [tea] will stop a heart attack in three minutes or less. A good tincture of cayenne (or drops of some of your stronger hot sauce) will also work.[15]

Dr. Richard Shulze, "master herbalist," described the following account of a gentleman cured of inoperable brain tumor by consuming cayenne pepper tea: the patient was given "a 5% chance of survival with chemotherapy." He refused chemo. Instead, he went home, "did a colon/liver detox and started a regimen of ten cups per day of cayenne pepper tea. In three months he returned to his doctor and his xrays showed a dried up, dead tumor in his head." Dr. Shulze explained that the high level of phytochemicals and other nutrients in the tea cleared the blood and boosted the immune system in the patient. Countries that consume spicy foods have much lower rates of cardiac disease and cancer than those who do not.[16] (Note that many people have used **hibiscus tea and rye bread** for lowering their blood pressure, cholesterol levels, and treating their anginal pain, as well as the vitamin, niacin.)

Chaparral & Brain Cancer

Chaparral tea is derived from an evergreen shrub called "the greasewood or creosote bush of the American Southwest...The active ingredient of the creosote bush is NDGA (nordihydroguaiaretic acid)...."[17]

When cancerous cells from a brain "glioma" were "incubated for just four hours with small amounts of this NDGA," it revealed anti-cancerous properties. It is very important if using chaparral tea, to purchase from a reliable supplier.[18] Trying to concoct home remedies of chapparal from unreliable sources is unsafe, since NDGA ingested in large amounts or combined with certain drugs can be harmful.

How Flax Oil Cured Inoperable Brain Cancer!

Many testimonials have been given of patients brought back from terminal illness to amazing health by the Johanna Budwig flax oil diet. Dr. Johanna Budwig, a "German biochemist and expert on fats and oils," was nominated seven times for the nobel prize **for her work in biochemistry**. In her research, she found that the blood of cancer patients is lacking essential "phosphatides and lipoproteins." Her diet revolves around very specific ingredients, including flax oil and cottage cheese.[19] These two ingredients as described at *www.healing-cancernaturally.com*, are combined as follows:

> For each tablespoon of flaxseed oil, add 2 tablespoons of low-fat cottage cheese (or quark) or 6 tablespoons of yoghurt. The flaxoil/cottage cheese or flaxoil/yoghurt mixture should be fully blended until no traces of oil remain visible, proving that the highly unsaturated fatty acids have become water soluble (a hand-held mixer or a blender works well).[20]

As you can see, the ingredients are very simple. It works because the flax oil reacts with the sulfuric contents of the cottage cheese and dramatically increases oxygenation at the cellular level. Fats "are only water-soluble and free-flowing when bound to protein; thus the importance of protein-rich cottage cheese." The body is also supplied with much needed natural "phosphatides and lipoproteins," without which "cancer cells grow wild and out of control."[21]

Note that this is not all of the famous Budwig diet. There are other facets included as well. For example: the diet forbids "animal fats…salad oils…meats… butter…margarine…" no sugar whatsoever, though "freshly squeezed vegetable juices" and "apple juice" are encouraged. Herbal teas are also recommended at least three times a day. Another variation of the Budwig diet is to combine in a blender "1 cup Organic cottage cheese (low fat, not too hard, best make your own) (or yogurt); 2-5 Tbsp. Of flaxseed oil - 1-3 Tbsp. of freshly ground up flaxseed (coffee grinder…works fine); enough water to make it soft [and] little cayenne."[22]

It is important to realize that the Budwig diet is a complete protocol involving a "lacto-vegetarian diet (except that fish is allowed), flaxseeds, fruit juices, vegetable juices, sauerkraut, sunshine, emotional and spiritual peace and stress control," as well as the ingredients above.[23] (See *www.healingcancernaturally.com,* for more specifics on the Budwig diet as well as chapter 17 of this book.)

Dr. Budwig described her work in the following way:

> And what do I actually do? I give cancer patients simple, natural foods. That is all. I take sick people out of the hospital, when it is said that they do not have more than an hour or two left to live, that the scientifically attested diagnosis is at hand and that the patient is completely moribund. In most cases I can help even these patients quickly and conclusively.[24]

There are many amazing cancer cures attributed to Dr. Budwig's flax oil diet. One example is that of "Sandy A.," who was diagnosed with "arachnoidal bleeding due to an inoperable brain tumor."[25] He was told that there was nothing that could be done for him, and "sent home to die." He started on Dr. Budwig's formula and says of the diet:

> My health improved so rapidly that I was soon able to return to work part-time. Shortly after that, I was again examined at the research center and my reflexes were completely normal. The Budwig diet saved my life! Ten years later, I was given a thorough examination at the Center as a follow-up. My incredible recovery has been written up in many medical journals...[26]

Ms. Budwig admitted that for those patients "who were diagnosed as being too far advanced for another operation to be of any help....Even in these cases health can be restored, usually within a few months, I would say in 90% of cases."[27]

The Budwig diet uses a natural formula that inhibits the formation of cancer. It is known throughout the world. Many people have followed this regimen, people who were terminal and "sent home to die." They were cured on the Budwig diet, and are now leading "normal healthy lives."[28]

Dr. Dan C. Roehm, M.D., F.A.C.P, said of this diet:

> Cancer treatment can be very simple and very successful once you know how. The cancer interests dont [sic] want you to know this. May those of you who have suffered from this disease (and I include your family and friends in this) forgive the miscreants who have kept this simple information from reaching you for so long.[29]

See Chapter 17 for more information on the amazing healing and curative properties of flax oil! Further details of the Budwig diet are also discussed in that chapter. Dr. Johanna Budwig authored several books, including *The Oil Protein Diet Cookbook*, which contains many recipes using the Budwig protocol. Her books are available in major bookstores and on *Amazon.com*.

Website: *www.healingcancernaturally.com*, contains a great deal of information on the Budwig diet, as does *http://www.barleans.com/budwig.html*. Be sure that you **never** heat flax oil and that you always keep it refrigerated. Also, if you choose the Budwig diet, be sure to use only certified organic dairy products! You may even want to consider soy yogurt! I have already discussed the problems associated with cow's milk and dairy products earlier in this book and in greater detail in chapter 25 as well. If you are fighting terminal cancer and someone tells you that you may have six months left, I would certainly recommend the Budwig diet. That choice is up to you. If you go with dairy, just be sure you use organic. The very last thing you need in your diet is the addition of hormones, herbicides and pesticides that are often found in non-organic dairy. These are the substances that may have caused your cancer! Read chapter 25 of this book before you include dairy products in your diet! You may want to switch to soy! (Fermented soy products, such as Haelan, can help remove harmful estrogens from the body in estrogen-receptor positive cancers.) Also, see chapter 35, *What To Do If You Are Already Ill*, for more information.

GLA & Brain Cancer Treatment

GLA, "Gamma linolenic acid" (found in "evening primrose oil and borage oil") has multiple "antitumor properties." In one study on brain tumors, it was discovered that "injecting GLA directly into a brain tumor (glioma) caused the tumor to regress." Not only does GLA destroy many types of cancerous cells, but it does not affect healthy cells![30]

In his book, *Natural Strategies For Cancer Patients*, Dr. Russell L. Blaylock, M.D., does not "recommend taking more than 2000 milligrams of GLA a day" because of the "narrow window of effectiveness" that they have. He believes that larger amounts may cause an "inflammatory reaction."[31]

Goldenseal Fights Brain Tumors

According to *Life Extension's* webpage, *www.lef.org*, "Goldenseal" and other herbs that contain an ingredient known as *"berberine"* (such as "...Barberry, Goldthread, and Oregon Grape"), are not only important as "anti-inflammatory agents," but berberine "is effective against bladder cancers." This herb has been known to suppress "colon cancer," cause "human leukemia cells" to self-destruct, and prevent "skin tumors" from developing! It has also shown "potent antitumor activity against human and rat malignant brain tumors..."[32] The website further explains just how powerful this ingredient is:

> Studies using goldenseal, which contains the alkaloid berberine, showed average cancer kill rate of 91% in rats, over twice that seen in BCNU (a standard chemotherapy agent for brain tumors). The preparation should be standardized to provide 5% hydrastine. Most herbalists recommend rotating goldenseal with other herbals, rather than giving it routinely.[33]

Berberine has been shown to prevent cancer cells in the liver from multiplying. However, you should not use herbs that contain berberine (such as "goldenseal, Oregon grape, coptis or barberry") with the following conditions:

> [I]f you are pregnant or have gallbladder disease. Do not take these herbs with supplemental vitamin B6 or with protein supplements containing the amino acid histidine. Do not use goldenseal if you have cardiovascular disease or glaucoma.[34] [Berberine can also increase blood pressure.]

Grapes (Resveratrol) & Grape Seed Extract

Read chapter two of this book for more information on resveratrol and its use in the prevention and treatment of many types of cancers! Remember too, that grape seed extract is a super anti-oxidant that has the ability to cross the blood-brain barrier! (Compounds that can cross the blood-brain barrier are important in the prevention and treatment of brain tumors as well as other disorders, such as Alzheimers.)

How Macrobiotics Cured Brain Cancer

Mona S. of Columbus, Ohio lost consciousness playing tennis when she "was 37 years old." She was told that she had "a brain tumor the size of a small grapefruit," and she was given "six to 18 months to live." Her story can be found in J. L. Eftekhar's book, *Heal Yourself*, from *Globe Digests™*. She gave up on traditional medicine (after only "three chemotherapy sessions") and started on a macrobiotic diet. She also developed a positive attitude, telling herself that "the tumor was decreasing."[34a] Four months after starting the diet, Eftekhar says that "a brain scan showed no evidence of cancer, and, incredibly, none have appeared since." She credits her healing to her "strong faith in God…many prayers…determination, a positive outlook…and carefully staying on the diet." She also used tapes and videos to reinforce her determination to get well.[35]

Macrobiotics, developed by "Michio Kushi" relies on "50 to 60% whole grains; 25 to 30% vegetables; 5 to 10% beans and seaweed; and 5% soups." Seafood and fish are allowed on the diet, as well as fresh fruits, "condiments and seasonings; beverages; and occasional healthy snacks."[36]

Though there are many health benefits to some of the ingredients in the macrobiotic diet, it is being included here for informational purposes only. I do not agree with all of it, especially the emphasis that it places on eastern philosophies, which I feel are in direct conflict with Christianity. I believe if one follows the diet advocated by Ann Wigmore, Dr. Kristine Nolfi, Rita Myers and George Malkmus, they will achieve the same results; a vegan diet, rich in fresh juices, raw vegetables and fruits, and giving thanks daily for everything to the Lord Jesus Christ, rather than resorting to eastern imagery and philosophies which do not glorify our Creator God. (Macrobiotics are discussed in greater detail in chapter 26 of this book for informational purposes only.)

In visiting natural health food stores you will often be bombarded with philosophies from eastern religions – Buddhism, Hinduism, and various new age doctrines. See chapter 35 in this book, *What To Do If You Are Already Ill,* for confronting these issues.

Marijuana Used Medically Destroys Brain Cancer Cells

When scientists from "Madrid" revealed very recently that "medical marijuana" ("Tetrahydrocannabinol…THC") could destroy "incurable brain cancer tumors in rats" when it was injected into the tumors, not a single newspaper in the United States reported the findings, and the story only ran one time "on the AP and UPI news wires, on Feb. 29."[36a] This was not "new" information. As far back as "1974," the "Medical College of Virginia" announced that medical marijuana "slowed the growth of three kinds of cancer in mice – lung and breast cancer and a virus-induced leukemia." This information was all documented in a book written by Jack Herer, *"The Emperor Wears No Clothes*….The government quickly shut down the Virginia Study."[37]

Cancertutor.com website reports that in 1976, then "President Gerald Ford put an end to all public cannabis research and granted exclusive research rights to major pharmaceutical companies…to develop synthetic" versions of marijuana that would not deliver the "high" that the natural plant induces. The pharmaceutical companies were not successful.[38]

Use of marijuana, especially over long periods of time has shown to be detrimental to overall brain health, however, I find it interesting that research studies proving that injections can cure "incurable brain tumors in rats," was aggressively suppressed by the government. Though I would never advocate any sort of illicit drug use, I am not against the use of medicinal marijuana for pain relief in cancer patients, as long as use is closely monitored, and the recipients are not out driving the highways while "relieving their pain!" (Of course, people who drink alcohol aren't supposed to be on the highways either, yet they are, and they are killing thousands every year!) Today, more than 30 years after former President Gerald Ford ended cannabis research, there is still a fight raging over the use of medicinal marijuana for pain control in cancer patients.

Melatonin & Brain Cancers

When a "clinical trial" was done involving "50 patients" and the use of "melatonin," some of them were given "supportive care" only, while others were given "supportive care" along with melatonin. At the end of "one year," those who received the melatonin had longer survival time, no tumor growth, and fewer adverse effects and "complications," as compared to those given "supportive care" only.[39] Melatonin is discussed in other chapters of this book, including potential side effects.

Mullaca Inhibits Brain Cancer (Gliomas)

Mullaca is another Rainforest herb toxic to gliomas (brain tumors). Clinical research is still going on with this fascinating herb, and preliminary laboratory and animal studies have shown it can boost the immune system, is deadly to many different forms of cancer cells, and kills microbes.[40]

Deanna K. Loftis, R.N., B.B.A.

Typical brain stem gliomas are usually found in children and are normally considered inoperable because they invade once healthy brain tissue that could end up causing paralysis and death if surgically interrupted. Most children with this diagnosis do not survive more than a year. Atypical gliomas, on the other hand, may carry a longer survival rate. A very ominous symptom children may first develop indicating the presence of this type tumor, is **double-vision.** As described at *www.braintumor.org,* other symptoms may include: "nausea, headache, speech or balance abnormalities, difficulty with swallowing and weakness or numbness of the arms or legs."[40a] Other types of gliomas described at the website above are: "ependymoma, ganglioneuroma, juvenile pilocytic, mixed glioma, oligodendrogliomas [and] optic nerve glioma."[40b] Some nonglioma types of brain tumors include: "chordoma, craniopharyngioma, medulloblastoma, meningioma, pineal tumors, pituitary tumors, pituitary adenoma, primitive neuroectodermal tumors, Schwannoma [and] vascular tumors."[40c]

Other types of cancerous brain conditions include: "CNS [central nervous system] lymphoma, meningeal carcinomatosis, pseudotumor cerebri [and] tuberous sclerosis."[40d]

"Extracts of mullaca" that inhibit cancer cells are phytosteroids [plant steroids] known as *"physalins."* They have shown impressive abilities during lab and animal studies in fighting many types of cancer, including "lung, colon, nasopharynx, liver, cervix, melanoma and glioma (brain)" cancers.[41]

Mullaca should not be taken by those on blood thinners, blood pressure medications, diabetic medications, or heart medications without the supervision of their physician since it "lowers blood pressure," affects clotting time, and has "hypoglycemic" effects.[42] For more information, contact Raintree Nutrition website at: *www.raintree.com.*

A Mushroom Extract Cures Brain Cancer!

Though *maitake* (a popular mushroom) and its healing properties are discussed in other chapters in this book, it is presented here because of its ability to fight **brain cancer.** One of the extracts from maitake known as *Maitake D-Fraction* has become popular as an immune-booster and cancer fighter!

In the book by Shari Lieberman, Ph.D., and Ken Babal, C.N., *Maitake Mushroom And D-Fraction,* the following amazing curative power of this mushroom is documented: "An egg-sized brain tumor in a 44-year-old male completely disappeared after taking maitake D-fraction for four months."[43] You can find this supplement in some health food stores as well as several internet sites, including *www.iherb.com.*

Pituitary Tumors

These type tumors, though rare, are found growing in "the pituitary gland, a small organ – about the size of a dime and located in the center of the brain."[43a] As described at website *http://www.ninds.nih.gov,* the pituitary manufactures "hormones that affect growth and the functions of other glands in the body. These type tumors are usually benign, which means they are non-cancerous, grow slowly and do not spread to other parts of the body." They can however, cause the body to "produce too many hormones, which can cause other problems in the body."[43b] There are many "symptoms of pituitary tumors," including: "headaches, vision problems, nausea and vomiting, or any of the problems caused by the production of too many hormones such as infertility or loss of menstrual periods in women, abnormal growth, high blood pressure, heat or cold intolerance, and other skin and body changes."[43c]

Tumors of the pituitary gland, though rarely cancerous are "best treated when they are found and diagnosed early." Current orthodox treatment includes "surgical removal of the tumor; radiation therapy, using high doses of x-rays to kill tumor cells, and/or drug therapy, using certain medications to block the pituitary gland from producing too many hormones. The most common treatment is surgery." Depending on "the type of pituitary tumor and the patient's age and general state of health, pituitary tumors are usually curable."[44] There are many types of alternative treatments for brain tumors given in this chapter, though surgery for pituitary tumors is usually very successful.

Poly–MVA for Brain Tumors

Poly-MVA is a high antioxidant nutritional drink which has several nutrients, including alpha lipoic acid. Wellness Directory of Minnesota's™ website says this is one cancer treatment that can even cross the "blood-brain barrier;" good news for those fighting brain tumors, and may be helpful in "reversing" other cancers such as "multiple myeloma" and "pancreatic cancer." Poly-MVA can be ordered at the main Poly-MVA website: *"http://www.polymva. net"*.[44a] (There are bogus forms of this formula floating around. The website above has the original formula.)

Taheebo Tea

Pau d'arco or "Taheebo tea" is discussed in other chapters of this book due to its antioxidant properties. Pau d'arco tea, which is produced "from the inner bark of a tree found in South American rain forests," is very popular.[45]

According to an article by Dr. Mowry on Karl Loren's website: *http://www.oralchelation.com/taheebo/research/page1.htm,* certain "groups of constituents of lapacho have….been found to suppress tumor formation and reduce tumor viability, both in experimental animal trials and in clinical settings involving human patients." This herb not only fights leukemia, but "some researchers feel that lapacho [pau d'arco] is one of the most important anti-tumor agents in the entire world."[45a] The testimonial below notes the power of this herb in fighting brain cancer, and is described at *www.oralchelation.com:*

> I had a large tumor in my brain. Traditional treatment produced only minor success. Then I began to use lapacho [pau

d'arco] tea. After several weeks a CAT scan showed that the tumor was totally gone. The doctors couldn't believe it because they had classified my case as basically untreatable.[46]

Taheebo tea (or pau d'arco) is sometimes referred to as *lapacho*, but lapacho is actually just one of the compounds extracted from pau d'arco. Since lapacho has blood-thinning properties, you need to discuss the tea with your physician before consuming large amounts.

Ukrain Effective Against Brain Cancer Without Toxic Side Effects

Ukrain is a product "developed in 1978 by Dr. Wassyl J. Nowicky," Director of the "Ukrain Anti-Cancer Institute of Vienna, Austria..." He effectively combined an herb known as "Greater Celandine," and an older "cytotoxic" drug known as *"thiotepa."* Given individually, they are toxic, but when combined, they are toxic only to cancer cells! Dozens of "scientific papers" have been written on this compound. It was tested by the NCI on 60 "different human cancer cell lines" and in nearly all of them cancer cell growth was repressed by "100 percent...."![47] Though it is an injection, thus not exactly "painless," it is discussed in several cancer specific chapters of this book because it is completely non-toxic and has been effective with so many different forms of cancer, including many of those considered *hopeless* and *terminal.*

Apparently, Ukrain aggressively congregates at the tumor "site" once administered. It boosts the immune system and promotes "anti-angiogenesis" (inhibits the formation "of new blood vessels at the tumour site"). Ukrain has been successful against many cancers, including rectal, colorectal, breast, pancreatic, bladder, prostate, bronchial, brain, testicular and neuroblastoma![48]

At the Ukrain website: *www.ukrin.com,* the following was documented on research studies involving Ukrain: A clinical human trial was done involving "363 cancer patients" having "47 different types of tumour...[who] were treated with Ukrain between September 1997 to January 2003 at the Villa Medica Clinic (Edenkoben, Germany)" by physician, "Dr. Aschoff." Every patient, without exception, had already "exhausted conventional" treatment without results. They were either progressing in their cancer or had relapsed.[49] (In other words, **all of them were *terminal***; conventional medicine had failed and there was nothing left to offer them!)

"The following rates of full remission were achieved" with Ukrain:

> breast cancer 31%, colorectal cancer 16.7%, bronchial ade-nocarcinoma 7.7%, small-cell bronchial carcinoma 21%, astrocytoma (brain tumor) 66.6%, neuroblastoma 60%, seminoma (testicular cancer) 75%, bladder carcinoma 50%.[50]

This compound repeatedly outperformed conventional medicine, and these are **humans** we are talking about, not lab mice! (Did you note that "66.6%" remission for "astrocytoma" and "60%" for "neuroblastoma," both of which are very deadly tumors?!) As described at their website regarding the late Dr. Atkins:

> Dr. Atkins regards Ukrain as the single best anticancer agent he has used to date. "Like chemotherapy, it kills cancer cells very well but, unlike chemotherapy, it spares normal cells, healthy tissue. If the medical community were willing to give it a try, Ukrain could replace chemotherapy in treating almost all cancers." – Robert C. ATKINS, M.D.[51]

You can visit their website at *www.ukrin.com,* if you are interested in more information. You can also contact them by email at *nowicky@ukrin.com.* See chapter ten for information about Dr. T. R. Shantha's clinic in Georgia. He also admnisters Ukrain therapy as well as intravenous vitamin C, and many other treatments.

Vassourinha & Anamu

These are two Rainforest herbs that have anti-tumor properties. "Vassourinha *(Scoparia dulcis)*" contains the plant compound "betulinic acid," which has undergone much recent testing for its "powerful, anticancerous, antitumorous, antileukemic, and antiviral (including HIV) properties."[51a] Raintree Nutrition at *www.raintree.com*, reports that it has been shown to be toxic to "malignant brain tumors, bone cancer and melanomas (without harming healthy cells)." This herb should not be used by pregnant women as it may cause uterine contractions. It has some "hypoglycemic" effects and it increases the effects of barbiturates and antidepressants, so be sure to consult with your physician before using this or any other herbal products, especially if you are on prescription medications or have a chronic illness.[52]

Anamu *"(Petiveria alliacea)"* has a pungent "garlic odor" and is sometimes referred to as "garlic weed," says Raintree Nutrition. This herb also has "antileukemic, antitumorous, and anticancerous" properties against many forms of cancer. Extracts from anamu were found (during in vitro studies) to be "toxic to leukemia and lymphoma cancer cells...liver cancer...[and] the growth of brain cancer cells."[52a] Apparently, the herb's sulfuric compounds are partly responsible for its potency. One animal study showed that anamu "increased natural killer cell activity by 100%..." This herb should not be used by pregnant women as it may cause "uterine contractions." Raintree also reports that Anamu has "hypoglycemic" effects and may interfere with blood coagulation, so be sure to consult with your physician before using it.[53]

Zyflamend

See page 79 for Zyflamend, used for prostate cancer. In lab tests, it also destroyed cancerous brain cells.

CHAPTER 14

PAINLESS CURES & PREVENTIONS FOR SKIN CANCER (MELANOMA)

"When I was in medical school in the mid-1960s, I was convinced that the medical profession was pure...Today, thirty years later, the profession embarrasses me. I now realize that the majority of physicians...particularly those in positions of power and authority, have no intention of investigating therapies other than those from pharmaceutical manufacturers..."

(Dr. Burt Berskson, M.D., Ph.D., from his book, *The Alpha Lipoic Acid Breakthrough)*[1]

Skin Cancer Types

As described at website *www.cancer-healing.com,* there are three main "types of skin cancer: basal cell, squamous cell, and melanoma.[2] Melanomas are derived from the melanocytes, or pigment cells, in the deepest level of the epidermis." If you are diagnosed with "basal cell" or "squamous cell cancers," these are normally found "on parts of the body exposed to the sun, such as the face, ears and extremities."[2a] These type cancers are "highly curable, especially if detected and treated early." However, melanomas are likely to be discovered in the form of "dark moles that spread over the surface of the skin," and they are more lethal," since they can spread so rapidly.[2b]

Vitamin A, C & E for Skin Health & Cancer Prevention

Antioxidants protect the skin against UV damage. If your skin is well fortified with the nutrition that it needs, skin cells will not usually transmute under normal sun exposure. According to author Maureen Kennedy Salaman in her book, *All Your Health Questions Answered Naturally,* scientists discovered that "topical vitamin C," when applied to "the skin of live pigs," protected them from "ultraviolet light at one to five times the dose" that would normally cause a "sunburn." Not only did it protect their skin from being burned, but it prevented damage at the cellular level. The shielding effect lasted a full "three days, even when the pigs were scrubbed with soap!"[3] Ms. Salaman says that other skin protectors are vitamin A and E. Apparently, ingesting over "100 units…of vitamin E (tocopherol) a day," (and applying it topically) can reduce cancer "risk" by "70 percent." Supplements of "more than 5,000 IU of vitamin A daily," reduces the risk of skin cancer by "90 percent…"[4] Other skin protectors are discussed later in this chapter.

If you are juicing beta-carotene rich foods such as carrot juice, the body converts beta-carotene into natural vitamin A.

Andiroba & Berberine Inhibit Skin Tumors

See chapter fifteen for more information on the herb, andiroba, used against sarcomas and skin cancers, and chapter seven for information on an important ingredient found in the herb Goldenseal, called *berberine,* which inhibits the formation of melanoma and many other cancers. (Also, see indications for when this herb should **not** be used.)

Azelaic Acid

In laboratory testing [topical] azelaic acid kills melanoma cells, but leaves normal cells unharmed. According to researchers, this compound caused regression in malignant skin cancers by not merely killing them, but inhibiting their growth as well. It has also been effective in treating acne and various skin problems due to its bactericidal properties. Azalaic acid was researched in over two dozen various "human melanoma cell cultures." It effectively inhibited further growth of cancerous melanoma in every single culture! Apparently, adding "the B vitamin, carnitine" to this ingredient enhanced its effect.[5]

Beta-Glucan Fights Skin Cancer

Beta-glucan is an extract from "brewers' and bakers' yeasts, and from oat and barley bran," as well as mushrooms "such as shiitake...and maitake..." It is available in supplement form at most health food stores.[5a] A report described at website *www.newhope.com* involving "a human study...on nine cancer patients" said that these patients had either "skin, breast, or lung cancer."[5b] When "beta-glucan [was] injected" directly "into their tumors...within five days" they shrank. Lentinan is a beta-glucan extracted "from the shittake mushroom." It is used in Japan to treat "advanced cancer patients," and when given "by intravenous injection," survival times can often be prolonged by "five or more years."[6]

Note that one website in particular promotes a beta glucan extracted from oats, *www.cancer-treatments.net/cancer.html,* which they claim is superior to "and more expensive to manufacture" than the "yeast beta glucan," which is most commonly found in health food stores. They explain that according to "recent research," this type beta glucan "will cause a three times greater production of Interleukin from the macrophage cell as compared to yeast beta glucan;" in other words, a greater immune boosting effect.[7] Note that according to this website, there is now available an even more potent "whole cell beta glucan made from baker's yeast." For more information see their web pages at: *www.cancer-prevention.net.*

Burzynski's Antineoplastons

See chapter 13 of this book for amazing cases of cancer patients completely cured of "terminal" cancers, people who were basically sent home to die, then chose non-toxic antineoplastons from the Burzynski Clinic in Houston, Texas *(www.cancermed.com).* Also, see many of the patient's own stories about their success in fighting cancer with antineoplastons at website: *http://burzynskipatientgroup.org/stories.html.* Many were "hopeless," very aggressive brain tumors, but several other forms of cancer are also treated successfully with antineoplastons.

Cansema Black Topical Salve for Skin Cancer

Cansema salve "contains zinc chloride and the herb bloodroot," and both of these ingredients combined "have the longest proven track-record of any [skin] cancer treatment." According to website, *http://www.cancertutor.com,* this salve is so effective that "the FDA recently shut down the largest seller of this product."[8]

Ground Ivy

Ground ivy (*"Nepeta hereacea,"*) or "Gill-Over-The-Ground," as it is sometimes called, has been studied for its potential use in treating melanoma due to its ability to suppress the formation of tumors.[9]

Chaparral Tea & Melanoma

Chaparral *("Larrea tridentata or Larrea diver-icata")* also called the *"creosote bush,"* has been around for years, popular as a medicinal tea for anything from common colds to cancer.[10] NDGA ("nordihy-droguairetic acid"), a highly potent "antioxidant" was extracted from chaparral in the early forties. *Curezone.com* reports that studies have shown that "NDGA attacks bacteria, yeast, viruses, fungi, and cancer cells..." without the toxic adverse reactions found in chemo drugs.[11] Scientists also discovered that NDGA works by preventing cancer cells from utilizing glucose, and cancer cells thrive on sugar. If you destroy their capacity to use glucose, they will die.[12]

Curezone.com also describes an article by "Drs. Dean Burk and Mark Woods...*NDGA The Penicillin of Quinones,"* which reports on the tumor inhibiting ability and basic non-toxicity of chaparral. They determined that "NDGA is one of the most potent cancer anti-meta-bolic agents in laboratory tests, in spite of its low toxicity." Although cancer cells function without oxygen, unlike "normal cells," they rely on huge amounts of sugar for their existence.[13]

One very impressive case study demonstrated the effects of chaparral tea on melanoma in an "85-year-old" man who had endured several surgical procedures for a "malignant melanoma of the right cheek." *Curezone.com* gives details:

> The cancer reappeared after each operation, and had spread to his neck. When he saw Dr. Charles Smart at the University of Utah, the lesion measured 3 x 4 centimeters...the patient decided to avoid further surgery and returned home. The patient began taking chaparral tea in November 1967, and by February 1968 the facial lesion had decreased to the size of a dime and the neck mass had disappeared.[14]

Seven months later, the patient was re-examined and the lesion was now "only 2-3 millimeters" in size.[15] His neck was free of any masses. His appearance was much improved, and he had even gained weight. He had brewed "7 to 8 grams of chaparral leaves to a quart of hot water. He drank 2 to 3 cups per day."[16]

Many people simply gather chapparal leaves and brew their own tea, but this can be dangerous if you consume too much. Chaparral grows abundantly in many western states. It has been reported that chaparral can cause liver damage if taken in excessively large amounts. It can also "cause nausea, vomiting, and abdominal cramps." It was recently removed from the marketplace by the FDA based on reports of four "cases of liver toxicity in users of the herb." *Curezone.com* says that the specifics from those four occurrences are not yet available.[17]

Did you note those **FOUR cases of liver toxicity** above? This is an HERB we are discussing, NOT a pharmaceutical drug. Did you notice how quickly the FDA acted to remove this herb from shelves in America? If you have read chapter one in this book, you already know that it is possible for a pharmaceutical drug to kill thousands of people before the FDA forces if off the market!

When more than two dozen cases of brain hemorrhage were reported to the FDA with the use of the drug PPA it was **NOT** removed from the market. Dr. Strand, in his book *Death By Prescription*, explains what happened:

The drug had been around for so long that everyone quickly dismissed reports of harm. An article that appeared in the New England Journal of Medicine, however, started to turn heads when it detailed more than thirty cases of hemorrhagic stroke (bleeding into the brain) that had been reported since 1979 in those having ingested PPA. Most of the reports involved adolescent girls or young women between the ages of sixteen and twenty-one who were using appetite suppressant drugs containing PPA.[18]

When reports of death began pouring in from the use of the drug Baycol, it was not removed from the market, but was prescribed to more than **half-a-million** patients! Dr. Strand also reports what happened with this killer drug:

More than fifty deaths were reported worldwide, and 1,100 reports of suspected cases of rhabdomyolysis were believed to be an adverse drug reaction to Baycol.[19]

Rhabdomyolysis is a devastating disease that destroys muscles! More than 300 people died before the drug Propulsid was finally taken off the market; many of them were children![20]

The drug, Vioxx, may have caused thousands of deaths before it was finally removed from the market (just recently), and now there are accusations that MERCK may have been involved in covering up data showing that the drug could cause fatal heart attacks. What is wrong with this picture? All the DRUGS mentioned above were controlled by huge pharmaceutical conglomerates! The drug companies were making millions off the concoctions and they fought to keep them in the marketplace regardless of the death reports pouring in!

The FDA had no "interest" in chaparral and there were no drug companies fighting to keep it on the shelves! And why the big "secrecy" about not revealing the details of the **four cases** of liver toxicity reported? The FDA would love to control every mineral, vitamin, and herb on the market. That is their ultimate goal! Their main concern is not the drugs manufactured by the pharmaceutical companies. They wait with bated breath for any minuscule report of some herb or vitamin preparation that gave somebody a sour stomach, headache or *buzz*, or isolated allergic reaction, so they can find an excuse to take away YOUR right to purchase herbs, vitamins, and alternative therapies!

Above is just one small sample of the blantant hypocrisy of the FDA. If you think that your safety is their ultimate concern, you are sadly mistaken. They are not concerned with keeping you safe, they are concerned with taking away your freedom and keeping you and your loved ones locked into a future of total dependency on multiple chemicals concocted by the pharmaceutical industry.

Chili Peppers

One of the main ingredients in these spicy little veggies, *capsaicin,* has demonstrated the ability to destroy cancer cells in laboratory testing. It is believed that they heat the cells from within, choking off the oxygen supply to the cancer cells. Problem is, researchers won't be sure if capsaicin can be used topically for skin cancers until more testing is done to determine the full effects on healthy cells. There are some capsaicin-containing skin creams on the market already, however, for other uses such as back and joint paint. It seems to me that if capsaicin was harmful to healthy cells, these other topical skin creams would have been discontinued years ago![20a]

Comfrey Plant

According to Dr. H. E. Kirschner, M.D., this plant (*"Symphytum officinale"*) saved the life of one of his patients who was dying from an "advanced externalized cancer."[21] The family was told to use "fresh, crushed-leaf comfrey poultices throughout the day," and within two days it was apparent that the patient was improving.[22] This continued over the next several weeks and all pain disappeared. There was also a "dramatic decrease in swelling." Dr. Kirschner believes that the "medical community has greatly persecuted this plant," probably due to "misuse of the leaves."[23]

Do not use comfrey except under the guidance of your licensed health care practitioner. This is one herb that should **NEVER be taken internally.**[24]

Espinheira Santa for Skin Cancers

Espinheira Santa ("*Maytenus* species") is an evergreen holly from South America, where the "bark or leaf of the plant" is allowed to soak "overnight in aguardiente (rum) and used as a household remedy for the relief of arthritis, rheumatism and back pain."[25]

Researchers have identified extracts from this plant for skin cancer treatment. It is believed that the "antitumor" qualities can be linked to the "triterpenes and antioxidants" found in the bark of this evergreen. The herb is available in "tincture" form or sold in bulk leaf tea format.[26] For more information on this herb, contact *www.raintree.com* or *www.herbs2000.com.*

Essiac Tea

See Chapter five for more information on the nurse who healed hundreds (perhaps thousands) of her cancer patients (many of them terminal) with an herbal tea containing four herbs, known as *Essiac tea.*

Garlic & Skin Cancer Prevention

Scientists in Japan have found that garlic inhibits the ability of skin cells to mutate. This according to Maureen Kennedy Salaman in her book, *All Your Health Questions Answered Naturally.* If you are looking for the best type of garlic to use, Ms. Salaman says it is "liquid aged garlic extract, which leaves out the agricultural chemicals, odor and burn."[27] Other important protectants against skin cancer, listed by Ms. Salaman are: "grape seed extract, ginkgo biloba and grass burdock extract..." (As well as aged garlic, topical vitamin C and E, and vitamin A taken orally, discussed earlier in this chapter.)[28]

I believe that Kyolic® is superior and is the aged garlic brand that I use. Kyolic® received an award from the National Nutrition

Foods Association, and uses a stringent manufacturing and aging process. When cooking, it is best to use fresh, organic garlic.

Green Tea Protects Against Skin Cancer

Scientists have discovered that the antioxidant protection in green tea is so formidable that using it topically on the skin of mice previously exposed to carcinogens, gave the animals "nearly total protection against tumor formation." The antioxidant nutrients in green tea "are found in the leaves."[29]

Hoxsey Formula & Skin Cancers

Though Harry Hoxsey was most famous for his tea recipe, he also developed a topical salve for skin cancer made primarily of "zinc chloride, antimony trisulfide and blood root" that is now used in a "related orthodox version" against skin cancer. "Mohs's microsurgery, is now standard for certain forms of skin cancers…Mohs reported…a 99 percent cure rate for all primary basal cell carcinomas he treated."[30] (This surgery for skin cancer involves shaving off the cancerous growth layer by layer, until it is completely removed.) The layers are reviewed microscopically.

Milk Thistle Protects Against Skin Cancer

Milk thistle, discussed earlier in this book because of its importance in protecting the liver, can also help decrease problems with psoriasis. It may even be important in treating endometriosis. It enables estrogen to be processed by the liver, helps "the flow of bile," and it may one day be considered an important anticancer herb for fighting melanoma.[30a] As noted in *The Healing Power of Vitamins, Minerals, and Herbs*, from the Reader's Digest Association: Cleveland scientists discovered "that when the active ingredient, silymarin, was applied to the skin of mice, 75% fewer skin tumors resulted after exposure to ultraviolet radiation."[31]

Pomegranate Fruit Extract for Skin Tumors

According to an article at Reuter's Health Information, "Pomegranate fruit extract (PFE)...inhibits skin tumor formation in mice...this from a "report in the January 20th issue of the International Journal of Cancer."[32] When "Dr. Hasan Mukhar and colleagues from the University of Wisconsin at Madison....tested the anti-cancer effects of PFE, a chemical with strong anti-inflammatory and antioxidant properties..." with "topical application" of the extract, "animals pre-treated with PFE" experienced "a substantial drop" in the development of tumors...in comparison to those not receiving the extract.[33]

Though these are animal studies only, it may not be long before you are able to purchase a sunscreen with natural pomegranate extract as a protectant against skin cancer! See chapter four of this book for a **human study described by Reuters Health, showing that drinking pomegranate juice** can help in the prevention of recurring prostate cancer.

Selenium Prevents Skin Cancers

Scientists exposed hairless mice to harmful doses of "ultraviolet rays," but gave three of the groups of mice selenium. Those mice receiving the largest doses of the mineral in their diet experienced the fewest malignancies. Further testing revealed that the mineral's anti-cancerous ability is probably because selenium enables the body to increase glutathione levels.[34] When researchers studied the effects of this important mineral on skin cancers, they found that insufficient amounts of selenium increased the participant's risk for "skin cancer...5.8 times..."[35]

Shark Cartilage Kills Human Melanoma Cells

Shark cartilage, discussed in several other chapters, has been shown to reduce melanoma cells in animal testing. In her book, *Nutrition: The Cancer Answer II*, Maureen Kennedy Salaman describes one study in particular where mice were given "human melanoma" cells;

half of them were also given shark cartilage supplementation on a daily basis. Within 21 days, says Ms. Salaman, mice receiving the shark cartilage had a reduction in the size of their tumors, while tumors in the control group grew twice as large without the shark cartilage![36] Shark cartilage is not for use with children, nor during pregnancy, or if you have recently had a heart attack, transplant, surgery, chemo or radiation. It is not for those with high blood pressure, pheochromocytoma (adrenal tumor which can cause excessively high blood pressure), liver diseases (though it has been used successfully to treat liver cancer), allergies to seafood, ulcers or circulatory diseases. More information on dosing is given in chapter six. Also, you should be consulting with a naturopathic health physician about your own individual dosing needs before taking this supplement.

Soy Heals a Precancerous Skin Lesion

Haelan is nothing more than "a fermented soy beverage," yet it has shown amazing abilities in treating different forms of cancer. An article from *Well Being Journal (www.wellbeingjournal.com)* by Donna Sage, M.S.S.A., tells the story of an eight-year-old who used Haelan to heal a "precancerous skin condition." The boy's family history was positive for melanoma. Drinking an ounce of Haelan per day caused the lesion to completely heal.[37] There are several websites that market Haelan, including *http://www.haelanpartners.com.*

Vassourinha – Betulinic Acid

Betulinic acid is one of the compounds found in the herb vassourinha. *Rain-tree.com* describes research noting that this compound has very potent "anticancerous, antitumorous, antileukemic, and antiviral (including HIV) properties." It was also able to kill "malignant brain tumor, bone cancer and melanomas [cells]," but was not toxic to normal cells![38] The herb can lower blood sugar, cause uterine contractions and increase the effect of any drugs having sedative or antidepressant effects, so should be used only with physician consult.[39]

Studies demonstrate that betulinic acid helps to seek out and destroy human malignant skin cells without harming normal cells, something chemo drugs fail miserably at, and it was also able to inhibit HIV I. The herb's affinity for skin cancer cells is remarkable, especially when the data was put alongside that of several toxic chemo drugs.

Wheat Grass Juice & Melanoma

Neva Whetzel from Virginia drank wheatgrass juice (along with a nutritious diet and herbs) to heal herself of melanoma. She refused the radiation and chemotherapy her doctor prescribed, allowing only the actual surgical removal of the melanoma. She not only used wheat grass, but barley grass, kamut grass and "the powdered grasses."[40]

A Word About the Pain of Psoriasis

Many people suffer their entire lives going from one dermatologist to another with painful psoriasis, which often manifests as patches of dry, scaly, itchy skin. Psoriasis, as mentioned earlier by Steve Meyerowitz, can be one of the emergency symptoms that you are dehydrated and need to increase your water and salt intake (see chapter 22). You also need to be getting extra EFA's (essential fatty acids) such as liquid flaxseed oil (3 tablespoons daily in with your salad dressings or mixed in with your fresh juices), as well as borage oil, avocados, and evening primrose oil. (If taking in supplement form, take supplements as instructed on the brand that you purchase.) Juice at least 3-4 glasses a day of fresh carrot juice. You need the vitamin A that you will be getting from the beta-carotene! Also be sure that you are taking at least 3 glasses a day of barley green (powdered drink) juice, or another green powdered drink such as Dee Simmon's *Green Miracle* (available at her website *http://ultimateliving.com*), and be sure that you are juicing greens from fresh kale, spinach, broccoli, cabbage, and celery on a daily basis! You should also include a good complete vitamin supplement daily, as well as a mineral supplement such as Maureen Kennedy Salaman's *Mineral Rich*®. Others have had great success using shark cartilage supplements for psoriasis as well as aloe and milk thistle! If you are a woman, you may also want to get on a NATURAL progesterone cream supplement for psoriasis help, such as *ProgestiMax®*. You can order *ProgestiMax®* (and *Mineral Rich®*) at Maureen Kennedy Salaman's website *www.mksalaman.com*. See chapter 21 of this book on hormone replacement therapy for more information about when you should (and shouldn't) take natural progesterone!

Poly–MVA (Palladium Lipoic Complex)

See chapters 9 and 13 for more information on this non-toxic nutritional formula that many cancer survivors are crediting to their complete recovery! Their main website is *www.polymva.net*. Many patients were sent home to die, using only Poly-MVA for alternative therapy, yet they recovered fully and are alive years later. Some combined Poly-MVA with other alternative treatments or conventional therapies. Some used Poly-MVA to treat secondary cancers that they received from prior radiation and chemo, or to treat more aggressive cancers that returned after they had already received radiation or chemo! Their testimonials can be read at website: *http://www.S94567060.onlinehome.us/survivors/testimonials.html.*

CHAPTER 15

PAINLESS CURES & PREVENTIONS FOR LYMPHOMAS & SARCOMAS

"A doctor whose patient had been diagnosed with terminal cancer, showed signs of recovery. When the doctor rang me he confirmed it was me who had helped the patient, then said, 'I will stop you from doing this to our industry'. Now that he has stopped the importation of this treatment he can now boast to his patients and colleagues that he has stopped cancer patients from purchasing Essiac in Australia."

– M. Costello.[1]

Sarcomas

Sarcomas usually begin in "supportive and connective tissues such as bones, tendons, cartilage, muscle and fat," and as described at *website, www.cancer-healing.com,* most commonly, they begin as a "painful mass on the bone." Types of "sarcomas" listed at the website are:

- Osteosarcoma or osteogenic sarcoma (bone)
- Chondrosarcoma (cartilage)
- Leiomyosarcoma (smooth muscle)
- Rhabdomyosarcoma (skeletal muscle)
- Mesothelial sarcoma or mesothelioma (membranous lining of body cavities)
- Fibrosarcoma (fibrous tissue)
- Angiosarcoma or hemangioendothelioma (blood vessels)
- Liposarcoma (adipose tissue)
- Glioma or astrocytoma (neurogenic connective tissue found in the brain)
- Myxosarcoma (primitive embryonic connective tissue)
- Mesenchymous or mixed mesodermal tumor (mixed connective tissue types)[2]

Hodgkins Vs. Non-Hodgkins Lymphoma

Lymphomas are cancers that arise from the body's lymphatic system, the "body's blood-filtering tissues that help fight infection and disease." There are two main forms of lymphoma: "Hodgkin's Disease," and "non-Hodgkin's lymphoma."[2a] Lymphomas of every kind, "except Hodgkin's disease are collectively known as non-Hodgkin's lymphoma."[3]

How does one determine which is which? The only way to tell them apart is to look at the cells under a microscope (usually done after a biopsy), as described at website *www.oncologychannel.com/nonhodgkins:*

> The lymphatic tissue in Hodgkin's disease contains specific cells – Reed-Sternberg cells – that are not found in any other cancerous lymphomas or cancers. [It is] These cells [that] distinguish Hodgkin's disease (HD) from non-Hodgkin's lymphomas (NHLs).[4]

Lymphomas are also staged according to their progression or severity, with Stage I being the least severe, meaning that the cancer is in at least one lymph node. Once the cancer has spread beyond the lymph system to other areas of the body, it is considered Stage IV. There are more than a dozen different types of non-Hodgkins lymphoma. How severe the lymphoma is depends on its type, location, whether or not it has spread, and how fast it is growing. Some cancers are aggressive, growing and spreading very rapidly; others grow very slowly.

A High Dose Vitamin C Regimen
Cures Hodgkins Disease

In a case study described by Maureen Kennedy Salaman in her book, *Nutrition: The Cancer Answer II*, when "Bernard Rimland, Ph.D.," world reknown for using nutrition for emotional and psychiatric disorders, was told that his teenage daughter had cancer ("a terminal type" of "Hodgkins disease, stage 4B"), he began her on a high vitamin C regimen. The cancer had aggressively attacked the teenager's "liver and kidneys." Doctors told him that they "had never seen anyone with kidneys so impaired" with the disease and she was given "six to eight months to live." Ms. Salaman says that her father immediately started her on high dose vitamin C every day – large doses – "40 grams" per day! He also gave her "a gram of niacinamide, 50 mg of the other B vitamins, 800 I.U. of vitamin E and 75,000 I.U. of vitamin A, as well as calcium, magnesium and other minerals in normal amounts."[5] The oncologists in his daughter's cancer ward had absolutely no faith in Dr. Rimland's nutritional supplement program, but his high nutritional regimen CURED his daughter's cancer. See chapter seven for more details on Dr. Rimland's vitamin C protocol that cured his teenage daughter![6]

Note that if you are taking high dose (oral) vitamin C and experience stomach upset, you can obtain buffered C crystals which have an alkaline pH and are less irritating to the stomach, or Ester-C. There are many websites that offer buffered C crystals. Natural health food stores also carry them. High dose vitamin C can also be given intravenously. (Taking the liquid C can be damaging to dental enamel, so use caution. This is why chewable vitamin C is not good for children! It can harm their tooth enamel.)

Andrographis & Non-Hodgkins Lymphoma

Andrographis is a plant that has been used for medicinal purposes for many years in Asia. Conclusive studies have shown it to be effective **(with very low toxicity)** against several different forms of cancer, including "non-Hodgkin's lymphomas." Very rarely, andrographis may cause "dizziness and heart palpitations," or mild to severe allergic reactions.[7] Andrographis can be purchased in a tablet form called *Androtech* that is standardized and produced by BioTherapies. They "combine it with Enchinacea and zinc."[8]

Ashwagandha, E. S., & Black Seed for Dalton's Ascitic Lymphoma

Dalton's lymphoma is a cancer of the T-cells. These are cells which help keep the immune system healthy, some directly killing pathogens and mutants. (If you get an organ transplant, these are the cells that will do their best to reject it!) The herb, Ashwagandha, was tested on mice with Dalton's ascitic lymphoma. The results are documented at *www.raysahelian.com/ashwagandha.html:*

> A significant increase in the life span and a decrease in the cancer cell number and tumour weight…in the tumour-induced mice after treatment with ashwagandha.…These observations are suggestive of the protective effect of ash-wagandha in Dalton's Ascitic Lymphoma.[9]

Another herb that has shown tumor inhibition against this type lymphoma is the leaves of "Elephantopus scaber" [abbreviated as E.S. above]. According to the *Indian Journal of Pharmaceutical Sciences,* "The antitumour activity of the leaves of Elephantopus scaber has been evaluated against Dalton's ascitic lymphoma (DAL) in Swiss albino mice." It extended the "survival time of mice with this cancer. Injections of the herb were found to inhibit tumour cell growth…"[10]

Black seed, sometimes referred to as black cumin has also demonstrated anti-cancer activity against Dalton's lymphoma cells. This herb contains essential fatty acids, carotene, and many nutrients. True black seed is also known as *Nigela sativa,* and is a very common spice in middle-eastern countries. This herb should not be used during pregnancy.

Beta-Glucan & Stage IV Non-Hodgkins Lymphoma

Beta-Glucan is a polysaccharide, a cultured extract derived from baker's yeast.[11] At website *AboutBetaglucan.com,* a victim of Stage IV non-Hodgkins T-cell lymphoma credits survival to beta-glucan supplements:

The doctors had given up on me after 3 years of chemotherapy and a stem cell transplant for my Stage IV non-hodgkins t-cell lymphoma. **In addition, chemo had destroyed my spleen which had to be surgically removed.** Since the standard medical community offered me no hope, I entered the world of researching alternative approaches.[12]

The patient describes the end of the ordeal:

When my health was restored through concentrating on simple things like beta glucan that anyone can do to...enhance immune function, my body went through a "reverse aging" process. I now appear young for my age especially for a person who has been through such an aging cancer ordeal.[13]

Beta-glucan supplements are available at natural health food stores and some internet sites. Another website promotes "oat" beta glucan, because "...research has demonstrated that oat beta glucan will cause a" three-fold greater immune response "as compared to yeast beta glucan. The oat product increases the production of interleukin." Interleukins are "used by the immune system cells to communicate with each other...to [help in] identifying and eliminating...cancer cells." Their webpage is at *www.cancer-treatments.net/cancer.html.*[14] Note that according to this website, there is now available an even more potent "whole cell beta glucan made from baker's yeast."[15] For more information see related website, *www.cancer-prevention.net.*

Burzynski's Antineoplastons for Lymphomas & Other Cancers

See chapter 13 in this book for more information on the non-toxic therapy of antineoplastons, which has brought many hopeless, inoperable cancer patients into total remission, even those with lymphomas and so-called "terminal" brain cancers, many of them children! The Burzynski Clinic website is at *www.cancermed.com.* Also, see the story of a woman diagnosed with fatal non-Hodgkins lymphoma treated successfully with antineoplastons at *http://www.can-cermed.com/patient_resources.php?table=patient_resources&page=8.* Her story is on Burzynski's website. When she was diagnosed, she was not expected to live. That was SEVEN years ago!

Chlorella & Bone Cancer

Refer to chapter eight for more details on the benefits of chlorella. Dr. Joseph Mercola of *www.mercola.com* states:

> It is not uncommon for people who have cancer to take as much as 30 grams of chlorella per day. One person with bone cancer showed tremendous results after 6 months of taking 20 grams of Chlorella per day....The specific dose and application of chlorella ideally should be monitored by a nutritionally oriented physician or a certified clinical nutritionist.[16]

How Flax Healed Hodgkins Lymphoma & Bone Cancer

Some amazing, even miraculous cancer cures have been attributed to flaxseed oil. Website *www.healingcancernaturally.com,* gives the case of an eleven-year-old boy, Timmy G., who was diagnosed with Hodgkins disease. After failure to respond to "24 radiation treatments...he was discharged as incurable...given six months to live and sent home to die..." Someone sent an article to his mother that led her to the use of the Budwig flax oil diet. Within "just five days" on the diet, her son's "breathing became normal for the first time in almost two years." He eventually returned to school and is now **18 years of age** and credits his life to Dr. Budwig's formula. The Budwig diet is very simple. The two main ingredients are flax oil and cottage cheese:

> For each tablespoon of flax oil, add 2 tablespoons of low-fat cottage cheese (or quark) or 6 tablespoons of yogurt. The flaxoil/cottage cheese or flaxoil/yogurt mixture should be

fully blended until no traces of oil remain visible, proving that the highly unsaturated fatty acids have become water soluble (a hand-mixer or a blender works well).[17]

See Chapter 17 of this book for more information on the healing powers of flax oil and details of the Budwig diet. (It is also discussed in greater detail in chapter 13 because of its success against brain cancer.)

Website *www.curezone.com* relates the story of an "incurable bone cancer cure" using the Budwig diet, however the patient used larger amounts of flax oil a day than the official diet calls for. He started out with 4 tablespoons of flax oil a day (plus the cottage cheese).[18] A few days later, he increased it to 8-10 tablespoons of flax oil a day combined with the cottage cheese. Three months later, all his lab work came back negative. His cancer was CURED! His physician was so incredulous that he ordered his tests three times, thinking there must be some mistake. There was no error. The patient, an **81-year-old grandfather, was in complete remission!**[19] (See chapter seven of this book for more information on natural treatments and cures for leukemia and multiple myelomas, and chapter 17.

Ginger & Willow Bark For Lymphoma

Ginger has apparent anti-cancer effects due to its immune-boosting abilities. When lab animals "with Dalton's lymphoma and Ehrlich ascites tumors" were fed ginger, the spice "extended [their] lifespan…by 11 percent."[20] Ginger also prevents dangerous clots by the "inhibition of platelet aggregation…platelets release growth factors that enhance tumor cell growth," and ginger inhibits "this process," thus it may keep cancer cells from spreading.[21]

One of the many components (out of hundreds) in ginger is geraniol. Geraniol is found not only in ginger, but rosemary as well (there are also "lesser amounts in corn and peas"). Apparently, it does not take much of this ingredient to inhibit cancer. "In tests only 0.1% of Geraniol increased the survival rate of rats with malignant tumors."[22]

Another herb that does this is willow bark. "Willow bark...contains salicin...a chemical precursor to aspirin." It can be used as a "pain reliever...to prevent heart attack," and this "same anticoagulant effect helps prevent cancer or more precisely, the spread of cancer..."[23] Be aware that you should discuss this herb with your physician, especially if you are already taking blood-thinners.

Graviola & Essiac Tea

See chapter two and chapter five of this book for information on the curative and healing properties of the herb, *Graviola,* and *Essiac tea.*

Green Tea Fights Non-Hodgkins Lymphomas

In an article on *Life Extension's* webpage, it is noted that green tea helps DNA "replicate naturally," and this tea prevented "the growth of non-Hodgkins's lymphoma cells...by 50%" when added to the diets of lab mice. A very popular chemotherapy drug, "*Cyclophosphamide,*" was also given to lab animals at the "maximum tolerable dose," **yet it "was unable to replicate" the same results as the green tea!** Researchers discovered that those cancers responding best to green tea were "breast, esophageal, liver, lung, skin, and stomach."[24]

Guacatonga & Andiroba – Two Herbs That Inhibit Sarcomas

Sarcomas are "rare types of cancer that develop in the supporting structures of the body. There are two main types: bone sarcomas and soft tissue sarcomas." As described at *www.cancerbacup.org,* Ewing's sarcoma, for example, "can start anywhere in the body. It usually develops in a bone, most commonly one of the bones of the hips, upper arm or thigh."[25] Other sarcomas can develop almost anywhere in the body. (See page 309.)

Guacatonga "*(Casearia sylvestris),*" also known as "*wild coffee,*" and a host of other common names, is a small bush or tree that grows in the Amazon and several Central and South American countries.

Multiple chemicals have been extracted from the leaves and stems, all showing impressive anti-cancer, anti-tumor properties. It appears that in some cases, it takes very small amounts of the herb to kill cancer cells. Guacatonga also contains "lapacho," a component found in pau d'arco tea.[26] Lapacho has blood-thining properties.

Japanese researchers discovered an extract from the leaf of the plant that showed very "strong antitumorous activity in laboratory mice with sarcomas…" There are no reported drug interactions or adverse effects in using this herb.[27] Contact *www.rain-tree.com* for more information.

Andiroba *"(Carapa guianensis)"* is a tree from the Rainforest that produces an oil-rich nut that looks much like "a chestnut." In 2002 researchers reported that the "seed oil could prevent and even reverse cervical dysplasia." In laboratory tests, several parts of the tree revealed "some activity against sarcoma cancer cells…." The oil is used to treat skin disorders, including skin cancers, parasites, rashes, and fungi. For more information, contact *www.rain-tree.com*.[28]

714X – Gaston Naessens

Gaston Naessens was a researcher who developed a very powerful microscope that allowed him to visualize living organisms in the blood. Gaston believed that diseases are not caused by germs, but that they come about because of disease processes. He believed that the human body with a healthy-functioning immune system will not produce diseases. From his work with *somatids*, Naessens later developed enzyme 714X to enhance the body's immunity. 714X, a combination of "camphor and nitrogen, is injected directly into the lymph system."[29] (Though 714X is not *natural* or *painless*, it is included here for informational purposes and because of its success treating various cancers.) 714X has been credited with many "cancer and AIDS" cures.[30]

For details on the amazing story of a young man who used 714X, Resperin Essiac tea®, and nutritional changes to cure his **Hodgkins lymphoma**, see website *http://www.grand-strand.com/suebest/boy-who.htm,* for "Billy's Story," as told by his parents Sue and Bill Best. You may recall seeing Billy on the news. In 1994 he was "diagnosed with Hodgkins Disease…[at] 16 years old." His parents explained that, "Not knowing any better, we took the advice of the oncologists and Billy started chemotherapy in July." He was treated until October, when he "ran away from home to get away from the chemo," leaving his parents a note "explaining that he felt the chemo was killing him rather than curing him."[31] Eventually, the news media picked up the story and it aired on two prominent TV shows in 1999. Once Billy came back home, "he was tested at the Dana Farber Cancer Institute in Boston." **The chemo had not helped him. His cancer was growing and worsening.** When his parents decided to opt out of any further chemo, radiation, or conventional treatments, the "hospital reported [them] to the Department of Social Services in Massachusetts as unfit parents and tried to have Billy taken away." However, the hospital lost, because the state refused involvement![32] The parents began alternative treatment which included using nutritional changes (e.g. no sugar or dairy products or carbonated beverages, no red meats), plenty of "fresh, organic produce…distilled water…[and] unprocessed natural foods." It was not a vegetarian diet, because he did eat "chicken, turkey and fish." They began using Resperin Corporation's Essiac tea ("nine ounces daily…for about six months…")[33]

Billy also used 714X "for 6 months," which is available from Canada at *www.cerbe.com.* Two and-a-half months later (after he began the dietary changes and the 714X injections), Billy's cancer had **completely disappeared** "(that was March 1995)" **and he has had no recurrence!** That was ten years ago! (He did continue to use the 714X for a total of 6 months.) He remains on the dietary changes, takes 4 ounces of Essiac daily, and occasionally does a "booster 21 day cycle of 714X…and gets lots of exercise with his favorite activity, skateboarding." Of chemo and radiation, his parents have this to say: "Chemotherapy and Radiation are man made and kill the body's immune system."[34]

You can read Billy's entire story at *www.grand-strand.com/suebest/boywho.htm,* and see photos as well. His parents were so impressed with Resperin Essiac®, they began taking it too and are now distributors for the tea! You can order Resperin Essiac® from their website above. He continues to do very well. In an email from his mom earlier this year (2005), she gave me permission to include part of his amazing story in this book. For those interested, 714X can be obtained from *www.cerbe.com.* The Centre expérimental de recherches biologiques de l'Estrie inc. (C.E.R.B.E. Inc.)

Hodgkins Disease & Hydrazine Sulfate

Though hydrazine sulfate is not a *natural* ingredient nor *painless* (unless given in pill form), it is embraced by many who promote alternative medicine, simply because of its effectiveness at treating so many forms of cancer (including lymphomas), and it is being included in this chapter for that reason.

Joseph Gold, M.D., of Syracuse, New York, tested and promoted the use of hydrazine sulfate as a cancer treatment.[35] Dr. Gold tested hydrazine sulfate extensively on animals before human testing. He found that with optimal dosing, he could kill cancer cells with very few adverse reactions. Not long after he published the results of the animal testing (while lecturing on the drug), a physician approached him asking for permission to use hydrazine sulfate on one of his patients whom he estimated had 3-4 days to live. Shortly after receiving the H.S., the woman improved remarkably. "Within a few weeks she was up and about."[36] H.S. was used in treating over a thousand cancer patients. Dr. Burk at the "government's cancer center," was very intrigued by Dr. Gold's results. He said that he had not seen anything comparable in his "forty-five years" working with "cancer" patients.[37] In 1973...Dr. Burk told officials at "Sloan-Kettering Institute" in New York of a remarkable cure of "Hodgkin's" disease using H.S. The patient had been bedridden for "seven weeks," had lost her appetite and was "paper-thin..." She was given the compound. As reported by Dr. Ralph Moss in his book, *The Cancer Industry*, seven days after taking the hydrazine sulfate, she was out "shopping...[and] five days later," she was outside working in her garden.[38]

Sloan-Kettering gave the drug to some of their "chemotherapists" for testing, however someone apparently dropped the ball. After the start of the study, Gold said that no one corresponded with him on the results. He "paid a surprise visit" to Sloan-Kettering and looked at records of some of the patients who had received the drug. The results were promising, but a controversy arose.[39] Gold claimed that the protocol given was inadequate and the entire testing was not conducted as he had recommended.[40] He said the study was flawed because dosing was not correct. Patients were either given double or triple the amount he ordered or they were given a few milligrams when the prescription was written for ten times as much, making it impossible to measure outcomes.

Eventually, SKI published a report that none of the patients responded effectively to the drug and the whole thing was shelved, however, in spite of all the opposition Gold experienced, H.S. was curing cancers. In one case, it was reported that a dentist not responding to conventional medicine for "Hodgkins's disease was able to return to work after only two weeks on hydrazine." He stayed in "good health" and continued to work for several years! (There were also cases of "prostate…cervical…brain…[and] lung cancer" treated with hydrazine sulfate, that went into remission.)[41]

The story of a cancer patient who used H.S. and suffered fatal liver damage was given much publicity recently, however, when you study the facts in cases like this, there is always missing information that is never given. For example, it is unknown whether or not the patient was ever told that H.S. is a MAO inhibitor. If not, and he ingested any medicines or foods that are strictly prohibited with MAO inhibitors, this could explain what happened. Also, you need to be sure that you are using reliable sources for any alternative therapies. If using H.S., be sure that you are seeing a reliable licensed natural health physician for this therapy, rather than trying to self-medicate.

When the "FDA raided" suppliers of "hydrazine sulfate," taking the drug as well as all the files connected with it, Gold was referred to as a "well-meaning zealot" whose "treatment has been lucratively promoted for two decades by 'alternative' practitioners." The drug is very in-expensive, however, as it retails for about "$20 for 100 tablets," so the treatment is hardly profitable as claimed! (Gold always believed that the tests done by SKI were skewed.)[42]

The entire story of Hydrazine Sulfate and the activity of the FDA in seizing the drug are reminiscent of others (e.g. Harry Hoxsey, Max Gerson, Gaston Naessens, and Rene Cassie), who spent a good part of their lives being constantly harassed and ridiculed by the cancer establishment, which was apparently upset that non-toxic treatments were curing more cancer cases than the toxic chemo drugs and radiation being promoted and forced onto the public. After all, why should they embrace natural, non-toxic cancer cures when doing so would mean certain death to their drug monopoly and the millions pouring into the pharmaceutical companies that many in the FDA held stock in?! And if you don't think that chemo drugs and radiation are being "forced onto the public," just try to refuse to allow a physician to give your young child toxic chemo drugs for cancer and see what happens! The state will do their best to take over custody of the child so that YOUR child can be FORCED to take chemo or radiation whether you like it or not! And forget about your *parental rights.* **You will have absolutely no say in the matter!** If you have a young child just diagnosed with cancer and you have no desire to see them go through toxic chemo drugs or radiation, you'd best be making plans to head for Canada or Mexico during the night (while you still can – or even Europe) where parents can still protect their children from American drug tzars, and the government does not try to take them away from you so that they can be given POISONS manufactured by the pharmaceutical industry! That is about the gist of your *freedom* now as an American citizen. And if you don't believe me, try it and see for yourself! (I am fearful that the day is soon coming when illegal aliens won't be trying to get across the border into America; Americans will be trying to get across the border OUT of the U.S.!)

As described at website *www.diagnose-me.com*, about 50% of the recipients who are given hydrazine sulfate in correct dosages "in the early stages of the disease, show an almost immediate weight gain and reversal of symptoms; in some instances the tumor eventually disappears."[43] The cancers that appear to respond most favorably to this therapy are "recto-colo cancer, ovarian...prostatic...lung (brochogenic)...Hodgkin's disease and other lymphomas, thyroid cancer, melanoma, and breast cancer." Other "less common types of cancer also benefit."[44] (See page 247 for Dr. Gold's address.)

Hoxsey Formula & Lymphoma

Harry Hoxsey developed an herbal tea that helped many people regain their health, yet he too was relentlessly hounded by the AMA and FDA. It is noteworthy that his herbal tea, "which contains red clover, buckthorn bark, stillingia root, barberry bark, chaparral, licorice root, cascara amarga, and prickly ash bark, along with potassium iodide...." has had good results against "lymphoma and skin cancer."[45] More details on Harry Hoxsey and his tea formula are given in other chapters of this book.

ICHT, IPT & Hyperthermia Cancer Treatments

ICHT ("Intra-Cellular Hyperthermia Therapy") according to website *www.heatkillscancer.com,* uses a new "patent pending, novel method that causes cells to be heated from the 'inside-out.'" (This is not the same as "conventional hyperthermia" which has also been used to heat the body "based on the fact that tumor cells reach lethal temperatures sooner than normal cells.") ICHT is "able to penetrate every cell in the body, including those in the brain. The net result of ICHT therapy is to convert mitochondria from efficient 'powerhouses' of energy production to 'chemical furnaces', heating cells from the 'inside-out.'"[46] (Though this is not what I would consider *natural* or *painless*, it is being included here for informational purposes.)

Cancer cells can not survive the heat generated in this process. Contact Dr. T.R. Shantha, M.D., Ph.D. and *Integrated Medical Specialists* at phone **#1-866-353-5315** *http://wehealcancer.org/contact.html* for more information. Dr. Shantha uses conventional treatments as well as alternative medicine. You can also obtain Ukrain therapy at Dr. Shantha's clinic, as well as high dose vitamin C intravenously, artemisinin therapy, chelation, laetrile, Hydrazine therapy, oral Poly-MVA, IPT therapy, and many other therapies. If you contact them, they will give you directions to their clinic in Georgia.

Again, IPT or Insulin Potentiation Therapy, is not a *natural* treatment, nor what I consider *painless,* because it is given intravenously, however, some alternative health physicians use it in combination with non-toxic cancer drugs such as Ukrain, making them work better. (As far as I know Dr. Shantha in Georgia is the only alternative medical physician that uses IPT/Ukrain therapy in combination, in the world. There may be others that I am not aware of.) Dr. Shantha says that he has used this combination to successfully treat nearly every imaginable cancer known, including pancreatic cancer, lymphomas, leukemia, myelomas, brain cancer, mesothelioma, and many others.

(Author's note: I am not affiliated with Dr. Shantha, nor can I vouch for the expertise of their clinic. This is just an informational note that you may want to research further, especially if you or a loved one are fighting a terminal cancer. I have read many success stories involving the use of Ukrain and more information is given on this amazing non-toxic compound in other chapters of this book. It appears that IPT therapy makes Ukrain work even more effectively than when given alone.)

IPT therapy uses insulin to treat cancer because insulin makes cell membranes more efficient in transporting nutrients and compounds into cells and also helps get medications across the "blood-brain barrier." First, the patient is given small doses of insulin IV, and a short while later, another medication of choice is given. Apparently, the insulin helps make the other medication given (whatever is chosen) work more effectively by getting it into the cells more rapidly. IPT also means that other drugs of choice can be given in smaller amounts, yet still be effective at killing cancer cells, while minimizing the adverse "side effects" that larger doses would cause (if they happen to be drugs that cause adverse "side effects!") IPT has been used to treat not only "many types of cancer," but "arthritis and related rheumatic syndromes…pancreatic cancer, multiple sclerosis, [and] paralysis after stroke."[47]

I do not advocate the use of chemo, though it is sometimes used with IPT therapy. If you are fighting cancer, whether or not you choose to allow your physician to "experiment" on you with chemo will have to be **YOUR** decision. Hopefully, the information on the many non-toxic alternative cancer therapies in this book will give you the background that you need to assist you in choosing the treatment you feel most comfortable with. Either way, be sure to read chapter 13 and 35 before you make that important decision!

Psoralea Seed & Osteosarcoma

Osteosarcoma is a malignant bone tumor. The herb psoralea (*"Psoralea corylifolia"*) contains compounds that may be important in keeping "osteosarcoma and lung cancer cells" from multiplying, and may help prevent the development of "secondary lung cancer." Psoralea seed can be found in capsule form. This compound causes an increased sensitivity to sunlight, so stay out of the sun if you are using psoralea. Use "Ginger tea…if mild stomach upset occurs."[48]

Shark Liver Oil & Hodgkins Lymphoma

In his book, *Miracle Food Cures From the Bible*, Reese Dubin discusses the case of a patient who developed an enormous mass on top of her heart. She was diagnosed with "Hodgkins lymphoma." She started out with standard medical treatment, but **did not respond**. Finally, in the last stage of the disease, she began taking "shark-liver oil with 30-40 percent AKGs, but with vitamins A and D removed to prevent overdosing on those vitamins." She began a gradual improvement. Within 7 months, says Dubin, she was "completely free of the Hodgkins lymphoma," and continues to take shark liver oil.[49] (Note that shark cartilage and shark liver oil are two entirely different supplements.)

Thymus Extract Successfully Treats Lymphomas

In an article at *cancertutor.com*, the results of a remarkable controlled study involving the use of "calf thymus extract" on humans with "fatal lymphocytic" tumors and "lesions (Letterer-Siwe disease, Hand-Schuller-Christian disease and esinophilic granuloma") were reported in the "New England Journal of Medicine…."[50] It was noted that "17" of the cancer "patients" in the study were injected on a daily basis with the "thymic extract." The control group, on the other hand, (a total of "20" patients) received "chemotherapy." Of the 17 people who received the extract, ten were in "full remission after one year." *Cancertutor.com* says that "Seven" either showed "no change" or worsened "after 28 days and therapy was discontinued." This "remission rate" was "statistically comparable" in those who received chemo, with ONE big difference! Those receiving thymus extract had **absolutely NONE of the side effects experienced by the group receiving chemo!** [51]

Thymus extract from calves is not a natural substance, and though I recommend natural substances over those that are synthetic or animal in origin, **whenever possible**, if I knew someone suffering from *terminal* lymphoma, I certainly would NOT tell them to avoid this extract, especially in comparison to something as toxic as chemotherapy and radiation!

Selenium & Vitamin C Heal a "Fatal" Lymphoma

According to website *DoctorYourself.com,* selenium and vitamin C are crucial in treating severe lymphoma. Dr. Abram Hoffer, M.D., Ph.D., in writing about the importance of these two supplements, believes that "the toxicity of selenium has been greatly exaggerated."[52] He recounts the experience he had in treating a patient from Chile, who had fatal lymphoma. The patient had surgery, but the cancer returned. **He received radiation and still the cancer returned.** He was told that he had "three months to live."[53] Dr. Hoffer started him on 600 **mcg** of selenium a day. However, the patient, thinking "like many patients…if 600 is good, more is even better. He came back and said he was taking 2 mg per day, or 2,000 mcg." Dr. Hoffer was, of course, alarmed about such a huge dosage of selenium:

> I became a bit concerned about that and suggested he cut down to 1,000. [mcg.] In any event, he recovered and he has now been alive for seven years. **There is no evidence of tumor**, and his major problem today is reorienting himself in a foreign culture.[54] [Remember that this patient was given THREE MONTHS to live and that was **SEVEN years ago**!]

Dr. Hoffer, as part of his cancer treatment program said: "I use selenium and I use a lot of it. I use some zinc, especially for prostatic cancers and I do use calcium-magnesium preparations." He also uses B vitamins, vitamin E, beta carotene and large dosages of vitamin C, of which he says:

> I am convinced today that vitamin C is the most important single nutrient that one can give to any person with cancer. The dose is variable. I find that most patients can…[take] 12 grams per day without much difficulty, that's the crystallin (sic) vitamin C sodium ascorbate or calcium ascorbate. They take one teaspoon three times per day. If they do not develop diarrhea, I ask them to increase it until this occurs [the diarrhea] and then to cut back below that level.[55]

Ewing's Sarcoma Cured

Dr. Abram Hoffer has also used high dose vitamin C in combination with large doses of niacinamide to cure a case of Ewing's sarcoma. His teenage patient had already been scheduled to have her arm removed due to the presence of Ewing's sarcoma. When she followed Dr. Hoffer's simple daily regimen of 1000mg of niacinamide and 1000 mg. of vitamin C after each meal, she rebounded completely, did not need the amputation, and went on to lead a normal life![56] Realize that if you decide to take a powdered form of ascorbic acid (that you mix with water), ascorbic acid taken this way is very hard on your teeth enamel! Another reason why chewable vitamin C is not good for children!

Dr. Hoffer has also had great success treating schizophrenia patients with niacinamide and other vitamins and minerals. (See his webpage at *www.islandnet.com/~hoffer* for more information.) Note that niacin causes your skin to flush, because of its ability to open up the capillaries in the body, increasing blood flow. You may also experience some itching with the flush, but this is all temporary and not harmful. It is actually good for the body. Niacinamide does not cause the flush, but neither will it open up the circulation like niacin. Niacin also has the ability to lower harmful cholesterol levels, something that niacinamide will not do.

Dr. Hoffer also reports that as far back as the late eighties, scientists knew the benefits of niacin in cancer prevention: "The 1987

Texas conference organizers have hypothesized that niacin prevents cancer. They treated two groups of human cells with carcinogens. The group given adequate niacin developed tumors at a rate only 10 percent of the rate in the group deficient in niacin." Dr. Hoffer says that "Very rarely niacin will cause obstructive jaundice which clears when the niacin is stopped."[57] If you are a physician, see his book, *Orthomolecular Medicine for Physicians.*

Ukrain

Ukrain is a **non-toxic** drug produced by combining two drugs that are toxic when given individually! Once combined, the drug is only toxic to **cancer cells**! There are several chapters in this book that discuss the remarkable ability of Ukrain therapy to bring about total remission in some cancer patients. Refer to them for more information on Ukrain. Also, recall the information above on Dr. T. R. Shantha, M.D., Ph.D., who uses Ukrain in combination with IPT at his clinic in Georgia, *Integrated Medical Specialists.* They can be reached at #1-866-353-5315. Their website is *http://wehealcancer.org/contact.html.* There are many alternative health physicians in Canada and Europe who administer Ukrain therapy, as well as others in the U.S. The main website for Ukrain is *www.ukrin.com.* It is the Ukrainian Anti-Cancer Institute.

How Wheat Grass Juice Cured Lymphatic Cancer

Dennis Lampron of "Chicago, Illinois" was given three months to live even if he took chemotherapy for lymphatic cancer. He began a disciplined regimen of wheat grass juice, raw foods, and fasting. Within six months, his illness was completely gone. Not only did he regain his health, his natural hair color returned. Premature gray hair was a family trait, but at 31-years-of-age, he was no longer gray![58]

Poly–MVA for Lymphomas & Sarcomas

See chapters 9 and 13 for more information on this amazing, non-toxic nutritional formula that many cancer survivors who were told they were "hopeless" are crediting to their complete recovery, many of them without ever resorting to chemo or radiation! Their main website is *www.polymva.net.*

CHAPTER 16

GOD'S GREAT GRASSES

"Pharmaceutical drugs are killing hundreds of thousands of people every year...In spite of that, they claim that two people were hurt with chaparral, so they have taken it off the market. And these claims aren't even substantiated."

—*Dick Shulze, N.D.*[1]

Wheat Grass – The Miracle Nutrient

Ann Wigmore was so impressed by the health effects of fresh wheat grass on her life that she not only wrote books about it, but she founded the *Hippocrates Health Institute* in Boston, where her guests were treated to a life of natural health living with a strict raw foods regimen. For years, many people came to the *Wigmore Mansion* as it was called, some with terminal illnesses. Many left cured of their illnesses, including Eydie Mae Hunsberger (a patient discussed earlier in this book in chapter three), who cured her breast cancer while on the Wigmore diet. Ann Wigmore healed her own body of many ailments by ingesting fresh wheat grass juice. In her own words: "The real proving ground was my own body, which was sickly and weak after twenty years of living and eating as an average American." She explains what happened next: "A few weeks after I started chewing and juicing young blades of fresh wheatgrass, and eating fresh sprouts and greens, a festering case of colitis that I had suffered with for months began to improve..."[2]

Ann notes that the colitis eventually healed up completely. Though she felt that a vegetarian diet of raw foods was very beneficial for health maintenance, she considered wheat grass juice "the most powerful and safest healing aid there is. Not because it can attack and destroy bacteria or malignant cells," but due to its stimulating effect on the body's immunity.[3]

Wheat grass juice is very rapidly assimilated into the body when taken. It does not need 30-60 minutes to go through the digestive process, since the nutrients are almost immediately absorbed into your cells. If you are fighting a debilitating illness, see chapter 35 for more information on why you need rapid assimilation of powerful antioxidants to heal your immune system. You need nutrition that is immediately available and not taxing on your body!

Wheat Grass Regimen Used Successfully To Treat Primary Peritoneal Cancer in 89-Year-Old

When an 89-year-old woman was diagnosed with "Stage IIIA, Grade 3, papillary serous carcinoma...in the left ovary and omentum" in October of 1999, she underwent surgery to remove the cancer, but refused the "traditional 6-round chemotherapy with paclitaxel and cisplatin" that her oncologist prescribed. Instead, she opted for a nutritional, alternative cancer remedy involving the use of wheat grass juice, even though her "oncologist...family physician...gynecologist, and a referred John Hopkins oncologist tried to convince her to "accept chemotherapy." (Her "CA–125" was "elevated" at "1040.")[4]

According to website *CancerLynx.com,* in their 7/8/02 article, the patient followed a nutritional regimen that included "Wheat grass, coenzyme Q-10, and bovine cartilage" post-surgery as follows:

100 mg of coenzyme Q-10, 2 grams of wheat grass, and 9 grams of bovine cartilage per day. The wheat grass was initiated within 1 week of surgery...100 milligrams of coenzyme Q-10 was added to the regime 1 week after the wheat grass, and 9 grams of the bovine cartilage followed 2 weeks later. By the end of the first month from surgery...the patient was receiving all three components of the nutritional therapy...the Q-10 dosage was increased to 150 mg per day approximately 9 months into the regime.[5]

As a result of this regimen, the patient began a gradual improvement in her health. She went from "111 pounds after the surgery to a high of 124 pounds, and she has maintained her weight at about 120 pounds for the past several months." Her "major organ functions have been normal since her surgery," and she has had "no pain."[5a] She has been "able to work around the house and yard." When she started having pain in July of 2001, it was found to be from arthritis, which was present before the surgery. The website notes that the last CA-125 test done on 8/21/01 was in "the low end of the normal range," at 8. What was the conclusion at the end of this case study in 2001? That "the primary peritoneal cancer is in remission...[and] has not metastasized." The patient continues on the nutritional regimen.[6]

An elevated CA-125 blood test may not necessarily be an indicator for ovarian cancer. CA-125, as explained at *www.labtestsonline.org*, "measures a protein in the blood that is elevated in about 80% of ovarian cancers derived from the surface cells," but "it is not specific enough to be used as a general screening tool."[6a] (Note that *labtestsonline* is a non-commercial website published by the American Association for Clinical Chemistry. For up-to-date information on clinical lab tests, visit their website: *www.labtestsonline.org.)*

High CA-125 levels are also "seen in other cancer, in hepatitis, pelvic inflammatory disease, and endometriosis as well as early pregnancy and menstruation. It is mainly used as a tumor marker to monitor ovarian cancer treatment and to help detect early recurrence of cancer." It can be used diagnostically along "with a transvaginal and/or pelvic ultrasound to help diagnose ovarian cancer."[6b]

Other tests used in conjunction with CA-125 to aid in diagnosing diseases such as ovarian cancer include "AFP (alpha feto protein) and hCG (human chorionic gonadotropin," levels of which are "often elevated in some ovarian cancers derived from the germ cells, but they are also elevated during pregnancy.... BRCA-1 and BRCA-2 are tests for two genetic mutations that have been associated with an increased risk of ovarian and breast cancer." If you have a genetic tendency in your family for "breast or ovarian cancer," your physician may choose any or all of these tests to diagnose or rule out disease.[6c]

Benefits of Purchasing a Juicer

For those of you who *are* already ill, one of the very first and most important things you can do is to purchase a juicer. Be sure that you obtain a juicer that has the capacity to juice not only fresh vegetables and fruits, but green foods like spinach, broccoli, and wheat grass, as well! Some juicer manufacturers will claim that their juicers can juice wheatgrass, but they do a very poor job of it. The juice will come out very foamy and warm, so that it has oxidized all its vital enzymes during the juicing process.

Types of Juicers

There are several good juicers on the market that will juice wheat grass as well as fresh vegetables and fruits. Four very good choices that juice wheat grass, vegetables, and fruits are the Samson juicer, the Green Star, the Green Power juicer, and the Omega 8003 juicer. These type juicers can sometimes be found at local natural health food stores, or they can be ordered or purchased on the internet. If your local health food store does not have the model you desire, they can usually order it for you. (The first large juicer I purchased was a *Champion*. I read on the internet that it did not do a good job of juicing grapes, but mine juiced grapes wonderfully. However, it juiced everything wonderfully EXCEPT greens!) There are manual juicers that juice wheat grass only that are very economical, as well as electric juicers made just for juicing wheat grass. However, if you buy one of these, you will need another juicer for your fruits and vegetables. An excellent manual juicer is the *Miracle* manual wheat grass juicer. *Miracle* also makes electric wheat grass juicers, but as stated earlier, if you get this type, you will need a separate juicer for your fruits and vegetables.

If you juice citrus fruits such as oranges and grapefruits in your main juicer, you will need to peel them first, or you can obtain a very inexpensive citrus juicer for about twelve dollars just for oranges, grapefruits, lemons and limes at your local department store or pharmacy; then, your main juicer can be one that does vegetables, other fruits (such as berries, apples, grapes, cantaloupe, etc.) and greens. Good choices of juicers that do it all are the four listed above. They will juice greens as well as veggies and fruits (without oxidizing the enzymes out of your greens), and the Omega 8003 is said to take 5 minutes for cleanup and costs about $259. Dr. Joseph Mercola at *www.mercola.com,* recommends and markets the Omega 8003 at his website.

A good rule of thumb to remember is that the softer the fruit you are juicing, the thicker the juice will be. You will get a much thicker juice from soft pears than hard pears. Strawberries, pineapples and berries will give you very thick, mushy-type juice. You can dilute it with water and other juices and drink it, or freeze it in popsicles, a healthy treat for kids! A general rule of thumb is that one pound of produce will give you approximately 6-8 ounces of juice. If you want an eight ounce glass of carrot juice, for example, be prepared to purchase about one pound of carrots. However, yield will also depend on the type juicer you choose as well. Some juicers extract more efficiently and you get more juice from your produce. The drier the pulp that comes out, the more juice you are getting. The 6-8 ounce rule does not apply to juicing greens. Yield depends on many variables such as the type of greens you are juicing and the type machine you are using. The Norwalk juicer is said to be the "cadillac" of juicers, but it is very expensive – about $2,000. I have heard users complain that it takes 30 minutes to clean after each use, but it gives an excellent yield and quality of juice, possibly 50% more than less expensive models. It is often used at health institutions, and you can order it on the internet.

What to Juice?

If you are seriously ill, purchasing a juicer that provides you with fresh wheat grass juice, vegetable and fruit juices is one of the most important **first steps** you can take for your health. You can also use green powdered drinks. If you want to boost your immune system and prevent sickness in the first place, juicing is not an option, it is a lifestyle that you will need to incorporate, along with fresh air, exercise, sunshine, and other tenets of health as described in this book. You will soon find that investing in a juicer has priceless benefits that far outweigh your initial cost!

Fresh wheat grass juice detoxifies the body so rapidly, only small amounts can be tolerated at a time. Start out consuming more than an ounce or two at a time and you will become nauseated or dizzy, simply because of the quick detox effect. You can gradually work up to larger amounts as needed. The same applies for beet root juice.

Wheat grass and other green juices are excellent sources of calcium and chlorophyll. Many people have been led to believe that we must get our calcium from milk, dairy products and supplements. This is not true. Even carrot juice is higher in calcium than milk! The best source of calcium is the SAME place that the cows and goats extract it! They get it from the soil – green plants in the soil! Your very best and most natural source of calcium is **green foods!** And you don't have to worry about whether or not your body is going to absorb the calcium when you ingest it in this format. The cells literally inhale it! (They know a good thing when they see it coming!) You can often purchase fresh wheat grass in trays at your health food store, or kits where you can try growing your own! It is also available in frozen cubes in many health food stores that you thaw and use as needed.

Grasses such as wheat grass are rich in 17 amino acids (including the 8 "essential" amino acids), as well as dozens of different enzymes. They are also rich in many vitamins, minerals, trace minerals, and essential fatty acids.[7] Because of this rich supply of nutrients, green foods and fresh juices are excellent for women who are pregnant.

It has been proven in many cases that cancer can be induced in laboratory animals by simply depriving them of specific minerals, vitamins or enzymes. Is it any wonder that fresh wheat grass juice with it's multiplicity of nutrients is so beneficial to the immune system?

Green Powders vs. Fresh

A word about green powders: there are some excellent green powders on the market. If you do not have the time to juice before leaving the house in the morning, powders are an acceptable alternative. You can even take the powdered drinks with you and mix them during the day for a healthy alternative to coffee and soda.

Dee Simmons' company, *Ultimate Living,* produces *Green Miracle*, an excellent green powder choice. Her green powder is advertised as pharmaceutical grade pure, containing 80 ingredients including: kamut, wheat grass, barley grass, spirulina, chlorella, flax seed, bee pollen, apple fiber, astragalus, reishi, papain, bromelain, curcumin, lutein, lycopene, carrot, beet, pepper powder and many other ingredients! You can find Dee's popular health food products at her website: *www.ultimateliving.com.*

Green Kamut® is a powdered wheat grass juice and *Just Barley™* organic green juice, and *Barley Green™* contain barley only. Many green powdered drinks on the market, such as *Green Miracle,* not only contain green grasses, but medicinal mushrooms, minerals, spirulina, chlorella, vitamins, enzymes, herbs, and fibers that you would not get merely consuming powdered barley, algae or alfalfa.

When possible, try to consume grasses (like wheat grass) in their most natural state while they are alive. Doing this in combination with an excellent green powdered drink will boost the immune system and ensure optimal health. (Note that whole leaf dried wheat grass actually has more chlorophyll than the fresh juice. This is because, once powdered, it is more concentrated.)

A few of the health food stores in the area where I live have fresh juice bars. You can order an ounce or two of fresh squeezed wheat grass and they will make it for you in minutes while you wait. They also juice fresh carrots, celery, beets, and smoothie mixes. Many people who can not invest in the time and expense of a juicer, obtain their fresh juices at a juice bar, though after a period of time, you will spend enough at a juice bar to pay for a juicer!

When using fresh wheat grass juice, it is best to consume it within ten minutes of the time it is juiced. After that amount of time (unless it is frozen), the living enzymes begin to oxidize rapidly. The same is true of any fresh squeezed juice. This is one reason why store-bought canned and bottled juices are no comparison to fresh-squeezed. By the time they are bottled, canned, packaged, homogenized or pasteurized, all of the LIVING enzymes in them have been zapped! You may get a few benefits from the Vitamin C (that is often added), but the syrups, sugars, food colorings and preservatives that may also be added, provide empty calories and possible carcinogens. It is possible to find bottled juices at health food stores that have no added sugars and preservatives. There are some brands that are even "flash pasteurized," but you have to check the expiration dates. They have a short shelf life. There are even a few commercial juicers that are finally getting the message that we don't want additives, food coloring, preservatives and sugar put into our juices, no matter how pretty the color, and a few of them are coming out with better quality juices.

There is ONE exception when it comes to consuming wheat grass immediately after juicing. The late "Dr. Virginia Livingston-Wheeler," who operated a "clinic that cured cancer patients," used a "vaccine…based on abscisic acid" [an ingredient in wheat grass juice], and according to her, "the hormone abscisic acid (ABA) is 40 times more potent **4 hours** after cutting the wheatgrass than it is at the time of cutting." As *cancertutor.com* website asks: "what do you do, eat it immediately or 4 hours after you cut it? Perhaps both." They suggest that you "drink most of it immediately," then "4 hours later you drink the rest of it."[8] In this manner, you are getting the benefit of live enzymes as advocated by Ann Wigmore in consuming the juice within ten minutes of making it, and you are still getting large amounts of the abscisic acid 4 hours later.

Fresh squeezed juices are also excellent for children. Be sure though, before giving them to young children, you check with their pediatrician. Infants and very young children do not have the intestinal maturity to assimilate many of the nutrients in raw juices that older children are capable of, plus many of them are too acidic. **Never give honey and other bee products to children under two years of age**. (Some pediatricians will let children <u>over</u> one-year-old take honey products.) The spores found in honey can not be assimilated by young children and babies. The result can be the formation in a child's intestines of **infant botulism,** a deadly toxin!

Sea grasses or *sea vegetables,* as they are sometimes called, belong to a family of *grasses* that will be discussed later in this chapter. Some of the sea vegetables recommended by Ann Wigmore were "arame, dulse, hiziki, kelp, kombu, nori [and] wakame." She recommended soaking sea veggies "in enough warm (not hot) water to cover, for 20 minutes or until they are soft enough to slice," then to pitch the water when you are done because it is "extremely high" in "sodium (salt) content."[9]

How Wheatgrass Juice Healed Gangrene & Colon Cancer

Ann Wigmore had good reason to trust in green grasses for vibrant health. She had first-hand experience about the miraculous healing powers of green grasses. As described by Steve Meyerowitz in his book, *Wheatgrass Nature's Finest Medicine*, Ann had a bumpy start in life. Born prematurely, she was not a healthy child. Her parents left her behind when they decided to travel to America to seek "a new life." She was taken in by "her grandmother, a self-taught naturalist," credited to helping Ann to regain "normal health."[9a] At 16, she traveled to the states to try to get an "education" and to "reunite with her estranged parents." Ann immediately adopted the "American diet" and later was diagnosed with "colon cancer," explains Mr. Meyerowitz. She was also involved in a tragic car accident that "shattered both her legs."[9b] When Ann developed gangrene, her physicians insisted on amputations to save her life, but she refused. Ann went back to her grandmother's diet of fresh "vegetables, grains, seeds and greens," and completely restored her health. "She picked wild weeds and greens," eating anything green she could find. When fresh greens ran out, she began sprouting them in her kitchen. Her gangrenous legs eventually healed completely, and "years later," she "ran in the Boston Marathon."[10]

Ann died at 85 years of age "of smoke inhalation in a middle-of-the night fire that destroyed" the "original *Hippocrates Institute*" that she founded, however, it eventually expanded to "six locations in the USA" and clinics in several other countries.[11]

Wheat Grass Treats Breast, Bladder, Colon, Liver, Throat Cancers, Melanoma, & Lymphatic Cancer

In his book, *Wheat Grass Nature's Finest Medicine*, Steve Meyerowitz, describes several cases of people who used wheat grass juice to regain their health after devastating illnesses:

See chapter 3 of this book for the story of Anne-Marie Baker, a "registered nurse" from "Ft. Meyers, Florida," who cured her own breast cancer without surgery, chemo or radiation, simply by switching to a raw food diet and using "6-9 oz." of wheat grass juice daily, along with "...supplements, exercise, and detox."[12]

Dorothy Naylor of "Naples, Florida," used wheat grass juice to cure herself of multiple bladder tumors. She purchased a "Green Power juicer," working up to drinking several ounces of wheat grass juice per day.[13]

Gary Garrett of "Gainesville, Florida" was given a poor prognosis when colon cancer metastasized to six lymph nodes and his liver. Physicians told him that chemotherapy and radiation would buy him **six months of life**. He refused both and began a wheat grass regimen. He lived another three years, then died while hospitalized for five weeks for a liver infection during a time he did not have access to fresh wheatgrass juice! His wife felt that had he been able to get access to fresh wheat grass juice during that time, he would still be alive.[14]

Neva Whetzel of "Singers Glen, Virginia" used wheat grass juice to heal herself of melanoma. She refused the "chemotherapy and radiation" that was recommended, only allowing the actual surgical removal of the melanoma itself, though her physician wanted to do much more extensive surgery. She not only used wheat grass, but "barley, Kamut...[and] the powdered grasses..."[15]

Dennis Lampron, of "Chicago, Illinois" was given three months to live IF he took chemotherapy for metastasizing lymph cancer. He took the chemo, then began a disciplined regimen of wheat grass juice, raw foods, and fasting. Within six months, his illness was completely gone. Not only did he regain his health, his natural hair color returned. Premature gray hair was a family trait, but at 31-years-of-age, he was no longer gray![16] (Ann Wigmore also stated that wheat grass restored her natural hair color after her fiftieth birthday.)

Wheat grass juice is not a panacea or *silver bullet* cure-all, though it may be close! Restoring health after a devastating illness is a combination of many factors. Nutritional juicing is just one of those factors. Wheat grass aids the body in healing itself. It is an amazing boost for the immune system. Cancer and autoimmune disorders happen when the immune system is ill. As Dee Simmons, Eydie Mae Hunsberger, Eric Gardiner, George Malkmus, Dr. Kristine Nolfi, and many others discovered, if you heal your immune system, your immune system will get you well! Ann Wigmore found that not only did wheat grass juice help cancer patients who came to her for help, but it also treated arthritis, emphysema, multiple sclerosis, and many other ailments.

Wheat Grass & Alkalinity

Wheat grass is very alkaline. Ann Wigmore said that it had been used to treat digestive problems, "ulcerative colitis...itchy or scaly scalp," sore throat, sore gums, sick pets, as an external poultice for skin problems, and a disinfectant, as well as for many other chronic health problems. It is high in chlorophyll.[17] Did you know that most of the expensive mouth washes and breath fresheners sold in your dentist's office merely use chlorophyll to kill the bacteria that cause bad breath?

Ann Wigmore advocated in the Hippocrates diet, raw fresh foods, fruits, vegetables, fresh juices, nothing cooked. (This was a total vegan diet, NO MEATS and no dairy products!) Sometimes cancer patients are so weak and debilitated that they can not tolerate a totally raw diet. It is easier for them to gradually convert to a totally raw diet over a period of time, however, in most cases, the sooner they make this total transition the better off they are, because, when facing a terminal illness, time becomes a very precious commodity!

Chlorophyll is one of the most important nutrients in fresh green juices like wheat grass. Stephen Blauer in *The Juicing Book*, describes chlorophyll as a "super blood and cell builder, cleanser, and overall regenerative tonic."[18] In fact, chlorophyll is so "similar" to the "hemoglobin molecule," it has been discovered that animals have the capacity to actually change "chlorophyll into hemoglobin..." Some scientists believe that we humans may have the same capacity![19]

What an amazing ability! Perhaps one day, patients needing blood transfusions, will be drinking chlorophyll products instead, thus eliminating all the potential complications related to receiving blood products. Is it any wonder that green drinks are so beneficial to leukemia patients and those with anemia and other blood disorders?

Deanna K. Loftis, R.N., B.B.A.

Seaweed

Seaweed is consumed in large amounts in Asian countries, but Americans rarely touch it. According to Dr. Earl Mindell in his book, *Earl Mindell's Soy Miracle*, there are many different types of seaweed: "*Nori,* a red seaweed, is used to wrap sushi." There are also "brown" algaes or seaweeds including "kelp, *wakame, arame* and *kombu."*[20]

Dr. Mindell also points out that there are ingredients in seaweed that may inhibit cancer formation. Scientists believe that these substances prevent cancer by boosting the immune system, and that they can prevent or "slow down the growth of cancer cells...seaweed also helps reduce cholesterol levels, and may help rid the body of toxic metals. *Nori* can be eaten right out of the package...or used as a seasoning in stews. *Wakame* is good in salads."[21]

Researchers conducted a study in 1974 which "showed that not only could **kelp** prevent the development of breast cancer, but it could also treat tumors that had already begun growing. Kelp slowed the progression of breast malignancies in 95 percent of test animals. Sixty-six percent of them went into complete remission."[22]

It is believed that a chemical in kelp, "fucoidan," contributes to its cancer preventative effects, but seaweed also has very powerful "antibiotic" effects, which means it may be helpful in "preventing or treating colon cancer" as well.[23]

As described by author J. E. O'Brien in *The Miracle of Garlic & Vinegar*, research done at the "University of Hawaii School of Medicine in Honolulu" revealed that "a dried version of...wakame" could help "cure and prevent lung cancer when injected into laboratory animals." Scientists have shown that an ingredient in seaweed has blood pressure lowering effects and that it "appears to act as an antidote to excess sodium consumption and may well help prevent strokes..."[24]

A word of caution: be sure to consult with your licensed health care practitioner before ingesting seaweeds such as kelp, especially if you have any sort of thyroid disorder, because of its iodine content.

Spirulina

"Spirulina," another green food, when taken as a supplement, is still considered a "whole food" because the entire plant is "contained in the supplement" that you take, not merely an extract of the plant.[25]

Dr. Mark Stengler in his book, *the Natural Physician's Healing Therapies*, says that most of the world's spirulina is produced by the "U.S...followed by Thailand, India, and China..."[25a] An ingredient in spirulina known as "Phycocyanin," is an important "phytonutrient" responsible for the "dark blue-green color" of the plant. It has the ability to increase the body's "red blood cells" in animal tests, and can fight cancer as well as viruses.[25b] It has also been used to treat "high cholesterol, hypertension, and diabetes," and it is believed to combine itself with toxic "metals" so that they can be eliminated from the system, explains Dr. Stengler. Spirulina helps the survival of "beneficial bacteria" in the intestines, and it is used in underdeveloped nations "to prevent blindness in malnourished children."[26]

There have been no known "toxic side effects" to spirulina, and even though it has large amounts of "nucleic acids and protein," Dr. Stengler says that it does not "cause problems for people who have gout." It is a helpful detoxifier, stabilizes blood sugar and appears to boost the immune system.[26a] "B12 deficiency anemia...a concern for strict vegetarians" can be prevented by supplementing with spirulina.[27] You can also take vitamin B12 as a sublingual tablet that dissolves under the tongue, or injections from your physician. You may want to check out Dr. Andrew W. Saul's recipe for a nasal delivery form of B12 at *http://www.doctoryourself.com/nasal.html.*

C. M. Hawken, in his book *Green Foods – "Phyto-Foods" for Super Health,* describes Spirulina's ability to boost the immune system by enhancing "bone marrow cells, killer cells, macrophages, and T-cells."[28] Thus, spirulina may be especially beneficial to those who are fighting blood disorders such as leukemia, anemia, or multiple myelomas.

Spirulina & Mouth Cancer

Spirulina has also proven useful in the treatment of mouth cancer. Researchers gave "tobacco chewers" with "oral leukoplakia…1 gram a day of spirulina" over twelve months. Almost 50% of the participants receiving the spirulina had significant "improvement," while a mere "3 out of 43 in the non-supplement group had any reversal of symptoms."[29]

Barley Grass Used to Heal Carcinoma

Researchers from Japan "discovered a protein, *P4-D1*– in barley grass juice," which appears to shield cells from dangerous "ultraviolet radiation." Using chlorophyll (such as that found in barley grass) as therapy has actually "saved limbs from amputation..," and one of the greatest advantages to using chlorophyll is that there are NO toxic side effects![30] (Recall that this is how Ann Wigmore cured her own case of gangrene!)

In *Miracle Food Cures From The Bible*, Reese Dubin describes the story of a "33-year-old Chinese-American…from Los Angeles," who was referred to an oncologist for a skin condition and diagnosed with a "rare form of melanocarcinoma…" Physicians wanted to treat her with "chemotherapy and radiation…" She refused because of their toxic effects on the body. Instead, she began drinking **barley juice** from Japan called "*bakuryokuso*….She took 1 teaspoon in a glass of juice or plain water with every meal…[and] within seven weeks [the] melanocarcinoma began subsiding."[31]

The power of green grasses has been attributed mainly to their chlorophyll content.[32] Chlorophyll is such a speed healer, that D. H. Collings proved that wounds took less time to heal when taking this nutrient than when using "penicillin, vitamin D, sulfanilamide, or no treatment." It has also been used successfully to treat many other diseases such as "endocarditis...peptic ulcers [and] pancreatitis," and poses no problems for individuals with "gluten allergies."[33] Chlorophyll increases clotting time, which helps to balance out the effects of vitamin K in green foods, which decreases clotting time.

Chlorella

Chlorella "*(Chlorella vulgaris),*" another green food "is a single-celled algae found in fresh water. It has the highest levels of chlorophyll of any plant: more than three times that of spirulina." This is reported by C. M. Hawken in *Green Foods "Phyto-Foods" for Super Health.* Due to its high level of chlorophyll, it is very cell-protective.[34]

Nutrient dense foods, such as chlorella, as well as fresh fruits and vegetables, can counter-attack free radicals and their insidious effects, thus wiping them out before they can harm us. Chlorella has the ability to remove toxic "metals like cadmium and uranium" from the body, and many studies have been done that support the ability of chlorella to boost the immune system.[35] Research has shown that chlorella can also halt the "progression of" and "even reverse" cancerous malignancies due to its ability to raise the body's levels of "interferon."[36]

Chlorella and other green grasses also enable the body to maintain a state of alkalinity, rather than acidity. A high acid environment generates free radicals and causes the leaching of calcium out of the bones to alkalize the blood. Keeping the body in a state of alkalinity fights free radicals and prevents this calcium leaching from the bones, thus preventing osteoporosis and other degenerative diseases.

Chlorophyll, found in all green plants, soothes the colon and rebuilds damaged intestinal cells, prevents the proliferation of harmful microbes in the intestines, heals "peptic ulcers, spastic colitis, ulcerative colitis...," purifies the liver, and increases bowel "regularity."[37]

Remember that there are many other "grasses" that are part of what we consider "green" foods, all of which are not discussed in detail here. Some of these include: "[d]ulse...broccoli, spinach, parsley...celery, kale, cabbage, kamut grass, rice grass, oat grass, and many others."[38]

Alfalfa

Though "not technically a *grass*," alfalfa has nutritive value comparable to "the cereal grasses" because it contains many of the same minerals and vitamins. Alfalfa sprouts are especially nutritious. As noted by C. M. Hawken in *Green Foods: "Phyto-Foods" for Super Health,* approximately one-half cup of sprouts has "double the calcium of lettuce and is extremely high in phosphorus." This green food also has all "eight essential amino acids."[39]

Individuals with a diagnosis of **lupus** should **avoid alfalfa products**, as alfalfa appears to have the ability to cause lupus to flare. Lupus is an auto-immune disorder. Auto-immune disorders are symptoms of a sick immune system. You may be told that if you have lupus, your immune system is too strong and it is attacking your own body, however, your body is being attacked, not because of an immune system that is too strong, but one that is SICK. When the immune system is ill, it becomes confused, attacking indiscriminately, causing debilitating diseases. See chapter 35 in this book on *What To Do If You Are Already Ill*, for help in healing the immune system.

Sprouts

Ann Wigmore was so convinced of the high nutritional value of fresh sprouts that she not only grew them for her clients, she incorporated them into her meals on a daily basis and wrote a book called, *The Sprouting Book!* In her words, "When used in abundance, sprouts have the power to keep your body young by giving your cells high-quality nourishment and helping to cleanse them of toxic wastes."[40]

Sprouts are so nutritious and easily digestible, that Ann Wigmore believed that when consumed, they are nearly capable of digesting themselves! They are very high in beneficial enzymes (that aid digestion), amino acids (plant proteins), and many vitamins. The human body has the ability to manufacture 14 essential amino acids, but there are "eight essential amino acids" that must be obtained through outside nutritive sources, and sprouts have all eight! In *The Sprouting Book*, Ann Wigmore said that "Right up until the moment you eat a fresh raw sprout, it is growing and increasing in nutritional value." This is not true with other living foods such as raw fruits and vegetables, whose nutrient value begins going downhill as soon as they are picked or cut.[41]

Ann Wigmore also said that an excellent source "of vitamin E" is wheat, but "sprouting wheat" actually causes the "vitamin E content" to triple that of the seed if left unsprouted. Also, "the type of E found in sprouted seeds, grains, and nuts...is at least ten times more easily assimilated by the body than synthetic E."[42]

Sesame sprouts are so high in calcium, they rival "cow's milk" for calcium content having more calcium "than almost any other plant food," and according to Ms. Wigmore, "almond, sunflower, alfalfa, and chick pea sprouts are also excellent sources of calcium."[43]

Sprouts are also high in chlorophyll, the benefits of which were discussed earlier in this chapter. They are so nutrient dense that they also enhance the immune system. Be sure that if you grow or purchase sprouts that you always buy organic. Sprouts can get contaminated with bacteria if not grown, handled and washed properly.

CHAPTER 17

FLAX – AN OIL OF GLADNESS

"I have the answer to cancer, but American doctors won't listen. They come here and observe my methods and are impressed. Then they want to make a special deal so they can take it home and make a lot of money. I won't do it, so I'm blackballed in every country."

– Dr Budwig[1]

The *oil of gladness* is mentioned in the Bible as being an anointing oil from the Lord (see psalm 45:7 and Hebrews 1:9). I am *borrowing* this phrase in speaking of flax oil, simply because it has so many amazing health benefits for those who use it!

Flaxseed Inhibits Cancer

Flaxseed has been in use for thousands of years. As described by Maureen Kennedy Salaman in her book, *Nutrition: The Cancer Answer II*, studies were done in 1986 in Canada "on the nutritional benefits of flax." Not only did they discover that it could reduce harmful blood lipids, but also inhibits cancer formation. Flax is rich in lignans, nutrients with "anti-tumor properties." Because of their antioxidant ability, they are important for inhibiting "breast cancer."[2]

Ms. Salaman further notes that two other essential fatty oils that showed the ability to destroy several types of "cancer cells in culture" without harming normal cells, were "evening primrose oil" and "borage oil."[3] The wrong kinds of fat not only depress the immune system, they transport cancer-causing chemicals into and throughout the body. She recommends that you avoid the use of anything that is "hydrogenated" or refined, including margarines. "Hydrogenation" creates "poisonous by-products…" that rob the body of "vitamin E." Obtain organic unrefined oils such as "nut oils from your local health food store."[4] Ms. Salaman says that even the FDA has recognized flaxseed oil as a cancer preventative![5]

Cold-pressed organic olive oil is also a good choice. (Note that most of the onion rings, french fries, fried chicken and other fried foods that are found in today's fast food restaurants are cooked with unhealthy oils.) The unnaturally high fats that Americans consume in popular fast food dishes are a primary cause of cancer. We need fats in our diet, but the RIGHT kind of fats. Refined, processed vegetable oils are contributing to the deterioration of the health of millions!

Flax has been called "the ideal survival food" because all the antioxidants in flax are enclosed "within a hard shell" that keeps the seed from spoiling for years. Once the outer shell is cracked or crushed, the oil inside is "exposed to oxygen" and will eventually spoil if not used immediately.[6]

In his book, *Fantastic Flax*, Siegfried Gursche lauds the many benefits of flaxseed as a healing food and nutraceutical:

Everyone will benefit from adding flax seeds to their diet, especially those who suffer from constipation, intestinal and digestive problems, high blood pressure, elevated cholesterol levels, cardiovascular problems and degenerative diseases.[7]

The importance of maintaining the body's alkalinity was noted earlier in this book and in a later chapter devoted to that concept. Mr. Gursche explains that flax can assist with sustaining a healthy state of alkalinity as it is "very alkaline." It is a good preventative for "heartburn" and excellent for "detoxification" and promotion of a correct acid-alkaline balance. He says that it forms a "thick mucilage" in the stomach, thus providing "an excellent remedy for stomach ulcers, as it covers the inflamed areas and protects them from the stomach acids."[8]

Essential fats are healthy. In normal amounts, they do not make people fat. It is all the non-essential fats that are being ingested that are causing the problem of obesity in America. Mr. Gursche described "Dr. Johanna Budwig," as "a pioneer in the field of health and nutrition research," who referred to flax as the "spark plug that cranks up fat metabolism in our bodies."[9]

Flax contains *lignans,* which are "plant estrogens (phytoestrogens) that may" play a vital part "in the prevention of breast, prostate, uterus and colon cancers," says Mr. Gursche. They also keep bones healthy and "prevent the formation of gallstones by binding with bile acids."[9a] He describes flax seeds as being so rich in lignans that they "contain 75 to 800 times more [lignans] than wheat bran, oats, millet, rye, legumes soybeans and 66 other foods tested." **They interfere "with tumor cell growth" by causing "excess estrogen" to be driven "from the body."** Mr. Gursche adds that lignans work by "attaching themselves to estrogen receptor sites and [taking] the place of estradiol and estrone, which are implicated in breast cancer." They also prevent "fatty tissue" from producing more estrogen.[10] (What this means is that all your cells have receptor sites where harmful estrogens can attach themselves and thus be absorbed into the cells. Lignans from flax take the place of the harmful estrogens, thus preventing them from being absorbed into your body!)

Flax is high in fiber and is "an almost perfect protein." (Note, when combined with cottage cheese or yogurt, as in the Budwig diet, it becomes a complete protein.) There are several varieties of flaxseed – "about six different kinds…of brown flax…[and] three different kinds of golden (or yellow) flax." There is little difference between the brown flaxseed and the golden, explains Mr. Gursche. "Golden flax has a higher protein content," but has less "oil," and is sometimes "a little more expensive…"[10a] He says that it is best not to purchase flax that has already been ground, unless it is in a sealed package and once opened, you keep it refrigerated and use promptly. It is preferable to purchase the flaxseed whole and keep it refrigerated, then grind in a coffee grinder the amount you need as you use it. This will prevent the flax from going rancid. The spoilage does not occur until after the seeds are crushed and left exposed to oxygen. When using flax oil, **never heat it,** and be sure to purchase organic flax from a reputable health food store.[11]

I prefer flax oil in salads, juices, cold dishes (such as chopped salads or avocados) or poured over a baked potato. (Just be sure the potato is not burning hot as flax oil should not be heated – ever!) If using fresh flaxseed, take 2 tablespoons of the seeds, grind them in a coffee grinder, mix them with 8 ounces of water, shake and drink for a breakfast drink. Or you can add the crushed (or cracked) seeds to cereals or salads. However, if adding to a drink, you must drink it quickly, because it thickens very fast! You may need to follow it with more water.

Dr. Johanna Budwig & the Margarine Battle

Dr. Johanna Budwig, a seven times Nobel prize nominee, famous for her work in isolating and identifying fatty substances in the blood, was appalled at the way margarine manufacturers took "good unrefined healthy oils" and transformed them "into processed and hydrogenated health-endangering margarine," and she was very vocal about saying so![11a] In *Fantastic Flax*, Siegfried Gursche says that "The orthodox medical establishment, the margarine manufacturers and the government" all attempted to prosecute Johanna "for claiming that trans-fatty acids and the hydrogenation process are harmful to humans."[12] (Does any of this sound familiar?) Johanna said the following about margarine: "[T]he process of artificially hardening liquid vegetable oils (hydrogenation) creates life-threatening fat molecules – the trans fatty acids."[12a]

The margarine industry brought legal action against Johanna. "She fought **twenty-eight court cases" winning every single one of them!** We see warnings everywhere today about the dangers of trans-fatty acids (like those in margarines) that contribute to "cancer, heart disease and...other degenerative diseases," (Emphasis, mine.)[13] and of course, we now know that it was the margarine manufacturers who were lying and not Johanna! Organic butter is actually better for you than margarine. (We can thank Johanna Budwig for exposing the truth about margarine and margarine manufacturers!)

"Flax oil is the highest single source of omega-3 fatty acid" at "48-64%." Be careful in purchasing flaxseed oil that you check the label for the words, "cold expeller-pressed" and "unrefined," and check the expiration date on the container![13a] Mr. Gursche recommends that you use the oil "within three weeks after opening," and always keep it refrigerated. You can use the flaxseeds in baking if you soak them "in water for at least an hour before using them..."[14] (Dr. Budwig's famous flax oil diet is given later in this chapter. She also authored several books on flax oil. One in particular, *The Oil-Protein Diet Cookbook*, has many of her recipes for a variety of ways to incorporate the Budwig diet into your menus.)

Flax Prevents Many Diseases – Helps the Heart, Kidneys, & Those with Lupus Nephritis, M.S., Diabetes, Colon Problems, & HIV

Research studies have found that flaxseed has an anticancer effect comparable to that of some chemotherapy drugs, but minus the toxic side effects. It is a well known fact that women having the highest levels of omega-3-fatty acids (such as those found in fish and flax oil) are the least likely to develop breast cancer. Flax has also been effective at treating skin disorders, and it is possible that it could extend the lives of patients with lupus who are fighting nephritis caused when the lupus attacks their kidneys.

Dr. Mark Stengler wrote in *The Natural Physician's Healing Therapies*, that "serious cancers such as those of the breast, uterus, and cervix may very well be prevented and to some degree treated with flaxseed and possibly flax oil lignan extracts."[15]

Dr. Stengler also believes that flax can be considered an important "preventative and...part of a comprehensive treatment for prostate cancer," as well as a prevention for "colon cancer," and treatment for "digestive disorders" such as "irritable bowel syndrome (IBS), Crohn's disease, ulcerative colitis, and constipation..."[16]

One physician in particular, "neurologist Dr. Roy Swank...has proven that a diet rich in essential fatty acids and low in saturated fat is key to the successful treatment of multiple sclerosis (MS)."[17] (If you have any of these disorders, or are taking prescription medications, be sure to consult with your licensed Naturopathic health care physician for appropriate amounts to take.)

In her book, All *Your Health Questions Answered Naturally*, Maureen Kennedy Salaman emphasizes the importance of EFAs in helping to metabolize dangerous blood lipids to prevent them from accumulating in blood vessels and tissues, causing disease. Some other sources of omega-3 oils (besides flaxseed) that she gives are:

"...cold water fish...[and] fresh dark green vegetables like broccoli, kale, collards and Swiss chard."[17a] Ms. Salaman lists one of the richest sources of "omega-6 fatty acids," as "borage oil." One researcher even discovered that the GLA in borage oil reversed some diabetic health complications, "especially retina problems."[18] (Another excellent source of essential fatty acids is the avocado.)

Researchers have shown repeatedly that omega-3 fish oil (the same type oil found in flax oil) in animal testing, actually shrank tumors and inhibited their metastasis. It also suppresses colon cancer and breast cancer in humans![19]

Studies also revealed that within just a few weeks, the proliferation of pre-cancerous cells would drop by "an average of 62 percent..." if "men with colon polyps" ingested "fish oil" supplements every day.[20] This according to Reese Dubin in *Miracle Food Cures From The Bible*. He also explains that "life expectancies of HIV patients [were] more than doubled" when they were fed "GLA [and] omega-3 fish oil."[20a] These essential oils have also been used to effectively treat rheumatoid arthritis patients. GLAs work by enhancing the body's ability to increase immune cells that kill pathogens and mutant cells in the body. Good sources of GLA are "evening primrose oil, borage, and black currants."[21]

Dr. Earl Mindell, R.Ph., Ph.D., reports in *Earl Mindell's Food as Medicine*, that flaxseed is also abundant in "alpha-linolenic acid" (ALA), another omega-3 fatty acid. "ALA" is one of the "good" fats, he says. "This omega-3 fat" prolongs clotting (or coagulation time) thus protecting against "dangerous blood clots" and lowering "the risk of heart attack and stroke."[22]

Flax is rich in "vitamin F," and, as described earlier, it provides very nutritious and healthy "mucilage," which helps detoxify and clean the colon.[23] Selene Yeager in *Doctors Book of FOOD REMEDIES* says that it has "75 times" the lignans of "any other plant food." As a comparison, you would have to eat 5 dozen "cups of fresh broccoli or 100 slices of whole-wheat bread to get the same amount of lignans that are in ¼ cup of flaxseed."[24] Ms. Yeager points out research from a study which showed that even with "estrogen-sensitive tumors...breast tumors in animals given flaxseed shrank by 50%

in seven weeks." She says that lignans apparently have the power to "block the effects of estrogen," as described earlier in this chapter.[25]

Heating oils to extreme temperatures changes their molecular structure and makes them unfit for human consumption. Fats that are artificially hardened, the fats that are bad for you, will be labeled *as* **"hydrogenated, modified, fractionated or partially hydrogenated...avoid all products that contain these dangerous fats."**[25a] (Emphasis, mine.) You will find these fats in processed food, in fast foods and in many places in your grocery store! Butter is actually better for you unless you burn it! Burning butter completely ruins it! Never eat anything cooked in butter that has been burned. It has become a harmful fat and will flood your body with dangerous free radicals.[26]

Refined oils are considered by Siegfried Gursche in his book, *Good Fats and Oils,* to be a "dead food" meaning they are deficient in "vital elements":

> These are the oils usually found in supermarkets...refined safflower, peanut, cottonseed, soya, grapeseed, canola... and even the "light" olive oils. "Olivera," for example sounds like an olive oil, but it is actually refined canola oil. "Light" olive oil is actually refined oil....These oils are highly processed and have a significant trans-fatty acids content.[27]

The same can be said of margarine and vegetable shortening. Organic cold-pressed extra virgin olive oil (unrefined) can be purchased at your local health food store. Another good oil (if organic, unrefined) is pumpkinseed oil (which has been shown to prevent prostate enlargement), but beware, some producers will "mix cheaper...pumpkinseed oil with another low-priced oil...to keep the price down," making you think you are getting a pure product.[27a] Mr. Gursche says that "you can test the oil yourself for purity. One drop of genuine pumpkinseed oil on a lettuce leaf will remain a solid drop, while mixed oil will disperse easily." This oil is famous for boosting the health of the "urinary tract" and "preventing prostate enlargement."[27b] Other good oils (if unrefined and cold-pressed), explains Mr. Gursche, are "walnut...hemp...hazelnut...almond...pistachio…avocado…macadamia nut…and coconut oil…in its natural state…" unrefined.[28] (Perilla oil and black seed (nigela sativa) are also a good source of these healthy oils.)

The Famous Budwig Flax Oil Diet

Johanna Budwig combined flax oil with cottage cheese as part of her anti-cancer program. I do not recommend cow's milk simply because many dairy products in this country are so tainted with hormones, pesticides and herbicides, and because cow's milk has been linked to juvenile or type I diabetes, and sometimes carries leukemia and lymphoma cells. If you insist on using dairy products, such as cottage cheese, I would recommend that you use only organic or better yet, soy substitutes. In the Budwig diet, you can use yogurt and there are some very good tasting organic soy yogurts on the market. Milk is not for children. It is for baby cows! Some studies indicate that giving cow's milk to babies under one year old causes milk allergies and may be the culprit in Type I diabetes! I do encourage the use of the Budwig flax oil diet in anyone battling a malignant disease, such as brain cancer or some other type of cancer, and as stated earlier, it can be done without dairy products. (Fermented soy products, such as Haelan, can help remove harmful estrogens from the body in estrogen-receptor positive cancers.) As described at *www.healingcancernaturally.com*, ingredients are combined as follows in the Budwig flax oil diet:

> For each tablespoon of flaxseed oil, add 2 tablespoons of low-fat cottage cheese (or quark) or 6 tablespoons of yogurt. The flaxoil/cottage cheese or flaxoil/yogurt mixture should be fully blended until no traces of oil remain visible, proving that the highly unsaturated fatty acids have become water soluble (a hand-held mixer or a blender works well).[29]

Flax Oil & Malignant Cancers

The type of GLA found in flaxseed as well as "evening primrose oil and borage oil," in laboratory testing, was shown to effectively "kill leukemia cells isolated from patients with alpha-cell chronic lymphocytic leukemia." As a matter-of-fact, their anti-tumor effects have been demonstrated against many different types of cancer, including deadly brain cancers.[30] (See chapter 13.)

Essential fatty acids work by protecting "cell membranes." The membranes work by allowing nutritious elements to enter, while blocking out harmful scavengers. This is why flaxseed is such an important antioxidant. It works to fight inflammations and pathogens, and it contains "plant-based estrogens (phytoestrogens)." According to *The Healing Power of Vitamins, Minerals, and Herbs*, a book by the Reader's Digest Association, flaxseed and flax oil have been used to treat "lupus and gout...skin lesions...arthritis...fertility problems... menstrual cramps...fibrocystic breasts...cold sores...shingles...constipation and diverticular complaints...angina and high blood pressure." It can also inhibit the development of "gallstones," and even "dissolve" them once formed.[31]

I have tried the flax formula with soy yogurt and there is no problem with taste, however I believe there is less risk in using organic soy than with dairy products! Because of the problems associated with dairy products (see chapter 25), I would certainly choose soy over dairy, and then only in moderation. Keep in mind that there is always the potential for soy allergies, just as with milk allergies.

The Budwig diet works by making important oils and lipoproteins easily available to the body at the cellular level, elevating oxygenation and energy. There is one website, in particular, that describes a new omega oil product known as "Omegasentials™" that it claims is "already water-soluble" and works the same way that the diet works. You can find more information on Omegasentials™ at website: *www.mnwelldir.org/docs/ cancer1/budwig.htm,* or you can email them at *info@mnwelldir.org* or email *info@integritydirectinc.com* for purchasing the product.[32]

Oxygenation & Flax Oil

Dr. Otto Warburg won "the Nobel prize in 1931" when he discovered that "cancer cells do not breathe oxygen. Cancer cells are anaerobic, which means that they derive their energy without needing oxygen....It turns out that cancer cells cannot survive" in a highly oxygenated environment.[33] See Website http://*www. mnwelldir.org/docs/cancer1/budwig.html*, which explains that this resulted in the advent of many types of cancer therapies providing tissue oxygenation, such as "hyperbaric oxygen...and blood ozonation." There is also "EWOT (Exercise With Oxygen Therapy)...doing light exercise, such as on a treadmill...while breathing pure oxygen."[34] This is probably one reason, among many, that regular exercise lowers cancer risk. It increases oxygenation at the cellular level. It was this principle of increasing the oxygen to the body at the cellular level that interested Dr. Budwig, and was part of the rationale behind her flaxseed oil, cottage cheese combination.

Dr. Budwig assisted many terminally ill patients in regaining their health through her simple diet of flaxseed oil and low-fat cottage cheese. Known as "Germany's premier biochemist" with "a Ph.D. in Natural Science," she was also trained "in pharmaceutical science, physics, botany and biology....German manufacturers of commercial dietary fats (margarine, hard shortening, [and] vegetable oils) went to extremes to prevent her from publishing her findings."[35]

Website *http://www.alternativehealth.co.nz/cancer/budwight,* gives a slight variation in the Budwig diet, (adding freshly ground flaxseed as well as the oil):

> 1 cup Organic cottage cheese (low fat...) or yogurt: 2-5 Tbsn. of flaxseed oil; 1-3 Tbspn. of freshly ground up flaxseed (use a coffee grinder); enough water to make it soft, and a little cayenne....Then it is advisable to "eat some of it every day."[36]

According to the above website, "Dr. Dan C. Roehm...oncologist and former cardiologist," studied the Budwig diet recently and said that, "this diet is far and away the most successful anti-cancer diet in the world." Dr. Budwig claimed that the diet not only prevented disease, but cured disease as well. She believed that "the absence of linol-acids [in the average western diet] is responsible for the production of oxydase, which induces cancer growth and is the cause of many other chronic disorders."[37]

Apparently, Dr. Budwig cured cancer by discovering that cancer patients were always found to be very deficient in certain "essential ingredients," including "phosphatides and lipoproteins...without [which]... cancer cells grow wild and out of control." What she found in her research was a completely natural way for people to obtain the missing ingredients they needed. As noted at The Cancer Homepage website *www.alternativehealth.co.nz/cancerbudwig.html* in an article by Robert Willner, M.D., Ph.D.:

> By simply eating a combination of just two natural and delicious foods not only can cancer be prevented, but in case after case it was actually cured. These two natural foods (organic flax seed oil & cottage cheese) must be eaten together to be effective since one triggers the properties of the other to be released.)[38]

Many testimonials have been given of patients brought back from terminal illness to amazing health by Johanna Budwig's diet. One example is that of Sandy A. who was diagnosed with "arachnoidal bleeding due to an inoperable brain tumor." He was told that there was nothing that could be done for him, and sent home to die. He started on Dr. Budwig's formula and explains what happened:

> My health improved so rapidly that I was soon able to return to work part-time. Shortly after that, I was again examined at the research center and my reflexes were completely normal. The Budwig diet saved my life! Ten years later, I was given a thorough examination at the Center as a follow-up. My incredible recovery has been written up in many medical journals...[39]

The parents of Eleven-year-old "Timmy G." were told that he had "Hodgkin's disease." After **failure to respond** to "24 radiation treatments," he was "given six months to live and sent home to die." His mother was told of the Budwig diet. Within "just five days" on the diet, she remarks that his "breathing became normal for the first time in almost two years." He eventually returned to school and is now 18 years of age and credits his life to Dr. Budwig's formula.[40]

Website *www.curezone.com* documents the case of an "incurable bone cancer cure" using the Budwig diet, however the patient used larger amounts of flax oil a day than the official diet calls for. He started "out with 4 tbl. [tablespoons] of flax per day," (plus the cottage cheese). A few days later, he increased it to "8-10 tbl [tablespoons] of flax [oil] per day" with the cottage cheese. Three months later, all his lab work came back negative. His cancer was CURED. His physician was so incredulous, that he thought there was some mistake and ordered his tests repeated **three times**. There was no error. The patient, an "81-year-old," was in complete "remission."[41]

Be aware that there are other components involved with the Budwig flax oil diet besides the oil and cottage cheese. For example: all "SUGAR IS ABSOLUTELY FORBIDDEN. Grape juice may be added to sweeten any other freshly squeezed juices." The following items are also strictly forbidden: "All animal fats…Salad oils (this included commercial mayonnaise)…Meats…Butter…Margarine…Preserved Meats." All "freshly squeezed vegetable juices are fine – carrot, celery, apple, and red beet." Tea is encouraged "three times daily," such as "peppermint, rose hips or grape tea – all sweetened as desired with honey."[41a] On a daily basis, "a glass of Acidophilus milk or [organic] Sauerkraut juice is taken…before breakfast…" Also, a large amount of flax is taken on the very first day of the diet. "No nourishment on day #1 other than 250 ml (8.5 oz) of Flax Oil with honey plus freshly squeezed fruit juices" (no sugar added). Note that many people skip that 8.5 oz. dose on day one and proceed to the main diet![42] Just be sure if using the Budwig diet that you are getting 2-5 Tbsp. of the flaxseed oil daily with ½ to 1 cup of organic yogurt, or cottage cheese (or a soy substitute) thoroughly blended. If you do not care for the taste of the flax oil, you can add fresh fruit to the mix and/or cinnamon, which hides the oil taste. Don't add fruit or cinnamon until after the oil and yogurt are thoroughly mixed!

Flax vs. Fish

Many nutrition experts will tell you that fish is the healthiest form of omega-3, but studies have shown that this may not be the case. FLAX is safer! For one thing, many of our coastal waters are dangerously polluted. There is much documentation available on mercury poisoning in fish.

Even if you are able to get untainted fish, while some fish may be good, "more isn't necessarily better," as noted by Selene Yeager in the *Doctors Book of FOOD REMEDIES:* when researchers completed a "30-year study of 2,000 men," they discovered that consuming over "8 ounces of fish a week" increases the risk of "stroke." While the Japanese do eat a large amount of fish in their diet, it is also true that "stroke and other cerebrovascular diseases are traditionally one of the leading causes of death in Japan."[43] During research studies, when mice received fish, flax or corn oil, and were then injected with cancerous breast cells, the only oil of the three that successfully retarded the growth of the cancerous tumors and their spread was the flax oil![44]

The Oil of the Green-Lipped Mussel

Another form of oil that should be considered for those fighting diseases such as cancer and arthritis is the oil from the green-lipped mussel known as *lyprinol,* an anti-inflammatory that some say is equivalent in potency to celebrex, but without the side effects associated with celebrex! As described at website *http://www.primohealth.com/PI Lyprinol.a.html* (reprinted with their permission):

> • Lyprinol® is a stabilized extract of lipids (oils) from the Green-Lipped Mussel of New Zealand. It contains a rare group of Omega 3 fatty acids. The mussel oil in Lyprinol® acts as an anti-inflammatory agent in the human body.

• Independent studies have shown that the oil from the Green Lipped Mussel is up to 350 times more potent than evening primrose oil and salmon oil and 400 times more potent than flax oil!

• Use Lyprinol® to help bring relief to rheumatoid arthritis, osteoarthritis, asthma, traumatic joint injury and Chronic Fatigue Syndrome.

• Non-steroidal anti-inflammatory drugs (NSAIDs), such as aspirin, cause gastrointestinal side effects and may damage your liver. Lyprinol® protects your gastrointestinal tract and has no side effects. One researcher found no toxic effects in seriously ill patients who were given 50 capsules of Lyprinol® a day.[45]

This supplement is marketed at the above website. I have also seen the green-lipped mussel extract in nutrient drinks on the internet and in health food stores.

Another healthy oil is a plant oil known as **perilla oil** discussed earlier. See Life Extension's website at *http://www.lef.org/magazine/mag98/nov98_perilla.html,* for more information on this heart-healthy plant oil.

CHAPTER 18

OTHER AMAZING ANTI-CANCER HERBS

"And God said, Behold, I have given you every herb bearing seed, which is upon the face of all the earth, and every tree, in the which is the fruit of a tree yielding seed; to you it shall be for meat."

(Genesis 1:29, AV 1611 KJV)[1]

The herb, *Graviola,* has already been discussed in chapter five as well as *Essiac* herbal tea for their anti-cancerous benefits. Many herbs that we call *grasses* (barley, alfalfa, wheat grass, kelp, etc.) have also been discussed earlier in this book, as well as garlic, saw palmetto (for prostate problems), and dozens of important preventative and curative herbs. However, there are many other herbs and herbal remedies used effectively in cancer prevention and/or treatment. Only a few of them are covered in this chapter.

There are so many medicinal herbs provided by our great Creator God for our benefit, it would be impossible to include them all in a book of this size, and new ones are being discovered every day! Carl C. Pfeiffer, M.D., Ph.D., a pioneer in researching the biochemical relationship of nutritive substances and their relationship to mental illness, as well as research on amino acids, believed that for each drug designed to benefit humanity, nature has already provided a natural ingredient that accomplishes much the same purpose, but without adverse effects! Quite a profound belief coming from a physician born in 1908!

I have taken what I believe to be some of the most important herbs related to cancer prevention and treatment and either listed them in this chapter or covered them elsewhere in this book in cancer specific chapters. (Be aware that many of these herbs have not yet undergone extensive testing in humans.)

If you are interested in pursuing more in-depth information about herbs and herbal remedies, a good book to begin with is *The Scientific Validation of Herbal Medicine* by Daniel B. Mowrey, Ph.D., and of course, the internet has a glut of information on herbs. There are also several very informative herbal books noted in my reference section, such as *Earl Mindell's Herb Bible*, by Dr. Earl Mindell, R.Ph., Ph.D., *The Herbal Drugstore*, by Linda B. White, M.D., and Steven Foster, and *Healing Power of Herbs*, by John Heinerman, as well as many excellent herbal websites, such as *herbs2000.com, rain-tree.com, planetherbs.com,* and *iherb.com.*

Remember that you should never give herbs or herbal preparations to children without consulting their physician, nor should you take them yourself without doing the same, especially if you are on prescription medications, are pregnant or nursing, or have a health condition that requires close monitoring. Prescriptions and even over-the-counter remedies may have adverse effects when combined with certain herbs or herbal remedies. (Even simple kitchen spices that may not affect you, may have an adverse effect on your baby if you are nursing or pregnant.)

There are hundreds of herbs that work as important anti-oxidants. I believe that for every ailment on this earth, there is a God-given remedy, for His word declares that He has freely given us every herb (as noted in the quote at the beginning of this chapter)! We have not yet "discovered" all those remedies, but everyday brings new ones! Below are just a few of those amazing herbs!

Actinidia Root

This herb, common in Chinese folk medicine, was discovered by research scientists to contain an extract, which was capable of halting the growth of hepatic tumors when placed into the peritoneum of test animals.[2] The rate at which some tumors were stopped was nearly 90% in one type of cancer and nearly 50% in another. Apparently the Chinese knew what they were doing when using this root for cancer treatment.[2a]

An extract from a Japanese fruit very similar to kiwi (in laboratory testing) revealed that it was able to suppress certain cells that had become leukemic.

Note that the common **KIWI fruit found in your grocery store is a type of actinidia, however, it is** *"Actinidia chinensis"* (not the same as the above fruit). Kiwi fruit has amazed scientists because it appears to be able to help prevent free radical (oxygen) damage to the DNA at the core of "human cells."[3]

According to website *www.whfoods.com*, studies on nearly nineteen thousand "children aged 6-7 in northern and central Italy," revealed that kiwi fruit, high in antioxidants, inhibited respiratory-related illnesses in the children who consumed the most fruit: at least "6-7 servings per week..."[3a] They also report that the fruit is high in fiber and may offer some "protection against asthma," and lowers the "risk for blood clots" and high lipids ("triglycerides)...making kiwi a delicious blood-thinning alternative to aspirin for protecting cardio-vascular health."[4]

Be aware that if you are taking blood-thinning medications, preparing for a surgical procedure, recovering from surgery or have a chronic disorder, including a blood dyscrasia, you should not eat excessive amounts of the fruit. If you are already taking an aspirin regimen, do not substitute the fruit for aspirin without first consulting your physician.

Do not consume excessive amounts of kiwi if you have a tendency to develop kidney stones or gallstones since it is a high oxalate food.[4a] (See chapter three.)

Aloe Vera

Aloe is a medicinal plant that has been used for thousands of years for many purposes such as: "Sunburn...Wounds...Digestive Problems...Hemorrhoids...Infections...Psoriasis...Abrasions...Stings by insects, Jellyfish, Stinging Nettle...Ulcers [taken internally]...Arthritis...Acne...Asthma...[and]...Sore Throat." According to Max B. Skousen in his book, *The Ancient Egyptian Medicine Plant Aloe Vera Handbook:* "There are many reports of total elimination" of skin cancers, simply by the topical application of "aloe vera juice...."[5] Be aware though, that if you have a suspicious appearing skin lesion, you need to seek professional medical attention immediately. Also, if you have problems such as ulcers, abdominal cancer, Crohn's or IBS, seek your physician's advice about using aloe products internally.

Aloe has been used to treat leukemia, and it is sometimes used to help increase the absorption potential of green juices and to soothe

the intestinal mucosa. (Dee Simmons uses an aloe-papaya preparation with her excellent nutritional products. See chapter three of this book. Her website can be found at *www.ultimateliving.com.*)

Note that papaya enzymes can have blood-thinning effects. This is one reason you should always discuss any new herb you are considering with your physician. Your physician will be able to tell you if the herb interferes with current medications you may be taking, such as anti-coagulants like coumadin. And of course, the same applies if you have any sort of chronic disease or condition, or if you are a transplant patient.

Artemisinin

Artemisinin, extracted from the wormwood plant, is gaining a reputation for being able to hunt down and destroy "breast cancer cells" without harming normal cells! In laboratory testing, the herb killed every single breast cancer cell it came in contact with and it took a mere 16 hours. As described in an article at website *www.herbtime.com*, researchers used it on a dog with osteosarcoma so debilitating that he was unable to "walk across the room." Within less than a week after receiving the treatment, the dog made a total recovery. His tumor had completely "disappeared!" At last check (two years later), the dog is still alive and well! Artemisinin has been used by the Chinese for "thousands of years" for treating malaria, but because of recent testing, is emerging as a potential treatment for tumors, especially those of the breast.[6] Dr. Hulda Clark used wormwood as one of her parasite-killing remedies, which is discussed later in this book in chapter 27. This herb is not recommended for those who are pregnant or nursing. Human testing is still being conducted.

Ashwagandha

Ashwagandha belongs to the same plant "family as the tomato" and can be found growing abundantly in several countries. *Herbs2000.com* reports that it has been used to treat "…Alzheimer's…arthritis…insomnia…stress," and libido problems.

Extracts from the herb have been known to put cancerous tumors into "regression."[7] This herb is also known as *"winter cherry"* and *"Indian ginseng."* According to Dr. Ray Sahelian, M.D., at *www.raysahelian.com*, it is "used therapeutically as an adaptogen for patients with nervous exhaustion, and debility due to stress, and as an immune stimulant in patients with low white blood cell counts."[8] As described by *"Life Science...*compounds isolated from the leaves of this herb inhibited "lung, colon, central nervous system and Breast human tumor cells lines." One compound in particular "showed...50% inhibition...[and] Preliminary studies" attributed the herb "with little or no associated toxicity."[9]

If choosing this herb, be sure that you get an extract "standardized with anolides." It is usually found "in capsule form." Do not use "ashwagandha oil" for cancer prevention or remedy, as this is a facial toner only, and avoid "ashwagandha berries as they can cause severe gastrointestinal pain." Do not use this herb if you are on any medications for "anxiety, insomnia, or a seizure disorder."[10] Dr. Sahelian's website has standardized ashwagandha herbal supplements available. For those interested, see website: *www.raysahelian.com.*

Aspilia

Aspilia, also known as "Wild Sunflower," not only kills parasites, but it acts much like an antibiotic. It has been shown to destroy cancerous cells in "solid tumors," especially those of the "lung and breast."[10a]

Astragalus

As noted by Dr. Earl Mindell in *Earl Mindell's Soy Miracle*, Astragalus is an immune stimulating herb that scientists have shown in animal testing, will increase the body's natural immunity. It has also been used to help stabilize "the immune systems" of **chemo patients who have had their immune system compromised by toxic chemo drugs.** It can increase the body's manufacture of "interferon," which helps destroy viruses. Researchers in Texas used a "purified extract" of the herb.[11] Do not use the herb during the presence of an infectious process.[11a]

Bromelain

Though not considered an herb, "bromelain" is a protein substance found naturally in pineapples, and it is being included here because it is often added to herbal remedies for digestive disorders, and to treat "osteoarthritis and rheumatoid arthritis."[11b] In one particular cancer study, the following results of a **human study** were reported from bromelain ingestion and described by Dr. Mark Stengler in his book: *The Natural Physician's Healing Therapies:* "12 patients with ovarian cancer and breast tumors were given 600 milligrams of bromelain daily for at least 6 months. (Some treatments continued for several years.)" Dr. Stengler said that "Resolution of cancerous masses and a decrease in metastasis was reported."[12]

Tumor cells are wrapped in a type of "coating" composed primarily of protein. This "coating" makes it difficult for cells from the body's natural immune system to recognize the cancer cell and destroy it. It is believed that bromelain dissolves this "coating" so that the body's "immune cells" can recognize the cancer cells and destroy them.[13] (Not for those with ulcers or blood disorders.)

Bupleurum

Bupleurum *("Bupleurum chinense")* is a wild herb that has been used in the orient for more than two millennia "as a liver tonic." It also helps rejuvenate a sluggish liver, much like milk thistle.[13a] "Sakosides" in this herb are very liver-protective, helping to enhance the productivity of the liver "even in" those with autoimmune diseases. It has been used to treat "bone cancer...hepatitis and other chronic liver problems."[14] This herb should not be used if you are running a temperature or if you are on prescription "antibiotics." It may cause epigastric discomfort, in which case your herbalist or natural health practitioner may need to lower the amount that you are taking.[15] It may also cause swelling, and it should not be combined with other medications. For more details on this herb, see website *http://www.herbs2000.com/disorders/cancer_bone.htm.*

Cascara Sagrada

Cascara Sagrada *"(Rhamnus purshiana)"* is known as a "champion colon cleanser and excellent laxative," and according to Marie Nadine Antol in *Healing Teas,* it may help combat "liver disorders, gallstones, leukemia, colitis and diverticulosis."[15a] It has been used for years to rid the body of parasites and increase "peristalsis" in the colon. It also has a "toning" effect on the intestines. Just be sure if buying the herb, advises Ms. Antol, that you purchase the "sacred bark," not the "purging buckthorn, *Rhamnus cathartica*," which is so much stronger in action, "it can be dangerous." Taking excessive doses of cascara can result in loose stools and "severe cramps."[16]

Cat's Claw

Cat's claw (also known as *Uno de Gato)* is discussed in many other cancer specific chapters in this book.

Chicory Root

"Chicory Root," commonly found in "herbal coffees, contains an anti-cancer carbohydrate known as inulin." **(Not insulin.)** According to *cancertutor.com,* researchers have found that this compound "prevented the formation of colon cancer tumors...in several animal studies." Their findings were recently described "in the British Journal of Nutrition."[17]

Chinese Asparagus

Chinese asparagus *"(Asparagus cochinchinensis)"* grows near the ocean and can be found in "Japan, China, and Korea..." It is also known as "Tian Men Dong," and is used as an "Antibacterial... diuretic...expectorant [for] fevers, [and] debility, sore throats...

diptheria, tuberculosis, bronchitis," and as a "folk remedy for cancer...[It] has shown antitumor activity in animal trials." See website http://*earthnotes.tripod.com/asparagus.htm#aspother* for more information on this herb.[17a] It is currently being investigated for use against "...lung cancer and lymphosarcoma."[18]

Cilantro

Cilantro is a mild herb that gets little attention, but according to website *www.mnwelldir.org,* this very "common" herb may "Save Your Life." The website has information from an article by Dr. David Williams from his newsletter *"Alternative (For the Health Conscious Individual),"* on the amazing ability of cilantro to act like a chelating drug to remove "heavy metals from your body."[19] (I.V. chelation therapy is common in alternative medicine as a way to get toxic metals such as aluminum, cadmium, mercury and other free radicals out of the body.)

A physician by the "name of Dr. Omura found that fresh cilantro removes heavy metals from the body in less than two weeks," and this is one chelation agent that you can take orally, rather than intravenously! The website above also gives recipes for using cilantro in a dressing and as a pesto sauce.[20]

Ciwujia

Ciwujia ("also known as Acanthopanax senticosis...or Siberian ginseng") has been tested in humans. It can be found in a supplement known *as Endurox™,* as well as by itself. It has strong "ginseng-like effects" with its powerful "saponin gylcosides," that, in animal studies, protect "against...arrhythmias, fibrillation and tachycardia." In **human studies**, according to K. Gilbert Udall in *Immune and Stamina Booster Cordyceps Sinensis*, ciwujia extract caused the increased production of "T-cells and...natural killer cell activity," thus it boosted the body's immune system! It is also being used to treat "chronic fatigue syndrome in humans."[21]

Cranberry

It is believed that cranberries protect against bladder infections by either acidifying the urine, destroying pathogens, or by preventing them from "sticking to the wall of the bladder."[21a] It is important to drink unsweetened cranberry juice because the bottled type of commercial juice generally found in your typical grocery store is usually loaded with sugar, corn syrup, and other additives. You may want to opt for supplements of "cranberry extract available in health food stores" in "capsule" form, which "are not only more potent but less caloric."[22] Some health food stores have unsweetened cranberry juice available, or you can always juice your own when cranberries are in season, using a natural herb such as *Stevia* for sweetening purposes. It will take a lot of stevia! Fresh cranberries are usually extremely tart. The berries are rich in antioxidants that can boost the immune system.

You may also want to check out Dr. Mercola's website at *www.mercola.com* for the *D-Mannose* supplement. *D-Mannose* is a nutrient extracted from peaches and berries such as cranberries, which is said to maintain urinary tract health without giving you the high sugar dose that is found in most bottled cranberry juices. (This nutrient will not destroy the "friendly" bacteria in the intestines.)

Curcumin (Turmeric)

Cancertutor.com webpage describes curcumin as a "natural substance so smart it can tell the difference between a cancer cell and a normal cell; so powerful it can stop chemicals in their tracks," and so potent, it has the ability to protect DNA from "lethal doses of radiation."[23]

Turmeric is a major component in curry powder, however, beware of buying curry products indiscriminately, especially the sauce! Try to purchase only from organic health food stores. Website *www.newstarget.com/001027.html* explains why:

Food safety investigators in the UK have found that the vast majority of curry sauce products sold on store shelves contain dangerous levels of artificial coloring chemicals which are linked to behavioral disorders such as ADD. The investigation names tartrazine – equivalent to FD&C Yellow No. 5 in the United States. This artificial food color, which is made from coal tar, is also widely used in the United States and is considered just one of many metabolic disruptors found in our national food supply.[24]

Curcumin is discussed in more detail in several cancer specific chapters of this book. Turmeric is safe when used as a spice, however, if you are taking turmeric in supplement form, do not use if pregnant, nor if you have gallstones, since it stimulates the gallbladder. Like garlic, turmeric can slow clotting time, so it should be used in caution by anyone taking anti-coagulant medications[24a] with blood disorders, or for anyone recovering from or contemplating surgery

Dandelion

Dandelion (*"Taraxacum officinale"*) is a great herb for detoxifying the body. It promotes bile secretion, "aids digestion," and has natural diuretic properties. Marie Nadine Antol in *Healing Teas*, says that it helps promote a healthy "pancreas, spleen, liver, bladder, and kidneys," and has been used to treat "anemia, gout, hypoglycemia, rheumatism, jaundice, cirrhosis, hepatitis, cramps, and constipation."[24b] It also lowers blood lipids "and uric acid, and may even help prevent breast cancer."[24c] Dandelion can increase bile and gastric acid, something to consider if you have gallstones, biliary disease, ulcers or other digestive disorders. As with any herbal regimen, consult with your physician.

D-limonene

D-limonene can be found in the part of the citrus fruits we humans usually throw away, the peelings! It can inhibit "mammary, liver lung, UV-induced skin cancer and [is] chemotherapeutic against both experimental mammary and pancreatic tumors." It fights "human pancreatic cancer, colon…prostate and lung cancer."[25] I have seen this extract in dried form for teas as well as in supplement form in health food stores. See *cancertutor.com* for more information. Do not indiscriminately ingest large amounts of citrus peelings. Doing so can be harmful. Moderation is always best. Many recipes call for small amounts of citrus peeling to enhance the flavor of foods.

Echinacea

According to Dr. D. B. Mowrey in *The Scientific Validation of Herbal Medicine,* "Echinacea, [the] purple coneflower," sometimes used in battling colon cancer, has a popular history of treating "typhoid, meningitis, malaria, [and] diptheria…" and is still being used for this purpose in modern times.[25a] This is yet another herb that helps boost the immune system by increasing white blood cells. It also prevents an enzyme from "dissolving HA (Hyaluronic acid)…the stuff that occurs in the tissues between cells to 'cement' them together," keeping germs out! It has an "anti-inflammatory" effect, stimulates the lymphatic system, and protects against viruses like "herpes, influenza, canker sores, etc."[26]

Dr. John Heinerman points out in the *Healing Power of Herbs,* that the best form of echinacea is not the one most popularized, *"enchinacea angustifolia,"* but the one known as *"echinacea purpurea,"* as this form of the herb increases the immune system's "production of lymphocytes and macrophages…."[27]

Forsteronia refracta (SL0101)

This very rare plant also comes from forests of the Amazon. The compound (above) that has been extracted from the plant was found (in laboratory testing) to suppress cancerous breast cells.[27a]

Ginseng

There are several different types of ginseng: "American ginseng *(Panax quinquefolius)*, Siberian ginseng (*Eleutherococcus senticosus),"* [and] oriental ginseng: "Chinese or Korean, (*Panax ginseng).*"[28] The Chinese have been cultivating and using it for thousands of years. Japanese researchers found that cholesterol levels dropped in test animals on "a high cholesterol diet" when given ginseng, and it raised the "beneficial, HDL cholesterol…"[29] This per Dr. Earl Mindell in *Earl Mindell's Herb Bible.* Recent studies revealed that ingredients "from panax ginseng not only inhibited the growth of cancer cells, but actually converted the diseased cells into normal cells."[30] (The big issue with cancer cells is that they do not differentiate. A cancer cell in the liver won't normally become a liver cell. If it did, it wouldn't be a cancer cell. The fact that this type ginseng actually caused the cancer cells to differentiate and turn back into normal cells is most remarkable.)

Dr. Ralph Moss in *Cancer Therapy* says that according to an article from "*Cancer Research*," scientists noted that a chemical isolated from ginseng had the ability to cause "melanoma skin cancer cells to revert to normal."[31]

Note that more than 5 to 10 grams of panax ginseng a day can cause nervousness and over-stimulation as well as problems with hypertension and "headaches."[32] It may also "cause vaginal bleeding in menopausal women" (very rarely). Taking "vitamin C can interfere with the absorption of ginseng." Because of this, do not take Vitamin C within "two hours before or after taking ginseng…"[33] As explained in Dr. *Earl Mindell's Herb Bible,* the only difference between red and white ginseng is that "…white ginseng is simply cleaned and dried;

thus, it retains it natural white color. Red ginseng is steamed with a solution of herbs and is considered of superior quality."[34]

Ginkgo Biloba

Ginkgo, another herb that has enjoyed prominence in China for several millennia, is the subject of intensive research throughout the entire world. It is excellent for overall circulation, helps to "improve memory and to relieve signs of senility…helps prevent blood clots," and is useful in treating "phlebitis (inflammation of a vein), and diabetic peripheral vascular disease." (PVD)[35] It also has blood pressure lowering effects.

Goldenseal

See cancer specific chapters in this book for details on goldenseal and berberine.

Gymnema Sylvestre

This is another herb that **has been tested on humans.** According to Dr. Ray Sahelian at *www.raysahelian.com,* the herb has been in use for many years for:

> Its therapeutic role in relation to diabetes mellitus, rheumatic arthritis and gout. [It] helps support healthy blood sugar levels. Gymnema sylvestre contains compounds known as gymnemic acids and triterpenoid saponins, gymnemasins A, B, C and D. Rodent studies indicate that gymnema may have the capacity to lower cholesterol and triglyceride levels…[36]

Gymnema sylvestre "did not show any toxicity" in animal studies.[37] Research was also done "of a leaf extract from Gymnema sylvestre in non-insulin-dependent diabetes mellitus patients…[in] Madras, India." In this study on **humans,** the participants ("22 Type 2 diabetic patients on conventional oral anti-hyperglycaemic (sic) agents" received "Gymnema (400 mg/day)…for 18-20 months as a supplement to the conventional oral drugs."[38] During this period of time, says Dr. Sahelian, those taking the herb were able to reduce their "conventional drug dosage" due to a "significant reduction in blood glucose, glycosylated hemoglobin and glycosylated plasma proteins…." The most AMAZING thing of all in this entire study was the following report described by Dr. Sahelian:

> Five of the 22 diabetic patients were able to discontinue their conventional drug and maintain their blood glucose homeostasis with Gymnena alone. These data suggest that the beta cells may be regenerated / repaired in Type 2 diabetic patients on Gymnema sylvestre supplementation. This is supported by the appearance of raised insulin levels in the serum of patients after Gymnema sylvestre supplementation.[39]

Further research with this herb on human testing (on both Type I and Type II diabetics) resulted in a decrease in all blood sugar levels including the HbA1c testing. No toxic effects were noted.

According to website *http://intelegen.com/nutrients/gymnema_ sylvestre_for _diabetes.htm,* a series of "published studies" on this herb came out in 1990, which showed that it was capable of:

> [R]egeneration of beta cells in the pancreas. In the words of the authors, 'This herbal therapy appears to bring about blood glucose homeostasis through increased serum insulin levels provided by repair/regeneration of the endocrine pancreas.' To my knowledge, this is the only compound that has shown the ability to lessen indicators of diabetes by directly repairing/regenerating the pancreas cells responsible for producing insulin."[39a]

This very same "team" of researchers found that "The control group used in this study not only didn't improve during the study period, they actually worsened." As for the "Type I diabetics," their "insulin requirements came down, together with blood glucose, glycosylated hemoglobin and glycosylated plasma protein levels. Serum lipids returned to near normal levels with GSE therapy." There were "no adverse side effects" except that many of the patients had lower blood sugar levels![39b]

Hoxsey Tea

Harry Hoxsey developed an herbal tea discussed earlier in this book, in cancer specific chapters. He was very much against the cancer establishment and even ran his own "Iowa radio station," where he boldly proclaimed a very "anti-AMA message" at every opportunity! He successfully operated several "cancer clinics" until he was eventually closed down "by the US medical authorities..."[40]

The Hoxsey Formula is still being used at his Mexico clinic, and a Hoxsey tincture with the following ingredients is described at website: *www.naturalopinion.com,* (reprinted with their permission):

- Arctium lappa (Burdock)
- Baptisia tintoria (Wild indigo)
- Berberis vulgaris (Barberry, Oregon grape)
- Glycyrrhiza glabra (licorice)
- Phytolacca decandra (Poke, pokeweed)
- Rhamnus frangula (buckthorn)
- Rhamnus purshiana (cascara)
- Stillingia sylvatica (Queen's root, Queen's delight)
- Trifolium pratense (Red clover)
- Zanthoxyllum clava-herculis (Southern prickly ash)
- 3% WV Potassium iodide: ¼ tsp. BID[41]

Hoxsey was ridiculed, made to look like a "snake oil salesman," harassed, and finally run out of the country when he claimed that his formula was curing cancer patients. However, in the years that followed his death, research into his herbal formula has shown that many of the compounds he used have powerful anticancer effects![42] Some of the herbs, (e.g. the pokeweed root and the burdock) can be dangerous if taken in excess amounts or improperly prepared. Burdock contains a substance that, "according to the World Health Organization," has "an 'inhibitory activity against HIV' virus..." Barberry extracts have "anti-cancer properties..."[43] The treatment that Harry Hoxsey received at the hands of the AMA was nothing short of criminal, and is described at website *http://www.getipm.com/personal/cancer-racket.htm*:

> It was not long before the infamous Morris Fishbein of the AMA heard about the Hoxsey treatment and wanted to buy sole rights to it, with some other AMA doctors. Hoxsey would only agree if it stated in the contract that everyone would have access to the treatments, not just a wealthy few. Fishbein refused and so began a 25-year battle, fought in the media, between Fishbein and Hoxsey. The mudslinging culminated in a lawsuit brought by Hoxsey against Fishbein. Much to everyone's amazement, Hoxsey won the case. Even so, in the late 1950's the FDA closed down all of Hoxsey's clinics.[44]

The Hoxsey formula is still available at their clinic in Tijuana, Mexico. They can be reached at: Bio-Medical center 615 General Ferreira, Colonia Juarez Tijuana, B.C. Mexico. Tel: 011-52-664-684-90-11 / Fax: 011-52-664-684-9744.

Iscador (Mistletoe)

Iscador is actually a type of mistletoe. It is used as an alternative cancer therapy in Europe, but not widely promoted or used in the U.S. It was given a flash of notoriety back in 2001 when actress Suzanne Somers announced to the world that she had refused chemotherapy for breast cancer and was using iscador treatments instead. She initially had a "lumpectomy" and "radiation," then refused chemo. Many people in the mainstream medical establishment criticized her immediately as though she had done something vile and unforgivable. Of course to them she had! After all, she was kicking their *untouchable* golden calf in refusing chemo, so naturally there were some upset people out there! Well that was four years ago and she is still alive and doing VERY well, having done just fine without the *golden calf* – yet you never hear any of the chemo pushers pointing that out do you!? You can read the details about this story at: *http://store.yahoo.com/annieappleseedproject/suzsomuseofm.html.*[44a]

Licorice

Licorice *("Glycyrrhiza glabra")* is soothing to the gastric system and has been used in treating ulcers. According to Marie N. Antol, in *Healing Teas*, it is also used to treat "colitis, diverticulosis, and gastritis...[and] is a noted expectorant and anti-inflammatory...."[45] It may be helpful for "PMS, allergies, hypoglycemia, stress" and other maladies. It has even been successful in treating "herpes simplex when used topically," says Ms. Antol, however, it is important if you choose to use this herb, to obtain "deglycyrrhizinated licorine or DGL."[46] Licorice that has not been deglycyrrhizinated can cause water retention, loss of potassium, and hypertension, and should not be used if you have "high blood pressure...or kidney problems, [or] if you are taking heart medication." Ms. Antol adds that licorice also has the unique ability to normalize "estrogen metabolism..,"[47] an important activity since **excess estrogen in the body has been linked to breast cancer.** Do not use un-deglycyrrhizinated licorice if you have glaucoma.

Milk Thistle

Milk thistle is so important in liver health and cleansing, it is discussed in chapter eight of this book for its use against liver cancer. See the report in that chapter on the patient whose *terminal* liver cancer completely disappeared while he was taking this common, non-toxic herbal treatment!

Olive Leaf Extract

Olive leaf not only boosts energy, but the immune system as well by enhancing the ability of white blood cells to destroy viruses and bacteria. It also has the "ability to directly penetrate infected cells and stop viral replication."[48] This nutrient, in supplement form, according to *www.drlam.com* website has been used to help in the treatment of:

> [I]nfluenza, the common cold, meningitis, Epstein-Barr (EBV), encephalitis, herpes I and II, human herpes 6 and 7, shingles (Herpes zoster), HIV/ARC/AIDS, chronic fatigue, hepatitis B, pneumonia, tuberculosis, gonorrhea, malaria, dengue, bacteremia, severe diarrhea, blood poisoning and dental, ear, urinary tract and surgical infections.[49]

Oregano

Oregano is another herb that has been used for centuries for many purposes, including toothaches, as an antiseptic, for candida, indigestion and ringworm. Oil of oregano has also demonstrated the ability to kill bacteria, parasites, fungi, even athlete's foot (used topically), and a myriad of other uses. Research using potent extracts from oil of oregano revealed that it even exerts some capacity at suppressing melanoma. (See page 512 for use with earaches.)

Parsley

Parsley ("*Petroselinum crispum*"), long known as a diuretic, is a very nutrient-dense anti-oxidant and cancer preventative. One of the ingredients found in this herb was shown to suppress cancer formation. It should not be used by women who are pregnant or nursing since it can cause premature uterine contractions and "dry up the milk supply." Do not use it in the presence of an "acute infection," particularly "if the kidneys are involved."[50] If you purchase dried parsley for tea, be aware that tea made from the root is going to be much more potent than if it comes from the leaf.

Parsley oil can cause skin irritations and is highly toxic.[51] Fresh, organically grown parsley (used in small amounts) is best!

Pau D'Arco

See other cancer specific chapters in this book for more information on this herb and its cancer preventative and healing properties.

Red Clover

Red clover is a mere "meadow grass," but it packs a punch when used in medicinal teas. In "the *Phrenological Journal* of December 1867," there was an account of Truman Woodford of "West Hartford, CT," who, in 1866, healed a "cancerous irritation that blinded his left eye and spread over his temple" by using a tea made with common red field clover. He drank it and also used it for an eyewash.[51a] As described by Dr. John Heinerman in his book, *Healing Power of Herbs*, "in less than two months" after Mr. Woodford began using the red clover, his "pain entirely ceased," and his eye and temple area healed. (Truman was "80 years old.")[52]

For fighting cancer, AIDS, or other types of illnesses, Dr. Heinerman recommends "red clover tea...Up to 8 cups or more a day, preferably on an empty stomach." He says that it is also "effective in capsule form," and if choosing capsules to use "four [capsules] at a time in between each meal...an average of a dozen capsules..." (taken daily).[53]

Linda B. White, M.D., and Steven Foster, in their book *The Herbal Drugstore,* describe an herbal combo composed of red clover in conjunction with "Astragalus, burdock, milk thistle...[and] yellow dock," that has been used as an alternative remedy in treating cervical dysplasia (though it is not claimed that it can reverse it). Red clover is very popular as a tea and is rich in "isoflavones that act as a mild form of estrogen." It is an herbal alternative for the treatment of "osteoporosis," combined with "Horsetail [and] stinging nettle."[54] Dr. White and Steven Foster also give a *"Typical dosage"* of red clover as "up to five 500-milligram capsules per day; or 2 or 3 cups of tea per day (steep 1 tablespoon of dried flowering tops in 1 cup of hot water for 10 to 15 minutes); or 15 to 30 drops of tincture up to four times per day."[55]

There are estrogen receptor sites in the body at the cellular level. As described earlier, the phytoestrogens in plants (such as red clover) lock onto these estrogen receptor sites thus preventing the **harmful, toxic forms of estrogen** from latching onto the receptor sites and being transported into the cells.[56]

Be aware that red clover has blood thinning properties, so should not be used without consulting your physician, especially if you are on prescription medications, and never use any form of **fermented** red clover.

Rose Hips

Rose hips are important simply because they are an excellent source of natural vitamin C, and vitamin C is critical in fighting cancer. In her book, *Healing Teas,* Marie Nadine Antol explains that there are "several varieties of rose hips" that are "sixty times richer in vitamin C than most oranges."[56a] They contain "the bioflavonoids that make vitamin C work better," and are much higher in vitamin C "than citrus fruits." They are also rich in several other vitamins and minerals, explains Ms. Antol. Rose hips are "a good blood purifier" and are "helpful against all infections," especially for those of the urinary tract. She says if you check roses "after the rose petals fall," you will see little "pods" that appear. These are the "rose hips."[57] (Many vitamin C supplements are made from rose hips.)

Triptolide for Cancer, M.S. & Lupus

Triptolide (*"Tripterygium Wifordii Hook"*) is a vine that the Chinese have been using for many years in treating "rheumatoid arthritis," yet as recently as "May of 1999....scientists at the Stanford University School of Medicine" found that triptolide "not only cooperates with TNF (Tumor Necrosis Factor) in killing solid tumor cells," but can also destroy tumors independently.[57a] Website *www.mnwelldir.org,* goes on to explain that "TNF-like compounds" kill tumor cells, but are toxic to healthy cells causing undesirable side effects, something **triptolide does not do!** Triptolide also kills "tumor cells…resistant to chemotherapy," and has been used to treat "multiple sclerosis and lupus."[58]

Wild Sunflower (Aspilia)

Aspilia *("Aspilia mossambicenisis")* is an anti-parasitic bush that has "antibiotic" properties with the ability to kill "cancer cells in solid tumors, such as those found in the lung and breast."[59] *Herbs2000.com* says that the leaves of the plant were first noticed because "chimpanzees in Gombe National Park and Mahale Mountains National Park of Tanzania" were swallowing "the leaves whole" and there would be "no visible evidence" that they had ever "passed through the digestive tract." It was noted that the animals also expelled large amounts of worms with the leaves![60] (Also discussed earlier in this chapter.)

Wolfberry

A "new discovery" for the West, though it has been used for hundreds of years in "inner Mongolia [is] called the Chinese wolfberry, also known by its Latin name, Lycium barbarum, or colloquial name, 'goji berry.'"[60a] It was found that the peoples consuming this berry live "over 100 years…[without] arthritis, cancer and diabetes." It is a very mild berry "with no known risk from continuous use."According to website *www.aroma-essence.com,* researchers in Beijing analyzed the nutritional components of the dried wolfberry fruit and found the following:

> The wolfberry contained over 18 amino acids (that is six times higher in proportion to bee pollen), 21 trace minerals, more beta carotene than carrots, and an astonishing 500 times more vitamin C by weight than oranges. It is also packed with vitamin B1, vitamin B6 and vitamin E. The

fruits and pedicels of wolfberry were effective in increasing white blood cells, protecting the liver and relieving hypertension.[61]

The website also says that when an alcohol extract of the fruit was tested in lab studies, it "inhibited tumor growth in mice by 58%, and the protein of wolfberry displayed an insulin-like action that was effective in promoting fat decomposition and reducing blood-sugar."[62]

In another study using **human** cancer participants, the following results were reported from taking the wolfberry: it "triggered an increase in both, lymphocyte transformation rate and white blood cell count…" It was also discovered that the berry may be useful in treating "Chronic Fatigue Syndrome (also known as Epstein-Barr)" and that it may "enable injured DNA to better repair itself and ward off tissue degeneration."[63]

Website *www.aromanotes.com/87/berry-young/* markets a bottled wolfberry juice that is a patent-pending combination of not only wolfberries, but "blueberries, raspberries, apricots, and pomegranates." (Pomegranate juice has "three times the antioxidant activity of green tea.") The drink is called "Berry Young Juice," and apparently is so high in antioxidants, that producers say you only need an ounce a day.[64] There are other websites that sell wolfberry juice, but some of them do not have the berry combination found in Berry Young Juice. Wolfberries are also known as "Lycium Berries…"[65]

Xi Shu: The "Cancer Tree"

Xi Shu *("Camptotheca acuminata")* is also known as the *"Cancer Tree…Happy Tree,"* and *"Tree of Joy."* It is yet another Chinese herb used for medicinal purposes to treat "diseases of the liver, gallbladder, spleen, and stomach," and it "has also been used to treat leukemia," thus giving it the name "the cancer tree."[66]

The FDA has approved two derivatives from this herb for treating cancer. The two drugs are "Topotecan" and "Irinotecan."[67] It is noteworthy that both of these drugs created by pharmaceutical companies are **toxic to normal cells,** having a variety of adverse side effects! Isn't it amazing that an herb safely used for centuries by the Chinese, once synthesized into chemo drugs by pharmaceutical companies, **becomes highly toxic to humans**!?

CHAPTER 19

MORE CANCER-FIGHTING
SUPER ANTIOXIDANTS

"Although Coenzyme Q10 represents the greatest potential breakthrough for cardiovascular disease and some other illnesses as well, the resistance of the medical profession to using this essential nutrient represents one of the greatest potential tragedies in medicine."

(Stephen T. Sinatra, M.D., from his book:
Coenzyme Q10 and the Heart)[1]

Coenzyme Q10 – A Miracle Worker

Many important antioxidants have already been discussed in this book, including vitamins A, C, E, grape seed extract (pycnogenol), resveratrol, garlic, beta-carotene, lycopene, ellagic acid, and Coenzyme Q10. Grape seed extract and Coenzyme Q10 are so powerful, that they are included in this chapter with a few other anti-oxidants that are noted cancer preventatives and fighters.

Cardiologist, Dr. Stephen Sinatra, M.D., F.A.C.C., in his book, *Coenzyme Q10 and the Heart* calls this super antioxidant **"a miracle in our midst."** He explains why he feels this way:

As a specialist, it is unthinkable for me to practice good cardiology without the help of Coenzyme Q10. And for the thousands of people with cardiac conditions so severe that they need a heart transplant, CoQ10 may be a suitable alternative that not only enhances quality of life but extends survival as well. For some, it serves as a potent medicinal while for others it may literally buy time until a donor heart is available.[2]

Dr. Sinatra is disappointed that although this nutrient is a great remedy for heart disease, most physicians have no idea it exists! It is useful for many degenerative disorders such as hypertension, cancer, gum disease, diabetes and many others.[3] (Even more amazing is the fact that the discovery of CoQ10 was accidental!) Dr. Sinatra recommends the following dosages of CoQ10 (Reproduced with permission of the McGraw-Hill companies) from his book, *Coenzyme Q10 and the Heart:*

- **30 to 100 mg daily** as a preventative in cardiovascular or peridontal disease and for patients taking Hmg-CoA reductase inhibitors. [These are cholesterol-lowering drugs].

- **90 to 180 mg daily** for the treatment of angina pectoris, cardiac arrhythmia, high blood pressure and moderate gingival disease.

- **180 to 360 mg. daily** for congestive heart failure, and dilated cardiomyopathy…For a severely impaired immune system, as in cancer, even higher doses of CoQ10 may be required.[4]

How do antioxidants like CoQ10 work? Apparently, cancer cells absorb substances in a different way than normal healthy cells. This according to Dr. Ray D. Strand in his book *What Your Doctor Doesn't Know About Nutritional Medicine May Be Killing You:*

Clinical research is revealing that cancer cells take up antioxidants differently than do normal cells. Normal, healthy cells will take up only the amount of antioxidants and supporting nutrients they need. This is a very important scientific fact when it comes to the principles of cellular nutrition. Cancer cells, on the other hand, continue to absorb nutrients without knowing when to quit. This intake of excessive antioxidants actually makes the cancer cells more vulnerable to cell death.[5]

In a nutshell – the right nutrients can kill them! Perhaps this accounts for why antioxidants like CoQ10, lycopene, resveratrol, quercetin, and ellagic acid are so powerful! It may also explain why Johanna Brandt's grape cure was so effective! Cancer cells thrive on sugar. The grape diet requires a few days of fasting before starting. Then when you start drinking the grape juice, the cells suck it up very rapidly in their "hungry" state! In the case of the grape diet, you are using a type of sugar that will kill the cancer cells, because they absorb more nutrients than they need, and in so doing, they also absorb excess antioxidants, sealing their own doom!

Antioxidants destroy free radicals, sometimes by giving up one of their own electrons in the process. Another way of looking at how antioxidants work is to remember that normally an "oxygen atom" is made up of 8 "electrons." Because of everyday stress (e.g. toxins in the environment, lack of sleep, vitamin deficiencies, etc.) and the normal aging process, the oxyen molecule loses "one of the electrons" and the result is a "free radical." This new renegade goes about "attacking other molecules," trying to steal an electron to substitute for the one that was "lost." Once it succeeds in stealing an electron from another molecule, "a new free radical is created," and "a chain reaction begins," a vicious cycle.[6]

This stealing of electrons starts to weaken the cell membrane and eventually the cell begins to deteriorate. After this happens, as explained by Lynn Keegan, Ph.D., R.N. in *Healing Nutrition*, "the cell surface is exposed to cancerous changes or a host of other ills."[6a] Anti-oxidants can enter cellular tissues and willingly "give up their electrons," but they do so without becoming renegades and "invading other cells." This puts a stop to the vicious cycle of electron theft, says Ms. Keegan, and the chain reaction comes to a halt. The cell wall is saved from destruction.[7] (Not all free radicals are bad. Some are essential to normal bodily processes.) Ms. Keegan further points out that no cell in your body "lasts longer than 7 years," and that you have "no blood cell…that is more than 14 days old." Your own body is able to "rebuild a new heart every 30 days." This means that once, at least every 30 days you get a "new start in life," to turn any bad habits around and provide your body with the nutrition to re-energize and regain your health![8] I believe that super antioxidants such as CoQ10 (and others discussed in this book) can help you to do just that. Just think of it this way: the quality of many of the body cells that you have a month from now will be the result of **what you are eating today**!

Deanna K. Loftis, R.N., B.B.A.

CoQ10 & Congestive Heart Failure

One of the largest research studies involving the effectiveness "of CoQ10 for the treatment of congestive heart failure is the Italian multi-center trial by Baggio, et al" using "2664 patients with heart failure."[9] It is described by Dr. Stephen T. Sinatra, M.D., F.A.C.C. in *Coenzyme Q10 and the Heart*. Participants in the study were given "50-150 mg for 90 days, with the majority of patients receiving 100 mg daily." After three months of taking CoQ10, patients experienced from 49% to 79% decrease in symptoms of "Edema...lung congestion...Liver enlargement...Venous congestion...Shortness of breath...[and] Heart palpitations..."[10]

One of Dr. Sinatra's patients was an "80-year-old" woman so severely affected with CHF, she was struggling to breathe and down to "77 pounds." She had a dysfunctional valve and an "EF of only 15 percent, barely enough to support a bed-to-chair lifestyle."[11] (EF or *ejection fraction* is a measurement of the heart's pumping ability. Normal is 70-80%).

Dr. Sinatra started her on "30 mg of CoQ10 three times a day (90 mg/day)," however she continued to deteriorate until something amazing occurred! Her son accidentally bought his mom "100 mg capsules instead of the usual 30 mg..." and she was taking 100 mg three times a day without realizing it. "Four weeks later," she was improving, so Dr. Sinatra kept "her on the 300 mg [a day] dose." 12 months from the time the patient started on the regimen, and "eight months after" Dr. Sinatra kept her on the "300 mg daily" of CoQ10, she "was shopping and visiting relatives," and actually overdid it to the point that "she fell down and fractured her hip!" She had an uneventful surgery. As a result of this case, Dr. Sinatra feels that if patients do not respond "to low doses of CoQ10," physicians should give larger doses and continue them, "over time," especially in those who are most severely ill![12]

These are not unusual case histories of the marvel of CoQ10. Dr. Sinatra is amazed at the widespread ignorance that prevails about nutritional medicine, and the severity of "bias against it," especially where CoQ10 is concerned, and he gives a possible reason for this bias:

The rejection of Coenzyme Q10 as a potent, nonpharmacological treatment defies the imagination. It is apparently difficult for highly trained medical personnel, well-versed in pharmacology and technology, to believe that anything so simple and so natural can be as effective as the highly engineered drugs modern medicine has to offer.[13]

Is it such a profoundly simple solution that mainstream medicine can not grasp it? Apparently so! It is also a fact that CoQ10 can not be patented, thus "there is no economic incentive for major pharmacological companies to develop or market it as a product."[14]

There are very few problems associated with the long term use of CoQ10. In a study of 5000 patients using the supplement, very minimal "adverse reactions" of gastointestinal upset, diminished "appetite...Nausea...Diarrhea...Elevated LDH (rare)...[and] Elevated SGOT (rare)," were reported.[15]

Dr. James F. Balch, M.D. in his book *The Super Anti-Oxidants* discusses the story of "Gina Ferguson," whose experience with CoQ10 was aired on a national news broadcast in a nutrition series. Gina was only 24 and dying from an "enlarged and weakened heart." She was so ill that doctors had given her "ten days" to live. Her physicians were ready to give up, having already tried various powerful pharmaceutical drugs that were not helping. Finally, they suggested she try CoQ10 supplements.[16] A month later, Gina was still alive and her heart had improved dramatically. Gina was happy with the results. In her words: "The end result is that I'm still here. I can still be a mother to my child and I can still be a wife. Co-enzyme Q-10 for me is my lifeline."[17] The mystery is why physicians don't recommend CoQ10 to their patients?

Dr. Ray D. Strand, M.D., also questioned this in his book, *What Your Doctor Doesn't Know About Nutritional Medicine May Be Killing You:*

The cost of taking CoQ10 in supplementation is about a dollar (US) a day. Not considering the reduced costs of hospitalization, this is substantially less than the $250,000 heart transplant for which most of these patients are waiting!

Furthermore, the use of CoQ10 has never shown any side effects or problems. In fact most of the studies show marked improvement within four months.[17a]

Dr. Strand was concerned that such a small minority of cardiologists are taking advantage of the healing benefits of this remarkable nutrient and admits why he believes this is so:

> Physicians are pharmaceutically trained. We know drugs, but we don't know about natural products. As much as we hate to admit it, the pharmaceutical sales representatives who come to our offices daily control much of what we learn in regard to new treatments.[18]

Although CoQ10 can be found in foods such as "organ meats, wheat germ, rice bran, and eggs," Dr. Ralph Moss says that you can not get enough of it for "therapeutic doses" without taking "it in the form of supplements…"[19] A few other natural sources of CoQ10 are "…mackerel, peanuts, salmon, sardines, and spinach."[20] (Note that organ meats have been shown to cause damage to the walls of the colon.)

Those who have a tendency to develop kidney or gallbladder stones should not consume large amounts of raw spinach due to its high "oxalate" content. Also, if you are taking "calcium supplements," wait "2-3 hours before or after" ingesting fresh spinach, since oxalates can inhibit calcium's assimilation by the body.[20a] (Though raw is best, cooking does destroy much of the oxalates.) See page 46.

High Dose CoQ10 Reverses Breast Metastasis

Author of *The Natural Physician's Healing Therapies*, Mark Stengler, N.D., explains that CoQ10 has shown dramatic effectiveness against breast cancer. There have been "Five cases of metastatic breast cancer" **completely reversed** by using "high doses of CoQ10 (390 milligrams)."[21] Do you know someone who has been battling breast cancer? Has their physician placed them on CoQ10 supplements? **If not – ask them – WHY?**

I believe we will soon see the day that patients will demand an explanation from orthodox medicine physicians for **keeping them in the dark** about powerful antioxidant supplements for fighting cancer, such as this one! (See chapter three of this book for more information on natural treatments for breast cancer.)

CoQ10, Multiple Myeloma & Pancreatic Cancers

See Chapters seven and eleven in this book for information on how CoQ10 can be helpful in fighting multiple myeloma and pancreatic cancers.

Ellagic Acid & Tangeretin

Ellagic acid, abundant in berries and grapes "neutralizes cancer and the toxins that cause cancer." They can also prevent cellular damage within the genes. One of the richest sources of ellagic acid is raspberries.[22] (Pomegranates are also a good source of ellagic acid.)

Tangerines contain a powerful antioxidant "phytonutrient called *tangeretin,*" which suppresses cancer metastasis.[22a] See other cancer specific chapters in this book for more information on these antioxidants. (For example, the amazing **prostate cancer prevention** ability of RASPBERRIES, described in chapter four.)

Grape Seed Extract – Pycnogenols

"Pycnogenols," also known as "OPCs" and "proanthocyanidins," for the purposes in this chapter, will include those found in grape seeds and pine bark. They have been used to reduce inflammation, increase "joint flexibility," and "decrease edema and swelling of the legs," as well as overall strengthening of the walls of blood vessels.[22b] According to James D. Krystosik, D.C., in his book, *Nature's Prescription for Over 60 Diseases – Grape Seed and Pine Bark Extract, they are also* used to:

[R]elieve the symptoms of "restless leg syndrome", reduce the symptoms and risks of varicose veins and phlebitis, improve vision and reduce diabetic retinopathy. They also improve the elasticity of the skin...increasing resistance to bruising...help to improve memory (even after a stroke), and reduce the effect of stress...[and] decrease the formation of histamines...[23]

Pycnogenols were probably first discovered when Cartier, "the French explorer...and his crew of a hundred men" were trying to keep from perishing during a rough "expedition in Quebec, Canada." All they had to eat were "Biscuits and meats..." explains Dr. Krystosik. They developed scurvy (rotting gums, swollen legs, and grotesque discolorations of the skin) due to a lack of "fresh fruits and vegetables..." It was not until they lost 25 fellow explorers to scurvy, (having "bled to death") with only "fifteen barely [still] alive," that Cartier ran into "a Quebec Indian" who gave him the answer to the frightful pestilence. Dr. Krystosik says that the Indian shared a tea that he had "brewed from the pine needles and bark of the 'Anneda' tree," and within seven days, "two men had recovered," and the rest of the crew rebounded shortly thereafter.[24]

It was much later in history (1865) that certain fruits and vegetables (e.g. "limes and lemons") were kept on board ships during long voyages to prevent this dread disease, but not until 1930 was a link discovered "between vitamin C and scurvy."[24a] Scientists discovered an ingredient in citrus fruit skins that could fortify the "walls" of "blood vessels," which would prevent the fatal bleeding found in "scurvy." They called "this substance 'vitamin P' for 'permeability.'" Dr. Krystosik futher notes that researchers have found that this vitamin "is a co-factor that strengthens the effect of vitamin C." Since these bioflavonoids are found in all plants and trees, obviously the tea from the pine needles and bark cured the explorers![25]

It was not until several centuries after the Cartier expedition that "Dr. Masquelier, Dean Emeritus of the University of Bordeaux," discovered these very peculiar "bioflavonoids found in nature." He called them "pycnogenols (pronounced pick-na-gen-nols)," and the best sources were found to be "grape seed extract and pine bark," though they can also be found in "peels, skins, pits, seeds, bark, and the leaves and blossoms of woody plants," usually the parts of the food that we humans pitch in the trash![26]

It was during "the International Conference on Pycnogenol Research," in 1990, that Dr. David White "of the University of Nottingham, England," disclosed that OPC's lower "LDL cholesterol." Dr. White called them "'the atherosclerosis antidote,'" and revealed that "it is the OPC's in…wine" that protect the heart. He believes that they are a "safe and effective alternative to taking aspirin to prevent heart disease."[27]

It is their fearsome ability at destroying free radicals that make grape seed extracts so important. Dr. Krystosik says that there is very little difference in the potency of the pycnogenols found in pine bark as opposed to grape seed extract except that "grape seed" is a little higher in "antioxidants," while "pine bark" extract is higher in "antihistamines."[28] (In most cases, you will find that pycnogenol from pine bark is much more expensive!)

Animals are able to manufacture their own "vitamin C" in their bodies (something humans are not capable of), giving them greater strength in "their blood vessels" than we humans have, and they usually consume the parts of plants we throw away (high in OPCs) such as peelings, pits and seeds. This is one reason why animals don't have heart attacks and strokes, only humans![29]

Cat's Claw – Pycnogenol Source

Another important source of "pycnogenol" is an herb known as "*cat's claw*." Though it is not as high in OPCs as grape seed extract and pine bark, cat's claw is emerging as an important antioxidant in the treatment of a vast array of disorders. A few of these are listed by Rita Elkins, M.H., in her book *Cat's Claw (Uno de Gato):* "Arthritis…Cancer…Crohn's…Intestinal Disorders…Lupus…Parasites… Ulcers…Viral Infections," and many other ailments.[30] This herb has also been used to treat acute leukemia. Scientific research on cat's claw showed that it can "specifically target cellular mutations such as leukemic cells and inhibit their development."[31]

Thus far, there have been no harmful side effects revealed for the normal use of cat's claw, however, it is not recommended for use "in autoimmune illness, multiple sclerosis, and tuberculosis," nor should it be given "with hormonal drugs, insulin, or vaccines," or taken during pregnancy or lactation.[32]

Which Grapes Are Best?

Though many nutritionists favor the red and purple grapes for their antioxidants, for higher OPC content, Dr. James F. Balch, M.D., recommends "green and white grapes rather than the red grape..."[33]

I believe the best advice, as given by Johanna Brandt, is to eat a **variety**, because you will get more **resveratrol** in the red, black, and purple grapes, yet more **OPC's** in the green and white grapes, and **you need both**!

Lycopene

See cancer specific chapters in this book for information on this powerful antioxidant.

Pomegranates

Pomegranate juice is very high in antioxidants that fight free radicals. One brand describes their juice (*POM Wonderful Pomegranate Juice)* as being very high in antioxidants.[33a] The research described at their website actually used the "Wonderful variety of pomegranantes." You can find *POM Wonderful Pomegranate Juice* in the refrigerated section of most grocery stores and some natural health food stores. For more information, see their website at: *www.pomwonderfulstore.com.*[34] The juice of pomegranates (as well as the seeds) have been shown to kill parasites.

Quercetin

Dr. James Balch, in *The Super Anti-Oxidants,* says that the very "potent flavonoid…found in onions, cayenne pepper, garlic, and green tea" known as *"Quercetin,"* has a very impressive "antioxidant" effect on the human body. It prevents the damage that free radicals can do to the entire cardiovascular system, and keeps blood platelets from gumming up and clumping together, thus protecting against "clots, strokes and heart attacks."[35] **Statistics collected not only from animal but human testing as well, reveal that quercetin suppresses cancer.**

Quercetin is one of the strongest anti-cancer agents known. According to Maureen Kennedy Salaman in her book, *How to Renew You,* this antioxidant "unleashes a one-two punch against cancer. It blocks cell changes that invite cancer and, if a tumor has already started, it stops the spread of malignant cells." One of the best sources is "Red and yellow onions."[36] See the cancer specific chapters in this book for more information on quercetin's powerful role against cancer.

ORAC

During the "early 1990s," Dr. Guohua Cao "and his colleagues" developed a way to measure the antioxidant potency of foods. It is known as "the Oxygen Radical Absorbance Capacity (or ORAC) test." Each substance on the list was compared in potency to that of a "standardized amount of vitamin E."[37] Of course, the greater the ORAC value, the higher the antioxidant power of the food!

If possible, try to get at least 10,000 or more ORAC points per day from the ORAC list (especially if you are struggling against cancer or some other life-threatening illness), and this is not hard to do! If you eat just 3.5 ounces of prunes, raisins, red grapes, kale, and onions in one day, you are getting OVER 11,000 ORAC points! (A sample copy of an **ORAC food list** is shown below.)

Various nutrient-rich drinks are being promoted that are high in ORAC content. One in particular is called *7 Essentials.* Their producers claim that one serving of their drink contains a whopping 21,010 ORAC units. As explained in an email from them, this "value was determined by Brunswick Laboratories according to the Tufts University method of rating." If you are interested, it is marketed at *www.healthy-living.org/html/essential_ seven.html.*[38]

The ORAC FOOD LIST

ORAC VALUES OF FRUITS & VEGETABLES
(per 100 grams, or 3.5 ounces)

ORAC values refer to the Oxygen Radical Absorbance Capacity of a food, as determined by the U.S. Department of Agriculture. By testing the ability of foods and other compounds to subdue oxygen free radicals, the DOA was able to determine each compound's antioxidant capability. The ORAC values in the following chart reflect these findings.

FRUITS	ORAC VALUE	VEGETABLES	ORAC VALUE
Prunes	5,770	Kale	1,770
Raisins	2,830	Spinach, raw	1,260
Blueberries	2,400	Brussels sprouts	980
Blackberries	2,036	Alfalfa sprouts	930
Cranberries	1,750	Spinach, steamed	909
Strawberries	1,540	Broccoli florets	890
Raspberries	1,220	Beets	841
Plums	949	Red bell pepper	713
Oranges	750	Onion	450
Grapes, red	739	Corn	400
Cherries	670	Eggplant	390
Kiwifruit	602	Cauliflower	377
Grapes, white	446	Peas, frozen	364
Cantaloupe	252	White potatoes	313
Banana	221	Sweet potatoes	301
Apple	218	Carrots	207
Apricots	164	String beans	201
Peach	158	Tomato	189
Pear	134	Zucchini	176
Watermelon	104	Yellow Squash	150
Source: Agriculture Research, February 1999			

This list and information is re-printed with permission from website *www.younga-gain.com/orac.html.*[39] The list originally appeared in the article "Can Foods Forestall Aging?" by Judy McBride, *Agricultural Research*, vol. 47, no. 2, February 1999, p. 14-17, published by the U.S. Department of Agriculture, Agricultural Research Service, Washington, D.C.

If at all possible, I believe it is best to obtain your daily ORACs from fresh, raw fruits and vegetables. If you can not do so, your next best choice would be nutrient-rich drinks (like the one above), and the green powdered drinks such as Dee Simmons' *Green Miracle* (available at *www.ultimateliving.com).*

Alpha Lipoic Acid

This important antioxidant has great protective benefits, especially for the liver. The late, "Peter Jennings on *World News Tonight*" said that "Alpha lipoic acid is probably the most potent…antioxidant known to man."[40]

Dr. Ralph Moss in *Antioxidants against Cancer* reports that Europeans have used alpha lipoic acid for years to "reverse the effects of mushroom poisoning." It also protects against "stroke, heart disease and cataracts," and increases "the body's" production "of glutathione by 30 to 70 percent." Its action in the human body is very much like that of "glutathione."[41]

Does your family have a genetic disposition toward some types of cancer? Dr. Moss explains that alpha lipoic acid has the unique ability of being able to "turn off the genes that accelerate cancer, without any signs of toxicity." Scientists are not sure why, but research proved that "people or animals with cancer absorb lipoic acid," and when lipoic acid was given to lab animals with cancer, their lives were "extended by 25 percent."[42]

According to Burt Berkson, Ph.D., in *The Alpha Lipoic Acid Breakthrough,* this vital nutrient is made by every cell in our body when we are children, then as we age, we produce less and less of it, however, the older we get, the more we need it to stay healthy! It is critically important because it appears to work by preventing cellular damage and when taken "in the correct dosage," there are "virtually no side effects…"[43]

Dr. Berkson takes 100 mg of ALA morning and evening. He also describes a few other amazing health benefits of ALA:

> [A]LA can inhibit the production of the AIDS virus...may prevent cataracts of the eye...protects the kidneys...insulates the pancreas from inflammatory attack and possibly prevents diabetes...keeps T-lymphocytes from committing suicide...enhances your immune system...increases helper T-cells in the blood...helps fight many disease processes, including cancer...prevents leukemia...can be used for treating diabetes...and serious liver disease...[44]

Alpha Lipoic Acid and Liver Transplants

Dr. Berkson has also treated several of his "hepatitis C" patients with ALA; patients who were told that they would DIE without "a liver transplant." After treatment with ALA therapy, all of his patients "except one," were "back at work or in school and feeling normal with increased energy levels."[44a] He believes that before anyone contemplates "liver transplant surgery...a doctor should prescribe a course of alpha lipoic acid." His treatment also included a nutritious diet, "a stress reduction program, and an exercise regimen...various vitamins...and silymarin" (milk thistle).[45]

ALA is also discussed in chapter eight of this book for its importance in treating liver cancer. A few natural food sources of ALA include spinach, potatoes, brewer's yeast and broccoli.

Acia Berries

There has been much recent publicity about *acia* berries. They are a high antioxidant berry taken from a palm tree in the Brazilian Rainforest. This berry is said to have twice the antioxidants found in blueberries and ten times more than those found in grapes. There are many websites that market acia berry juice. It is also available in capsules as a supplement.

Glutathione & Glutamine

"Glutathione" protects the brain and "the stomach lining" (against toxins), and overall, it is a "master antioxidant" important due to its protective functioning in strengthening the immune system. It is not easy for the body to assimilate glutathione if taken in supplement form unless your levels are severely depressed. If you do use supplements, it is best to combine them with "selenium and vitamin B2" since they enhance its function.[46]

The very best way to increase your levels of glutathione is to take those supplements that boost the levels of glutathione in the body, supplements like NAC or N-acetylcysteine (an amino acid).[47] Milk thistle also raises glutathione levels in the body and vitamin C preserves it.

For natural sources of glutathione, use raw "fresh green, yellow and red vegetables...Canned and frozen vegetables lose all of their glutathione in processing."[48] Cooking also destroys much of the glutathione. Another reason to consume your veggies and fruit raw, their most nutritious state! (See the graph in chapter nine for many natural food sources of glutathione. It also shows you how much glutathione is destroyed in cooking.)

Animal studies have revealed that several spices and plants can raise glutathione levels in the body. Scientists concluded from their studies that these phyto-compounds can play a role in the prevention and suppression of cancer. (e.g. the next time you bake bread, you may want to add some poppy seed or flaxseed! Flaxseed can be used for cooking, if you soak them "in water for at least an hour before using them...")[48a]

Avocados are very rich in glutathione. They also contain "beta-carotene," and "more potassium than bananas...Scientists believe that avocados may also be useful in treating viral hepatitis (a cause of liver cancer), as well as other sources of liver damage."[49] They are also high in lutein!

Another nutrient known as "glutamine," functions as a "protein building block." Tumors feed on glutamine to grow.[50] They seem to need excessive amounts of this amino acid and absorb it to the extent that the patient's own body is depleted of the nutrient. Because of this the patient wastes away, a disorder commonly found in cancer patients called "cachexia.'"[51]

Glutamine appears to boost immunity. As a matter of fact, rats with tumors had a "40 percent" decrease in "tumor growth" after receiving "seven weeks" of "glutamine supplements..."[52] Beans, fish, and whey protein contain glutamine. This amino acid is also available in supplement form at health food stores.

Antioxidants Not Merely For Cancer Prevention & Treatment

Antioxidants not only protect against debilitating and deadly diseases such as cancer, they also protect the rest of the body and its vital functions. One example is the xanthophylls, zeaxanthin and lutein, and also bilberry, which protects valuable eyesight from free radical damage. Studies show that people with the "highest intake of lutein and zeaxanthin – abundant in spinach, collards, and other dark, leafy greens – had **57% less risk** of developing macular degeneration." Bilberry has also been used "in treating cataracts and helping to clear vision...[and] Italian scientists recently found that a dried leaf extract" of bilberry lowered blood sugar in laboratory animals. Bilberry has even been used to lower harmful "LDL cholesterol...reduce hypertension...alleviate symptoms of diabetes ...as a remedy for diarrhea and indigestion," and in treating ulcers.[53]

Help for Multiple Sclerosis, Downs Syndrome & ALD

More and more research is pointing to the fact that diseases like multiple sclerosis and muscular dystrophy are preventable as well as treatable through nutrition. Even the severe problems encountered by those born with the genetic disorder, Downs Syndrome, can be helped with nutrition.

Nutrition & MS

A physician by the name of Hinton D. Jonez used nutrition to bring about incredible results with MS patients, and they are described by Maureen Kennedy Salaman in *All Your Health Questions Answered Naturally*. She explains that Dr. Jonez described his protocol in a book he wrote, *"My Fight to Conquer Multiple Sclerosis*, and an article in the *Journal of Postgraduate Medicine,* outlining his nutrition regimen (which included 8,000 mcg of vitamin B12, omega-3 and omega-6 essential fatty acids, and intravenous minerals)."[54] Also recommended by Ms. Salaman for MS patients is the use of "Lorenzo's Oil" as well as "borage oil...which contains up to 26 percent GLA."[55]

See chapter five of this book for the amazing results obtained by one physician when he merely placed his M.S. patient on a nutritional supplement program! Also, see website *http://kinsman.epix.net/water/ Multiple.htm*, for the story of M. Fox, who claims that all her symptoms of M.S. disappeared when she went on Dr. Batmanghelidj's *Water Cure*. His water cure is also discussed in chapter 22 of this book. It is noteworthy as well, that vegetarian diets and low fat diets significantly reduce the risks for M.S. Research has also shown that curcumin may be beneficial in fighting M.S. because it appears to have a protective effect on nerve cells. (Curcumin does have blood-thinning effects and can increase bile and gastric acid output, something to consider if you have gallbladder disease or ulcers.)

ALD

Lorenzo's Oil was the name of a movie in 1992, the true story of a child battling a rare disease "ALD (Adreno-leukodystrophy)," which is described by the National Institute of Neurological Disorders and Stroke (NINDS) at their website: *http://www.ninds.nih.gov/disorders/adrenoleukodystrophy/adrenoleukodystrophy.htm:*

(ALD) is one of a group of genetic disorders called the leukodystrophies that cause damage to the myelin sheath, an insulating membrane that surrounds nerve cells in the brain.

People with ALD accumulate high levels of saturated, very long chain fatty acids (VLCFA) in the brain and adrenal cortex because they do not produce the enzyme that breaks down these fatty acids in the normal manner. The loss of myelin and the progressive dysfunction of the adrenal gland are the primary characteristics of ALD....The most common symptoms are usually behavioral changes such as abnormal withdrawal or aggression, poor memory, and poor school performance.[56]

The problem with the disease is that the body is not able to correctly assimilate fats. This results in abnormal fat deposits where they don't belong! The results can be disastrous, eventually causing brain damage. The National Institute of Neurological Disorders and Stroke says of Lorenzo's oil that it is composed of "a mixture of oleic acid and euric acid," and that it "can reduce or delay the appearance of symptoms.."[57]

According to website: *www.jr2.ox.ac.uk/bandolier/booth/neuro/lorenz.html*, Lorenzo's oil is "a mixture of glycerl trioleate (C18:1) and glyceryl trierucate (C22:1). It is used to reduce the concentration of longer chain fatty acids in the body, and the hope is that it also reduces demyelination and clinical progression" of the disease.[58] Lasting effects of the oil are uncertain. The main problem with the oil is that it does not "cross the blood-brain barrier," so it can not "replace the very long chain fatty acids in the brain," though it can "delay onset of symptoms." However, it does not appear to be able to reverse them or prolong them indefinitely.[59]

The MS Patch – Prokarin™

During a phone conversation with me on May 26, 2005, Elaine DeLack, a registered nurse, told me that she was diagnosed with M.S. in 1988 though her symptoms actually began in 1984. She said that when the symptoms first began, she would wake up in the middle of the night and could not move her left leg. After her son was born, the symptoms extended to her left hand. Initially she was in denial until the day that she was carrying her young son and her left leg gave out on her, causing her to fall. She consulted with a physician in her home town, who sent her a prescription for vitamin B-12 and adenosine monophosphate injections. She improved and was able to finish nursing school. Ms. DeLack did a great deal of research and felt that histamine should be added to the vitamin B-12 and adenosine monophosphate. The end result of her research was a treatment for multiple sclerosis, a histamine patch known as Prokarin™ that she says has even enabled some M.S. sufferers to leave their wheelchairs behind.

The actual formula for Prokarin™ is proprietary information. Ms. Delack has had amazing success treating herself with this product. She said that she has remained symptom free while on this medication. This is remarkable when you consider that she was diagnosed 17 years ago! Although the FDA has not approved Prokarin™ for treating MS, your physician can still write you a prescription for Prokarin™, but you have to request it. Studies are currently continuing on the compound.

Help for Muscular Dystrophy

As described by Maureen Kennedy Salaman in *All Your Health Questions Answered Naturally*, muscular dystrophy has also been attributed to nutritional deficiencies. It is a disease where the "muscles atrophy and degenerate, eventually being replaced with fat." It differs from MS in that "nerves" deteriorate in MS and in muscular dystrophy, the "muscles" deteriorate. CoQ10, a powerful antioxidant, has been very effective "in treating muscular dystrophy."[60] Ms. Salaman further explains that scientists believe the muscle degeneration is linked to a lack of "choline" in the body as well as "vitamin E." In fact, she says that they actually "caused" the disease "in rabbits" simply by feeding them a vitamin E deficient diet, but they later found that it was a lack of choline that "caused the dystrophy."[61] Natural sources of "choline" are: "Cabbage…Cauliflower, Egg yolk, Garbanzo beans…Kale, Lentils, Oatmeal, Peanuts, Soybeans, Soy lecithin, [and] Wheat germ."[62]

Also noted by Ms. Salaman was another study in Sweden which showed that improvement in adult muscular dystrophy occurred with "high doses of vitamin E and selenium…" Not only that, but keeping the muscles healthy requires the essential fatty acids, as well as minerals and amino acids.[63] Ms. Salaman has an easily absorbable, good-tasting liquid mineral drink that I use and highly recommend, called *Mineral Rich®.* You can find it at her website *www.mksalaman.com,* and in some health food stores, along with her many other excellent nutritional products and books.

Help for Downs Syndrome Children

For parents with Downs syndrome children, Ms. Salaman suggests calling "(504) 769-TRIS. Representatives there say you'll get all the information you need to either convince your doctor to try nutritional therapy, or do it on your own" for your "Downs' Syndrome" child. She suggests that you may also want to check into "live cell therapy," which has been effective with some of these children. "Contreras Oasis Hospital in Tijuana, Mexico" practices live cell therapy (Their "ph# (800) 700-1850"), as well as "Claus Marten's Four Seasons Clinic and Health Resort at Fareerweg, Rottach Egern, W. Germany, phone: 80-222-6780-24041."[64]

Soy Products

Though the benefits of soy products have been discussed earlier in this book, there is some controversy about soy. My suggestion would be to use soy products in moderation. I would certainly choose organic soy over dairy products. Fermented soy is fine!

Soy contains "a substance called the protease inhibitor," which, according to Don Colbert, M.D., in his book, *Walking in Divine Health*, is "actually the seed's defense against destruction." Though the seed can be swallowed by birds, it can not be digested, nor "broken down. Researchers are highly interested in these phytochemicals because they have been able to use them to reverse cancerous cells back to their original precancerous state."[65] (Fermented soy products, such as Haelan, can help remove harmful estrogens from the body in estrogen-receptor positive cancers.)

CHAPTER 20

MORE CAROTENOIDS THAT CURE & OTHER HEALING FOODS & NUTRIENTS

"A few days ago on a national television show, I saw an oncologist (a conventional cancer specialist) discussing cancer. She said, 'We still don't know what causes cancer. But we have surgery, chemotherapy, and radiation to treat it.' I could only shake my head and ask myself, Where has she been for the last twenty years?"

(Burk Berkson, M.D., Ph.D., from his book,
The Alpha Lipoic Acid Break-through)[1]

I. Carotenoids

Carotenoids give fruits and vegetables their wonderful colors. They are what give the deep colors to peppers, "carrots...and tomatoes..." Jack Challem, in his book, *All About Carotenoids Beta-Carotene, Lutein & Lycopene,* reports that there are actually "600 different plant pigments" included in this group, yet very few of them are known to be important to our health.[1a] There are "around fifty carotenoids...in the foods" we ingest, yet "only fourteen have been identified in the bloodstream," he says, meaning that there are very few actually "absorbed by the body." Even though some of the others are not absorbable, they may play vital health roles that we are not yet aware of. All of them are "fat-soluble," meaning that they should be eaten along with some form of fat such as olive oil or flax oil, rather than water.[2] What all this means (in a nutshell) is that if you are eating a fresh veggie salad with lettuce, diced tomatoes, peppers, onions, summer squash, broccoli, and carrots, your salad dressing should be oil-based. (A good choice would be organic flax oil or olive oil, or dice up an avocado and include it in the salad!)

How Carotenoids Fight Cancer

Beta-carotene makes the monocytes (white blood cells that hunt for and kill cancer cells and pathogens) more powerful at what they do. According to Jack Challem, in order to be able to tell "a cancer cell from a normal" cell, "monocytes" have a type of sonar protein located on the "surface of the cell." This sonar is called "MHC II". As soon as "the MHC II protein detects a cancer cell," it sends an SOS signal to related immunity cells, which surround and zap the intruders! If the monocytes are deficient in these sonar or "radar" proteins, cancerous cells slip by undetected, then begin their harmful replicating.[3]

David A. Hughes, Ph.D, and "colleagues at the Institute of Food Research, England," discovered that the amount of "MHC II proteins on monocytes" can be increased by the consumption of "beta-carotene..."[3a] In his research, he found that when he gave "15 mg...supplements...[of] beta-carotene" to a group of "healthy men" for one month, the result was a dramatic increase in "cancer-detecting MHC II proteins on their monocytes." He also discovered that the men taking beta-carotene had an increase in "tumor necrosis factor alpha (TNF-a), an immune system molecule, that like a heat-seeking missile, zeroes in on cancer cells and destroys them." The control group received a placebo and did not have the same results.[4]

Mr. Challem, in *All About Carotenoids,* also discusses research showing that beta-carotene has reversed "precancerous" mouth lesions:

> There is evidence based on a number of human studies conducted at the University of Arizona, Tucson, and other research centers that beta-carotene can help reverse a condition called oral leukoplakia, a precancerous lesion of the mouth or throat that often leads to full-blown oral cancer if left untreated. Vitamin A and vitamin E can also reverse oral leukoplakia...[5]

Organized medicine, in their bias against alternative cancer treatments, will now admit (after years of denying it) that good nutrition can prevent cancer, however, they will not admit that it can reverse cancer, though there are many case histories (e.g. documented in this book) that prove this to be true.

Numerous research studies have been done to prove that beta-carotene can protect against many types of cancer, including those difficult to treat such as pancreatic cancer. Mr. Challem explains that a prolonged deficiency in beta-carotene "over many years may increase the risk of rheumatoid arthritis," as well as "lupus." This nutrient also helps asthma sufferers, prevents visual problems, reduces the risk of heart disease, lowers cholesterol, and protects against sunburn![6]

When it comes to taking beta-carotene, it is best to take natural, rather than synthetic beta-carotene. Natural beta-carotene can be found in "lettuce, parsley, sweet potatoes,[7] apricots...asparagus, broccoli, cantaloupe, carrots...kale...pumpkin, spinach, watermelon," and many other foods.[8]

While synthetic vitamin A can be toxic in large doses (because it is stored in the liver) beta-carotene in natural form (e.g. carrot juice) converts into natural vitamin A in the body, in a slow process that prevents system overload!

According to H. Winter Griffith, M.D., in *Vitamins Herbs, Minerals & Supplements*, the liver normally stores "a 2-year supply" of vitamin A. Once that supply is gone, deficiencies will show up as "Night blindness, lack of tear secretion...eventual blindness...dry, rough skin...poor bone growth, weak tooth enamel, diarrhea...acne, insomnia, [and] fatigue," and a host of other health problems.[9] If you have any of these health problems, you may need to start juicing fresh carrots immediately!

Papaya & Guavas

Papaya has important enzymes that are useful in treating cancer, but without toxic side effects. Scientists have been studying the effects of enzymes like those found in papaya for the treatment of illness for nearly twenty years. In his book, *Papaya The Healing Fruit,* author, Harald Tietze describes the anti-cancer effects of this amazing fruit:

There are many reports of cancer sufferers being healed by drinking a concentrate made from papaya leaves...South American natives have used papaya leaves and fruit to treat tumors for hundreds of years. After an application of papaya remedy, the tumor wounds are reported to heal and the pain immediately subsides.[10]

In modern times, the use of papaya for cancer treatment is "backed by scientific study." Research has shown that cancer cells contain "a type of fibrin," permitting them to travel through the "immune system...undetected," thus their insidious attachment to the walls of blood vessels.[10a] After sticking to the wall, Mr. Tietze says that the cancer cell then forces itself "through the wall" and attaches "to the nearest organ" to begin replicating. "The founder of modern enzyme therapy...Dr Wolf, discovered that people with cancer lack protein-splitting enzymes called proteolytic enzymes," which work by splitting up the fibrin to "prevent cancerous cells...from forming."[11] (Be aware that papaya enzyme preparations can increase blood coagulation time. If you are taking blood-thinners, your physician should know if you plan to use papaya enzymes.)

Harald Tietze tells the story of a Swiss homeopath's experience in "November 1996" using "papaya concentrate [on] a female patient," who had metastasizing cancer, and was given "two weeks" to live. The patient began taking a "high daily dosage of the papaya concentrate and her condition improved." Her physicians were baffled. By "the end of September 1997," her symptoms had nearly disappeared and she had returned to work.[12] **(This was almost a _year_ after doctors had given her two weeks to live!)**

Mr. Tietze also reports that "papaya leaf concentrate, [and] Kombucha-papaya extract" have been "successful" in treating "skin cancer." Papain itself proved effective in laboratory testing when "50 percent of rats given papain survived a normally lethal dose of radiation."[13]

Papaya not only tastes good, it is very nutritious, having "more vitamin A than carrots and more vitamin C than oranges." It hinders "the growth of human breast cancer cells," cleanses the body by removing toxins, and increases metabolism. Every part of the plant is useful for "medicinal and nutritional" purposes. Hens are even fed "papaya fruit" to give egg yolks a deeper "orange-yellow" color![14]

The next time you consume a meal high in protein, remember that papaya has important enzymes that help digest proteins. It is actually more nutritious for this purpose when the flesh is mature but still a little on the *green* side. When fully mature, most papayas are yellow.

There are teas available that are made from the leaves of the papaya plant. If you see a tea called "Dried Paw-Paw Leaves" from "The Kombucha House in Australia," this is actually a papaya tea, however, a "pawpaw in North America with the Latin name *Asimina tribola* is in no way related to the papaya."[14a] There is a pawpaw "in Australia and New Zealand" called "*Carica papaya*," which **is** a papaya. Just be aware that if something is called "pawpaw," it may not necessarily have anything to do with papaya. Check the label of contents![15]

It is noted that the carotenoids in papaya "can quite literally, save your life. [They]…are extremely powerful antioxidants. Many fruits and vegetables contain carotenoids, but papayas are way ahead of the pack."[16]

The papain found in papaya is very much like the digestive enzymes that occur "naturally in the stomach," making papaya an important digestive aid if you eat it raw either "during or after a meal." Selene Yeager in *Doctors Book of FOOD REMEDIES,* says that it may also be important as an anti-ulcer food. This was demonstrated when researchers gave test animals large amounts of papaya "for several days," then fed them "stomach-churning drugs…The animals fed papaya were much "less likely to get ulcers…"[17] The "unripe…fruit, skins, leaves, seeds…." should not be eaten by "pregnant women…"[18]

According to website *http://alternativecancer.us/pawpaw.html,* an extract from pawpaw, "a cousin of the Graviola, guanabana, and soursop trees," has ingredients that have anti-angiogenesis properties, that is, they prevent new "blood vessels" from growing, thus cutting off the nutrient supply to tumors (This is also what shark cartilage does).[18a] They also "inhibit the growth of MDR (multiple drug resistance) cells." There is "no other alternative or conventional cancer treatment (except treatments from trees similar to pawpaw)" that "has shown any effectiveness against MDR cells," says the website, and about 2% of tumors are made up of MDR cells which remain even after chemo. This is one reason why a tumor that initially appears to respond to chemo, often returns a short time later. Problem is, when the tumor returns, all of the cells that make it up will now be MDR cells and no amount of chemo (or radiation) will kill them! "**PawPaw is the only cancer treatment that has shown effectiveness against MDR cells**."[19] (Emphasis, mine.) During **human testing**, when "100 cancer patients" were studied, pawpaw was effective in 50% of them. Website *alternativecancer.us/pawpaw.htm* suggests four capsules of the supplement per day "evenly spaced out during the day, and taken with some food." They recommend that you do not take pawpaw at the same time that you take other nutrient supplements such as CoQ10 and SOD. For a full list of the non-compatible nutrients see their website.[20] The above website also has ordering information for the extract, or you can contact any distributor from *Nature's Sunshine* to obtain pawpaw for you. It can also be found in health food stores.

As for side effects, Selene Yeager explains that "some people have reported...nausea. For this reason it is recommended to take pawpaw with food."[21] She also says that guavas are sometimes mistaken for papayas, but they are very different. The thing that makes guavas significant is that they are very rich in "lycopene," averaging "50 percent more lycopene in a single fruit" than do tomatoes, plus they are very rich in fiber, having "about 9 grams per cup."[22] (So, the next time you grab tomatoes for their lycopene content, you may want to add a few guavas to your cart as well!)

Peas & Beans

Peas are rich in chlorophyllin...(cousin to "chlorophyll..."), which has such a unique "molecular shape" that it can latch onto carcinogens and stick to them, preventing their assimilation by the body![23]

Beans (legumes) carry nutrients that inhibit cancer, and regulate serum glucose, an important benefit for diabetics. Besides being fiber-rich, they also contain "protease inhibitors," which appear "to be extremely effective in blocking the formation of certain cancers including colon and breast."[24] This is explained in Charmaine Rivers' *Manna from Heaven – Healing Foods From The Bible.*

Other Carotenoids: Alpha-Carotene, Cryptoxanthin, & Astaxanthin

A very close relative of beta-carotene, "**alpha-carotene**," is found in "carrots" and "pumpkins," and as described by Jack Challem in *All About Carotenoids Beta-carotene, Lutein & Lycopene,* research conducted by "Michiaki Murakoshi, PhD.," and "his colleagues at the Kyoto Prefectural University" found that this carotenoid can slow down or inhibit many types of cancer cells such as "those of the brain, pancreas, and stomach."[24a] Another study involving **human subjects** in "New Jersey" had an impressive outcome: male smokers, some diagnosed with cancers of the respiratory tract ("trachea, bronchus, or lung") had their diets compared to "diets of healthy men of comparable age. It was found that those men who" ate diets high in alpha-carotene had lower risks of "developing these cancers."[25]

Cryptoxanthin [a] "carotenoid...found in papayas, peaches, tangerines, and oranges," says Mr. Challen, also has anti-cancer properties. In research that involved "a fifteen-year-long study of 15,000 women," he says that it was revealed that women who ate foods high in this carotenoid greatly decreased their risks for "developing cervical cancer."[26]

Astaxanthin, another "carotenoid," is found in marine animals like "salmon and trout." Sometimes carotenoids, such as this one, are mixed with the diets of "farm-raised fish," says Jack Challem, to heighten their color and marketability. This particular carotenoid was found "to be more protective...against UVA light" (exposure to which, can result in melanoma and "sunburn") "than beta-carotene and lutein."[27] Mr. Challem has a new book out: *Feed Your Genes Right: Eat to Turn Off Disease-Causing Genes and Slow Down Aging.* It is described in detail at website *www.feedyourgenesright.com.*

II. Other Healing Food Nutrients

Apples & Figs

The "natural acids" found in apples may be their main weapon against cancer, but to get the full benefit, it is best to "eat the whole thing, skin and all." The skins have most of the "pectin fiber" which decreases harmful "cholesterol…[and] blood pressure," normalizes "blood sugar," and inhibits "cancer."[27a]

According to Charmaine Rivers in *Manna from Heaven Healing Foods From The Bible*, Figs contain "benzaldehyde…[an] anti-cancer" compound, which has been tested on animals and **humans.** During **human** testing, says Rivers, "Of the 55 patients in the test group, seven went into complete remission, 29 into partial remission," and most remarkable of all was that the compound **actually performed better** "on human malignant tumors than on experimental tumors in mice."[28]

Artichokes & Asparagus

Research has revealed that a compound in "artichokes" not only inhibits cancer but it can also reverse liver damage! The compound is "silymarin," also shown in animal studies to "prevent skin cancer…" Artichokes are merely "the immature flower of the thistle plant."[28a] (Silymarin is the main ingredient of the herb, milk thistle. Milk thistle is so important for liver health, it was discussed in greater detail in this book in chapter eight on liver cancer.)

Selene Yeager, et al., in *Doctors Book of FOOD REMEDIES,* explains that "Asparagus" protects against colon cancer and "spinal cord birth defects (called neural tube defects)" due to its high folate content. It is one of the richest sources available of natural glutathione and it also contains vitamin E. In an analysis of "38 vegetables," researchers placed "freshly cooked asparagus" at the top of the list due to "its glutathione content."[29] This vegetable is so alkalizing to the body, it retains some alkalinity, even when it is cooked!

Barley, Buckwheat & Bulgar – Cancer Fighting Grains

Barley is an excellent way to get your daily supply of natural tocotrienols. "Like vitamin E, Tocotrienols, are antioxidants," which protect the heart and help the liver cut cholesterol level! Barley is a rich source of antioxidants, "lignans...selenium and vitamin E."[30]

Buckwheat, high in flavonoids, as well as "quercetin and rutin," keeps "cancer-promoting hormones from sticking to normal cells." If carcinogenic substances do enter the cells, quercetin and rutin can keep DNA from being injured further. Rutin inhibits dangerous clot formation, and can lower total cholesterol levels. Buckwheat is "the best known grain source of high quality protein." (Once "roasted," it is referred to as "Kasha.")[31]

Selene Yeager says that **bulgar** is nothing less than wheat "in its whole form." Nearly everyone is familiar with nitrates (cancer-causing compounds used excessively in highly "processed foods.") Once nitrates enter the body, they are chemically changed into "nitrosamines," which cause cancer.[31a] Ms. Yeager further explains that bulgar has a substance known as "ferulic acid," which prevents the body from changing nitrates into dangerous nitrosamines. It also has "lignans," notable for their anti-cancer properties.[31b] Bulgar wheat is important for diabetics in that "it has a low glycemic index," meaning that during digestion, its sugar content is not dumped rapidly into the bloodstream, but "released...slowly," assisting in blood sugar stability. This grain can "go rancid" rapidly, so it should be kept in your refrigerator until you plan to eat it.[32]

Celery Inhibits Tumor Growth & Relieves Hypertension

Celery has the ability to inhibit cancer and relieve hypertension. When a hypertensive patient was told by his physician to cut back on his salt intake, "he began eating a quarter-pound (about four stalks) of celery per day. Within a week his blood pressure had dropped from 158/96 to 118/82." However, you can overdo the celery, since it does have natural sodium.[32a] Celery may cause sun-sensitivity in some people. (Sometimes, this can be countered simply by being sure that you clean "celery thoroughly before eating it...to remove fungi," which may be responsible for the problem, however, any raw fruit or vegetable should be cleaned "thoroughly" before consumption!)[32b] Celery also contains anti-cancer ingredients called "acetylenics," which can halt the growth of "tumor cells." It is best to consume celery with the leaves, where many of the vitamins and minerals are most concentrated.[33] (Another natural nutrient, besides celery that can lower blood pressure is rye. Baking rye bread from rye flour, or even purchasing ready-made rye bread and eating it, can help lower blood pressure. Be sure, if baking, that you add plenty of limonene-rich caraway seed!)

Chinese Red Yeast Rice

Though promoted mostly for its ability to lower cholesterol levels, Rita Elkins, M.H. in her book, *Chinese Red Yeast Rice*, says that this substance has demonstrated anti-cancerous properties. It is a fermented extract containing valuable compounds such as "mevinolin, also known as lovastatin," capable of lowering blood cholesterol.[33a] Even though "extracts of red yeast rice have been used in prescription drugs like Mevacor," some of the extracts are now available in natural health food stores. Ms. Elkins says that during "one of the clinical studies...at the College of Pharmacy of Nihon University" in Japan, the "red yeast rice pigment referred to as *Monascus* pigment, was able to inhibit the growth of malignant tumors in laboratory test mice."[34]

IP-6: The Anti-Tumor Pill

IP-6 may be a significant nutrient for fighting cancer. It has demonstrated anti-cancer properties, and is a natural extract derived from soy and grains. Testing thus far has shown that IP-6 can suppress cellular mutations better than green tea without harming normal, healthy cells. Many believe that IP-6 can cause abnormal cancer cells to revert back to their healthy state. Studies have shown that the extract has the ability to inhibit several types of cancers. Several websites market IP-6 and most natural health food stores do as well. See chapter eight of this book for more information on this supplement. Check with your physician before supplementing with IP-6 since it does have blood-thinning properties.

Indoles – DIM – The Phytonutrient
That Prevents Cancer

DIM *(diindolymethane)* is a plant compound that appears to have impressive anti-cancer effects by blocking harmful estrogens from being absorbed into the body. DIM can be purchased as a supplement at most natural health food stores. This plant nutrient is most abundant in all of our cruciferous foods such as cabbages, broccoli, kale, kohlrabi, turnip greens and others.

Nutrition at the Cellular Level

The advocates of *Orthomolecular Medicine* (discussed elsewhere in this book) use a nutritional approach to disease, stressing the importance of megavitamins such as vitamin C, and megaminerals such as niacinamide, selenium, and amino acids like lysine.

Some natural sources of lysine are: "eggs…potatoes…and brewer's yeast."[35] (note that lysine can also be found in many other foods including fish, avocados and whole wheat bread.)

Another proponent in favor of high dose vitamin C supplementation for cancer prevention was Dr. E. Cheraskin, M.D., D.M.D., author of *Vitamin C Who Needs It?* In his book, he discussed a research discovery by "the Albert Einstein College of Medicine in New York City," showing the importance of vitamin C intake for women:

> [W]omen whose intake of vitamin C was less than 30 mg daily (only half the RDA and equal to about half a medium orange or two ounces of juice from concentrate) had a risk of developing cervical dysplasia ten times greater than that of women whose intake was higher.[36]

See chapters seven and fifteen of this book for an amazing account of how a teenager was healed of "terminal" Hodgkins disease with a high dose vitamin C regimen! Chapter seven also explains how people are sometimes misdiagnosed with leukemia when they don't have leukemia at all. What they have is scurvy, or dangerously low vitamin C levels in their body! Levels so low that they can't even be measured! (Sometimes they have dangerously low levels of B12.)

Oils for Cancer Prevention (& A.D.D.) – Evening Primrose Oil

Evening primrose oil is a rich source of gamma-linolenic acid (GLA), discussed earlier in this book. It has been used with some success in treating diseases such as multiple sclerosis, and it demonstrates aggressive anti-cancer properties.

The late "Dr. David Horrobin," notable for his studies involving essential fats, believed that (as he discovered in his research) GLA could help children with ADD (Attention Deficit Disorder).[37] In fact, as detailed at website *www.absolutelythepurest.com,* the "American Journal of Clinical Nutrition (Oct. 1995) reported on a study which found that 53 boys diagnosed with Attention Deficit Disorder had significantly lower levels of essential fatty acids in their brain tissue."[38]

Dr. Horrobin's research also demonstrated the importance of GLAs in cancer prevention. He and his colleagues believed "that cancer cells cannot make a substance that converts linoleic into gamma-linolenic acid," and that "providing" GLA might "normalize malignant cells and reverse cancer's growth," a totally "non-toxic" treatment.[39] He suggested using it in "cancer cases for which no other viable treatment was available." When scientists tested his theory, they found that "GLA supplements" reduced "the growth rate of "human liver cancer cells in the test tube, up to 87 percent..."[40] Dr. Ralph Moss in his book, *Cancer Therapy,* says that "Horrobin and colleagues" published in a prestigious medical journal that "polyunsaturated fatty acids killed human breast, lung and prostate cancer cells at concentrations which had no adverse effects on normal human cells..."[41]

Other studies showed that "GLA…suppressed the growth of four kinds of nerve cancer cells…Normal cells were not killed, but their rate of division slowed." Dr. Moss believes it is possible that GLA works by causing the development of "deadly free radicals in cancerous – but not in normal – cells."[42]

CHAPTER 21

PRESCRIPTION HRT – THE GREAT TRAGEDY OF THE 20th CENTURY

"Yes, you were right: HRT the way your doctor prescribes it can increase your risk of breast cancer. If you were one of the millions of women who refused to take HRT, or questioned your doctor about it, or felt queasy about taking it because you were afraid of getting breast cancer, you were right..."

(From *What Your Doctor May Not Tell You About Breast Cancer* by John R. Lee, M.D., David Zava, Ph.D. and Virginia Hopkins, M.A. Copyright © 2002 by John R. Lee, M.D., Virginia Hopkins, M.A., and David T. Zava, Ph.D., by permission of Warner Books, Inc.)[1]

Hormone Replacement Therapy & Cancer – How the Public was Betrayed

There are several different forms of estrogen, however estrogen is merely "the name of the *class* of hormones with estrus activity...not the name of one hormone, but the name of a group of similar hormones."[1a] These different types of hormones are described by the late Dr. John R. Lee, M.D., et al., in *What Your Doctor May Not Tell You About Menopause.* One form of estrogen known as "*estriol,*" is actually a natural estrogen hormone found in nature. He explained that synthetic estrogen, created in the laboratory and dispensed by pharmaceutical companies is either "*estradiol*" or "*estrone.*"[1b] (There is night and day difference between natural estrogen and synthetic estrogen!) There are also "phytoestrogens" or plant estrogens that have "estrogen-like activity," said Dr. Lee, but weaker forms of "one's own estrogens," though they "compete for the same estrogen receptors throughout the body." Thus, they can often help alleviate issues involving "too much estrogen."[2]

Other types of estrogens are the "Xenoestrogens," harmful estrogens that come from toxins and pollutants in our environment that have such powerful "estrogen-like" effects, they are very detrimental.[3] Are you aware that estrogen is even being put into hair products, such as shampoos? As noted at website *alkalizeforhealth.net*, "Dr. David Williams in *Alternatives* Newsletter, June 2002" states:

> It shocks me that no one is alarmed that 14-month old babies can grow pubic hair and develop breasts simply from using shampoo....I would certainly suggest that you check the labels of your shampoos, hair conditioners, skin creams, and facial products to see if they contain placenta, a common source of estrogen in these products. Some may list 'estrogen,' 'estriol,' or 'natural hormones' as an ingredient.[4]

The late Dr. John Lee left behind a remarkable achievement in his studies and contributions, including several health books that he authored and co-authored, clearly pointing out the dreadful aftereffects that women are facing from synthetic HRT (hormone replacement therapy). He (along with David Zava, Ph.D., and Virginia Hopkins, M.A.) discussed the safe estrogen, the estrogen that occurs in nature, in their book: *What Your Doctor May Not Tell You About Breast Cancer:*

> Most conventional medical doctors in the United States don't remember from their medical school biochemistry classes that there's an estrogen called *estriol;* nor do they know how to get it, or what its benefits are. Estriol isn't even listed in the *Physician's Desk* Reference (PDR), because no pharmaceutical company in the United States sells it commercially...[5]

This found-in-nature-estrogen ("estriol") has about the same benefits of the pharmaceutically created "estradiol and estrone," however, it does not have the toxic "side effects." It is very common for "European" physicians to give their female patients, natural estrogen.[6] Yes, there is a form of natural estrogen made by our Creator that does not have the toxic side effects of the *freak-of-nature* synthetic estrogen created by pharmaceutical companies – and most doctors know nothing about it!

Synthetic Estrogen Replacement –
A Double-Edged Sword

As noted above, there are vast differences in the types of estrogen on the market today. Dr. Lee believed that it is possible that so-called estrogen-deficiency is "largely a myth." His studies and research revealed that most women are **"estrogen dominant"** rather than estrogen deficient.[6a] This is because, as he explained, estrogen is manufactured in fat cells. Women naturally have a higher ratio of fat cells than men and the more fat cells a woman has, the more estrogen she produces. A thin women before menopause may actually make less estrogen in her body than an obese woman does after menopause, yet the woman who is obese will still have a "problem with hot flashes."[6b] Not only that, but most Americans consume a lot of meat. It is no secret that our meat and dairy supply (including fowl) is tainted with hormones, herbicides, and pesticides! Also, many women have received estrogen in prescription form.[7] Dr. Lee believed that the main culprit in "estrogen dominance in menopausal women is the estrogen almost universally prescribed to them" by their physicians. He also believed that it is primarily responsible for the high incidence "of breast cancer in women over age 50."[8]

For women who are pre-menopausal, "estrogen dominance" will show up in them as "a lack of ovulation…(not enough progesterone is made after ovulation)."

The problem with *"estrogen dominance…*a term coined by Dr. Lee in his first book on natural progesterone," is that regardless of a woman's estrogen level, even if her estrogen levels are low, if she has no progesterone in her body, she will still be estrogen dominant![9]

There are many symptoms of "estrogen dominance." A few of these according to website *Diagnose-me.com* are:

> Weight gain, headaches, bad temper, chronic fatigue and loss of interest in sex…breast cancer…fibrocystic breast disease…[it is] a prime cause of osteoporosis…fibroids…menstruating [becomes] irregular…Endometrial cancer…high blood pressure…risk of stroke and heart disease is increased dramatically…[10]

To these, Dr. Lee, added the following:

Allergies…asthma, hives, rashes, sinus congestion; Anxiety…Auto-immune disorders…lupus…Hashimoto's thyroiditis…Cold hands and feet…Fat gain, especially around the hips and thighs…Headaches…Increased blood clotting…Infertility…Insomnia…Polycystic ovaries…Water retention, [and] bloating.[11]

Estrogen replacement hit a snag as far back as 1975 when it was discovered that women taking ERT were getting "uterine (endometrial) cancer at a rate **four to eight times greater** than" those not taking estrogen.[12] A main problem of "estrogen dominance," explained Dr. Lee, is that once estrogen "becomes the dominant hormone and progesterone is deficient, the estrogen becomes toxic to the body…"[13]

According to Dr. Ray D. Strand in his book, *What Your Doctor Doesn't Know About Nutritional Medicine May Be killing You,* drug companies convinced physicians that their patients needed HRT despite the hazards:

In 1997 the New England Journal of Medicine reviewed several studies involving women who took estrogen replacement for more than five to ten years. The results shocked reviewers, revealing more than a 40 percent increase in breast cancer. The pharmaceutical companies quickly responded to this negative report by convincing the doctors that the benefits of HRT far outweighed the risks…[14]

Research also shows that, contrary to earlier belief, women do not have to take synthetic hormones for long periods of time to increase their risks! As reported on website *www.natural-progesterone-advisory-network.com:* in an article by Catherine P. Rollins:

The Million Women Study, of whom about half used or had used HRT, indicated for the first time that the increased risk [of synthetic HRT] started between one and two years of

HRT use dashing any suggestion that increased cancer risk only developed after long-term use. But the risks grew larger the longer the HRT treatment continued...[15]

Dr. Lee et al, in *What Your Doctor May Not Tell You About Breast Cancer,* said that when researchers began pouring over "records of more than 16,000 women [they] concluded that combined HRT tends to make breast cancer tumors more aggressive and harder to detect, reducing the chances for successful treatment."[16]

Estriol, the NATURAL form of estrogen found in nature, is free of the toxic side effects found in prescription HRT. However, "estriol" was competing with a "tough rival, Premarin," a synthetic estrogen "patented product" extracted "from pregnant mares' urine..."[16a] As Dr. Lee pointed out, premarin had the backing of a pharmaceutical company that had invested millions to study, promote, and market it. Once it was given FDA approval, this meant that a well-equipped "trained sales force" from the drug company would ultimately use high pressure sales reps to talk thousands of physicians into using it for their patients![17]

Lest you are unaware of how successful this campaign was, "22 million prescriptions" for Premarin were issued during 1996. C. Norman Shealy, M.D., Ph.D., in his book, *Natural Progesterone Cream, Safe and Natural Hormone Replacement,* suggests that maybe they should call it "Horse Replacement Therapy?!" Even more alarming is the fact that Premarin causes a **"43 percent increase of breast and/or uterine cancer,"** as well as many other dangerous side effects.[18]

I wonder how many women taking Premarin were told by their physicians: *"This prescription I am writing for you comes from the urine of pregnant horses and, oh, by the way, it can increase your risk of breast or uterine cancer by 43%!"* Do you think this happened? Are YOU or a loved one taking Premarin? Did your physician ever tell you this?

How did this happen? How is it that there is a NATURAL form of estrogen without the toxic side effects of the synthetic form, yet millions of women were never offered the natural form, but given instead, the synthetic form produced by a pharmaceutical company that brought with it a deadly cloud of adverse side effects? It is because drug companies have no vested interest in a natural substance like estriol, regardless of how "safe and effective it is," because natural substances can NOT be patented! If they cannot patent a product, anyone can sell it, thus they cannot get exclusive rights to market it and make millions in profits![19]

Synthetic estrogen has many other potential deadly risks and side effects besides those already listed. Some of them are listed at http:*//www.ninds.nih.gov,* (the National Institute of Neurological Disorders & Stroke)*:* "…blood clots, nausea, abdominal pain, breast tenderness, irregular bleeding, headache…hair loss…edema, weight gain, hot flashes, mood swings and acne," and it can also "increase the risk of uterus cancer."[20]

There were many professionals, however, who realized that *natural* estrogen *(estriol)* was a safe form of estrogen replacement therapy. "Professor Henry Lemon" had been advocating this for three decades. In "a 1966 article published in the *Journal of the American Medical Association,"* Dr. Lemon said (in a nutshell!) that **natural** estrogen combined with **natural** progesterone could **prevent** breast cancer and uterine cancer![21]

Estriol (NATURAL estrogen), according to Dr. Lee in *What Your Doctor May Not Tell You About Breast Cancer* is vastly different from the synthetic form:

> [It] protects against breast and uterine cancers…prevents vaginal atrophy and urinary tract infections…helps protect your bones…relieves hot flashes and night sweats without stimulating uterine growth…doesn't cause blood clots [as synthetic estrogen does...and] protects the skin from aging…[22]

It appears that only small amounts of "an estriol cream" are needed! Studies reveal that only "0.5 mg" of estriol "every other day for two weeks is adequate for most women."[23] As a matter-of-fact, this is the dosage most commonly prescribed by European physicians to their patients.[24] Apparently, the body does not assimilate estriol as rapidly as with "other estrogens; one dose lasts for two days," and using it topically as a skin cream is "20 times more efficient than" taking it by mouth.[25]

You should not be taking any type of estrogen treatment without consulting with your physician, especially if you have a history of unusual bleeding, any sort of liver disorders, or a history of cancer, nor is it recommended during pregnancy.

As always, if you are nursing or pregnant, you should consult your physician about any medication, herb, or hormone you are contemplating. However, if your physician is planning a hysterectomy for you, I would recommend that you read both books by Dr. John R. Lee, et al. *(What Your Doctor May Not Tell You About Menopause,* and *What Your Doctor May Not Tell You About Breast Cancer),* as well as a "book by Dr. Stanley West – *'The Hysterectomy Hoax.'* Dr. West is the Chief of Reproductive Endocrinology and Infertility at St. Vincent's Hospital in New York City." This, according to website *safemenopausesolutions.com.* Dr. West believes "that 90% of all the hysterectomies done in the U.S. are medically unnecessary."[26] (Website *www.safemenopausesolutions.com* also has a women's hormone profile test that you can take if you have more questions about natural hormone replacement. They explain that many menopausal and pre-menopausal symptoms can be caused by a deficiency of natural progesterone in the body!)

Natural Progesterone

Dr. John R. Lee called natural progesterone "the great protector," and for good reason. **Natural** progesterone has the opposite effects on the body that are seen with the synthetic hormones![27] Chances are that if you are going through menopause, or even if you are several years pre-menopausal, you may already be "estrogen dominant" and in need of natural progesterone, rather than estrogen!

It was only after years of putting women on prescription estrogen that the medical profession finally admitted that synthetic estrogen was causing many adverse side effects, as well as being implicated in deaths from blood clots, strokes, heart attacks and cancer! Studies were done to back up their suspicions. It finally dawned on them that the ovaries make two major hormones, not one! Their patient's needed progesterone!

Not to be outdone, it did not take the pharmaceutical companies long to change a molecule (or two!) in natural progesterone and develop the SYNTHETIC form of progesterone (known as *progestin*), just as they had done with estrogen! (Are you smelling a RAT yet?) Physicians then began prescribing HRT to their patients that included both **synthetic** estrogen and **synthetic** progesterone.[28]

The BIG problem was that the synthetic progesterone *(Progestin)* was also found to have some very ominous side effects, many of which are listed at website: *www.rxlist.com/cgi/generic/medrox_ad.htm:* including: "hirsutism...pulmonary embolism [clots in the lungs], breakthrough bleeding...change in weight...changes in cervical erosion...depression, pyrexia, insomnia, nausea...cerebral thrombosis [brain clot or stroke]...retinal thrombosis...nervousness, dizziness, edema...jaundice...acne, alopecia [loss of hair]...vaginitis...convulsions...anemia...tachycardia...changes in breast size, breast lumps...paralysis...scleroderma, osteoporosis...cervical cancer, varicose veins...thrombophlebitis, deep vein thrombosis," and infertility.[29]

There was a glut of HRT being prescribed in the U.S. up until 2000, that is, until the study done by the "National Cancer Institute...in January 2000," which discussed the fact that HRT could cause a dramatic rise in the risk for "breast cancer."[29a] Since that data was made public, Dr. Lee said that "conventional physicians" are not quite as hasty "to insist" on the drug, but they still "pressure" their patients "to use it."[30]

A study done by *"The Women's Health Initiative...*sponsored by the National Institute of Health...found that women on hormone replacement therapy of combined estrogen plus progestin (PREM-PRO)," as noted on website *www.safemenopausesolutions.com* experienced the following (reprinted with their permission):

*A 41% INCREASE in strokes
*A 29% INCREASE in heart attacks
*A 100% INCREASE in the rate of blood clots
*A 22% INCREASE in total cardiovascular disease

*A 24% INCREASE in breast cancer
*A 100% INCREASE in the rate of Alzheimer's Disease
(in women over 65)[31]

Apparently, those women who use HRT for several years are at a greater risk over those who use it for shorter periods of time. *Safemenopausesolutions.com* describes the reaction of "Dr. Marcia L. Stefanick of Stanford University," to HRT. Dr. Stefanick stated that the risk for cancer increased according to the amount of time women used HRT. She explained that women who had been taking HRT the longest, were at the greatest risk.[32] (The website above also has information on how safe, NATURAL progesterone can help with male menopause problems.)

Dr. Lee believed that it was very supercilious of drug manufacturers to assume that they can change the chemical structure of something like natural progesterone, make a synthetic form they can patent then presume that the body will assimilate it and that it will accomplish the same purposes as the natural substance!

Do you see how the public has been duped? There is also a **natural progesterone** available, and if you are on prescription hormone replacement therapy, I could win a bet right now that your physician has never told you that natural progesterone exists (so does natural estrogen), and it does not have the toxic side effects associated with *progestin*!

Natural progesterone has many of the EXACT opposite effects on the body that **synthetic** estrogen and **synthetic** progesterone have! As noted by C. Norman Shealy, M.D., Ph.D., in the book, *Natural Progesterone Cream*, this natural hormone is:

Essential for development of [the] fetus, Prevents Osteoporosis....Prevents fibrocystic breasts...[is a] Natural energizer/antidepressant, Normalizes Blood sugar, zinc and copper, Cell oxygenation, Helps burn fat and prevent obesity, Optimizes libido, [and is a] Natural diuretic.[33]

Since progesterone relaxes the body, **using excessive amounts** of the hormone can cause "sleepiness, depression... [or] digestive problems…"[34] "…swelling, bloating, constipation," nausea, diarrhea and "upper respiratory tract infection,"[35] though these are not common! Some people can have allergic reactions to this hormone, which would be manifested by "Breathing problems or tightness in your throat or chest, chest pain, skin hives, rash, or itchy or swollen skin."[36]

Any time you experience breathing problems or tightness in your chest immediately after takng a medication, food, herb, vitamin, hormone, or mineral, this could signify a severe reaction and you need to seek help immediately. Side effects with natural progesterone only occur with excess dosing and are very extremely rare! Compare this to the deadly array of side effects from the synthetic drug, *Progestin*!

According to website *www.healthtouch.com*, you should not take natural progesterone if you are pregnant or breast feeding, if you are taking "Doxorubicin (Adriamycin), Conjugated Estrogens (Premarin), Ketoconazole (Nizoral), [or] Red Clover," and you should ask your physician before taking natural progesterone if you have any of the following conditions:

[I]f you have or have had cancer of the breast or genital organs…liver problems…an abortion that has failed…if you are allergic to peanuts…if you have a bleeding or blood clot disorder, thrombophlebitis, or cerebral apoplexy…if you have vaginal bleeding that hasn't been seen by a doctor….If you have epilepsy (seizure disorder), migraine headaches, asthma, heart problems, or kidney problems use caution taking Natural Progesterone, because it might make your condition worse…Do not take if you have depression."[37]

Note that this website recommends using natural progesterone with caution in those with migraines, however, Dr. Lee was an expert on natural progesterone, having used it in his own practice for many years, and he used the cream successfully to treat migraines! (More information on that is given later in this chapter.)

According to website *safemenopausolutions.com*, **normal dosages** of natural progesterone have "NO known…side effects!"

According to many doctors, when used in amounts no greater than what the body normally makes, there are **NO natural progesterone side effects**. Fortunately, you don't have to worry about side effects of progesterone cream. Just use it in the "psysiological doses", which means use it in the same quantities as what the body makes, or 20 to 40 milligrams per day of natural progesterone cream. *Natural progesterone side effects* have never been reported by women using it for more than 30 years.[38]

Even though natural progesterone is actually developed from Mexican wild yam, it is identical to the progesterone found in nature, human progesterone, so it is considered natural! Being a natural product, it could not be patented. Dr. Lee said that snythetic and natural progesterone are so vastly different that **natural** progesterone protects "the fertilized egg," but the **synthetic** prescription "progestins…can be used to abort a pregnancy in its early days," as well as "cause birth defects."[39]

Natural progesterone can be found in health food stores in a cream form that is applied topically to the skin and absorbed through the skin. It is a very effective mode of delivering the hormone.

In her book, *How to Renew You*, Maureen Kennedy Salaman describes why a research study on HRT was brought to a halt:

> On July 9, 2002, the National Institutes of Health announced that it had halted a major study, stating that the long-term use of estrogen and progestin significantly increases the chances of invasive breast cancer, blood clots, and heart attacks.[40]

After just **one year** of using this **synthetic**, prescription estrogen-progestin, the women in the study were at an increased risk for heart attacks, breast cancer, and strokes![41]

Ms. Salaman's company, *Maximum Living,* produces a natural progesterone cream called *ProgestiMax®*. More information on *Progestimax®* and Maureen's other vital health products can be found at *www.mksalaman.com.*

If you are wondering where pharmaceutical companies obtain the raw materials to "create" synthetic progesterone, they manufacture if from NATURAL progesterone. That's right! They purchase NATURAL progesterone (which is derived from Mexican wild yams or soybeans) and then "chemically alter its molecular form" to create their synthetic and potentially deadly hormone![42]

Are You "Estrogen Dominant"?
(Do You Have Too Much Estrogen?)

If you are a woman who is pre-menopausal and you are having problems with "weight gain, headaches, bad temper, chronic fatigue…fibrocystic breast disease…fibroids…irregular [periods]…breast cancer…endometrial cancer…high blood pressure…[and] heart disease," you may very well be estrogen dominant.[43] These are ALL problems associated with too much estrogen and a deficiency of progesterone![44] (See website: *http:www.diagnose-me.com.*)

Be aware that you should not purchase products with "wild yam extract" thinking you are getting natural progesterone! You will need to read the label of contents. To get natural progesterone, the label must say: *"USP Progesterone"* in the list of ingredients. If you purchase a two ounce container, for example, it will tell you the exact dosage of progesterone you are purchasing. There are many products on the market that contain black cohosh and wild yam for example, and while some users claim that they can relieve hot flashes and other menopausal symptoms, they may contain no natural progesterone at all in them! Also, be alert for the "medium" that your natural progesterone is found in. If you obtain a product that uses "mineral oil" for a "medium," topical absorption will be inhibited. As Dr. Lee explained, other products not "properly stabilized" will "deteriorate over time with exposure to oxygen, and by the time you get to the bottom of the jar, you aren't getting any progesterone."[45]

A few of the many brands Dr. Lee and Virginia Hopkins discussed in *What Your Doctor May Not Tell You About Menopause,* that do contain natural USP progesterone ("400-600 mg. progesterone per ounce…") are: *"BioBalance…FemGest…NaturalProg… Progest…ProgestaCare…Pro-Osteo-All…Supra-Gest…Endau…[and] ProCreme Plus,"* among others. If you use a progesterone cream that has a higher or lower dosage than the above, "you'll need to adjust your dosage accordingly…begin with the physiologic dose (approximately 15-20 mg per day) and adjust from there for your own body as needed."[46]

Dr. Lee and Virginia Hopkins also noted that "estrogen dominance" does not automatically begin with menopause! Here in the U.S., many women who are "10- to 15" years pre-menopausal are having problems related to "estrogen dominance," yet their physicians "are giving them more estrogen."[47]

Women who are menopausal and are placed on HRT for irregular bleeding, hot flashes, insomnia, weight gain, etc., often worsen in their symptoms, going on to develop severe uterine bleeding with clots and lumpy breasts AFTER being on synthetic HRT! They are then told that they will need hysterectomies or lumpectomies! No one is putting two and two together and figuring out that it was the prescription HRT that probably CAUSED their excess uterine bleeding and lumpy breasts to begin with, but who is going to point it out to them when it is making a gold mine for the surgeons doing the hysterectomies and lumpectomies? What is wrong with this picture? Their bodies are still making estrogen, but not enough progesterone. The very last thing any of them need is more estrogen, but that is often exactly what they are given! Many of these same women go on to develop severe osteoporosis, degenerative hip disease, degenerative disc disease and subsequent back pain and disability, and numerous other ailments, when all they ever needed to begin with was progesterone, NATURAL progesterone and no estrogen! Natural progesterone helps balance the rest of the hormones in the body. If you are having menopausal symptoms, find a good licensed naturopathic physician who is knowledgeable about natural progesterone or a conventional medicine gynecologist that believes in natural progesterone, and prescribes it!

Natural progesterone will help in the replacement of bone! Estrogen helps slow bone loss, but only briefly, and it does nothing to replace the bone that has already been lost.[48]

It's Never Too Late to Start!

It is never too late to begin a natural progesterone regimen. Dr. Lee was "paid a visit by Dr. George Moraes, a gerontologist from Sao Paulo, Brazil." He had started "his ninety-one year old mother, who had been consigned to a nursing home because of weakness and senility," on the "progesterone cream for her dry, fragile skin and osteoporosis." The next time he paid her a visit, she had improved significantly in her "socializing abilities – skills that had deteriorated in the preceding years."[49]

Fibrocystic Breasts, Uterine Fibroids, Infertility, & Miscarriages

Many women who lack sufficient progesterone also develop fibrocystic breasts and problems with uterine fibroids. Instead of trying them on natural progesterone, their physicians are performing hysterectomies that are often totally unnecessary! Lack of sufficient progesterone has also been linked to problems with infertility and miscarriages. Countless women have been put through needless fertility studies and agonizing months and years of infertility, when all they really needed was a safe, simple regimen of **natural** progesterone. Dr. Lee treated a number of his patients complaining of infertility with natural progesterone, and recommended that when treating infertility, they should not use the cream until "after" they had "ovulated each month."[50] (Women can determine when they are ovulating by taking their basal body temperature every morning before arising.) Specifics on exactly how to read and record those results can be obtained from your physician. It can also be found on many websites and in books on infertility.

If you ask your physician about taking natural progesterone, many of them will not have a clue what you are talking about, because many physicians still have no idea that there is such a thing as NATURAL progesterone that is delivered topically and has no toxic side effects! They will immediately begin writing you a prescription for SYNTHETIC progesterone! Why? Because most con-

ventional doctors have been trained to serve the interests of a mecha-
nized multi-million-dollar pharmaceutical industry that has no interest in natural substances that they can not patent and sell for a profit!

Dr. Lee emphasized the fact that "many physicians mistakenly
believe (thanks, in part, to misinformation from drug company reps)
that synthetic progestins are merely different forms of progesterone.
None of them is progesterone."[51]

Your doctor may be very insistent about putting you on prescription *progestin,* possibly even quoting all the reasons from the fliers
that he has received from drug companies bragging about the wonderful benefits of their synthetic hormones! This is one opportunity
where your physician can learn from you!

How Much Progesterone Do You Need?

In his book *What Your Doctor May Not Tell You About Menopause,* Dr.
Lee recommended the following dosage of progesterone cream: "1/8
to 1/2 teaspoon of natural progesterone cream per day, or three to 10
drops of the oil…"[52] Proper dosing will relieve your symptoms. Some
of the natural progesterone creams are available in individual pre-
packaged dosages, so there is no guessing as to measuring. Factors
influencing how much you take depend on whether you are "pre-
menopausal…menopausal…[or] post-menopausal" and whether or
not you are currently taking HRT, and whether or not "you have had
a hysterectomy."[53] Dr. Lee and Virginia Hopkins explained that if you
are taking prescription estrogen, you should wean from it slowly,
never all at once, however, they had no problem with stopping
"Provera abruptly." Remember that when you start taking NATURAL
progesterone, you will no longer need to be on the synthetic form of
the hormone! Be sure to discuss this with your doctor and express
your concerns about being on synthetic hormones![53a]

Many women are apprehensive that if they are menopausal and
take **natural** progesterone that they may start having periods again.
This usually does not happen, however, if this does occur after you
have been taking natural progesterone for a "week or two," this is due
to the high estrogen level in your body. Dr. Lee's recommendation
was to "stop taking the [natural] progesterone for a week and then

start up again for three weeks," just as though you "were still menstruating":

> The cycle should be three weeks on progesterone and one week off. During the week off progesterone, there may be some bleeding. This is due to the persistence of estrogen production, which will diminish over time. This is the advantage of stopping progesterone for one week each month. It allows the estrogen-induced blood buildup to be shed.[54]

Later, when you are no longer having monthly bleeding, "the progesterone can be continued on a calendar basis: 24 days of progesterone and then stopping for the remainder of the month..." Naturally, if you are having "persistent spotting or vaginal bleeding..." you should always seek professional medical help.[55]

Note that in the quote above, 24 days on the cream is recommended, which is a little over three weeks. This is because of the day difference in months. The simplest way to remember is to always go off the cream the last seven days of every month, regardless of how many days there are in the month. (This way you would always start using the cream on the first day of every month.) Always check with your licensed health care practitioner to verify proper dosing and advice regarding hormonal creams.

Migraines: Natural Progesterone & Other Natural Treatments

Natural progesterone cream has been used successfully to stop migraine headaches. One website promotes such use and Dr. Lee also recommended progesterone cream for migraines.

As described at website *www.mcvitamins.com/migraine.htm*, research has shown "that high daily doses of riboflavin – 400 mg a day – sharply reduced the number and severity of migraine attacks for over half the participants," and *"The Lancet"* reported that headache relief could be obtained by most of these victims if they would simply abstain from any foods to which they were "allergic."[55a] Also, patients taking "between three and six 1,200-milligram capsules" of "lecithin… when they felt a headache coming on had fewer, milder migraine attacks." The website above also suggests that you include "exercise…alternative hot and cold showers, and taking [the herbs] feverfew & hyssop," for migraine headache relief.[56] Also see chapter 22 in this book regarding the connection between dehydration and migraines.

Testing For Low Hormone Levels

Be aware that if you are using a progesterone cream and your physician orders a blood test to check your progesterone level, he or she may tell you that the hormone is not being absorbed adequately. This may not be the case, simply because a serum test for progesterone is not reliable. It will tell a woman how much progesterone her ovaries are making, but won't be an accurate measurement of how much of the progesterone cream she is actually absorbing!

Some physicians argue that progesterone isn't well-absorbed when delivered topically.[57] At his website *www.johnleemd.c*om, Dr. Lee explained that some practitioners are using a "report" that was published in the *Lancet,* (casting doubt on the absorption of topically used natural progesterone cream) to argue that taking natural "progesterone [in the cream form] is not well-absorbed" by the body.[57a] However, Dr. Lee called the report in *Lancet* "erroneous," because he said that its "authors did not understand the significant difference between serum and saliva progesterone levels."[58] Most of the progesterone produced by the ovaries is bound to protein. "Only 2 to 5 percent of serum progesterone is 'free' or non-protein bound," and Dr. Lee explained that this is "the progesterone available to target tissues and to saliva." Therefore, the progesterone that is "measured by serum levels is mostly a measure of progesterone that is not going to be used by the body."[58a] On the other hand, topical progesterone skin cream "is a highly lipophilic (fat loving) molecule that is well absorbed through skin into the underlying fat layer…" and Dr. Lee said that from there it is picked up by "red blood cell membranes in capillaries passing through the fat."[58b] This progesterone…"readily available to all target tissues and to saliva…is completely bioavailable," he explained, and quite easily "measured by saliva testing. Only a small fraction of it is carried by the watery serum." This is why blood levels are not an accurate measurement of topical "absorption."[59] (You can order saliva testing kits from Dr. Lee's website: *www.johnleemd.com*, as well as a few other websites on the internet.)

Normal Saliva Levels of Progesterone

If a woman is "ovulating normally," her "saliva hormone assay" progesterone level should be "0.3 to 0.5 ng/ml…. Under usual circumstances, there should be no reason to exceed that range."[59a] According to Dr. Lee, the amount of progesterone cream that is needed to give you this "saliva level of 0.5 ng/ml is commonly only 12 to 15 mg per day. For creams containing 900 to 1000 mg per 2-oz. container, 12-15 mg a day for 24 days would use up only about one-third of a 2-oz. container."[60] (Thus you can see that a small jar of progesterone cream could easily last 2 – 3 months, depending on the dosage.) However, you may want to take slightly higher amounts, not only because most women are more likely to be estrogen dominant, but because the ovaries normally make an average of "22 milligrams" of progesterone a day before menopause, depending on the menstrual cycle.[61] Everyone is unique and your dosage will vary according to your own bodily needs. Find a knowledgeable, licensed, alternative health care practitioner, if your conventional medicine physician is not up-to-date on natural progesterone creams.

There are also times when it is beneficial to have higher levels of progesterone in the body. For example: during "PMS… [and] stress….Stress increases cortisol production." Cortisol has the ability to block progesterone from reaching its destination and/or to prevent it from functioning.[61a] Dr. Lee believed that you may need higher amounts of the natural cream in order "to compete with this cortisol blockage…[as much as] 30 to 40 mg/day is sometimes initially required…."[61b] The same holds true for "women with endometriosis, the goal is to increase progesterone levels to that found in women two months pregnant." Dr. Lee explained that in order to get this level, you may need "topical progesterone…in a range of 30 to 50 mg/day from day 8 to day 26 of the menstrual cycle."[62]

See website *www.johnleemd.com* for more information on endometriosis and natural progesterone cream. Read the "July 98 issue of the John Lee Medical Letter." He emphasized that what you are trying to do in endometriosis is to get "the right dose…that results in progressive decrease of endometriosis pain." Once your pain "is largely gone, levels can be decreased gradually over time…"[63]

Estrogen Dominance & Cancer

Why has there been such a tragic rise in breast cancer in women? Dr. Lee believed that it was probably due to the "prescription of unopposed estrogen…to menopausal women," especially during "the early 1950s to the mid-1970s." Even though "the medical community acknowledged that this practice caused endometrial (uterine) cancer," he said that they "never admitted that it also caused breast cancer."[64]

Think back, how many of your loved ones have died of uterine and/or breast cancer that had a history of taking prescription hormone replacement therapy? Your mom, perhaps? Your grandmother? A sister, a daughter, or a favorite aunt?

What was the response of the medical community to the rise in breast and uterine cancers? They actually claimed that breast cancer rates were falling and tried to attribute this to the use of tamoxifen, a chemotherapy agent given to breast cancer patients. However, the late Dr. Lee was very scornful of tamoxifen:

> We hope that those promoting tamoxifen remember to mention how many women taking it suffer from blood clots, deterioration of vision, and diminished quality of life (hot flashes, night sweats). Also, how many women have been forced to have a hysterectomy due to a particularly aggressive form of tamoxifen-caused uterine cancer? It's rarely mentioned that women actually die of tamoxifen-induced uterine cancer.[65]

Do you see how the statistics are manipulated to make chemo drugs look *attractive*? A woman with breast cancer is given tamoxifen. She develops **uterine cancer (a side-effect of the tamoxifen)** and dies, but the statistics say that she didn't die from breast cancer, she died from uterine cancer, making it APPEAR that the tamoxifen HELPED her breast cancer, because after all, the breast cancer didn't kill her, the uterine cancer did, right? Thus, the drug company prints up a lovely rainbow-colored chart for everyone to see how effective tamoxifen is at curing breast cancer – I mean – just **LOOK at the statistics**! The tamoxifen cured the patient, course she is dead, but at least she didn't die from breast cancer! Right? The exact same thing happens when a patient has liver cancer and they take chemo or radiation therapy. They may develop a severe blood disorder from the chemo (such as leukemia!) that kills them. Well, the liver cancer didn't *kill* them, so the chemo or radiation must have HELPED their liver cancer, right? Well, that is exactly how the statistics are done, and how drug companies dupe the public into believing that chemo is an effective cancer treatment! **(Can you see the insanity of this type of reasoning?)** This is exactly how some drugs get pushed through quick approval by the FDA, based on statistics that are often manipulated just like this – to make them look successful and favorable!

Dr. John Lee received a letter from a woman who had declined the use of tamoxifen on his advice. She expressed her great appreciation for his being "gusty enough to tell" her about his concerns with this drug. He had advised her against using it, giving her as she put it, "the courage to buck my very pushy oncologist who wanted me to take it." Since refusing the tamoxifen and starting on progesterone cream, she said that her follow-up mammograms were perfect and the breast that initially had the lumpectomy appeared "normal and benign," as she explained to Dr. Lee:

> I am 56, postmenopausal, and am using progesterone cream. You reassured me it was safe even for a woman like me with high estrogen and progesterone receptors, explaining this means progesterone can get in and do its job of stopping the cancer when the receptors are present. When I heard the flap about the "hazards of progesterone" I knew…that it was

probably a botched reporting job that really referred to the synthetic progestin…M.H.[66]

Writer and "T.V. personality…Dr. Bob Arnot" in his book, *"The Breast Cancer Prevention Diet…"* was scathingly criticized by U.S. media moguls "for using the word *prevention*," however, he never stated "that diet was a cure-all." He was made to look like an idiot for even hinting that perhaps a healthy diet could fend off breast cancer! Dr. Lee explained what the real issue was behind the controversy involving the author and his book:

> Arnot was an unfortunate victim of the intense breast cancer political establishment, which savagely attacks those who stray outside conventional medical boundaries and dare to suggest that something besides surgery, chemotherapy, radiation, and tamoxifen might be helpful.[67]

If you will recall in chapter three of this book, Eydie Mae Hunsberger, Rita Myers, and Dr. Kristine Nolfi all proved **that a healthy diet and lifestyle changes can CURE breast cancer**! There are several examples given in chapter three of breast cancer **CURES** using natural means!

Remember that another major culprit in the cause of "estrogen dominance" is environmental factors. For example: the FDA **allows** farmers to inject cattle with synthetic "estrogen pellets to fatten them up for market! This estrogen is still in the meat when it gets to your table."[67a] At one time, cattle were allowed to freely roam, but now are often kept in tight, huddled quarters, making them more susceptible to disease. They are given large amounts of antibiotics that also end up in the meat that ends up on your table! This is one of the many reasons for all the new antibiotic-resistant strains of microbes baffling scientists![68]

The fact that estrogen causes water retention, salt retention and fat retention has been a *gold mine* for the cattle industry. All they have to do is shoot the cattle up with estrogen hormones, they gain weight rapidly, go to market sooner, bring bigger bucks and we consume the stuff every time we feast on hamburgers, steaks, sausage, hot dogs, chicken (yes, fowl too), and roast beef sandwiches. Is it any wonder that our teenagers, who consume fast-food hamburgers and other meats are struggling with acne, insomnia, weight problems, difficulty concentrating, irritability, and – later in life – develop problems with infertility, irregular menses, and high blood pressure? And don't forget that dairy products too, are contaminated with hormones! We are pushing milk on youngsters, not realizing that cow's milk has been linked to autoimmune disorders, insulin-dependent childhood (Type I) diabetes, and a myriad of other ailments to which I have devoted chapter 25 of this book.

If you truly want to win the battle against estrogen dominance, stay away from meats and dairy products. (If you do keep them in your diet, for your health's sake, only use certified ORGANIC meats and dairy products that have been certified to be free of hormones, herbicides, and pesticides, and you can always substitute soy products for dairy. (Fermented soy products, such as Haelan, can help remove harmful estrogens from the body in estrogen-receptor positive cancers.) Taking natural progesterone to balance out your hormones will be of little benefit to you if you are consuming estrogen in a diet high in meat and dairy products!

How Safe is Natural Progesterone?

In an article by Catherine P. Rollins, at *www.natural-progesterone-advisory-network.com,* she reminds us that "research has shown natural progesterone is safer than all over-the-counter pain medications currently available, and there has **never been a single case** of anyone being admitted to [a] hospital due to a poisoning from this natural-to-the-body hormone." She explains that: "We are now learning that 'too little' progesterone (needed to oppose estrogen in our body) is more risky" than "applying 'too much.'" (Catherine Rollins is author of *A Woman's Guide to Using Natural Progesterone* and Director of the website above.[69]

Breast Cancer Awareness Month?

What about the "much-hyped...*Breast Cancer Awareness Month?*" Are you aware that *Breast Cancer Awareness Month* that "occurs every October," is mostly "sponsored and funded by the drug company that makes tamoxifen?"[69a] Dr. Lee thought it very ironic that this same company produces chemo drugs that contribute to "breast cancer." There is little emphasis in October on prevention or "raising funds for independent research," and he felt that maybe it should be called "Breast Cancer Unawareness Month." Especially since the main focus is about being aware of ONLY those breast cancer treatments recognized and pushed by today's cancer industry![70]

Natural Progesterone & Autoimmune Disorders

A lack of sufficient progesterone in the body has the ability to throw the thyroid out of whack, resulting in hormonal disarray with a debilitating effect on the immune system. (How many women do you know on thyroid medication post-menopause?) It is very odd that during the time of their lives when they are most likely to be estrogen dominant, is when women fall victim to autoimmune diseases such as "rheumatoid arthritis, Sjogren's syndrome (dry eyes and dry mouth), Hashimoto's thyroiditis, Grave's disease, lupus...and rosacea."[71]

This was a troubling fact to Dr. Lee. He documented that many of his "patients with autoimmune disease" that he placed on "natural progesterone...reported that their disease symptoms also gradually abated." He wondered if autoimmune disorders were "an unrecognized symptom of estrogen toxicity...."[71a] He felt it was very possible from evidence with his own patients, to "suggest that progesterone protects against autoimmune disorders caused by excessive estrogens."[72] In fact, Catherine Rollins points out at her website (*natural-progesterone-advisory-network.com)* that new "studies have shown that women who use hormone replacement therapy containing estrogen are more likely to get lupus! Birth control pills also cause autoimmune diseases by causing the body to form antibodies to its own hormones."[73] (This ominous trend is especially insidious when you realize that many more WOMEN succumb to autoimmune disorders than do men, and the fact that they do not occur in such dismal proportions in areas outside the U.S, where estrogen dominance and HRT are unheard of!)

When purchasing natural progesterone, always look for creams that contain *USP Progesterone* on the label. The cream is used as described by Rita Elkins, M.H., in her book, *Natural Alternatives to HRT*:

> The cream should be applied where the skin is the thinnest and where multiple veins are visible...the wrist, the back of the hand, and breast tissue are the best areas for maximal absorption. The thighs and abdominal wall are poor receptor sites because the skin is tougher, thicker and has more layers of fat with fewer visible blood vessels.[74]

Natural progesterone cream has also been successfully used to treat cases of rosacea and psoriasis when applied topically to the affected areas.[75] Be sure when applying the cream, you give it time to be absorbed so that most of it does not end up in your clothing instead of in you.

Osteoporosis – How to Prevent it, How to Reverse it

Dr. Lee, in his own practice, proved that natural progesterone had the capacity to dramatically **REVERSE bone loss in patients who came to him with advanced osteoporosis.** He was perplexed by the obstinacy with which the current medical industry insists on using synthetic "estrogen as the mainstay of osteoporosis treatment for women," because, as he explained, scientific validation for it does not exist![76] He pointed to an article in a "1995 issue of the *New England Journal of Medicine*" that documented "eight years" of research involving close to 10,000 elderly "women" in the "United States." What Dr. Lee found so disturbing about this study was the fact that even though the participants were all more than 65 years of age and taking estrogen, it did absolutely nothing to protect them from hip fractures![77]

Dr. Lee discovered and taught that while estrogen may slow down the loss of bone, "progesterone will actively increase bone mass and density and can *reverse* osteoporosis." In his own practice he observed that using natural progesterone along "with proper diet and exercise" was very beneficial in the fight against osteoporosis, and he explained why:

[It[steadily increases bone density regardless of age, there's no reason for any women to have to take estrogen for osteo-porosis... The makers of Premarin and other estrogen man-ufacturers would have us all believing that estrogen loss is the major hormonal factor in osteoporosis for women. If that is so, why does significant bone loss occur during the 10 to 15 years before menopause, when estrogen levels are still normal?[78]

Many of Dr. Lee's patients came to him suffering with osteo-porosis in various degrees of severity. He was soon to discover that while "estrogen therapy may have slowed their bone loss...it did noth-ing to reverse the disease." Even when his patients "took calcium, vitamins D and C and...quit smoking, their bone loss continued."[79] He placed his patients on "natural progesterone" cream and they enjoyed "a 15% increase in bone mass over a period of three years with no negative side effects."[80] (Eventually, his patients had a return to what is considered normal bone density.)

How serious is osteoporosis? In the book *Remifemin: Herbal Relief for Menopausal Symptoms*, author Frank Murray explains that "25 million Americans – 80 percent of them women," suffer from this disease.[81] Osteoporosis has been linked to the cause of "about 1.5 mil-lion fractures each year..."[82]

As noted in her book *How To Renew You*, Maureen Kennedy Salaman says that "natural progesterone cream can be used by both men and women for prevention of bone loss and osteoporosis. Natural progesterone has no feminizing effects."[83] Ms. Salaman also lists some excellent natural sources of vitamin D. These are "...sardines, sunflower seeds...cottage cheese, and bee pollen."[84] (Remember, if you are taking calcium supplements, you should be using a brand that includes magnesium, and boron, and if it does not include vitamin D, you need about 10 - 20 minutes of sunshine every day (without sunscreen!) to give your body an adequate amount of vitamin D! It is best to get your vitamin D from the sun! (This sun exposure should not be during the hottest times of the day, and never while you are on herbs or drugs that increase sun-sensitivity. Check with your physician first if you or your immediate family members have a prior history of melanoma.) (See chapter 25 regarding dairy.)

Be sure that you are not taking excess calcium, which has been linked to clogged arteries! (Also, recall that you can get your **calcium** from the same place the dairy cows and the goats get it – not from milk, but from the soil, in the form of green leafy vegetables!) See the note in this book regarding the high amount of calcium in fresh carrot juice, and page 160 for calcium in dried barley grass juice!

Another ingredient that is gaining popularity in bone and joint health is the combination of "glucosamine" and "chondroitin sulfate," commonly used for arthritis patients. In *How To Renew You*, Maureen Kennedy Salaman points out that chondroitin sulfate actually "works better than heparin in preventing blood clots and without the dangerous side effects,"[85] yet very few physicians prescribe chondroitin over heparin for this purpose.

Menopause & Weight Gain

It is important to realize that when women become estrogen dominant, they get caught up in a vicious cycle. A high fat diet increases estrogen levels in the body, but fat cells also make estrogen, and as discussed earlier, we consume synthetic estrogens in our diets. We also get toxic estrogens (xenoestrogens) from substances we use everyday. A good example is plastic. If you do not want to get additional estrogen (or dioxin) in your food, avoid plastic containers and pots for your foods, and using plastic wrap in the microwave. There are times this is unavoidable, such as purchasing frozen fruit that usually comes in plastic bags!

Fat accumulates in breast tissue, the body makes even more estrogen from this stored fat, the estrogen causes the body to accumulate even more body fat, and then more estrogen is produced.

Women find themselves caught up in this vicious cycle of finding it not only more and more difficult to lose weight as they get older, but they keep gaining more weight as their estrogen production rises and their progesterone levels drop out of sight! They do not understand what is happening to them, especially if they haven't changed the amount of calories they ingest and they can't account for the weight gain. Many try one fad diet after another, or one exercise regimen after another, only to fail in the end. Regaining a normal hormone balance between estrogen and progesterone is sometimes all that is needed to win this battle.

Note that your physician should be checking your progesterone levels with a saliva test, which gives a much more accurate reading than a blood test, as discussed earlier in this chapter! Be sure to find a reliable, licensed, alternative health care physician, knowledgeable about natural hormones! See the sample list of practitioners at *http://altmedangel.com.*

Phytoestrogens

There are many plants and herbs that mimic the action of natural estrogen in the body. Black cohosh is one of them. These are called "Phyto" or plant estrogens. As noted by Rita Elkins, M.H., in her book, *Natural Alternatives to HRT*:

> In premenopausal women they block high estrogen levels, while in aging women they boost estrogenic actions. These...*isoflavones* give a plant its estrogenic action. Researchers at the Department of Obstetrics and Gynecology at the University of Bari, Italy, have concluded that phyto-estrogens increase bone density and reduce cholesterol....They may be helpful in preventing post-menopausal cardiovascular disease as well as osteoporosis.[86]

Soybeans and all soy products (such as tofu) are sources of "isoflavones." There are also many herbs available that contain "phytoestrogens." A few of these hormone-friendly herbs are "Red

Clover...Black Cohosh Root...Dong Quai...Chaste Berry (Vitex)...Licorice Root...Gotu Kola, Ginkgo and St John's Wort."[87]

A word of caution: be sure to discuss any of these products with your physician. St. John's Wort should not be taken by anyone on anti-depressants especially MAO inhibitors! Some herbs interfere with anti-coagulant medications or with other medications that a patient may be taking. Red clover and black cohosh root should not be used by children, nor by women who may be nursing or pregnant. (Fermented soy products, such as Haelan, can help remove harmful estrogens from the body in estrogen-receptor positive cancers.) Licorice can raise blood pressure (unless it is deglycyrrhizinated). It should only be used under a physician's direction.[88] You should realize that while these natural forms of estrogen may be beneficial by blocking out harmful estrogens in the body, all the plant estrogens in the world won't help if your main problem is a lack of progesterone, or if you are consuming large amounts of synthetic estrogen in meats and dairy products every day!

CHAPTER 22

WATER – THE DESPERATE THIRST

"It is estimated that 12 million children suffer from asthma, and several thousand die every year. Let us declare an end to asthma in less than five years. Let us save children from the constant fear of suffocation because they do not recognize they are thirsty for water!"

(F. Batmanghelidj, M.D., from his book:
Your Body's Many Cries For Water)[1]

If You're Already Thirsty, it's Almost too Late!

Chances are you've been thirsty enough at some point in your life to know what it means to crave an icy, cold drink! The problem is, the very **LAST symptom** that your body gives for dehydration is usually thirst! This means that once you hit the actual point where you are physically thirsty, you may already be seriously dehydrated. It is important to make sure that you are providing your body with enough water that you never reach the point of being overly thirsty (apart from unusual circumstances such as running a high fever, grueling exercise, excess salt consumption, illness, diarrhea, etc).

Scientists are only recently making the connection between long-standing dehydration and the onset of chronic, degenerative diseases. Most people drink a few cups of coffee during the day, soda, juice, or tea with their meals, and are convinced that they're getting their quota of fluids. Unless you are drinking 8-10 (8 ounce) glasses of WATER per day, (depending on your body weight), you are STARVING yourself for water and risking your health.

To determine how much water your body needs, you should be drinking approximately half your weight in **ounces** of water each day. (For example: if you weigh 100 pounds, you need about 50 ounces of water every day. If you weigh 200 pounds, you need about 100 ounces of water each day.)[1a] Caffeinated drinks are diuretics – they strip valuable water from your body! If you can't seem to stay away from them, then you will need more water to make up for their dehydration effects on your body!

It is critically important that the water you drink should NOT contain fluoride or chlorine. "Dr. John Yiamouyiannis," in an article at *website www.health-science.com/fluoride_toxicity.html* on "Fluoride Toxicity," estimates "that 30,000 - 50,000 people die from flouride (sic) poisoning each year," and "In his book, Fluoride: The Aging Factor," he attributes this chemical to "'collagen breakdown, genetic damage and/or disruption of the immune system.'"[2] It has also been shown by "Dr. Takeki Tsutsu and co-workers of the Nippon Dental College in Japan," that fluoride is responsible for causing "genetic damage, [and] was also capable of transforming normal cells into cancer cells." Research done by "Dr. Dean Burk, former Chief Chemist of the National Cancer Institute showed that 10,000 or more fluoridation-linked cancer deaths occur yearly in the United States."[3]

In his very informative book, *Your Body's Many Cries For Water,* the late Dr. F. Batmanghelidj, M.D., insisted that "You Are Not Sick, You Are Thirsty," and that you should not "treat thirst with medications."[3a] Dr. Batmanghelidj, born in "Tehran, Iran," was incarcerated there "at Evin prison" during the days of the brutal "Iranian revolution…1979" and it was during this time in prison that he discovered a treatment for stressed inmates who were developing peptic ulcers. The only thing he had to give them was water! The government of Iran was so impressed with his findings and subsequent article, they published his work in "the Iranian Medical Council Journal in 1982," and he was eventually released in June of that year. His article also appeared in "the science section of *The New York Times.*"[4]

Dr. Batmanghelidj had "treated more than 3000" of his "peptic ulcer" patients by merely increasing their water intake! He published his findings on "treating dyspeptic pain with water" in the *"Journal of Clinical Gastroenterology* in June of 1983." He claimed that "dyspeptic pain is the most important signal for the human body. It denotes dehydration. It is a thirst signal of the body." He also believed that "Chronic and persistently increasing dehydration is the root cause of almost all currently encountered major diseases of the human body."[5]

Just as we have a hunger stimulus when we get hungry, Dr. Batmanghelidj taught that our "'thirst pain' signal in the body" is called "dyspepsia," and treated "with all sorts of medications until there is local duodenal or stomach tissue damage from the metabolic complications of dehydration." He also taught that the consumption of "antacids for the relief of this pain," is like "slow poison..."[6]

It is very alarming that antacids are high in aluminum content. The accumulation of "excessive aluminum" in the brain has already been linked to "Alzheimer-type" disease. A good example is from an island "in the Western Pacific – Guam island."[6a] At one time there was such a high level of aluminum in Guam's drinking water, the entire population on the island (including "the younger people") were afflicted with a mental "dementia" (very "similar to Alzheimer dementia"), however, once the "problem was recognized and the water purified," the statistics for this dementia began to decline![7]

Dr. Batmanghelidj believed that "aluminum toxicity is a secondary complication of dehydration," and that "chronic dehydration" is what actually causes "*Alzheimer's disease.*" He also believed that in most cases of "Colitis Pain...False Appendicitis Pain...[and] Hiatus Hernia..." these are actually "thirst signals," and results of starving the body for water![8]

There is clinical evidence presented in *Your Body's Many Cries For Water* to link the pain of "Rheumatoid Arthritis," back and neck pain, and angina (as well as problems with allergies and asthma attacks) to chronic dehydration, and in some instances, inadequate salt intake.[9]

Help for Asthma Patients

Dr. Batmanghelidj discovered, almost by accident, exactly what causes asthma. He even tried to present his discovery to the American Medical Association (in a letter to then "President" of the "AMA...Dr. C. John Tupper, 1990"), but Dr. Tupper's response a month later was evasive and non-committal. Basically, he promised to share the information with others, and that was the last Dr. Batmanghelidj ever heard from him! Nothing was ever done with the information he gave them! However, his asthma cure was "aired on June 5, 1995, by Paul Harvey News for the first time."[10]

The treatment Dr. Batmanghelidj received by the AMA isn't at all surprising! It is the typical treatment that anyone gets when they promote a NATURAL CURE for a disease that is treated conventionally with a whole gamut of *acceptable* pharmaceutical drugs! How happy do you think it would make all those producers of asthma medications (and inhalers) if the public suddenly realizes that there is a natural, inexpensive treatment for asthma apart from the use of multiple pharmaceutical drugs?!

Dr. Batmanghelidj pointed out that adults and children with asthma and allergies have a high level of histamine in "their lung tissue." In a nut shell, histamine regulates water and "bronchial muscle contraction."[10a] Asthma is caused by chronic dehydration! This lack of water in the body causes the body to increase histamine production so that water will be conserved (sort of like an emergency stop-gap in a water crisis!) A great deal of water is lost through the lungs everyday, just from breathing![10b] Since the body is already starved for water, the histamine tries to conserve what little is left by CONSTRICTING the bronchioles to keep water from evaporating through breathing! What is the end result? ASTHMA, choking, suffocating, inability to breathe! This is also the reason for many allergies. Dr. Batmanthelidj very successfully weaned his asthma patients off asthma medications, simply by having them increase their WATER and their SALT intake![11] However, he warns that not taking enough water for months or years can not be compensated for in a day or two. You should increase your water intake if you are suffering from allergies and asthma, but you can not "OVERDRINK thinking you can undo the damage of many months or years of dehydration by excessive intake of water in a few days." You should take the normal amount recommended ("eight to ten 8-ounce glasses")... "until full hydration of the body is achieved over a longer period of time." He also recommends not drinking more than "one, or at most two, glasses a day" of "orange juice," due to its "high...potassium content," which can increase the body's histamine, especially with asthmatics.[12]

When You Need Extra Salt

For every two quarts of water that you drink every day, you need to add 1/2 tsp. of salt to your diet.[13] Salt plays a crucial role in asthma, because any time your body is dehydrated it automatically begins to hoard salt. "Salt is a natural antihistamine. People with allergies should begin to increase their salt intake to prevent excess histamine production," if their physician does not have them on a salt-restricted or water-restricted diet.[14] As explained by Dr. Batmanghelidj in describing what happens with **asthma**:

> It is a physiological adaptation of the body to dehydration and salt shortage. It will recur anytime sufficient attention is not paid to regular water and salt intake. A pinch of salt on the tongue after drinking water fools the brain into thinking a lot of salt has arrived in the body. It is then that the brain begins to relax the bronchioles. Alcohol and caffeine contribute to severe asthma attacks. People with asthma should slightly increase their salt intake.[15]

Dr. Batmanghelidj describes several case studies in his book, *Your Body's Many Cries For Water*, on the effects of increased salt and water intake for asthma patients. One case in particular was a "10-year-old" boy who was taking "five different medications to treat his asthma."[15a] After following Dr. Batmanghelidj's advice, the child was able to come off every single one of his asthma drugs, and this was not an isolated case! Another child was able to come off all of his asthma medication after only one month of sufficient water and salt treatment.[16]

If you are the parent of a child with asthma, think about this – do you KNOW how much water your child is taking in every day? You can NOT count pop, tea, juices, coffee, and soups! If for example, you have a 7-year-old in the second grade and you send them off to school after a breakfast that includes a glass of orange juice and milk, do they go the entire remainder of the day with NO water? What about lunch time? What do they drink for lunch? Milk? Soda? Soup? Water? Most school children go their entire 12 years in school chronically dehydrated! Schools have water fountains, but how much water do you think your child gets from a water fountain during the school day, rushing between classes? Many people believe that drinking extra water means too frequent trips to the bathroom, however (even though this happens initially when you begin increasing your water intake), once your body adjusts to the extra water, those frequent bathroom trips soon taper off.

Banish Back Pain & Prevent Autoimmune Disorders

Dr. Batmanghelidj authored several books and videos on the importance of water consumption for banishing back pain and autoimmune disorders like lupus and rheumatoid arthritis. It is important to realize that much of the degenerative disc disease that we encounter as we age is because of the fact that the discs in the spinal cord are composed mostly of water, and chronic dehydration over many years will shrink the discs, causing degeneration and herniation, resulting in severe back pain and disability.[16a] He pointed out that "75% of the weight of the upper part of the body is supported by the water volume that is stored in the disc core" of the "5th lumbar disc." It is this disc that is so critical to back health. Many patients that experience low back pain are told by their physicians that the problem involves their "5th lumbar disc."[17]

The M.S. Symptoms That Vanished!

Dr. Batmanghelidj also taught that months and years of starving your body for water can lead to autoimmune disorders ("multiple sclerosis…rheumatoid arthritis…lupus"), high blood pressure, diabetes, and many other ailments.[17a] At website *http://www.watercure2.org,* the story of Marilyn Fox, who suffered for five years with multiple sclerosis, is described. All of her M.S. symptoms disappeared after following the water cure. She said that she had been diagnosed with M.S. for "about 5 years" and that her symptoms included "being confined to bed for a month [and] retaining fluid so badly" that she was unable to walk.[17b] She also said that for her height she was overweight, and she "could hardly talk as well." Marilyn had no idea what was happening to her. She also had chronic problems involving her bladder and bowels and "was told" that she would eventually have to undergo "a colostomy." An LPN for 44 years, she had already been through a trial of several different medications. She did not begin the "water cure" until her disease was "very severe," and she explains what happened once on the "water cure":

All the medicine that I was taking, I stopped taking. I had seen such an improvement in my intellect, memory, coordination, breathing, [and] upper respiratory problems were gone as well. My bowel and bladder were stagnated, but they now are starting to function the way they should. I hadn't seen my doctor for a couple of months. When I walked in, he couldn't believe what he saw. "YOU LOOK WONDERFUL", is what he said to me. He asked what I was doing. I told him that I'm on Dr. Batmanghelidj's Water Cure, the water & salt cure! He asked what that was all about. I told him that everyone needs to drink two (2) quarts of water daily and add 1/2 tsp. of salt as seasoning on his food. He said evidently it does work because he could see the results in me and said, Marilyn, you have never been in better health.[17c]

Marilyn further describes her physician's reaction to the change in her medical status:

He thinks it is the greatest thing that he has ever heard…He even tried it himself and has now lost a lot of weight thanks to the Water Cure. He said that this therapy is so simple and unique that it has to get out to the people. In the Bible, you see salt & water…salt & water. If we would all…do the things like Jesus did when he was on this earth, and we all know he drank water and we all know that he must have eaten salt. We are the salt of the earth. And if it is good enough for him, it's got to be good enough for us. This has SAVED MY LIFE![17d]

According to Bob Butts at the *www.watercure2.org* website, "This is the 5th report of a person losing all symptoms of M.S. after going on the WATER CURE. All were ambulatory."[18] (Be aware that vegetarian diets and low fat diets can significantly reduce the risks for M.S. Research has also shown that curcumin may be beneficial in fighting M.S. because it appears to have a protective effect on nerve cells.)

Cancer & Dehydration

As for cancer, Dr. Batmanghelidj believed that "chronic dehydration in the human body is a primary causative factor for tumor production."[18a] You can find his books and products at his website: *www.watercure2.com*, or from Global Health Solutions, 8472 A Tyco Rd., Vienna, VA 22182, USA. They are also available at many natural health food stores.

Banishing High Blood Pressure

When the body is deprived of water, it hoards salt, leading to high blood pressure (as well as high cholesterol!) Dr. Batmanghelidj believed that many physicians are currently misleading their high blood pressure patients by putting them on salt-restricted, water-restricted diets, since the majority of high blood pressure problems are nothing more than what he referred to as "the result of an adaptive process to a gross body water deficiency."[19] He explained that "The present way of treating hypertension is wrong to the point of *scientific absurdity*." Due to dehydration, the body is actually trying in its desperate state to conserve water, so what do physicians do? They give their patients diuretics to get RID OF WATER![20] In his experience, Dr. Batmanghelidj said that, "Water by itself is the best natural diuretic..." If patients having hypertension, **who have sufficient urinary output**, will "increase their daily water intake, they will not need to take any diuretics." He advises in cases of heart failure problems, this water intake has to be done very gradually.[21] If you are on a water-restricted or salt-restricted diet, discuss this with your physician. Note that you should not discontinue any medications you may be taking without consulting your doctor. To do so could be harmful! (I highly recommend Dr. Batmanghelidj's books and videos; information you may want to share with your physician!)

Water & Oxygen

Remember, if you are fighting any chronic illness, diseases (such as cancer) can not survive in a highly oxygenated environment, and the main component of water is OXYGEN! Starving your body for water = intracellular oxygen starvation and deprivation. Cancer patients are dehydrated. Inadequate oxygen at the cellular level promotes cancer!

How Much Water Do You Need?

As noted earlier, you need ½ your body weight in **ounces** of water daily (if you weigh 200 pounds, you need about 100 ounces of water every day) for optimum hydration.[21a] You also need "¼ teaspoon of salt in every quart of water" that you drink or about ½ teaspoon for every **ten** (8 oz. glasses) you drink every day.[22] You will need more water during times of illness (e.g. fever, vomiting, diarrhea, stress, etc.), or excessive perspiration. Don't wait until you are thirsty! Drink water throughout the day (not all at once), and get used to carrying a water bottle around with you to develop a habit of drinking more water. A lack of salt may also contribute to osteoporosis, because if there is not enough salt in the blood, your body will remove salt from your bones to make up the deficit.[23] [24]

If your kidneys are not functioning correctly, and you increase your water and salt intake, you will start swelling up. Dr. Batmanghelidj's remedy (if you accumulate fluid in your skin and ankles) is to "Reduce salt intake for a few days, but increase your water intake until the swelling in the legs disappears," and increase your activity![25] However, you should have your regular physician involved at the very onset before you ever begin a new water/salt regimen, or if you experience any type of swelling as noted above!

Steve Meyerowitz, in his book, *Water The Ultimate Cure*, describes a "dehydration epidemic," which certainly is true for most people! Humans are composed of "67% water." If you lose just "2%" of this content, you will suffer weakness. If you lose "10%," the result will be "significant health problems," and if you lose more than this, it "can be fatal!"[26]

It is best NOT to drink water and other fluids while you are eating because they dilute the hydrochloric acid in the stomach needed to digest your food! The exception to this, of course, is times when you will swallow vitamin/mineral supplements that go with meals, or if you are taking medications that are supposed to go with meals.

Water Hydration & Cancer

Being chronically dehydrated "renders the immune system ineffective and unresponsive," robs the body of much needed antioxidants (due to the toxic buildup of acids), lowers the body's pH, and contributes to many degenerative diseases, including cancer![27]

Steve Meyerowitz identified progressive levels of dehydration: "Early Signs" may include "Fatigue, Anxiety, Depression, Cramps, [and] Headache." Some "Mature Signals of Dehydration" include "Heartburn, Joint and back pain, Migraine Headaches, Fibromyalgia, [and] Constipation/colitis…" A few "Emergency" symptoms that you are lacking water include: "Asthma and Allergies, Old Age Diabetes, Hypertension, Autoimmune Disease, Lupus, [and] Psoriasis…"[28]

Chronic dehydration has become "a risk factor for getting colon, breast, and urinary tract cancers…" The "immune system cells" cannot reach cancer cells to destroy them in a dehydrated, poorly functioning circulatory system![28a] One study in particular revealed that women who consume "more than five glasses of water per day" can cut their risk for "kidney and bladder cancer by 45 percent," and women also slash their chances of getting "breast cancer by 79%," simply by increasing their water intake.[29] (Research studies have also shown that men can reduce their risk of bladder and colorectal cancers by **increasing** their water intake!)

How Pure Is Your Drinking Water?

Much of the water provided in our city water supply systems is full of chlorine and fluoride (and most city water systems allow certain levels of bacteria in the water supply). This does not include the potential poisons from the plumbing the water runs through before it ever gets to your glass![29a] Bottled "spring water" may not be as clean as you are led to believe! If possible, "filter your own water" with a "high-quality filter." You can find out which filters are best and exactly what they filter (and don't filter) at "The National Sanitation Foundation (*www.nsf.org*)," which is "a non-profit, independent testing agency that rates most of the leading filters…"[30]

Another alternative is steam-distilled water. It usually has a "pH" of "7.0," so if you are slightly acidic, it will help bring up your pH.[31]

Be wary of the container your bottled water comes in. If you are drinking out of plastic bottles and tasting plastic, you are consuming dangerous toxins! Glass is best, but bottled waters using glass are expensive too. As noted by Steve Meyerowitz in *Water The Ultimate Cure*:

> Polycarbonate plastic is strong and rigid and is the kind most often used for 5-gallon water cooler jugs. It is highly inert, and imparts no taste and has been used for water bottles, baby bottles, and food storage containers for 35 years. **Look for #7 in the triangle** on the bottom of the bottle.[32] [Emphasis, mine.]

Some health food stores sell empty polycarbonate bottles in various sizes for water storage.

Heartburn & Reflux Disease

According to Dr. John R. Lee and Virginia Hopkins in their book, *What Your Doctor May Not Tell You About Menopause,* despite what you are being told by "the makers of Tums, Rolaids, Mylanta, Pepcid, Zantac, and Tagamet…heartburn is rarely caused by too much stomach acid."[32a] It is "most often caused by *too little* stomach acid." The older we get, the "less stomach acid" we make. When you have too little stomach acid, your food just "sits there," without digesting. It begins to ferment and this is the source of your esophageal irritation and "heartburn," or "gastroesophageal reflux," another fancy word for "heart-burn."[33] If you have too little stomach acid, Dr. Lee recommends one treatment that many people resort to: "a tablespoon of apple cider vinegar in one-third of a cup of water before a meal." Since the "vinegar is highly acidic," it may give you just enough acidity for "quick, easy digestion." Just be sure you don't take the vinegar during an "active case of heartburn," because it will only make it worse![34]

You may find help from chewable papaya extracts as well (available in health food stores). Most taste delicious, or you can try eating fresh papaya with your meals! There are also enzyme supplements available that aid in digestion. Maureen Kennedy Salaman has helpful digestive enzyme supplements available at her website *www.mksalaman.com:* **Enzyme Ease®, and Multi-Enzyme.**

Be aware that papaya enzymes can have blood-thinning properties, something you should discuss with your physician, especially if you are already taking anti-coagulant medications, or other prescription drugs.

Asthma & Mushrooms

See the information in chapter 24 of this book regarding Cordyceps Sinensis mushroom and asthma.

CHAPTER 23

PREVENT CANCER WITH OXYGEN, EXERCISE, REST, & SUNSHINE

"Cancer is increasing at such an alarming rate that about 40 percent of Americans will develop cancer, but only 14 percent of Americans who exercise regularly will develop cancer"

(Don Colbert, M.D., from his book:
Walking in Divine Health.)[1]

Oxygen Therapies for Cancer

The importance of oxygen in cancer prevention was discussed briefly in chapter 22. According to Ann Wigmore in *The Wheatgrass Book*, "Otto Warburg, M.D.," won a "Nobel prize" by showing that "cancer cells thrived in an oxygen-poor environment." He ultimately saw cancer as a "process of cell mutation caused by oxygen deprivation on the cellular level."[2] Even though Dr. Warburg's discovery is over "fifty years" old, it has never been disproven. Healthy ways to increase your cellular oxygen is with fresh vegetable and fruit juices, "deep breathing" exercises, adequate water intake, regular physical exercise, and green foods that increase chlorophyll in the body; foods like wheatgrass, barley juice, and other green drinks.[3]

One cancer treatment that seeks to get more oxygen into the body at the cellular level is **ozone treatment**. You can purchase ozonators at some health food stores, but they are rather expensive. Ozone is another form of oxygenation, important to all body cells.

Hydrogen peroxide is given intravenously for increasing the body's oxygenation. Many patients claim that they have been cured using an intravenous form of hydrogen peroxide given by Naturopathic physicians, even though the mainstream media has presented it as controversial by claiming that ONE patient was harmed with this ingredient! However, there never was any evidence substantiating that this alternative therapy harmed the patient in question. I saw the case as presented on a popular T.V. news program. It was just another example of the bias against Naturopathic practitioners. Though I do not consider this a *natural* or *painless* treatment (since it is given intravenously), you will see it promoted by some alternative health practitioners, and many people claim that it has brought their cancers into complete remission. (What we need are T.V. programs highlighting all the THOUSANDS of cases of people who are fatally harmed with toxic chemo drugs and radiation every year, but their surviving family members would have to provide the documentaries since the witnesses are all dead!)

According to Conrad LeBeau in his book, *Hydrogen Peroxide & Ozone*: an "owner of a health food store" in "Sonora, CA," said that she was able to shrink "a large tumor with adhesions" when she used a **topical** "hydrogen peroxide based gel."[4] The tumor, "the size of a hen's egg," shrank "to the size of a half-dollar," plus she reported that her pain had disappeared.[5]

R.N. Cures Her Pancreatic Tumor with Dietary Changes & Topical Hydrogen Peroxide Gel

Also described by Conrad LeBeau is the story of "a registered nurse" from "Scottsdale, AZ" with "inoperable cancer" (pancreatic tumor), who cured her cancer on a "vegetarian diet." She also used "½ tablespoon of a hydrogen peroxide based gel three times a day. (She absorbed about 67 drops of 37% H2O2 into her skin each day,)"[6] This was a **topical** application; it was not taken by mouth. Her story is extraordinary because her oncologist had given her "3 months" to live! "He was surprised to see her" walking into his office a year later for a "catscan and physical….The catscan showed her blood to be normal and that the mass of tumor in the pancreas area was gone, leaving a small indentation. Her doctor said; 'this is amazing.'"[7]

Mr. LeBeau describes another account of a patient who was able to shrink a tumor by "mixing 1 part of 35% H2O2 with 5 parts of aloe and applying it directly on the tumor" (topically), and a patient from Ohio who said that she was "rid of her rheumatoid arthritis which she had for 17 years," after she began "using hydrogen peroxide **externally**." In a fourth case study, another patient used "Peroxy Gel" which led to "a complete remission" from "breast cancer."[8] This too was topical, NOT internal! **Never take peroxide internally** unless you are ordering or purchasing a type of peroxide that is manufactured and sold for oral consumption. If so, it should be clearly stated on the label!

Hyperbaric Oxygen Therapy

Hyperbaric oxygen therapy is used to increase oxygen levels in the body. It is often resorted to in cases of severe oxygen deprivation such as CVA's. It is also finding popularity as an alternative cancer therapy. Orthodox medicine uses hyperbaric oxygen therapy extensively. This therapy is often prescribed after delicate microsurgery for increasing cellular oxygen in cases where fingers or entire limbs have been re-attached after traumatic injuries. (It was not unusual for my patients to receive hyperbaric oxygen therapy when I worked on a hospital surgical floor, and this was several years ago.)

In getting more oxygen to your cells, remember that you need FRESH AIR every day! Cancer cells grow faster in stale air that is poorly oxygenated.

Exercise & Cancer

One of the quickest ways to oxygenate your body is with regular exercise. Studies have shown that exercise on a regular basis (at least 30 minutes 3 - 4 days per week) greatly reduces the risk of all types of cancers.

Exercise need not be overly "strenuous" or exhausting to reap its "health benefits." For example: "30 minutes of brisk walking" will accomplish the same thing for you that "15-20 minutes of jogging" will do. According to Valerie Saxion in her book, *How To Feel Great All The Time*, A "twelve-year study" of "17,000 Harvard alumni...recently released," showed that as exercise increases, so does "life expectancy," however "exercising more than...3,500 calories per week" appeared to be "counterproductive."[9]

Scientists have recently discovered a relationship between routine exercise and cancer prevention. A survey was done resulting in data from over two decades, which revealed that colon cancer can be prevented with routine exercise. Merely riding a bike or taking walks every day could very successfully cut the risk of colon cancer in half! A woman's study also confirmed that regular physical exercise can prevent breast and uterine cancers. The more exercise the women undertook, the less likely they were to develop cancer.

Adequate Rest Keeps the Immune System Healthy

If you are not getting adequate rest at night, you may be doing significant damage to your immune system. (If I know that I am going to be up working late, I take extra vitamin C to help my immune system!) Insuring that you get adequate amounts of sleep can slash your risk of cancer! For optimal health most of us need about eight hours of sleep every night. A very important hormone is produced by the body during sleep, known as *melatonin.*

The importance of this hormone is described in Maureen Kennedy Salaman's book *How To Renew You.* She explains that melatonin is very crucial in the human "circadian rhythm – the sleep-wake rhythm" cycle. "It is increased in the blood" during "hours of darkness" as we sleep. Levels decrease during the day.[10]

Because of this wake-sleep melatonin cycle, and the way growth hormone is released in the body, it is most important to get several sleep hours before midnight. Going to bed at nine PM and rising at 5 AM is much healthier for you than staying up until midnight and getting up at 8 AM, where all of your sleep hours occur after midnight! (Note that some people require 8-9 hours of sleep every night, rather than the usual 7-8. If you require **much more than that**, you are either a teenager or pregnant, an infant or young child, breastfeeding, 85 years old, the parents of a newborn, or you have a medical problem!)

As described by Ms. Salaman, the only time that human growth hormone (HGH) is produced is when you drop into "the deepest phases of sleep." Since it is referred to as the "anti-stress hormone" (because it "regulates the rhythms of other hormones"), failure to get adequate rest at night will rob you of much needed HGH (and mela-tonin), and eventually your overall health will suffer.[11] It is not unusu-al for nurses, other healthcare workers, and industrial workers who do swing shifts, to have problems later in life with insomnia when they try to get back to sleeping at night, rather than in the daytime! Many of them don't realize at the time, that working these odd hours can cause them problems years later when they try to readjust their sleep pattern for nighttime hours. (This has happened to me many times, even years after working hospital night shifts!)

Sufficient Sunlight Prevents Cancer

Everyone has been so brain-washed by the health community and news media that sunlight is so bad for you, that new cases are arising every day of children with ricketts, a disease where the bones are soft and malformed from vitamin D deficiencies. This is a disease that we thought had long ago nearly vanished in America. What is happening? Parents are over-reacting to the hype about skin cancers and the sun, bundling their children up against **all sunshine exposure**, slathering them with globs of sunscreen and sending them outside to play. Since the best source of **natural vitamin D is SUNSHINE**, children are suffering from vitamin D deficiencies from not getting adequate sun exposure! When sunshine hits the skin, a chemical reaction occurs that creates natural vitamin D in our bodies. People who live in north-ern states often have problems with vitamin D deficiencies (more so than those living in the south) because of less sun exposure in colder climates.

Dr. Joseph Mercola, author of the *Total Health Program* (see his website at: *www.mercola.com),* believes that inadequate "exposure to ultraviolet radiation" is putting us at increased risk for "cancer in Western Europe and North America."[12] A study in the journal, *Cancer,* supports this belief. When researchers studied "506 regions," they found a "close inverse correlation between cancer mortality and levels of ultraviolet B light." It is believed that the body needs ultra-violet B light in order to produce vitamin D.[13] The author of the study, "Dr. William Grant…says northern parts of the United States may be dark enough in winter that vitamin D synthesis shuts down completely."[14] This study, though more "focused on white Americans," found the very same "geographical trend affects black Americans, whose overall cancer rates are significantly higher." Apparently, people with darker skin "require more sunlight to synthesize vitamin D," as much as "10-20 times" more "sun exposure" to get "the same amount of vitamin D" as those with lighter skin.[15] There were 13 different malignant cancers that were affected by this sunlight phenomenon, but the ones most affected were "breast, colon, and ovarian cancer." Others included "tumors of the bladder, uterus, esophagus, rectum, and stomach."[16] As further explained by Dr. Mercola:

> Most people believe that sun exposure causes cancer. Nothing could be further from the truth. As this study published in the prestigious Cancer journal indicates, exposure to sun actually decreases cancer rates...the solution is not to slather sun block on. Sun block can be quite toxic and should be avoided by most people. The sensible approach is to limit sun exposure so you never get sun burned.[17]

Dr. Mercola believes that skin cancers are linked to the high amount of "omega-6 fats in most diets," which increase cancer risk during excess sun exposure. He says that "you can't have it both ways. Avoid the sun and don't change your diet and you will lower your risk of skin cancer, but **increase your risk of far more common and deadlier cancers**."[18]

Perhaps you are thinking you will just get your vitamin D from milk and supplements, after all we see commercials about milk and its vitamin D content plastered everywhere to make us **think** that milk is actually good for us, right? As described in H. Winter Griffith's *Vitamins, Herbs, Minerals & Supplements:* the vitamin D you find in milk and vitamin supplements is "synthetic...D2...also called *ergocalciferol,*" and it's a poor substitute for the one that comes from natural sunlight "or natural food sources...vitamin D3 or *calciferol.*"[19] Other sources of vitamin D (besides sunlight) are: "...Egg substitutes...Herring, Mackerel, Salmon, Sardines...[and] Tuna..."[20]

There is no way that mankind, hard as he tries, can improve on what our Creator God has given us in its natural state! Vitamin D from natural sunshine is one of God's many *health gifts* to us, intended for our nourishment and well-being.

As described at *www.mercola.com*, vitamin D is critical in maintaining "normal blood levels of calcium and phosphorus."[21] One reason for the rampant osteoporosis in this country is because people are not getting adequate vitamin D from sunshine! It regulates our body's absorption of calcium, assisting with the body's maintenance of a strong skeletal system. Taking all the calcium supplements in the world will not help you if you are deficient in vitamin D! Vitamin D is fat soluble, meaning it can be stored in the body, so overdosing with synthetic forms can be dangerous! This is another reason why getting vitamin D through sunlight (rather than taking supplements) is preferred.[22]

Caroline Ryan of BBC News, in her article at website *www.greatestherbsonearth.com*, discusses the advantages of sunshine in preventing cancer. She says that Professor Michael Holick, from "the Boston University School of Medicine...suggests that Caucasians spend five to 10 minutes in the sun, unprotected, two to three times a week."[23] Ms. Ryan further explains that an "independent researcher from Virginia...Dr. William Grant...estimates there have been 23,000 deaths from cancer per year...which could have been prevented if people had had enough vitamin D. He suggests this figure could be 30,000." He estimates that in the UK "a quarter of breast cancer deaths...are a result of vitamin D deficiency." In Boston he estimates that as much as "40 to 50% of adults over 50 were vitamin D deficient."[24]

Just consider someone you know that may be elderly. How much sunshine are they exposed to every day? What about those who spend their time in nursing homes? How much sunshine do you think THEY get every day, if any? Fresh air?

Ms. Ryan further noted that "Professor Holick's team...isolated a key enzyme, or body chemical," crucial "in the processing of vitamin D," and it was located "in the colon." It is this "active form of vitamin D [that] prevents colon cells from proliferating and prompts them to change into more mature cells which are less capable of becoming cancerous," **thus the reason why vitamin D deficiencies will lead to colon cancer!**[25]

Sunshine has also been proven to boost the immune system, lower blood pressure and relax the body. This is why it is so easy to fall asleep on the beach in the sun! Have you had YOUR dose of sunshine today? What about fresh air (oxygen), and exercise? As noted earlier, if you yourself have a history of melanoma, or a strong hereditary background of familial melanoma, always consult with your physician about sun exposure.

CHAPTER 24

MUSHROOMS – FANTASTIC FUNGI
THAT FIGHT CANCER

"In Japan their most powerful chemotherapies come from mushrooms and are nontoxic. They use our pharmaceutical chemotherapies only when all else has failed, as a last resort...They treat disease with nutrition first, medicine second. They practice preventative medicine."
(From website: Wellness Directory of Minnesota™ – *www.mnwelldir.org)*[1]

Several different mushroom varieties have already been discussed in this book. There are many others, barely mentioned, with amazing healing properties. This chapter is devoted to some of those.

Agaricus Blazeil Murill

Agaricus mushroom is described at website: *www.mnwelldir.org/docs/Newsletters/01_Aug.htm*, as "The most powerful chemotherapy in Japan today." According to them, the healing properties of this mushroom are amazing:

> Found in Brazil, this mushroom is producing spectacular results, results heretofore never obtained by any other substance or chemotherapy...In Brazil there is a health practitioner who raises these mushrooms and has sent out an open invitation to physicians throughout the world to come down and witness people being cured of deadly cancers using only this mushroom. He will put them up and feed them, all they have to do is get there. So far, only the Orient has responded to his invitation.[2]

Apparently, when researchers visited the area where this mushroom grew, they found that the "local natives" were free of disease with many of them "living well over 100." Since that time, it has been discovered that "the polysaccharide" found in this mushroom is "effective against Ehrlich's ascites carcinoma, sigmoid colonic cancer, ovarian cancer, breast cancer, lung cancer and liver cancer as well as against solid cancers."[3]

Agaricus mushroom is "80% more effective than the world's number one cancer drug, PSK," in Japan. (Note that this excludes the U.S., where PSK is not promoted as a cancer treatment.) This mushroom, in animal studies, destroyed "all cancerous tumors in 90% of the experimental mice." It was also effective as a preventative.[3a] When mice were fed ABM then "injected with a very powerful cancer causing agent (Sarcoma 180), 99.4% of them showed no tumor growth. **Conventional medicine has nothing as powerful as this.**" (The Japanese "studies were so successful that today Japan is now buying over 90% of the available ABM from Brazil.")[4]

You can order this mushroom in capsules ("freeze dried extract") from *"http://www.hplus.com/a36.html."* It is also available in bulk "wholesale from China" at *"http://www.abmcn.com."* One of the "largest suppliers in the world is *www.agaricus.net*."[4a] If you need them fast, at the very best prices, order from *"www.mitobi.com."* Note that this mushroom is "also known as Himematsutake and can be used in your cooking the same way as other mushrooms are." *Wellness Directory of Minnesota*™ website recommends taking vitamin C with your mushroom supplements for better absorption.[5]

Cordyceps Sinensis

Cordyceps Sinensis is considered "one of the most valued medicinal fungi…in all of Chinese medicine and among the most potent." Kate Gilbert Udall in her book *Cordyceps Sinensis,* states that "It has been helpful in curing asthma and other respiratory ailments." An extract from this fungi known as *cordycepin* (in a study in 1989) revealed "that cordycepin inhibited the…spread of HIV infection."[6] (Note that the common table spice "curcumin from turmeric" also inhibits HIV.)

Cordyceps sinensis, says Ms. Udall, is reported to have the capacity to "…control the division of cancer cells, delay the diffusion of cancer cells and increase the engulfing abilities of T-cells in the human body," thus enhancing the immune system's ability to fight cancer![7]

Coriolus Versicolor

An important cancer fighting extract comes from this mushroom, called "PSK," discussed earlier in this chapter. Many "studies have suggested that PSK can improve survival rates in people who have stomach, colon, or lung cancer."[7a] Also, lab studies have shown that coriolus versicolor "might be able to overpower HIV in the test tube." Further testing is needed to see if it will function the same way in humans! When this mushroom was used in "cancer patients" they were "remarkably free of adverse side effects."[8] (However, as noted earlier, agaricus appears to be even more powerful than PSK.)

Enoki

In an article at website *www.rwood.com/Articles/Mushrooms _Detoxify.htm,* Rebecca Wood reports that "enoki," mushrooms can "inhibit tumor growth and may prevent liver disease and stomach or duodenal ulcers." They are best "with light cooking."[9] It is interesting that the "area of Japan" where this mushroom grows in abundance is "known to have the **lowest incidence of cancer in the country.**"[10] You can often purchase fresh enoki in health food stores.

Hoelen

This mushroom known as *hoelen ("Poria cocos")* can be found underneath "the roots of pines and other trees." *Herbs2000.com* explains that some of them grow to a size of "fifteen and twenty pounds" and are sometimes "ground" and used in a form of bread known as "tuckahoe bread." They are an excellent "source of potassium," and have been used for "kidney ailments…lowering blood sugar and controlling stomach acids." An ingredient in this mushroom (poriatrin) appears to be especially effective at helping "people with autoimmune kidney disease" such as in "lupus." Best results are obtained from actually ingesting the mushroom, rather than "taking extracts."[11] (It is always safest to cook mushrooms.)

Kombucha

You may have tasted kombucha tea, but it's not from a mushroom. "Kombucha" isn't exactly a mushroom, "not technically." According to *www.drlam.com*, it is actually a "group of yeasts (simple fungi) and bacteria," but it contains many similar "healing properties" as found in mushrooms. Kombucha boosts the immune system by increasing "levels of interferon."[12]

Maitake

Dr. Ralph Moss reports in his book, *Cancer Therapy*, that maitake mushrooms have successfully "stopped the growth of tumors" in many animal tests. In one study in particular, ten mice were fed "maitake powder one month after tumors had been implanted." They had a decrease in their "tumor growth...by a remarkable 86.3 percent....[and] Four of the ten mice were totally cured."[13]

In his book, *Alternative Cures*, Bill Gottlieb says forget the "chicken soup," because these mushrooms outperform the soup when it comes to combating the common cold![14] Maitake is also known as "hen of the woods or the dancing mushroom." The extract taken from them, "beta-glucan or D-fraction, has been highly effective in shrinking tumors in laboratory animals," and is discussed in other cancer specific chapters of this book. Most nutritionists recommend cooking mushrooms, because, as noted by Selene Yeager in *Doctors Book of FOOD REMEDIES,* there are "toxins" in the raw fungi that are destroyed at high temperatures.[15]

Morels

Morel mushrooms, described by *www.rwood.com*, vary from "thumb to fist size," and can be "black, brown, ivory or yellow," and their caps are very spongy with "pitted...hollows." Used as a "digestive tonic," they also have the ability to suppress "the formation and growth of tumors...."[16]

Oyster Mushrooms

These mushrooms demonstrated a "75.3 percent tumor inhibition" when animals "with sarcoma cells were given injections of...water extracts" from them, however, Dr. R. W. Moss at *www.ralphmoss.com*, reports that shiitake appears to be more potent than oyster mushrooms! Extracts from shiitake resulted in even better results with "80.7 percent...tumor inhibition." The "Shiitake white powder" produced inhibition rates of "81.1 percent..." The power of the mushrooms apparently came from "polysaccharides" extracted from them![17]

Reishi Mushroom

According to Deanne Tenney in her book, *Medicinal Mushrooms*, "Reishi" mushroom *("Ganoderma lucidum")* comes in "many different varieties," each one being a different color. They are "Akashiba (red reishi), Kuroshiba (black reishi), Aoshiba (blue reishi), Shiroshiba (white reishi), Kishiba (yellow reishi), and Murasakishiba (purple reishi)."[18] Studies from the "Cancer Research Center in Moscow" prove that this mushroom can enhance immunity and inhibit "the growth of tumors."[19] Dr. Earl Mindell says that "Reishi," in Japan is known as "*kisshotake* or the 'lucky fungus.'" In his book, *Earl Mindell's Soy Miracle*, he explains that compounds in reishi boost the immune system, act as "natural antihistamines...lower blood cholesterol...and prevent the formation of dangerous clots."[20] As discovered by one researcher, you can greatly enhance the "anti-cancer effects" of this mushroom "by combining it with high dose vitamin C."[21] (Be aware that as with any other mushroom or herb that has anti-clotting properties, if you are on prescription medications or have a chronic condition requiring frequent monitoring, before taking in large amounts, you should discuss them first with your physician.)

Shiitake

Shiitake mushroom, already mentioned earlier, increases "interferon" in the body, and as described by Jean Carper in *The food Pharmacy*, it has been "amazingly successful in fighting cancers." **Human testing** has been done in China on "leukemia patients" and on "human breast cancer in Japan." Shiitake can also lower blood cholesterol.[22] *Doctors Book of FOOD REMEDIES* by Selene Yeager reports that an extract from shiitake, lentinan, has been used in fighting cancer. Lentinan injections are discussed in cancer specific chapters elsewhere in this book. Scientists discovered that they could add "lentinan...in the form of dried mushroom powder to [the diets of] laboratory animals with tumors, [and] inhibit tumor growth by 67%."[23]

It was during the 1980s that researchers from Japan discovered the ability of this extract in halting "the growth of liver cancer in mice."[24]

Suehirotake & Yamabushiitake Mushrooms

Extracts from suehirotake mushroom (for example, SPG) are being studied for their effects in fighting cancer as well as chronic fatigue syndrome. See page 540 for information on MGN-3 which contains several mushrooms, including this one! Yamabushiitake (Lion's Mane mushroom) is also being studied for its potential at inhibiting the onset of senile dementia.

Wood Ear Mushrooms

When you see this mushroom in dried form, it resembles "black leather," but it looks elastic when fresh. Website *www.rwood.com* describes it as being able to "clear the body of free radicals, support brain function and relieve constipation."[25]

CHAPTER 25

MILK – DON'T GET IT! PITCH IT!

"Learn the truth about the foods you consume. Don't be dissuaded by the media and other influences within our capitalistic society where money has become more important than human welfare."
(Robert Morse, N.D., from his book: *The Detox Miracle Sourcebook)*[1]

Are the Risks Worth That Dose of Calcium?

Our culture has been so brainwashed by the media into believing that drinking milk is absolutely essential to strong bones and teeth, most parents are shocked when they are told that cow's milk is actually for baby cows (CALVES), not humans! Though humans do need some calcium, there is controversy about the amounts actually needed and the best sources!

"But, doctor, what will happen to my teeth and bones if I stop drinking milk?" is a question asked of Dr. Frank A. Oski in his book *Don't Drink Your Milk!* His reply? "Nothing. Nothing that wouldn't have happened anyway."[2]

Do you realize that you can get your daily calcium needs from the same place the cows and goats get it? From the soil! Green foods! Some excellent sources of calcium listed by Dr. Oski are: "collards… turnips…rhubarb…kidney beans, broccoli, soybeans, almonds,"[3] carrots, and just about any GREEN food you can think of. Wheat grass, barley grass, kale, spinach, chlorella, dandelion greens, and celery all have calcium. After all, what do cows and goats EAT all day? GREEN FOODS mostly, that is, if they are left to their choice of grazing out in a field as our Creator intended. Have you ever known of a cow with osteoporosis, brittle bone disease, or heart disease?! (On the other hand – if you really want to foul things up, something we humans are so-o-o GOOD at – just grind up some dead animal parts, add that to the grain you feed your cows – and give them MAD COW disease, but that's another story!) Also, see page 160.

Other excellent sources of calcium as described by H. Winter Griffith in *Vitamins, Herbs, Minerals & Supplements*, are "Almonds, Brazil nuts…Kelp…Sardines…[and] Tofu."[4] (Salmon is also high in calcium.) However, you don't need milk or meats to get your calcium! As noted by Deborah Lee in *Juicing: Your Liquid Nutritional Supplement,* an 8 ounce glass of carrot juice will give you "two-and-a-half times **more calcium** than a comparable glass of milk." (Emphasis mine.) Besides that, you also get a huge dose of beta-carotene that is much healthier than all those hormones in the milk given to the cows to "make them produce more milk."[5]

Maureen Kennedy Salaman agrees wholeheartedly that it isn't milk that we should be getting our calcium from! In her book, *How To Renew You,* she explains:

> Everybody knows that calcium strengthens bones. That's why we drink milk, right? Wrong! You've seen billboards pronouncing "everybody needs milk?" They should change it to read: Everybody needs…sesame seeds, kelp, spinach, chard, brewer's yeast, sardines, carob, caviar, soybeans, almonds, torula yeast, parsley, Brazil nuts, watercress, salmon, chickpeas, egg yolk, and beans.[6]

If you still aren't convinced that milk is NOT the place to get your calcium, 80,000 nurses that participated in a research study done by Harvard are! As described at *hsiealert.com,* here's why:

> [The] Harvard study of 80,000 nurses showed that a high intake of commercial milk appeared to actually increase the risk of bone fractures. Other studies have shown mounting evidence that milk may play a role in a variety of health problems, including prostate cancer, rheumatoid arthritis, atherosclerosis, anemia, MS, and leukemia.[7]

When an investigation by the "Consumers Union examined milk as a product and evaluated it for taste, bacterial contamination, and undesirable additives…Their findings should frighten even the milkaholics away from their local dairy bars." Dr. Frank A. Oski,

M.D., summarized those findings in his book, *Don't Drink Your Milk!* "Not only is there very little evidence that cow milk is of nutritional benefit to humans, but it…may be contaminated with bacteria, and can contain substances that are actually hazardous to your health."[8]

Many people think (erroneously) that cow's milk is "sterile" due to the pasteurization process. Nothing could be further from the truth! Even the milk of "a healthy cow will always contain some bacteria," says Dr. Oski. This normally comes from "fecal matter that has contaminated the cow's udder and teats." Farmers know this; they are around cows all the time, so they know about cleaning off the cow "before and after milking" in order to remove any traces of fecal matter.[9] (Are they doing this efficiently? Most of them probably are, but if so, WHERE is all that bacteria coming from?)

According to the U.S. government, explains Dr. Oski, once milk has been pasteurized, it "should contain no more than 20,000 bacteria per milliliter of milk and no more than ten organisms of the coliform species in each milliliter. (…there are 5 milliliters in a teaspoon…)"[10] Do the math! That comes out to **100,000 bacteria allowed in every teaspoon of milk that you drink!** (I don't know about you, but I think that's a pretty hefty dose of allowable *bugs.*)

So you see, it isn't expected that the milk will be sterile after pasteurization, just that the "number of bacteria will be kept at a respectable minimum." Of course, if the milk isn't kept cold, the bacteria begin to multiply like mad! Dr. Oski reveals that the investigators (mentioned above) from the "Consumer's Union found that seven samples tested had bacterial counts in excess of 130,000 per milliliter. One sample had almost 3 million and some had too many to count."[11]

Of even greater concern perhaps, was that some of the milk samples tested by "Consumers Union" also contained pesticides and "chlorinated hydrocarbons," however, realize that "The FDA operates on the notion that a little bit of cancer-producing material won't hurt you."[12] (You do remember the FDA, don't you – from chapter one? You know – that august, designated, staunch, elite government body that is concerned with your welfare, right?)

What did the "Consumers Union" testers have to say about all of this? Dr. Oski summarized their findings: "The Consumers Union expert milk consultant 'considers the milk supply throughout the five-state Midwestern area covered in our tests to pose a potential hazard.'"[13] Now **that** should greatly enhance your ability to sleep well tonight, along with that warm glass of milk…right?

Milk to Die For!

One scientist in particular, after being diagnosed with breast cancer, going through chemo, then having it return, found that her cancer completely disappeared when she finally eliminated all dairy products from her diet.

Dr. John R. Lee, et al., in the book, *What Your Doctor May Not Tell You About Breast Cancer*, attributed the hormone given to cows to raise their milk production "(rBGH)" as a culprit that "may increase the risk of breast cancer," and he explained why:

> According to cancer risk specialist Samuel Epstein, M.D., this biotech hormone induces a marked increase in levels of insulin-like growth factor (IGF-1) in cow's milk. There's little doubt that if you have too much IGF-1, it can play a role in causing breast cancer.[14]

And if that isn't enough to scare you from dairy products forever, consider this fact from Maureen Kennedy Salaman's *All Your Health Questions Answered Naturally*: if you are a woman, dairy products can also increase your risk of ovarian cancer![15] Physician Daniel W. Kramer from the "Harvard Medical School in Boston," a "gynecologist," has "linked galactose consumption with an increased risk of ovarian cancer."[16] He wasn't the only one concerned! According to website *http://www.hsialert.com,* scientists from the "National Institute of Environmental Medicine in Stockholm, Sweden," were also suspicious of a connection between milk consumption and ovarian cancer. They studied the "medical records of more than **61,000 women**, aged 38 to 76 years who were cancer-free at the outset of the study." They followed the participants for "about 13 years." During that time, "more than 260 subjects were diagnosed with epithelial ovarian cancer, and 125 of those cases were considered 'serious.'" After compiling all their information, they concluded from their study the following (quoted from *www.hsialert.com* with their permission):

> Lactose intake was associated with serious ovarian cancer risk. Women who consumed approximately four daily servings of dairy products had twice the risk of developing serious ovarian cancer compared to women who consumed less than two daily servings of dairy.
>
> The dairy product most strongly associated with serious ovarian cancer was **milk**.[17] [Emphasis, mine.]

You've seen the ads. You know, the kids (and adults) wearing the cute white milk mustache? Health Sciences Institute prefaced the above article on their webpage with the title "One dangerous moustache (sic)."[18]

Maureen Kennedy Salaman further warns about the additives in milk in *All Your Health Questions Answered Naturally*:

> Let me warn you about the vitamin D in milk. An intake of dairy foods fortified with vitamin D, like milk, results in decreased magnesium absorption. This is because the so-called vitamin D added to milk is actually a hormone – and a synthetic one…it can actually contribute to aging by depositing calcium in the soft tissue at the surface of the skin. Get your vitamin D from foods and sunlight instead.[19]

Also, are you aware that the majority of the people in this planet (at least "70 percent" of them) are located near the equator? Dr. Lee and Virginia Hopkins in *What Your Doctor May Not Tell You About Menopause*, reported that this is the area "between the tropic of Cancer and the tropic of Capricorn," with a warm climate where people harvest living plants "year round," and they do not consume milk from dairy cows! Most of them "have better bones than we do" in the more developed countries![20] Not only that but "several years ago, the now former U.S. Surgeon General, C. Everett Koop, M.D., told the world: 'Dairy products are bad for you.'"[21] **(Why has no one LISTENED to him?)**

The Calcium Myth

According to Deborah Lee in *Juicing: Your Liquid Nutritional Supplement*, "Milk Is an Imperfect Food," because "We all grew up being taught that milk is the best source of calcium. It is not. Heavy metals, detergents, antibiotics, viruses, and other toxins have been found in milk."[22] Even though "calcium and phosphorus" are important in our bones and teeth, "cow's milk contains ten times the amount of calcium and three times as much phosphorus as human milk." This unbalanced ratio "actually causes the calcium to be leached from the bones and can lead to the weakening of the bone structure and osteoporosis."[23] In a nutshell, **cow's milk does NOT prevent osteoporosis, and may even CAUSE IT!**

Ms. Lee also reports that large amounts of an enzyme responsible for heart disease "xanthine oxidase" is found in "commercial milk." Homogenization makes it possible for this enzyme to be "absorbed through the" gut and this is what damages arterial walls leading to coronary artery disease.[24]

How Not To Give Your Child Juvenile Diabetes, Leukemia, Lymphoma, or Multiple Sclerosis

Besides the obvious link to breast cancer noted above, cow's milk has also been singled out as one of the culprits responsible for the rising statistics in the United States of juvenile diabetes! Dr. R. M. Kradjian in a report at *www.notmilk.com*, says that researchers believe that during the "first year of life" infants produce "antibodies…against the milk protein" in cow's milk. Since the milk protein is very similar to the protein in the pancreas cells that produce insulin, those same antibodies that the child has made, attack the pancreas cells, resulting in juvenile or Type I diabetes![25] Do the facts support the theory? YES! Did you know that the biggest consumer of "dairy products" in the world is the country of Finland? "Finland" also has the **"world's highest rate of insulin dependent diabetes."** As Dr. Kradjian further notes, Finnish scientists followed "'142 Finnish children with newly diagnosed diabetes. They found that every one had at least eight times as many antibodies against the milk protein as did healthy children, clear evidence that the children had a raging autoimmune disorder.'"[26]

Burt Berkson, M.D., Ph.D., agrees that there are problems associated with milk and diabetes in his book *The Alpha Lipoic Acid Breakthrough*: "Fewer cases of type I and type II diabetes are reported in countries with low milk consumption…" He also notes that "Vegetarians who eat sensibly appear to be free from type II diabetes mellitus."[27] (Dr. Berkson recommends that anyone with diabetes avoid dairy products.) From what I have read, you should be avoiding them to PREVENT you from getting diabetes in the first place! Once you already have diabetes, is it then too late?

Still unconvinced that milk is not for children (or adults for that matter)? According to Gabe Mirkin, M.D., at *www.drmirkin.com*, "In Puerto Rico, almost all babies get cow's milk. In Cuba, almost all babies are breast fed. Puerto Rican babies are more than **10 times more likely to suffer juvenile diabetes," than babies in Cuba!** (Emphasis, mine.)[28] Now, it doesn't take a rocket scientist to add two and two together to get the big picture here, does it?

This is HUMAN babies we are discussing, not animal studies, however, Dr. Mirkin says that even animal testing bears this out! "Among animals bred to develop diabetes, infant animals given cow's milk have a much higher incidence of diabetes."[29] (Except of course, baby calves fed raw unprocessed, unpasteurized milk from their mother cow!)

Are you aware that the "bovine leukemia virus is found in more than three of five dairy cows in the United States? Dr. Kradijian explains that this involves about 90% of dairy herds." When "raw milk samples" were "randomly collected" and analyzed, "the bovine leukemia virus was recovered from two-thirds."[30] Do the statistics support that states having the highest incidence of leukemia in humans also have the highest incidence of bovine leukemia? YES! These states in the U.S. are "Iowa, Nebraska, South Dakota, Minnesota and Wisconsin." It is also true, says Dr. Kradijian, that "Dairy farmers have significantly elevated **leukemia** rates."[31]

Not only may cow's milk promote juvenile diabetes, but according to Dr. Russell Blaylock in his book, *Natural Strategies For Cancer Patients*, it has been shown to harbor a large "number of cancer viruses, primarily those responsible for leukemia and lymphoma, two of the most common diseases in cattle."[32] In the U.S. alone, says Dr. Blaylock, "approximately 60 percent of the herds examined were infected." Research has even shown a statistical "increase in the incidence of acute lymphoid leukemia" in populations where the herds "have a high incidence of infections."[33] Even though "pasteurization" is supposed to destroy many of these viruses, Dr. Blaylock emphasizes that the milk will still contain a large amount of "white blood cells," and it is these cells that "contain the viruses."[34] He even advises against mothers drinking milk while they are pregnant since they can transfer these viruses to their baby![35] (Ever wonder about the rising statistics of young children developing leukemia and lymphoma? Why are so many **very young children** coming down with leukemia and type I diabetes? I know of parents who have to give their one and two-year-olds insulin, and I have seen many children under five-years-old diagnosed with leukemia!

When researchers followed "1422 individuals…for 11 and a half years" in Norway, Dr. Kradjian says the results revealed that consumers of "2 or more glasses of milk per day had 3.5 times the incidence of cancer of the lymphatic organs. (British med. Journal 61:456-9, March 1990.")[36]

It isn't just diabetes, T.B., leukemia, and lymphoma that we need to be concerned about! As noted at The Food Web: *www.anarac.com/milk_and_dairy.htm,* giving your kids milk may also increase their risk for multiple sclerosis:

> An article in the April 2001 issue of the *Journal of Immunology*, written by a team of researchers…reported that, "Multiple sclerosis and juvenile diabetes may be different manifestations of the same disease." They also suggest that "a diet that includes cow's milk…may also increase the risk of developing MS for those genetically predisposed to that disease."[37]

For you moms-to-be out there, new research shows that getting adequate sunshine while you are pregnant (for vitamin D production in the skin), may be an added measure you can take to prevent your child from developing multiple sclerosis. [37a]

To Homogenize or Not to Homogenize

Besides killing pathogens (something it is supposed to do), homogenization and pasteurization of milk may have some very undesirable effects most of us are not aware of! A retired veterinarian, Earl D. Smith, D.V.M., tells what happened when he tried to use pasteurized and homogenized milk:

> I doctored horses and cattle for 25 years and then I did only the small animals...When the farmers kept a milk cow on the farm to feed the weaner calves, there were few digestive problems. But when no dairy cows were available they went to the local store and got "Store Bought" milk for the calves to drink. Soon the calves died with diarrhea. I thought milk was milk but I soon found out that the Pasteurized and Homogenized milk could not be digested by these calves. Homogenization broke the fat globule into such a small bit that it wouldn't curd in the stomach and passed directly into the small intestine where it created severe inflammation. I called it toxic enteritis.[38]

Dr. Smith explains how he countered this problem: "I learned to treat these cases with goat's milk which has the largest fat globule of any milk found on the farm. The calves made a quick recovery if the patient hadn't gotten too debilitated."[39]

Dr. Smith then goes on to explain what happened when he himself started drinking processed milk:

> I too drank a lot of milk when we milked cows on the farm. I never had any adverse effects from drinking a quart or more at one time. When I went on to college and I was using "store bought milk" I got so I drank very little milk and what I did drink reacted in my system like poison. I was told I was allergic to milk. Now 50 years later, a friend, who has a milk

cow out in the country, asked me if I could use some milk. I accepted and for three years now I can drink milk like I did when I lived on the farm. I have no adverse side effects. This milk is raw milk, also not Homogenized.[40]

Naturopathic physician, Dr. Robert Morse agrees with Dr. Smith. He writes in *The Detox Miracle Sourcebook*: "What happens to a baby calf if you feed it pasteurized milk instead of its fresh, raw mother's milk? It dies."[41] Ask yourself this question: **if pasteurized, homogenized milk KILLS BABY CALVES when they drink it, what in the world are we doing giving it to <u>our children</u> to drink?!**

The Mucus Myth

Dr. Robert Morse also attributes much of the upper respiratory ailments we suffer to dairy products, and he explains why:

> Colds, flu, mumps or any lymphatic respiratory condition can be largely attributed to congestion from dairy products. Dairy products are highly mucus-forming and constipating. When you have a cold or respiratory problem, where do you think that…mucus comes from? Or lymph node swelling, especially swelling of the tonsils?[42]

Are your kids plagued with constant ear infections, colds, sore throats, tonsillitis, and sinusitis? You may be able to rid them of these type problems forever, simply by taking them off milk and all dairy products! Dr. Don Colbert, M.D., in his book, *What You Don't Know May Be Killing You*, agrees that dairy products cause many of these ailments with children:

> Most children I see with chronic ear infections, chronic sinus infections and many other conditions have dairy sensitivities. I take these youngsters off dairy products and substitute soy or rice milk; many times the problems clear up.[43]

He also reminds us that "man is the only species in the animal kingdom to drink milk as an adult."[44] Also, cooking milk (heating it in the pasteurization, homogenization process) changes it from "alkaline to acidic...this can create stone formation, muscular weakness, GI tract inflammation, and other conditions."[45] Apparently, there is more to processed milk than *meets the eye!*

Pass Me the Hormones n' Cream, Please!

Dr. Gary Null believes that it is best to avoid dairy products completely if you want to cut your risk of disease. In his book *The Complete Encyclopedia of Natural Healing,* he explains another risk in drinking milk, one that women in particular should be concerned about: "Dairy products contain large amounts of estrogen." He believes this may account for the dramatic difference in breast cancer rates between U.S. women and those in Japan. Milk simply is NOT a major component of the diet in Japan. Not only that, but he says "a recent Environmental Protection Agency report on dioxin [which has been found in milk] concludes that common levels of exposure may threaten human health by causing cancer, as well as fetal, immune-related, and reproductive problems."[46]

See chapter 21: *Prescription HRT – The Great Tragedy of The 20th Century,* for more information on the many health problems estrogen is causing for women in this country (in the hormones given to cattle)!

Neither are excessive amounts of hormones healthy for men! Dairy products have been linked to prostate cancer! If you are wondering about the addition of hormones (found in cow's milk) consider this note in *The Milk Letter: A Message To My Patients,* from Dr. Robert M. Kradjian, M.D., at website *www.notmilk.com*: "Fifty years ago an average cow produced 2,000 pounds of milk per year. Today the top producers give 50,000 pounds! How was this accomplished? Drugs, antibiotics, hormones, forced feeding plans and specialized breeding; that's how."[47]

Mother's Milk

Everyone knows by now that breast feeding provides the best milk for human babies, however, if you are convinced that "mothers' milk is pure," guess again! Dr. Kradjian discussed a large study revealing that "human breast milk in over 14,000 women had contamination by pesticides." What was the source of this contamination? "Meat and— you guessed it—dairy products." Interestingly enough, a "subgroup" study of breast feeding moms who were "vegetarian" revealed 50% less "contamination" levels in their milk![48]

CHAPTER 26

ORTHOMOLECULAR MEDICINE, MACROBIOTICS, PROBIOTICS, MOLASSES, & SEED FOODS

"In one case where complete remission was achieved in myelogenous leukemia...the patient took 24-42 gms vitamin C per day...it is inconceivable that no one appears to have followed this up...without the scurvy, leukemia may be a relatively benign, non fatal condition. I wrote a paper...in an attempt to have the therapy clinically tested. I sent it to 3 cancer journals and 3 blood journals...it was refused by all...Two without even reading it."

—Irwin Stone, Ph.D.[1]

Orthomolecular Medicine

Orthomolecular Medicine uses megadose vitamin and nutrient combinations to heal the body. This type treatment is responsible for many complete cancer cures but is not given the publicity that it deserves! See chapter one in this book for more information about how the current cancer establishment has deliberately suppressed this valuable treatment. Many cancer patients are never informed about this safe, non-toxic alternative treatment for cancer!

Dr. Abram Hoffer, M.D., Ph.D., F.R.C.P.(C), and Linus Pauling, Ph.D., in their book *Healing Cancer – Complementary Vitamin & Drug Treatments,* describe Orthomolecular Medicine and give an excellent comparison between Orthomolecular Medicine and synthetic drugs:

> The practice of othromolecular medicine...recognizes that most acute and chronic diseases are due to a metabolic fault which is correctable in most patients by good nutrition, including the use of large doses of vitamins and mineral supplements. In sharp contrast, drugs are synthetics which are not naturally present in the body and for which the body does not have ready made mechanics for their destruction

and elimination. They are called xenobiotics – that is, foreign molecules.[1a]

I highly recommend Dr. Hoffer's books for anyone wishing to pursue Orthomolecular Medicine and/or complementary treatments. Dr. Hoffer has authored many books that deal with Orthomolecular Medicine, including: *Putting it All Together: The New Orthomolecular Nutrition; Orthomolecular Treatment for Schizophrenia;* and *Vitamin C & Cancer: Discovery, Recovery, Controversy,* and several others!

As for those who are against any type of complementary treatment, Dr. Hoffer has this to say:

> One of the main criticisms of complementary medicine (conventional plus orthomolecular) is that it denies or delays the use of standard treatment. I think that this argument is not based on fact for nearly every patient. In my experience, patients seeking complementary medicine have already been treated by conventional methods, usually unsuccessfully. Failures provide the main reservoir of patients seeking help outside the [conventional] medical profession. Even if it were true, there is little proof that for most cancers standard treatment prolongs life or even improves its quality.[2]

See chapter nine in this book for the case of a lung cancer patient who was cured with Orthomolecular Medicine. Also, see chapter eleven for the story of a patient completely cured of pancreatic cancer using this therapy, as well as chapter fifteen for information on a teenager who was miraculously cured of Hodgkins lymphoma with megadose vitamin C therapy! Be aware too, that megadose vitamin C therapy has been used successfully in curing polio, shingles, and other diseases! Also see Dr. Robert F. Cathcart's website at *www.orthomed.com* for his opinion on how vitamin C might be useful in treating other immune-threatening diseases!

Macrobiotics

The word "macrobiotic" means "long life." Dr. Ralph Moss in *Cancer Therapy* says that this diet was initially introduced to the Europeans and Americans by "George Ohsawa in the 1950s," however, "its best known proponent...has been Michio Kushi."[2a] Cancer and other diseases were basically blamed on the "typical Western diet," and macrobiotic followers believe "cancer, when it strikes, is a kind of" payback for errors that we make in our life style choices.[3] Many people with cancer have claimed that this diet cured them.

Lynn Keegan, Ph.D., R.N., in her book *Healing Nutrition*, explains that the diet itself is a combination of "low fat, high...complex carbohydrates and fiber, and nearly cholesterol free..."[4] The "goal" is "to eat foods that are more balanced within themselves and to one another." Those who follow the diet try to get food in "its most natural state: fresh, locally grown, when possible," what we would consider organically grown, Ms. Keegan says. The use of "dairy products and highly refined carbohydrates are discouraged."[5]

Macrobiotics is also based on Chinese philosophy and harmony within nature. The diet allows many natural grains, fresh vegetables, soups, tofu, certain fish, and some teas. Animal foods are not allowed in the diet, or at least extremely discouraged! Foods should be natural and organic as much as possible. Multiple websites have specifics on this particular diet and there are reams of books in health food stores on macrobiotics!

Gary Null, Ph.D., in *The Complete Encyclopedia of Natural Healing*, explains that advocates of macrobiotics claim that many terminal cancer patients following this diet have had "full recoveries."[6] This is understandable because of the many antioxidants provided by this diet. It is also low fat, and a low fat diet has been linked to lower levels of all cancers, however, they also believe that you should take fluids based on how thirsty you are, something I disagree with. By the time you are actually thirsty, you are probably already dehydrated at the cellular level.

Dr. Null also says that: "Best results with the macrobiotic diet are seen with endocrine-related cancers, such as cancer of the breast, prostate, pancreas, uterus, and ovaries."[7]

As a Christian, I do not support some of the philosophical tenets promoted by those who use macrobiotics, especially oriental astrology, or any type of astrology, for that matter! Just be aware that if you are a Christian, many promotions for oriental diets are steeped with mysticism, astrology, Buddhism and other "isms" that you should avoid!

Probiotics

You can eat the healthiest foods in the world, but if your intestines are sick and unable to digest and absorb the nutrients from that food, it will do you little good! As described by Dr. Joseph Mercola in "The Benefits of Probiotics 9/29/04," We humans are host to at least "100 trillion bacterial cells from at least 500 species, not including viruses and fungi.[8] These bacterias (probiotics) are referred to as 'friendly' bacteria and are responsible for several important biological functions."[9] These "friendly" bacteria should flourish in the intestines, unless they've been zapped with harmful enemies such as antibiotics and processed sugars! "Probiotics are defined as 'live microorganisms which, when administered in adequate amounts, confer a health benefit on the host,'" and, as explained by Dr. Mercola, having sufficient amounts of these "friendly" bacteria in the intestines, will help in the "prevention or control of" the following disorders (from his website *www.mercola.com,* with permission):

- Food and skin allergies in children
- Bacterial vaginosis
- Premature labor in pregnant women
- Inflammatory bowel disease
- Recurrent ear and bladder infections
- Chronic diarrhea[10]

Killing these vital organisms or keeping the body in a state that prevents their survival can create havoc in the human body! Just restoring the body's natural flora can bring about maximum health and wellness and banish disorders such as Crohn's disease, ulcerative colitis, and irritable bowel syndrome (IBS). Dr. Mercola has a wide variety of health products available at his website: *www.mercola.com.* His website also markets *Primal Defense™* probiotics.

A good example of someone who successfully overcame bowel disease is the case of Dr. Jordan Rubin of Palm Beach Gardens, Florida, author of the book *The Maker's Diet,* also discussed earlier in chapter five.

Dr. Rubin was diagnosed with Crohn's disease at age 19, and it nearly killed him. "For more than two years [he] experienced between twelve and 30 usually bloody bowel movements per day," sometimes during the night as well.[11] Dr. Rubin's weight rapidly declined from 180 pounds to a sickly 104. He was able to finally "regain his health by supplementing the small amount that he could eat with homeostatic soil organisms (HSOs™), which reversed the degenerative process of his Crohn's disease. The HSOs™ detoxified Jordan's intestinal tract, increased his ability to absorb nutrients from food, boosted his immune system..," and got him well.[12] These "friendly" organisms are "super probiotics (the opposite of **anti**biotics)." HSOs™ are in a new product Dr. Rubin was instrumental in developing known as Primal Defense™[13] He also developed a diet plan based on biblical principles from the Old Testament, described in his book, *The Maker's Diet.* However, before he was able to begin taking in nutrients, he had to restore the health of his colon. He did this with probiotics. Many probiotic supplements on the market will not survive the acid in the stomach. The HSOSs™ are supposed to be formulated to do so! You can order Primal Defense™ at some health food stores and internet sites, as well as Dr. Mercola's website discussed above! Once you have restored your colon health to enable you to digest and absorb the foods that you eat, you can keep the "friendly" bacteria healthy and happy by giving your body the foods that these "friendly" flora thrive on. A raw food alkaline diet, including green foods such as wheat grass juice, barley grass juice, chlorella and other nutrients promote colon health.

As further noted by Dr. Rubin in his book, *The Maker's Diet:*

Even human intestines – an environment most people consider pretty familiar – are home to perhaps 10,000 kinds of microbes....[Researchers are] now looking at how these largely unknown microbes might play a role in Crohn's disease...[14]

There are other nutrients and herbals that promote colon health. (See chapter five of this book for more information on Dr. Rubin's dietary program or see his book, *The Maker's Diet*).

Http://www.molocure.com, of Molo-Cure Research in Florida, developed *A.M.P. Molo-Cure®* "(Aloe Mucilaginous Polysaccharide), a...highly concentrated healing agent extracted from the aloe vera plant" that has shown effectiveness at healing those with intestinal disorders and other ailments. Aloe vera has long been popular as an aid in establishing and maintaining healthy intestinal flora. Be sure to discuss an aloe regimen with your physician.

Molasses

Molasses, particularly blackstrap molasses, is being mentioned here because it is one of the few sweeteners richer in nutrients than it is in calories, and because of its anti-cancer properties.

According to C. Scott and John Lust, Naturopath, in their book: *Crude Black Molasses, The Natural "Wonder Food"*, A physician known as "Dr. Forbes Ross drew attention to the value of Molasses in connection with cancer..." prior to WW I. It was he who noticed and "pointed out that workers on sugar-cane plantations who were constantly sucking the crude sugar, seldom if ever were known to suffer from that dread disease [cancer]." He believed that it was due to the high level of "potassium salts in unrefined sugar-cane," and he believed that cancer was primarily due to a potash deficiency.[15]

Authors Cyril Scott and John Lust also describe an account of "James Persson," over sixty years old, from "New Zealand," who was incapacitated with a bowel growth, heart disease, bronchial congestion, digestive problems, "pyorrhoea, sinus trouble and weak nerves."[16] He was also "losing weight, and his hair had turned white."[17] When he discovered that a neighbor of his, a Mr. S. had been sent home to die with a terminal colon cancer and cured himself completely by drinking crude black molasses, he decided do the same. "[N]ot only did the growth in his bowels disappear, together with all his other troubles…but his hair, which was white when he started the treatment, actually regained its original color."[18] The authors of the book also state that "numerous" other cases of cancer have been "cured solely by Molasses-therapy," including "growths of the uterus…breast…intestinal growth…[and] numerous cases of growths of the tongue, diagnosed as malignant."[18a] Another patient, a "Mrs. M.," had been diagnosed with "breast cancer" and "given two months to live." She began taking molasses and "the growth disappeared," with no relapses.[19]

It is recommend that molasses be taken "before meals…one tea-spoonful" dissolved in a few ounces of hot water, then add enough "cold water to equal a total of 2/3 cup. Drink it warm. For children, half the dosage." For those with "growths," not only is the molasses taken "during the day [but] last thing at night and on rising," as well.[20] There is night and day difference between processed white sugar and molasses! So much so, that processed white sugar is acid-forming, while crude black molasses is alkaline![21]

Besides being high in potassium, "Crude Blackstrap Molasses" is also high in several other minerals and vitamins.[22]

Seed Foods

Seed foods, according to Jean Carper in her book, *The Food Pharmacy*, are important because they contain substances called "protease inhibitors," which are antioxidants capable of passing through the digestive tract and coming out intact. One physician proved this by making them "radioactive" and tracing them through the colon in animals! They're also important because they "squelch the activity of proteases," some of which promote cancer," says Ms. Carper, hence the name *protease inhibitors.*[23] She also reports that "Dr. Walter Troll, professor of environmental medicine at New York University…" believes that these compounds "can slow down the very late stages of cancer progression" similar to the way that "chemotherapy does, but in a much more targeted, less toxic fash-ion."[24] Dr. Troll does not believe that they will help much once metas-tasis occurs, but if used before that, he believes they may stop cancer from ever spreading in the first place.[25]

It has also been proven that protease inhibitors "retard the growth of human breast and colon cancer cells." Researchers were unable to promote skin cancers in mice, even when they treated their skin with carcinogens, as long as they added "protease inhibitors" as well![26] Ms. Carper lists some excellent examples of foods that contain these cancer fighters: "...nuts...sweet potatoes...banana...spinach... pineapple [and] cereal grains," though she warns that cooking will destroy much of the "protease inhibitors in potatoes."[27]

CHAPTER 27

FLUSH THE BUGS!

"In September of '94, the following story appeared on TV: City Officials have discovered that a tiny parasite, cryptosporidium, has become immune to chlorine and has infested 50% of our drinking water. The eggs are so small that 33% slip through the testing process. The TV broadcast went on to say that many large cities are infested, specifically mentioning San Francisco, Milwaukee, and New York"

(Hanna Kroeger, from her book: *Parasites The Enemy Within*)[1]

If you still think that your tap water is safe to drink, and you do not believe that getting infested with this type parasite is very alarming, consider this: several victims of this parasite lost their kidneys and ended up on the kidney transplant waiting list after the organism attacked their kidneys.

Parasites & Cancer

If your immune system is sick, it will not be able to fight off parasites, yet there are some physicians who believe that cancer itself may be caused by parasites. Dr. Hulda R. Clark, Ph.D., N.D. is one of them. In her book, *The Cure For All Cancers,* she describes the parasite she believes is responsible for cancer:

> [A]ll cancers are alike. They are all caused by a parasite. A single parasite! It is the human intestinal fluke. And if you kill this parasite, the cancer stops immediately. The tissue becomes normal again. In order to get cancer, you must have this parasite.[2]

Now if you are a citizen of the United States or another industrialized country, you may have been brainwashed into believing that we don't get parasites in the developed nations. This isn't true. Do you own a pet? Do your children keep hamsters for pets? Mice? Guinea pigs? Parrots? Lizards? Cats? Dogs? If you own a pet, you probably have parasites, plain and simple. Even aquariums contain parasites. You can take your pet to the vet and get shots to fight parasites, but they never get ALL of them, especially if you have animals that run about outdoors (e.g. dogs and cats)! Even indoor cats scratch around in litter boxes that are full of parasites. Raw food, such as uncooked meat is full of parasites! If those fresh vegetables you are eating have been fertilized with cow manure, and they have not been thoroughly cleaned, they will be full of parasites! Soft cheeses and processed lunchmeats can also become infected with parasites. If you are eating at a fancy restaurant, the food you eat is only as "safe" as those who are preparing it! If the workers are not washing their hands often, especially after bathroom trips, they could be serving you parasites with that dinner dish! And don't think you are any "safer" dining at a fancy restaurant as opposed to a fast food burger joint! Anytime you eat out, you may want to carry a few capsules of milk thistle and cinnamon to swallow along with the meal, as well as 3-4 fresh cloves to chew on! This will help, but may not give you a full jump on some nasty bug that you ingest along the way, depending on what it is and how many there are!

Have you or a loved one ever been hospitalized for an ailment such as dehydration from diarrhea? A very common lab test your physician will order is called a test for "O & P", which stands for *Ova and Parasites!* When your physician orders this test, **he or she is checking you for worms and their eggs!**

According to Dr. Hulda Clark, the intestinal fluke does not cause cancer in the intestines, but if it travels, for example to another organ, like the liver and "establishes itself" there, it will "cause cancer!" As long as it just stays in the intestines, you may end up with an intestinal disorder such as "colitis, Crohn's disease, or irritable bowel syndrome," or you may be unaffected.[3]

Dr. Hulda Clark also links many of our health issues, such as arthritis, cancer, and auto-immune diseases to the metal dentistry that we allow in our mouths. Have you ever noticed that when you have a mercury filling removed from your mouth, your dentist will put it in a "hazardous" material waste box, yet tell you that when it is inside your mouth, not to worry, that it won't harm you? This does not make sense, because all polymers and metals eventually deteriorate and begin seeping; dental ingredients and appliances are no exception! Not only that, but clostridium bacteria thrives in dental fillings and caps.[4] If you don't believe this, the next time a cap comes loose from a tooth and you take it back to have it replaced, before you do, have the black stuff that has formed on the top of it cultured at a local laboratory! It will most likely be swarming with clostridium bacteria!

Because of all the dangerous chemicals that can leach into our bodies from plastic and metal dental fillings and teeth, Dr. Clark believes we are giving ourselves diseases like cancer due to the way that these chemicals suppress our immune system. She suggests that "If you are in a wheelchair without a very reliable diagnosis, have all the metal containing teeth removed from your mouth."[5]

If you are interested in the dangers of metal in dentistry, a very good book on the subject is by Dr. Frank J. Jerome, D.D.S., *Tooth Truth – If You Want to be Healthy Don't Metal With Your Mouth.* Other good books are: *Root Canal Cover-up* by George E. Meinig; *Elements of Danger: Protect Yourself Against the Hazards of Modern Dentistry*, by Morton Walker; and *Dentistry Without Mercury*, by Sam Ziff and Michael F. Ziff, D.D.S. If you ask your dentist NOT to put a mercury (silver amalgam) filling in your mouth, he or she will give you the usual spiel about how it is perfectly safe and harmless, exactly what the dentistry profession has been telling us for years! There are some dentists, however, who are speaking out and telling the truth about these hazards!

According to Sam Ziff and Michael F. Ziff, D.D.S. in *Dentistry Without Mercury,* it takes very little mercury to make you seriously ill:

> Scientific research has already demonstrated that mercury, even in small amounts, can damage the brain, heart, lungs, liver, kidneys, thyroid gland, pituitary gland, adrenal glands, blood cells, enzymes and hormones, and suppresses the body's immune (defense) system.[6]

These dentists have a survey that was done showing 221 patients who had all their mercury fillings removed, and as a result, the majority of them were cured of allergies, blood pressure problems, fatigue, migraines, multiple sclerosis, insomnia, memory loss, skin disorders, and thyroid problems, to name a few![7] Even Alzheimer's has been linked to mercury fillings! A word of caution though! If you decide to have all your metal fillings removed, if not done properly, it can cause you more harm than good!

Dr. Hulda Clark not only blames parasites on dentistry metal (as well as pets), but isopropyl alcohol as well. She recommends that once you rid yourself of parasites, stay away from isopropyl alcohol, because once it gets into the body, it enables flukes to multiply in some people. She also recommends getting all toxic chemicals, cleaners, etc, out of your home environment; very good advice, because we are often inundated with toxins simply in the everyday cleaners, shampoos, soaps, sprays and even toothpastes that we use! Each item alone, may have little affect on your health, but if your immune system is already compromised, the combination of all of them can be overwhelming!

Getting Rid of the Bugs

Dr. Hulda Clark, Ph.D., N. D., recommends three main items (taken in combination) in her de-parasitization program: *"Cloves, black walnut, and wormwood."*[8] All of these items can be obtained at local health food stores (and at various websites), but she says that you must be sure in purchasing black walnut hull tincture that it is still pale GREEN. Once it turns from green to black, it has lost its effectiveness.[9] She provides instructions in her books for making your own tincture if you happen to have a black walnut tree in your back yard. Dr. Clark has an information website at *www.drclark.net*. She has clinics in California and Mexico. I have heard much criticism as well as much praise about her cancer treatments. She has certainly been controversial, to say the least. She lists many testimonials of cancer cures at her website above, as well as many professionals that also use her therapy or parts of her therapy, that you can read and judge for yourself. She also uses an electrical frequency generator device that she says can eliminate pathogens.

Wormwood comes from the artemisinin herb and has been discussed in chapter 18 of this book for its effectiveness at fighting cancer, especially breast cancer. If cancer can be caused by parasites as Dr. Clark believes, this would account for artemisinin's effectiveness. It isn't unusual for parasites to be found in tumors that have been removed from patients. Dr. Clark has an 18 day program for taking the clove, wormwood and walnut hull. The "Parasite Cleanse Handy Chart" showing exactly how to combine these 3 ingredients can be found on her website at *www.drclark.net/info/p_chart.htm*, as well as on page 23 in her book *The Cure for All Cancers*. Be sure if you are using cloves, they are freshly ground, or they will not work at killing parasites. Once the cloves are ground up, the compounds released kill the parasites. In order for the wormwood, cloves and walnut hull to be effective, Dr. Clark says that they must be taken together.[10]

Where Do All Those Bugs Come From?

There are many reasons for the increase in parasite infestation in the U.S; a few of which are pointed out by Ann Louise Gittleman, M.S. in her book *Natural Healing For Parasites:*

> The rise in international travel [we are going overseas to many "remote" areas and bringing parasites back with us.]...Contaminated water...Day-care centers...Immigrants [Some are bringing parasites from their former countries with them]...Exotic foods...Household pets...Antibiotic use...Changes in sexual partners...[and the] Spread of AIDS[11]

To help get rid of parasites and "sweep" them out of the digestive tract, Ms. Gittleman recommends using items such as "psyllium husks, agar-agar, flax seeds...beet root...citrus pectin and papaya extract."[12] Also, in order to kill parasites and keep them from coming back, there are many natural substances that she recommends:

> Fresh pineapple and papaya...the seeds from papaya, pumpkin and lemon...eat one handful of raw or roasted [pumpkin] seeds...twice a day for one week...Repeat in two

weeks...Lemon seeds should be crushed and taken with honey once a day for five days....[repeat] in two weeks...[13]

(Remember that honey and honey products should never be given to children under two years of age. Some physicians set this restriction to those one-year-old and younger.)

Other natural "foods that have anti-parasitic properties, according to Ms. Gittleman are: "onions, carrot tops, radish roots, kelp, raw cabbage, ground almonds, blackberries, pumpkin, sauerkraut, and fig extract."[14]

There are also many herbs and herbal teas that kill worms and parasites. One example described by *herbs2000.com* is *"Aspilia (Aspilia mossambicenisis")*, also known as "Wild Sunflower." Not only does this herb kill parasites, but it acts much like an "antibiotic." It has been shown to destroy cancerous cells in "solid tumors," especially those of the "lung and breast."[15]

There are many other herbs, nutrients, and spices too numerous to mention that have parasite-killing abilities. A few of these are: cinnamon, pomegranate juice, honey, grape juice, cayenne pepper, wild oregano oil, ginger, curcumin, parsley, barberry, buckthorn, cajueiro, gentian, horseradish, cascara sagrada, slippery elm, violet, marshmallow, golden seal, dandelion, catnip, chickweed, coptis, pau d'arco, quassia, sage, swedish bitters, glutamine, myrrh, and grapefruit seed extract. (Grapefruit seed extract is so potent at killing pathogens that some hospitals use it to keep infectious organisms out of their respirator equipment.) You can find GSE at health food stores.

A T.V. program announced not long ago that "a homoelytic parasite (blood parasite) was found in all cancer patients. It was so tiny, the announcer said, that many hundreds could live in a drop of blood." According to Hanna Kroeger, Ph.D., N.D., an excellent way to fight such parasites is with "Calmyra figs." Apparently these figs contain within "their skins and kernals a substance which rips the skin of worms."[16] Most health food stores sell organic Calymyra figs.

Remember that if you keep your immune system healthy, it will destroy invading parasites in your body before they can ever start multiplying in the first place!

CHAPTER 28

BEE POLLEN, PROPOLIS, HONEY, & ROYAL JELLY

"While pure honey is a potent vitamin-mineral food, it is pollen that is preferred by researchers as a means of health building and cancer fighting because it contains a high concentration of valuable nutrients and substances not found in honey. Pollen appears to be a miracle food in the battle against cancer."

(Carlson Wade, from his book:
Carlson Wade's New Fact/Book on Bee Pollen and Your Health.)[1]

Be advised that if you have severe allergies, are an asthma sufferer, or have other chronic illnesses, consult with your physician about using honey, bee pollen, propolis, or related products. There are rare cases of individuals who have had severe reactions to these products. Never give them to children under two. If giving to older children, consult with their physician for advice on dosages beforehand, especially if they have asthma, allergies, or other respiratory ailments. Do not take bee pollen supplements if you are allergic to bee stings.

Bee Pollen

Bee pollen, as well as honey, has been used as a medicinal for thousands of years by nearly every civilization on the earth, yet not until modern times are scientists discovering exactly why these ingredients are packed with so much healing power.

The pollen bees gather actually comes from the "male element of a flower," which they accumulate in near "microscopic amounts and bring it into the hive for food." The insects will gather only the best for their hives, passing up inferior "pollen."[2] (See precautions earlier regarding those who are allergic to bee stings.)

Human testing using bee pollen has brought some amazing results. Some health problems that were found very responsive to bee pollen, often when other remedies failed, were "chronic constipation...colonic infections...[and] chronic diarrhea." If you have allergies or asthma, note that there is daylight and darkness between the pollen you inhale that is irritating and the bee pollen collected by bees.[2a] Bee pollen has actually been used to strengthen the "respiratory" system, "heal and even prevent allergies. By taking one teaspoon of bee pollen daily, resistance to wind-carried pollen is slowly built up and the sensitivity to allergy is reduced."[2b] The property of bee pollen to be able to "immunize the body against allergies," was noted several years ago in the "*Florida Farmers Bulletin* (October 15, 1969)," from the article: "Doctors Recommend Raw Honey Treatment for Allergies."[3] The popularity of bee pollen has since grown, as well as raw honey.

Dr. Mark Stengler, N.D., author of *The Natural Physician's Healing Therapies,* admits that though he had been able to help his own allergy-suffering patients, when he developed severe allergy problems himself one spring, nothing worked for him. When some of his "colleagues, and even a number of patients," told him that they had been relieved or even cured of "their allergies" with bee pollen, he started taking "8 capsules daily." He explained that "by the sixth day," he was nearly free of most of his "hay fever symptoms."[3a] He continued to take the pollen, reducing the dosage. Later, he states that "the hay fever was gone for good." He does not, however, recommend bee pollen for anyone allergic to bee stings. He recommends that you start slowly, placing a very "small amount of the powder on your tongue," and if any type of allergic reactions occur – "such as wheezing or a rash – don't take any more." The usual dosage is "2 capsules daily (equivalent to 500 to 1,000 milligrams)."[4]

As described by Jean Carper in *Miracle Cures*, it took many years of taking antihistamines before "Senator Tom Harkin, Democrat of Iowa," found a better treatment for his hay fever. After a friend suggested "a bee pollen-herb tablet called Aller-Be-Gone," he began taking the supplement, which he said "cured my allergies. It's a miracle. It's the best thing I've ever seen."[5] (I have seen this product on the internet spelled *Aller-Bee-Gone*.)

The power of bee pollen in cancer prevention isn't new. As explained by Carlson Wade, it was known at the turn of the last century. An article in the "*Journal of the National Cancer Institute,* October 1948," described an animal study where "bee pollen" was given to "test animals bred to develop tumors." The scientists were surprised to learn that the bee pollen "could delay and control the appearance of cancerous tumors."[6]

Scientific studies on lab animals given "standardized pollen extract [revealed that] mice with lung carcinomas survived almost twice as long" as those not given the bee pollen.[6a] C. Leigh Broadhurst, Ph.D., in *Health and Healing with Bee Products*, explains that it was believed that the pollen worked by boosting the "immune system." Bee pollen has also been shown to prevent liver injury, and to "reduce pain, inflammation and the risk of prostate cancer."[7] According to Carlson Wade, there are many medical reports of patients not responding to antibiotics for "prostatitis" being helped with bee pollen supplements! Dosages are usually about "six tablets" per day of bee pollen.[8] (See precautions given earlier in this chapter.)

Carlson Wade also describes bee pollen as the "perfect food." This is because it is a "complete food" containing "every nutrient required to sustain life in addition to substances added by the bees..." Researchers have determined "that a person can live indefinitely on a diet consisting of Bee Pollen and water alone...without the least sign of distress."[9]

In her book, *Bee Pollen Royal Jelly Propolis and Honey*, Rita Elkins, M.H., says that honey may even prove to be a new weapon in the fight against ulcers caused by H. Pylori bacteria. Laboratory research showed that honey outperformed "several other antimicrobial agents."[10] It is actually sweeter than sugar and a healthy alternative. The best honey is organic honey found at health food stores.[11] Be sure you check with your physician about using bee products, especially if you have allergies and/or diabetes. Diabetics can not safely consume large amounts of honey or royal jelly.

In an article from *Reuter's Health Information* by Amy Norton, researchers are also discovering that it isn't necessarily just bee pollen that inhibits cancer. Testing in "Croatia" showed that "bee products ranging from sting venom to sweet honey were able to prevent tumors in mice from growing and spreading, and in some cases even shrunk the tumors."[12] Ms. Norton explains that scientists "led by Nada Orsolic of the University of Zagreb tested...honey, propolis, royal jelly, bee venom and caffeic acid – an antioxidant found in propolis –

on tumor cells implanted in mice," and they discovered that all of the bee products had "some anti-tumor effects, depending on the route and timing of the dose:"

> [P]ropolis and caffeic acid, both given orally, appeared to slow tumor progression, while oral honey impeded tumors from spreading to other sites in the animals' bodies – but only when given before the tumor cells were implanted...bee venom was able to shrink tumors when it was injected directly into them. Three of the seven animals given bee venom showed a complete remission, according to Orsolic's team.[13]

In *Health and Healing with Bee Products,* C. Leigh Broadhurst, Ph.D., says that the "caffeic acid" in propolis (in lab studies) "strongly inhibited the growth of skin and colon cancers in cell cultures...[The] Phytochemicals [in propolis] are thought to prevent cancer development because of their antioxidant, detoxifying and antimutagenic activities."[14] (Recall that in chapter two, caffeic acid is also found in grapes!)

Be certain that you **never** give honey or other bee products to babies and children under two years of age. Always check with their physician! There are spores in honey that can cause deadly botulism in very young children due to their immature digestive systems.

Royal Jelly

Royal jelly is an enigma to researchers who find it "extremely difficult...to completely breakdown its components or to synthesize its compounds" due to its complexity, and it certainly can not be duplicated! So says Rita Elkins, M.H. in *Bee Pollen Royal Jelly Propolis and Honey.* Although honey, if stored in a sealed container, will not spoil, royal jelly will spoil. Mixing it with honey will preserve it.[15] A prominent "endocrinologist and specialist in live-cell therapy...Dr. Paul Niehans...concluded that royal jelly vitalized the glandular system," much like "an injection of fresh endocrine cells" would do.[16]

Propolis

Ms. Elkins calls propolis (another bee product, rich in bioflavonoids) "Nature's Penicillin" because it is a "natural antibiotic," so much so, that the "only insect to have been found free of bacteria" is the bee, because of the "antibiotic action of Propolis."[16a] Bees "use Propolis to protect the hive from contamination," probably one reason why it is sometimes effective at fighting bacteria that has become resistant to mainstream antibiotics, yet without the side effects that antibiotics often bring with them![17]

In *Health and Healing with Bee Products*, C. Leigh Broadhurst, Ph.D., reports that propolis comes mainly from "resins exuded from leaf buds and the bark of certain trees."[17a] Honeybees collect these resins and use them as a sort of "putty for sealing cracks and openings in the hive and to strengthen and repair honeycombs," as well as to "mummify" insects that have been killed trying to invade their hive, says Broadhurst. When used "topically," propolis has powerful healing properties.[18] It is such a powerful anti-inflammatory, Broadhurst further explains that it is often effective in the treatment of "arthritis, boils, acne, asthma, dermatitis, ulcers...inflammatory bowel diseases such as Crohn's disease, irritable bowel and chronic diverticulitis...." A "more severe inflammation" may require as much as "six to ten capsules of propolis per day..."[19]

Propolis has demonstrated anti-cancer effects, possibly due to its content of caffeic acid. In **human studies**, "cancer patients" in "Romania" were given propolis, which caused them to go into remission! Another recent study suggested that propolis may inhibit colon cancers.[20] Be sure that in purchasing propolis, you do so from a reliable health food provider to ensure that you are getting a pure product!

Honey

Honey is also effective at killing bacteria and is often used for packing wounds just for this purpose. As explained by Jean Carper in *The Food Pharmacy*, honey will relieve asthma and diarrhea, and it is often combined with "lemon juice or vinegar" for "cough syrup." Ms. Carper tells of a surgeon in Great Britain who appalled his fellow physicians when he admitted to them that he "regularly used honey on open wounds after vulvectomies (cancer surgery)." He explained to them that the wounds healed quicker with "less bacterial colonization than wounds treated with ordinary antibiotics." His fellow physicians were amazed when they did an experiment using honey in "test tubes against a wide range of infectious organisms..." Every one [of the pathogens]...without exception, was destroyed by the honey.[21]

Ms. Carper further describes an experiment "at the University of Natal, Durban, South Africa," which proved honey's effectiveness against gastroenteritis. Half the children with "acute gastroenteritis" were given "fluids with sugar and another group fluids with honey." Those children with the "*bacteria-caused* diarrhea," receiving the honey, "recovered forty percent faster."[22]

Manuka Honey

A very potent honey as far as bacteria-killing ability is the honey made from the pollen of flowers that are found on the manuka plant. Honey that comes from the pollen of this plant (which grows prolifically in New Zealand) has the capacity to kill deadly staphylococcus aureus germs (and many other pathogens) and is becoming a popular treatment for diabetic sores and leg ulcers. Many health food stores carry manuka honey.

CHAPTER 29

ALKALIZE & STAY THAT WAY!

"No matter how you got there, or how deep you're in it, a healthy, plant-based diet and low-stress lifestyle will keep you in acid/base balance and housing only helpful microforms. Eating the right kind of foods is the single most important thing you can do for yourself and your health."
(Robert O. Young, Ph.D., and Shelley Redford Young,
from *The PH Miracle*, Copyright © 2002 by Robert Young, Ph.D.,
By Permission of Warner Books, Inc.)[1]

Alkaline is Best

Undoubtedly, the reason that the organic raw foods diet is so successful at cancer prevention and cures is because it keeps the body in a state of correct acid base balance, on the side of alkalinity. If you've ever owned a fish aquarium, you know that once the water gets acid, the fish sicken and die unless you change it periodically to maintain its alkalinity! We humans can not tolerate an acid system in our body either. Most chronic, degenerative diseases and even cancer can be traced to a body that has high levels of toxic acid. Cooking foods increases their acidity. If you eat a diet primarily of cooked meats and few vegetables, your body's acidity will increase as the foods are digested. This may account for the fact that cancer is much less seen in vegetarians than it is in meat eaters. In their raw state **most foods** are more alkaline than they are acidic, thus eating a raw food diet will help keep your body in an alkaline state, which is optimum for health. Worms, parasites, bacteria, molds, and fungi are more apt to attack and take up residence in a body that is highly acidic, rather than alkaline. This is another reason I believe that the high carb diet is not healthy. Its emphasis on meat and other high proteins keeps the body in an acid state. This is why adherents to this diet, check their urine for acidity levels. According to the diet, if the urine is acidic, you are burning fat, however you are also losing valuable calcium from your bones (as well as other minerals) in the process. When your blood is acidic, the body tries to balance it out the best way it knows how and that is to rob your bones of calcium. The calcium raises the pH! But remember this – the body does not care WHERE it takes the calcium from in order to raise the pH of the blood. It will steal it from anywhere it can get it! Other minerals that your body will rob to alkalize the blood are potassium, magnesium and sodium.

What Causes Excess Acidity?

According to Dr. Theordore A. Baroody, N.D., D.C., Ph.D, C.N.C., in his book *Alkalize or Die*, foods have different minerals in them that, once they are "metabolized" by the body, either "throw off alkaline or acid residues in the urine."[1a] Generally, foods that contain "Calcium, Magnesium, Sodium, Potassium, Iron, and Manganese" are "alkaline-forming," because when passing through the body, "they bind acid toxins and leave alkaline-forming ash in the urine." Foods that are high in "Phosphorus, Sulphur, Chlorine, Iodine, Bromine, Flourine, Copper, and Silicon," normally produce acidic "residue."[2]

Dr. Baroody further explains that "From the standpoint of pure energy, pH is the measurement of electrical resistance between negative and positive ions in the body," or "how much the negative ions…and positive ions…push against one another." A healthy saliva and urine of 6.4 is "best for human body function."[3] The pH scale goes from 0 to 14. Seven is neutral. If your blood pH is below seven, you are on the acid side. If it is above seven, you are alkaline.

If you have **blood** drawn by your physician, they like to see a serum pH of 7.35 - 7.45. When your pH starts dropping, your oxygen levels also decrease. This is why your physician may start you on oxygen if you are in the hospital and your lab tests show an acid blood pH that has dropped drastically. He or she will also be doing other diagnostics to determine the cause. Sometimes the cause is quite obvious, for example, someone having an asthma attack with wheezing and difficulty breathing will very rapidly develop dangerous blood acidity.

Once your blood is overloaded with too much acid, it begins dumping the "excess acid…into the tissues for storage," and it often ends up right back "in the blood, creating a vicious cycle of drawing out still more basic minerals…stressing the liver and kidneys" as well.[4] This whole process is described by Robert Young, Ph.D., and Shelley Young in their book, *The pH Miracle Balance Your Diet, Reclaim Your Health.* Unfortunately, the end result leads to many chronic disorders, such as the pain of arthritis from the "irritation and inflammation" due to acid build-up in the joints and tissues. It also invites other conditions such as candida infections, fungus, parasites, and worms (as noted earlier).[5] (Another reason that a vegetarian diet is better for the joints!)

In order to keep your body in a healthy state that "sustains your alkaline reserves," Dr. Baroody suggests that you "follow the rule of 80/20 – which means to eat 80% of your foods from the alkaline-forming list and 20% from the acid-forming list."[6] On an acid/alkaline scale, the higher the number, the more alkaline, the lower the number, the more acidic. For example "dried figs (7.0)…grapes (6.0)…all varieties of melons (7.0-7.5)…papaya (7.0)…endive (6.5)… Kelp (7.0)…[and] asparagus (6.5)," are all very alkaline-forming foods (provided they are not cooked of course! Once they are cooked, they become more acidic!) "Cranberries (3.0)…basmati rice (2.5)…white rice (1.5)…lentils (3.0)…corn (2.0) …[and] pumpkin (3.0)," are acid-forming foods.[7] There are many nutrition books on the market that list the pH values of foods. Dr. Baroody provides such a list in his book *Alkalize or Die,* as do Robert Young and Shelley Redford Young in *The pH Miracle.*

If you keep your body in an optimal state of alkalinity, you are much less likely to get cancer and chronic, degenerative diseases. There have been many cases of people curing their cancer by **reversing their body** from acidic to alkaline. Many have done this simply by changing their diet! This is what happened with Eydie Mae Hunsberger, Eric Gardiner, Rev. George Malkmus and others discussed in this book who were able to cure their cancers by a change in diet and life style. Remember too, that it is not only food that determines your body's pH state. Stress will increase the acidity of your body. It is also possible to become much too alkaline, which is just as dangerous as high acidity, but this is very rare in our nation of fast-food addicts!

How Raising pH Cured a Stage III Bladder Cancer!

In *The pH Miracle*, Dr. Robert Young and Shelley Young related the story of a bladder cancer patient diagnosed with "Stage III" (possibly "Stage IV") bladder cancer, who cured his cancer by reversing his body's acidity. The malignant bladder tumor had already "blocked one of Pete's "ureters."[8] After he underwent "two months of chemotherapy," **without any change in the tumor**, his physicians recommended complete surgical removal of his bladder. Pete came to see Dr. Young, who found his blood to be highly acidic, which Pete says came "from years of eating garbage and ignoring my health." He refused the surgery and completely changed his diet, beginning with a "ten-day fast, with vegetable juices and soups."[9] A mere "three months into the program, there was no sign of any cancer spread." Pete's physicians still wanted to do the radical bladder removal, however, diagnostic testing revealed that the tumor had shrunk dramatically and "was suspended on a stalk to the bladder wall, no longer fully attached."[10] His ureter was no longer blocked by the tumor. All of the remaining tumor (what was left of it) was removed with a minor surgical procedure that left all of his organs intact! Furthermore, all diagnostic testing showed no further traces of bladder cancer. Even after all this, Pete was amazed that his physician still wanted to completely remove his bladder! Of course, he refused.[11] (I am sure that Pete's physician simply wanted to be on the safe side in removing the bladder, however, it is very typical of some surgeons to want to remove entire organs in situations where only the surgeon benefits, certainly not the patient!)

This may seem contrary, but it is possible for highly acidic foods to have "a very alkaline effect on the body." Harald Tietze explains why in his book *Paypaya The Healing Fruit*. He says that a good example is limes, which are "extremely acid with a pH reading of 1.9, but this fruit increases the alkalinity of the body." Not only is it important to know which foods are alkaline and acid-forming, but also to know how the body reacts to certain foods.[12] (The best way to stay alkaline is with raw foods and juicing!)

Keeping your body in a state of alkalinity will increase oxygen at the cellular level. Website *www.cancer-healing.com* explains why:

a solution that is mildly alkaline "can absorb over 100 times as much oxygen as a mild acid."[13] This is why oxygen is "driven out of the body" when acidity increases! "According to Nobel Prize winner, Otto Warburg," keeping the body in an acid level increases the likelihood of cancer![14] (This information is discussed in chapter 23 of this book, including oxygen treatments that are being given to cancer patients to increase oxygenation at the cellular level.) Also, see chapter 22 on water drinking! Remember that water is mostly composed of OXYGEN. When you rob your body of water, you are cutting off a major oxygen supply for your cells!

The reason a vegetarian diet promotes alkalinity is because most raw vegetables and fruits are alkaline and alkaline-forming, with a few exceptions. All MEATS, including RAW meats are acidic with **NO exceptions**!

Juice-fasting

One of the best ways to restore your body's proper alkalinity is with a juice-fast. While fasting is discussed in chapter 34 in greater detail, juice-fasting is being mentioned here simply because it is so important in establishing alkalinity and detoxifying the body. Dr. Don Colbert in his book, *Toxic Relief,* agrees and explains that even though a total fast (water only) will detoxify the body, a juice-fast "can be even more beneficial, and it is far less strenuous, since it supports detoxification, alkalinizes the body and supports the liver," plus, juice-fasting will usually maintain your energy level, something water-fasting will not do.[15] (Also see chapter two for more information on the grape juice diet, which brings the body into alkalinity and is very detoxifying!) Remember too, that with any type of fasting, your body still needs WATER! I never recommend a total fast where even water is not permitted. You should never go for days without water, a total fast is dangerous!

CHAPTER 30

SPICES TO SAVE YOUR LIFE

"We have a multi-billion dollar industry that is killing people, right and left, just for financial gain. Their idea of research is to see whether two doses of this poison is better than three doses of that poison."
—Glen Warner, M.D. oncologist. [Speaking of chemotherapy][1]

There are many spices that fight cancer. Several of them, such as turmeric, garlic, cloves, and cayenne pepper have already been discussed in this book. Some herbs are what we consider our most popular seasonings and spices. Those discussed here are high in antioxidants that help boost immunity to fight cancer and other illnesses and disease.

Basil

According to Selene Yeager in the *Doctors Book of FOOD REMEDIES*, there are several compounds in basil that are responsible for its ability to, not only "calm your stomach," but lower your risk of developing cancer as well! Animal testing revealed that increasing amounts of basil in the diet, raises enzymes in the body that have the capacity to neutralize substances known to cause cancer. Basil also contains "eugenol," which alleviates painful "muscle spasms."[2]

Cinnamon

This is one spice that doesn't just enhance the flavor of food. It may one day save your life! Studies have shown that it functions as a food preservative as well as a tasty additive to many dishes and treats! In one experiment done by "Kansas Sate University microbiologists," when testing various ingredients for their effectiveness in killing "one of the most virulent bacterial causes of food poisoning, E.coli type

0157," they discovered something truly amazing, as described at the New Agriculturist website *www.new-agri.co.uk/02*:

> The Kansas researchers found that cinnamon added to apple juice that had been contaminated with E.coli, was able to kill 99.5% of the bacteria within three days, at room temperature. They also did tests on meat and sausage, and found that cinnamon, cloves and garlic all had a powerful ability to stop the growth of bacteria. Other microbiologists in Tennessee have found that oils extracted from oregano, coriander and basil, also have strong anti-microbial properties.[3]

What does all this mean? The next time you and your family eat out and you are concerned about getting food poisoning (and well you should be), it might behoove you to take a small spice jar with some cinnamon (or garlic, or cloves) with you to add a bit to your food! (Cinnamon also has some capacity to lower blood sugar.) You may also want to include a milk thistle capsule! (Unless you have ulcers.)

Cloves

When cloves are ground up, the substance that is released from them is powerful at killing worms and parasites, as discussed in chapter 27. However, the most important role of this spice may not be in its ability to kill dangerous vermin, but its role in neutralizing the effects of asbestos. An "extract from cloves *(Eugenio caryophyllata),* eugenol, may provide an answer to the hazards posed by asbestos." Asbestos was commonly used as "a fireproof material in buildings, until it was discovered that the mineral's fibres, (sic) when inhaled, caused lung cancer."[3a] Website *www.new-agri.co.uk* explains that "Italian chemists" found that "when this clove extract comes in contact with asbestos, it hardens into a polymer, trapping the fibres, (sic) and potentially making the asbestos 'safe'…Good news for asbestos removers."[4] The chemists were mainly looking at whether or not coating asbestos fibers in the extract might make it safe so that it could be left in buildings.

Ginger & Willow Bark

Ginger is a very healing, protective herb with many advantageous properties including "Analgesic [and] Anti-diabetic." It also prevents blood clots, inhibits ulcers, supports the body's immunity, kills pathogens, and suppresses tumor formation.[5] It is such a powerful anti-inflammatory that Paul Schulick, in his book, *Ginger Common Spice & Wonder Drug,* describes the account of a "rheumatoid arthritis" patient who began consuming "fifty grams of fresh ginger daily after light cooking along with vegetables and various meats" for a period of "30 days." The patient was "50 years old." After following the above ginger regimen for 3 months, he "was completely free of pain, inflammation or swelling. He has continued to perform his job as auto mechanic without any relapses of arthritis for the last 10 years," as reported by "Dr. K. C. Srivastava, Danish Researcher."[6] (I have also known people to use fresh ginger successfully for their migraine headaches.)

Mr. Schulick also notes the failure of "Modern medicine [in] treating arthritis, the nation's primary crippler..." He explains that ginger offers tremendous hope to these individuals. "In two clinical trials conducted in Denmark, ginger actually reversed many of the subjects' arthritic symptoms and did so without side effects."[7] (These were HUMAN trials!) Many other clinical trials have been done showing ginger to be superior to aspirin and NSAIDS as an anti-inflammatory. According to Dr. K.C. Srivastava:

> Ginger produced better relief of pain, swelling and stiffness than the administration of NSAIDS...Some of our (arthritis) patients have observed added benefits on taking Ginger, and they include relief in cold sores...fewer colds....[and] Amelioration of stomach irritation and constipation.[8]

Mr. Schulick also reports that ginger has apparent anti-cancer effects due to its immune-boosting power. When lab animals "with Dalton's lymphoma and Ehrlich ascites tumors" were fed ginger, the spice "extended" their "lifespan...by 11 percent."[8a] Ginger also prevents dangerous clots by the "inhibition of platelet aggregation...platelets release growth factors that enhance tumor cell growth," and ginger inhibits "this process." By doing so, it may "actually help to prevent the spread of cancer."[9]

Ginger also has the power to protect the digestive tract from ulcers, hardly good news for the pharmaceutical giants, when you consider that ("for 1992"), "three of the twenty top-selling drugs in the U.S., Zantac, Tagamet and Pepcid..." exceeded "sales of $2.8 billion annually." As Mr. Schulick concludes from all this, "It is easy to understand why these drug companies would prefer the benefits of ginger to remain in the books or databases."[10]

One of the many components (out of hundreds) in ginger is geraniol. Geraniol is found not only in ginger, but rosemary as well (there are also "lesser amounts in corn and peas"), and apparently, according to website *www.earthnotes.tripod.com*, it does not take much of this ingredient to inhibit cancer. "In tests only 0.1% of Geraniol increased the survival rate of rats with malignant tumors."[11] There is another herb that does this and James Duke, Ph.D., and Michael Castleman describe it in their book *The Green Pharmacy Anti-Aging Prescriptions*. It is willow bark. Willow bark "contains salicin, a compound that's a chemical precursor to aspirin." It can be used as a "pain reliever...to prevent heart attack...[and] this same anticoagulant effect helps prevent cancer, or more precisely, the spread of cancer..."[12] Because of the ability of ginger and willow bark to affect blood coagulation, if you are on prescription medications, awaiting surgery, or just recovering from surgery, be sure to check with your physician before using ginger or willow bark. The same holds true for those who are pregnant or breast feeding.

Horseradish & Grapefruit Seed Extract

"Horseradish *(Armoracia rusticana)*" root, described at *herbs2000.com*, is a very pungent herb (or spice) that has long been considered a medicinal treatment in many cultures. A popular "home remedy for hay fever" is a "sandwich of freshly grated root." It is also used for "fevers, colds, and flu."[13] The horseradish root is very potent. It is not for small children or pets. Excessive amounts of the root "can cause vomiting or excessive sweating," and, as further noted *by herbs2000.com*, it "contains chemicals that can interfere with the thyroid gland's production of hormones, which can result in an enlarged thyroid gland."[14] This is not a problem for those who are "healthy," but the root should not be used excessively for "people with thyroid conditions."[15] (As always, check with your physician.)

Fresh horseradish, grated up with cooked beets (also grated) is a concoction that spices up many European dishes! I have been able to kill a cold within 72 hours just by eating a tablespoon a day of horseradish sauce (with meals) for 3 days in a row. I wouldn't recommend it on an empty stomach though! Always take with food. I sometimes just purchase the grated horseradish sauce that you can find at your grocers or local health food store, and use that alone, or combine it with the grated beets.

Another ingredient that quickly kills germs is grapefruit seed extract, which can be purchased in pill supplements, drops, or even in a nasal spray. As mentioned earlier, the extract of grapefruit seed is so powerful at killing germs, some hospitals even use it in their respirator equipment. If you are fighting sinus infections that keep recurring, you may want to try this germ killer. Grapefruit extract nasal spray can be purchased at most health food stores.

Miscellaneous Spices

Researchers have found that many different spices can increase the body's glutathione levels, one of the most valuable antioxidants needed by the body. They determined that these spices could protect against the formation of cancer. Many of those tested were common everyday spices used in cooking such as basil and cinnamon. The best advice when cooking is to use a variety of spices for their antioxidant effects! Foods such as avocados are high in glutathione as well as many other vegetables and fruits. Taking alpha lipoic acid will also raise your glutathione levels. When glutathione levels drop, the results are devastating to the overall health of the body.

Oil of Wild Oregano

This pungent spice has also been discussed earlier. Website *www.cancertutor.com* revealed that "Greek investigators, publishing in the *Journal of Agriculture and Food Chemistry,* determined that oil of wild oregano" could destroy "human cancer cells."[16]

From my own experience, I have found oil of wild oregano to be an excellent earache remedy. Just a drop or two of the oil in the affected ear has very quickly cleared up earaches! Do not use for children unless you have consulted with their pediatrician, especially if there is the possibility of eardrum perforation or allergy to this herb. I use only organic oil of wild oregano, which is available in a small dropper bottle at natural health food stores.

Paprika

Paprika may be significant for cancer prevention. It is derived from a red pepper that is carotenoid-rich. Researchers discovered, in laboratory testing, that this popular spice has powerful tumor-prevention abilities as well as the capacity to inhibit certain viruses. In animal tests, it also suppressed not only skin cancers, but lung cancer as well.

Rosemary

Rosemary contains a compound that inhibited cancer in animal testing. It apparently blocks a substance that promotes the formation of cancerous breast cells. Do not use this herb excessively since it can raise blood pressure.

Saffron

See chapter seven for information on saffron's ability to kill cancer cells.

Other Spices & Herbs That Inhibit Cancer

Many herbs and spices have anti-cancer effects. Ginger and fennel help suppress colon cancer, cumin and fennel inhibit prostate and bladder cancers, coriander fights breast and liver cancers, and mint is high in limonene, which has anti-cancer properties.

CHAPTER 31

TEAS FOR ILLNESS PREVENTION & HEALING

"To make a good cup of medicinal tea, here's a good rule of thumb. Start with boiling water and steep your medicinal herbs until the water is cool. If you like to drink it hot, reheat the tea gently."
(James A. Duke, Ph.D., from his book: *The Green Pharmacy)*[1]

Several teas with healing, curative powers have already been discussed in this book, including *Essiac* tea and *Hoxsey* tea. There are many other teas that can be important in boosting immunity and fighting cancer. A few of those are discussed here.

Be aware that sometimes you will be told that the NCI, FDA or some other institution has tested compounds, for example those in pau d'arco, and flatly announced that they do not help cancer. However, what you usually are not told is that often when a tea is tested, it isn't the whole tea with ALL of its components that are tested by the institution. They will extract one or two compounds from the tea and use that extract to test it. Common sense would tell anyone that this does not always work because teas (e.g. Essiac, pau d'arco, green tea) need to be taken as a whole, without breaking them up into ten different compounds and only using one or two of their main ingredients for the test, then expecting it to perform miracles!

Chaparral Tea

Dr. Ralph W. Moss in his book *Cancer Therapy*, describes an ingredient in chaparral tea known as "NDGA (nordihydroguaiaretic acid)," which was shown in tests on animals to prevent "colon cancer." It also inhibited the formation of "breast tumors" in animal studies. In vitro testing of NDGA prevented leukemia as well as "glioma (i.e. brain cancer)."[2] There was one report from Canada of a consumer having symptoms of "liver damage" after she began ingesting a product "called Chaparral Leaf for several months."[3] As mentioned earlier in this book (chapter 14), the FDA reported a total of 4 cases of liver toxicity from this tea. It was taken off the market, but many people still make their own chaparral tea as it grows wild in some states.

In a human study done by scientists in the western U.S., Dr. Moss tells of a patient with melanoma who "experienced a 95 percent regression" after taking chaparral tea. Research conducted by the "NCI" revealed "that 'this was a very active agent against cancer,' as explained by Dr. Charles R. Smart, associate professor of surgery at the University of Utah Medical Center."[4] In another remarkable case, "an 85-year-old man [was] diagnosed as having melanoma on his right cheek at the University of Utah. He refused surgery." Instead, he began self-treating with chaparral tea. Dr. Moss explains that the patient came back to his physician "eight months later, with marked regression of the cancer..."[5] (I would not advise someone with melanoma not to have surgery, because sometimes surgical removal alone will cure melanoma, depending on the stage it has reached. However, as discussed in earlier chapters, unless you make different lifestyle choices, taking aggressive cancer prevention measures, the cancer may recur.)

Dandelion Tea

Marie Nadine Antol, in her book *Healing Teas*, reports that this herbal tea works to cleanse the liver and blood and helps treat "anemia, gout, jaundice, hypoglycemia, rheumatism...cirrhosis, hepatitis, cramps...reduces uric acid," and has been used in "breast cancer" prevention.[6] (Dandelion has diuretic properties. Using this herb excessively can cause dehydration.) Also, be aware that dandelion herb and dandelion greens can promote bile secretion and increase gastric acid, something to consider if you have gallstones, biliary disease, ulers, or other digestive problems.

Essiac Tea

See chapter five for more information on this amazing, healing herbal tea.

Ginger Tea

In Dr. *Earl Mindell's Food As Medicine*, ginger tea isn't just for stomach upset, morning and motion sickness. One study in particular discovered that women given ginger capsules following "general anesthesia" experienced less symptoms of nausea and vomiting than those given an "antinausea drug." Not only that, but they were able to "recuperate without any additional medication for stomach upset." This herb has also been under close investigation because of its "anticancer properties."[7] I have known of people who successfully use fresh ginger for their migraine headaches.

See the story (in chapter 30 of this book) about a rheumatoid arthritis patient who began ingesting fresh ginger with his meals, which totally eliminated his pain and arthritic symptoms. He has been pain free for the last ten years and he credits his recovery to ginger!

Green Tea

Drinking several cups of green tea a day may be the most important thing you can do to prevent and fight cancer! In one research study described by Dr. James F. Balch in *The Super Anti-Oxidants*, this tea slashed pancreatic cancer by 50% in the group drinking it! More and more data is supporting the use of green tea as a major preventative in "digestive" cancers, esophageal, breast, colon, skin, lung, liver cancers and leukemia![8] A very "promising" study revealed that ingredients in green tea "inhibited proliferation of AML [acute myeloblastic leukemia] cells in *all* cases examined."[8a] Dr. Balch also explains that green tea may be one of the most important developments in treating leukemia, because "It is almost impossible to find anything in medical research that works in all cases," as the study above revealed! Green tea "tells mutant (cancer) cells to die." It apparently causes the cancer cells to "die early," and prevents them from "reproducing…"[9] If you see "Golden Green Tea" at your local health food store, it is merely green tea combined with "lemon grass." Research shows green tea can even prevent dental caries and halitosis.[10] (I would recommend decaffeinated green tea since caffeine is so dehydrating!)

Kombucha Tea

Kombucha tea *("Fungus Japonicus")* is derived from a popular fungus that resembles a mushroom. According to Marie Nadine Antol in *Healing Teas,* there are "reports – primarily anecdotal" – that kombucha has been shown to enhance the body's immunity, attack "cancer and AIDS," lower blood lipids, neutralize toxins, stabilize "blood pressure," attack acne, reduce wrinkling, promote hair growth, help restore natural hair color, "ease arthritis," and energize the body.[11]

Liver Tonic Tea

In *The Green Pharmacy*, Dr. James A. Duke, Ph.D suggests the following tea combination for liver health: "licorice, dandelion, chicory, turmeric and ginger…you can also add anise, caraway, celery seed, dill, clove, fennel, peppermint, rosemary and vanilla bean."[12] You can add the herbs "to taste," but it is always best to mix them dry and keep all ingredients dry until ready to use.[13] A word of caution: licorice, unless it is deglycyrrhizinated (DGL), can raise the blood pressure. Do not use undeglycyrrhizinated licorice if you have "glaucoma, high blood pressure, or disorders affected by estrogen." Always consult with your physician first. If you take this herb, also "take a potassium supplement daily…"[14] (You can purchase DGL licorice in health food stores. If you get the chewable wafers, they taste like coffee beans!) Also be aware that some of these herbs have blood-thinning properties. You should not take them if you are already on prescription medications such as coumadin, or if you have not yet discussed them with your physician. If you are a transplant recipient or waiting for a transplant, never start a new herbal regimen without consulting with your doctor. (Rosemary can raise blood pressure.)

Oolong Tea

This tea, a favorite in China, is partially fermented tea. It is high in anti-oxidants, but has half the caffeine of green tea. If using oolong tea, sip with food, rather than drinking it on an empty stomch.

Parsley Tea

Marie Nadine Antol in *Healing Teas*, describes parsley *("Petroselinum crispum")* as a natural diuretic and overall cleanser, with enough vital "nutrients" to make it an important antioxidant and "preventative."[15] Scientists have recently discovered a substance in parsley that "inhibits the development of cancer cells." If you buy it dried, be sure to find out if it came from the **leaf or roots**. Tea made from the roots will be much more potent than leaf tea. Parsley tea can help the body in "the removal of all stones, including gallstones, if they are not too large."[16] It can also cause uterine contractions, so should not be used during pregnancy, nor during nursing as it "can dry up the milk supply." It should not be used during an "acute infection or...inflammation...especially if the kidneys are involved."[17]

Rooibos Tea

Rooibos tea is harvested in South Africa and is quickly gaining popularity in the West. It is high in antioxidants and flavonoids such as rutin and quercetin and some claim that it demonstrates greater anti-cancer activity than that found in green tea. You can purchase rooibos in fermented form, which has no caffeine, or the unfermented rooibos. There are many internet sites that market this tea and some health food stores carry it.

Sir Jason Winters Tea

Sir Jason Winters had a "large, cancerous growth [that] appeared on the side of" his "neck...in 1977." He went the conventional medicine route, but refused major surgery. Nothing happened to the growth. He was sent home and "told to prepare to die," and given "three months to live." As described at his website: *www.sirjasonwinters.com*, what happened next is nothing less than miraculous! He traveled to three different continents and developed a tea blend containing red clover, herbalene (a Chinese spice), and Indian sage that he combined and began drinking religiously. The cancer began shrinking until it disappeared completely! Today you would never know that he was once a cancer patient! The tea that he used is called his *Classic Blend Tea*, Jason Winters Tea.[18] When the "mixture was tested by Dr. Ian Pierce of England, it was said that the Herbalene acted as a catalyst to make the other two herbs in the tea 27 times stronger." According to their website above, "Hashimoto, the former Prime Minister of Japan, considers Jason Winters Tea to be THE HEALTHIEST DRINK IN THE WORLD!"[19]

Jason Winters' book, *Killing Cancer,* is available at his website, along with his *Classic Blend Tea*, and several other teas that he offers. His website reports that he has "won awards from six foreign governments and the U.S...for his work in the health field,"[20] I would certainly recommend *Jason Winters Tea* for anyone fighting cancer!

Alphabet Tea Blend

See chapter 35 for my own recipe of a multiple tea blend that contains many nutrients and antioxidants that I use for its herbal variety! The recipe makes approximately seven cups of dry tea mix that will last one person several weeks, depending on how many times a day it is used.

CHAPTER 32

THE OPPOSITION & CLINICAL TRIALS –
THE "GOLD STANDARD" (OR IS IT?)

"With today's modern medical science, 'we need a double-blind, controlled study published in a peer-reviewed medical journal to prove that apples fall from trees before we can accept the concept of gravity.'"
(Hans Selye, *Clinical Trial vs Clinical Judgment*
from the book *Left For Dead*, by Dick Quinn)[1]

I. The Opposition to Alternative Cancer Treatments

There is much opposition to alternative cancer treatments, most notably by the AMA, the FDA, some insurance companies, medical schools, many cancer research and treatment centers, and the pharmaceutical industry. As soon as a *new alternative therapy* with much promise is publicized, it is immediately attacked by organized medicine. As a nurse, I do realize that there are always going to be unscrupulous characters promoting their own contrived inventions with unfounded claims that they cure this or that, however I also know that the powers that be (the cancer establishment) have grown into a beauocratic monstrosity with tentacles reaching everywhere, making millions by marketing chemotherapy drugs, radiation treatments, and diagnostic and surgical procedures. They do not like it a bit when someone or something comes along that could threaten their wallets! All you have to do is read about Essiac tea, Burzynski's antineoplastons, Hoxsey tea, Ukrain, or Dr. Joseph Gold, to realize that this is true. (Did you know that one of the AMA board members **who tried to shut Hoxsey down, eventually became one of his patients?**)[2]

There are websites on the internet dedicated to criticizing and defaming every alternative cancer therapy that does not advocate the use of toxic drugs or radiation as part of its regimen!

One such website even criticizes *the Grape Cure* diet, saying that there is very little actual nutritional value in grapes, however, this is not true! Grape juice (including the seeds of the grapes which

Johanna Brandt recommended), besides resveratrol, also contains: "ellagic acid, catechin, quercetin, oligomeric proanthocyanidins (OPC)…pycnogenol…pterostilbene, selenium, lycopene, lutein, laetrile (amygdalin or vitamin B17)…beta-carotene, caffeic acid and/or ferulic acid…and gallic acid." (This is described in detail at *www.cancer tutor.com.*[3])

Another website critical of alternative medicine, expresses total disbelief in the possibility that any type of oncology treatment or diet can enhance the body's immunity; this even in light of the fact that the American Cancer Society is now putting on their printed literature information that a diet high in fruits and vegetables and low in fat can reduce your risk of cancer!

Apparently the alternative medicine critics at this particular website have never read anything of the 1997 *JAMA* article either, (which Dr. Ralph Moss describes in his book, *Antioxidants against Cancer),* which states: **"The era of nutrient supplements to promote health and reduce illness is here to stay…There is overwhelming evidence of immunological enhancement following such an intervention."** (Emphasis, mine.)[4]

This same website has a writer's forum where those who feel they have been victimized by alternative therapies can write to complain. There is one case of a patient with a breast tumor that visited an alternative practitioner who charged her thousands of dollars up front before she could be seen. This should have set warning bells off in anyone with an ounce of sense, however it should be mentioned right about now, that if you are going to a conventional medicine physician to get a bone marrow transplant, or a solid organ transplant, or even another type of major surgery, most of them won't look at you either until they know for sure that you (or your insurance carrier) are going to be able to PAY them the several hundred-thousand-dollars that some of these transplants and surgeries cost! How many doctors' offices have you visited lately that wanted their co-payment OR the entire office visit payment *up front* before they would even see you? If you don't have the money, or your insurance won't cover it, forget about a transplant. It won't happen! (Some people have fund drives to pay for transplants, etc., but the transplant still isn't done until they are sure they will be paid!) They want to be sure if you die, they don't get stuck with an unpaid bill!

Another writer to the website complained about a doctor who was promoting an alternative cancer cure (because the doctor herself was living proof that it worked). The writer said that this particular doctor was promoting her cure with a television marketing program and thereby profiting from the suffering of other people.

Did you know that a recent issue of a *Reader's Digest* magazine with 204 pages in it (exluding the back cover), had **THIRTY-EIGHT pages that were FULL PAGE ads by pharmaceutical companies?** WHOSE suffering do you think they were profiting from? Where do you think pharmaceutical companies get the kind of money to put 38 FULL PAGE ads in a major monthly magazine?

Another writer to the site already had metastasizing cancer to the liver and was going through another round of chemo. This writer voiced the opinion that they had complete confidence in their physician. And my question to this writer is *why would you place complete confidence in your physician? Why would anyone?* Granted, you should have some amount of confidence in your doctor, or be looking for another one, but you should never place *complete confidence* in any physician! You should be questioning your doctor routinely, especially if you have uncertainties about any of their treatments. There are a lot of people who had *complete* confidence in their physicians who would still be alive today, if they had **NOT placed complete confidence in their physicians** and asked a few more questions before they took Vioxx, Rezulin and Baycol! Ask their widows and surviving children! (If your doctor puts you on a new prescription, do you research it before you blindly take it? Do you read about the potential side effects and interactions with other medications and foods? Do you check to see if the drug can be toxic to your kidneys or liver, or do you just gulp it down, without question?)

Another writer commented that they believed the ability to create pharmaceutical drugs and medicine was wisdom given by our Creator to those who make them. While I believe that our Creator DOES impart wisdom and knowledge to individuals for the development of pharmaceuticals that will BENEFIT mankind, there is a mighty big difference between making aspirin for headaches or insulin for diabetics, than making a chemotherapy drug that you know will kill the patient, lying about the clinical trials, and purposely withholding evidence of negative results so that you can get the drug approved faster and make a huge profit at the expense of human lives! In going along with the type of bizarre reasoning that the above writer used, I am sure that all the family members of those patients who died with heart attacks while taking Vioxx will certainly be comforted to know that, according to the above writer, it was *God* who was responsible for the brains behind the drugs that killed their loved ones!

We've also been given the **wisdom** (and I use the term very loosely here) to develop alcohol, crack cocaine, heroin, highly efficient ways to commit abortion, and pornographic videos, so what are we to do? Blame God for all the suffering that these developments have caused? What ridiculous reasoning!

(Maybe there should be alternative sites for people who are victimized by chemotherapy and radiation quackery; like when they take Tamoxifen, then find out that it gave them uterine cancer, or leukemia caused by radiation! Some sites are beginning to spring up out there that do have such testimonials. The problem however, with all the chemo and radiation horror stories is that so many of the "victims" **don't live long enough to tell them!**)

II. Double-Blind, Randomized, Placebo-Controlled Clinical Trials – The "Gold Standard"

There are many alternative therapies for cancer, with new ones being discovered every single day. Some of them are not supported by clinical trials on humans, and of course, that is one of the big arguments that organized medicine gives against alternative therapies. However, there is something you should know about the *gold standard* of the modern medical profession. *Double-blind, randomized, placebo-controlled clinical trials* ARE their gold standard! However, the results of clinical trials are often manipulated by those doing them and many times, they are simply lied about or the results are concealed. For example, if a drug company is in a hurry to get their *promising new drug* approved by the FDA (and they usually are), there are subtle ways (and some not so subtle!) that they can make sure that the results of their *clinical trials* come out favoring their drug! This is done in a variety of ways:

If you want to be sure that the participants testing a new blood pressure drug have excellent results, be sure that all the people in your group using the new drug do not have multiple co-morbidities, and choose participants in your control group that do! That way it will ensure that those on your new drug are more likely to stay healthier than the control group, making your drug APPEAR to be very beneficial. Also, your new drug testers won't die off and the drug get the blame! (Even though the drug might be responsible for their deaths!) If someone using your new drug drops dead from heart failure, for example, just replace that person with a live body, or dismiss the death as *unrelated,* so it does not show up as one of the adverse effects when you are reporting results of the study to the FDA! Or just start a new trial and hide the unfavorable results of the old trial from the FDA. You are living in *la-la land* if you think this isn't being done. It's done, all right, and on a regular basis!

Put the worst adverse effects of the drug in very **tiny** microscopic print in your drug warning label on line 165, in complex technical jargon that even a trained doctor can't decipher, ensuring that no physician (in his or her right mind) is ever going to read it, understand it, or warn their patients about it!

As noted by Dr. Thomas A.M. Kramer, M.D., in "Understanding Clinical Trials in Context," "[M]ost clinical trials are six weeks long. Most patients take their medication considerably longer than that. Who is to say that what is true in 6 weeks will remain so?"[5]

Get the drug approved for treating one illness, but have the drug reps PUSH physicians to prescribe it for *off-label* usage for a dozen other problems! (e.g. it is approved to treat hypertension, but convince the docs that it is also good for insomnia, anxiety, edema and gastritis, thus expanding the sales and profits for the drug company!) This push to use a drug for off-label use is what happened with the drug propulsid, discussed in chapter one of this book. It was supposed to be for adults, but ended up being prescribed to babies. Over 300 people, many of them infants, died before this one was taken off the market![6]

Admit (also in very fine print) on the drug label that the drug's effectiveness had not been fully determined through clinical trials, so it is important that doctors prescribing the drug routinely determine whether those patients who are to receive it will benefit.[7] (Oops! Did you see **how THAT ONE WAS DONE**? You are left hanging out on a limb this time! Suddenly, the responsibility for evaluating this drug's *effectiveness* falls in the lap of (you guessed it!) your friendly, neighborhood, physician!) Six months go by and ten people die from taking the drug and the drug manufacturer points the guilty blood-stained finger at your physician for not conscientiously evaluating the drug's *effectiveness!* (Nothing like *passing-the-buck,* is there!?)

Lie about any unfavorable results, or simply cover them up, or pay an outside investigator to conduct the trials for you. If they do five studies for you and only two studies favor the drug you want approved, bury the three studies you don't like and ship the other two to the FDA with your new drug application. (Ah yes, there are ways around the "system" and you can be sure most drug companies have figured out every single one of them!)

You can read the reports any time you like. A good example is the cover-up that went on with Prozac. Just go to *http://www.prozac-truth.com/*:

> June 29, 2004 – Today, New York Attorney General Eliot Spitzer requested Forest Labs to supply information of the non-disclosed clinical trials for Celexa and Lexapro and the promotion of their products. Eliot Spitzer is concerned Forest may be in violation of New York state law. This follows the Attorney General filing suit against GlaxoSmithKline for non-disclosure of negative clinical trials with their antidepressant Paxil.[8]

You may wish to read that last sentence again, about the suit "against GlaxoSmithKline for non-disclosure of negative clinical trials with their antidepressant Paxil." What happened with this drug is nothing new and it has happened before! The drug company deliberately withheld the results of some of their clinical trials because they were "**NEGATIVE!**" They LIED to the FDA in order to get the drug approved and on the market! And did you note the remark about Forest Labs being "requested...to supply information of the non-disclosed clinical trials" for two of their drugs? [9] How willing are YOU to trust the results of clinical trials on that new drug your doctor just prescribed for you? How TRUSTING are you?!

This is just the *tip of the iceberg*! Website *www.prozactruth.com* describes an article by Elizabeth Shogren from the *Los Angeles Times* 4/6/4 where she describes how the "FDA kept suicide findings secret" concerning antidepressants prescribed to children:

> When the government scientist filed his report last winter...his bosses decided to keep it secret – even though it found that children who took the drugs were twice as likely to be involved in serious suicide-related behavior as those who did not. Instead of revealing the findings, senior FDA officials ordered more studies...They also squelched plans to have the author, Dr. Andrew Mosholder, present his conclusions to an FDA advisory committee....Mosholder's report still has not been made public.[10]

Because of the uproar over the antidepressant drugs, the fact that they increased the likelihood of suicide in young people taking them and the cover-up involving those side-effects, "Senate and House committees have ordered the FDA to hand over documents that might illuminate what the agency knew about the possible link between the drugs and suicidal behavior."[11]

The above litigation came about primarily because of a "whistleblower" working for the drug company. The story was reported on "NBC NEWS" on "July 11" on "NBC's John Hockenberry reports," when whistle blower "David Franklin" admitted that "I was trained to deceive, to lie to doctors." When John Hockenberry asked him: "Who would train and then pay someone to mislead doctors? Scientist David Franklin says pharmaceutical company Warner-Lambert paid him to do that back in 1996." His job as verified by Mr. Hockenberry was "to find trust, and exploit it, to produce more sales for Warner-Lambert."[12]

Isn't this amazing? Especially when you consider the pompous claims that many drug manufacturers display on their drug commercials! Yet, let a health food store owner try to make similar claims about a natural herbal remedy that has no toxic side effects, and the FDA will scream *FOUL* and shut them down! In Canada, Rene Cassie suffered constant surveillance and harassment when she said that her herbal tea was curing cancer without toxic side effects, yet the U.S. FDA is no different! They will remove an herbal tea from American shelves, classifying it as dangerous and harmful for you, because four people (out of 700,000) had adverse reactions to it, and in the same breath, tell you that it is entirely safe to give your child with brain cancer a chemotherapy drug that has already **killed 700,000 people!** Maybe they died a little slower, but they are still dead! This is sanity? Well of course it isn't, but think about it, because our entire medical system of treating cancer is based on this type of insanity! As a matter-of-fact, if your physician wants to give you or your loved one some "new" chemo regimen, do this – **ask him or her to first provide you with the studies showing how many people were CURED or had their lives extended significantly after taking the same drugs that they are wanting to give YOU!**

If you still have doubts about the objectivity of clinical trials, consider **who** it is that does most of these trials! According to Dr. Thomas A. M. Kramer, M.D:

> Most clinical trials are sponsored by **pharmaceutical companies**. Although they are often presented in independent journals as objective scientific research, they almost always show results that are **favorable** to the sponsoring company. It is important when reading the results of a clinical trial to take note of **who paid for it** so as to appreciate the **potential bias. Pharmaceutical companies ensure favorable results in a number of ways.**[13] [Emphasis, mine.]

In his book *Healing Cancer – Complementary Vitamin & Drug Treatments*, Dr. Abram Hoffer, says of double-blind studies:

[D]ouble-blind experiments influence the medical-political world only when they are conducted by and reported by establishment institutions and published in establishment journals. Other double-blind experiments of equal or even greater worth unsupported by the establishment are ignored. Most clinicians know this.[14]

In view of all this, remember the above when you are considering a safe, non-toxic alternative therapy and someone (who thinks they know something you don't) tells you that the therapy you are contemplating is not backed up by *scientific double-blind, randomized, placebo-controlled clinical trials*! Just smile, shake your head, and ignore them completely! They are wasting your valuable time!

CHAPTER 33

MISCELLANEOUS ALTERNATIVE CANCER THERAPIES

JAMA 1949: *"There is no scientific evidence whatsoever to indicate that modifications in the dietary intake of food or other nutritional essentials are of any specific value in the control of cancer." JAMA* 1997: ***"The era of nutrient supplements to promote health and reduce illness is here to stay...There is overwhelming evidence of immnological enhancement following such an intervention."***

(Ralph W. Moss, Ph.D., from his book: *Antioxidants against Cancer)*[1]

Some of the alternative therapies given in this chapter have cured cancer, others are preventatives only, or they may promote the health of certain organs such as the liver. Some are not *natural* or *painless* since they may be given through injection or other invasive means, however, the majority of them (with one or two exceptions) do not involve the use of toxic chemo drugs and radiation therapy, and many have helped cancer patients to survive the disease and extend their lives. They are being included here for informational purposes only. In choosing alternative therapies, the choices you go with will ultimately have to be your own decision.

ALA – Alpha Lipoic Acid

This nutrient was discussed earlier, especially in relation to liver detoxification and health. It is a very powerful antioxidant and occurs normally in the human body in small amounts! When Dr. Burt Berkson, M.D., Ph.D., was asked to treat two victims of acute mushroom poisoning (from the "Destroying Angel mushroom Amanita verna)," he did not actually see them until "24 hours after their mushroom meal," because they had been misdiagnosed (but not by him)![2] Because of their lab results, he knew that both patients already had acute liver poisoning. The hospital told him there was no way for them to survive. He treated them with ALA, alpha lipoic acid infusion. He obtained the ALA from a physician at "National Institutes of

Health," who express-shipped it to him within a few hours. Both patients recovered completely. Seven days later, the exact same thing happened; another couple came to the hospital with the same diagnosis, their livers in worse shape than the previous victims had been! Dr. Berkson said that the hospital "ordered" him "not to use ALA." The "pharmacists had never heard of the drug…and it was not on the hospital formulary list."[3] He ignored the order, used the ALA that was left over from the prior weekend and within a few days, both patients were recovering, eventually to be discharged home! This, in spite of the fact that "hospital authorities" had told him the same thing they told him the weekend before, "that these people had no chance of living." Dr. Berkson was "eventually awarded the Food and Drug Administration (FDA) investigational drug permit for intravenous ALA therapy," however, the hospital that had ordered him not to use the ALA "was furious" with him.[4] (Dr. Berkson did not identify the name of the hospital, I'm sure due to legal ramifications, but I can guarantee you, if I ever found out who they were, I would NEVER go there, nor recommend them to anyone! Would you?) Do you think what happened to Dr. Burkson in the above story is an isolated incident? It is an excellent example of what happened to Dr. Burzynski, Dr. Koch and Rene Cassie! This is one case only, **but it is a microcosmic example of the BIG PICTURE of our modern U.S. medical system of treating cancer which says to cancer patients – in essence:**

We could care less that this new treatment is non-toxic and will cure cancer, if it isn't approved by <u>our</u> <u>system</u>, you can't use it! You can only use these drugs for your cancer, because WE approved them – Oh – and never mind the fact that they are so toxic that they may kill you before your cancer does!

ALA is available in supplement form. Most natural health food stores carry this nutrient. Potatoes, broccoli, brewer's yeast, and spinach are natural sources of alpha lipoic acid, however you would have to eat enormous amounts to get the ALA equivalent in one 100 mg supplement capsule!

B-17 – Laetrile

There is still much controversy about laetrile and possibly will be for some time to come. Probably because so many people were cured of deadly cancers taking laetrile! Some researchers believe that insufficient amounts of B17 in the diet are responsible for diseases such as sickle cell anemia and various cancers. Though B17 has never been given the FDA's kiss of approval as a vitamin, the body still needs it in small amounts, nonetheless. Some reports even claim that cells can take B17 and make their own supplies of B12, thus preventing megaloblastic anemia. (B12 injections can also be given by your physician or taken as sublingual tablets (under the tongue). You may want to check out Dr. Andrew W. Saul's website at *http://www.doctoryourself.com/nasal.html,* for his recipe on a nasal delivery form of B12.

Animals seem to have instincts that we humans could learn from. When a deadly tsunami killed thousands in Asia, in December 2004, it was reported that very few animal bodies were found. Apparently, the animals, sensing something amiss, scrambled for higher ground, saving their lives. Animals often know what is best for them, even when it comes to choosing their food (if they are out in the wild, that is!) God gives imparted knowledge to animals to help them survive, something we call *instinct.*

When Maureen Kennedy Salaman's "beloved Siamese cat…was diagnosed with…terminal…cancer," she describes what happened in her book, *Nutrition: The Cancer Answer II.* She said that she began "crushing Laevalin (laetrile) tablets into his food." She also included in his diet "ground beef, ground apricot seeds, garlic and millet. Within six months, the veterinarian" told her that the cat was free of cancer! He lived for "another five years, dying at the ripe old age of 19, but not from cancer."[5] Ms. Salaman recommends that you should watch what your pet does when they are ill. Many times they will stop eating altogether, or they will scrounge around in your garden and start nibbling plants. You should take notice of what your pet chooses to eat if they forage outdoors, especially when they are ill. Watching what animals eat when they are ill is one way that scientists have been able to select plants we now know to be "therapeutic."[6]

Ms. Salaman further notes that "Indians" from "Taos, New Mexico…Pueblo Indians…eat many foods rich in amygdalin." ("B17" or "laetrile" is derived from "amygdalin").[7] It is noteworthy that "cancer is rare among this population." She says that the Pueblo Indians gave her a delicious recipe that she sometimes drinks: "In a glass of milk or juice mix a tablespoon of honey with a quarter ounce or two dozen freshly ground apricot kernels, or one kernel for every ten pounds of body weight." Ms. Salaman said that when they gave her this recipe, she initially drank it daily and "On the third day a funny thing happened. Two little benign skin growths on my arm, which were formerly pink, turned brown. By the seventh day, they were gone." Though apricot seeds are one of the richest sources of B17, sweet potatoes also have this nutrient as well as many other foods and seeds.[8] (In this recipe, I would use juice instead of milk!)

Ms. Salaman recommends Amygdalin B17 as "The most important supplement in the metabolic program of cancer control…six to nine 500 mg amygdalin tablets should be taken daily, specifically two or three after meals when there is food in the stomach."[9] She explains that the best tablet found in the U.S. is Laevalin. Many others available may be "totally ineffective." With the tablets, she also recommends "10 to 15 (apricot) kernels a day to…enhance the action of the Laevalin" for patient's who are in "crisis," as well as eating the kernels routinely for cancer "prevention."[10]

Interest was sparked in B17 foods when a group of people living in isolation in the "Himalayan Mountains of Pakistan…the Hunzakuts," were discovered. The late Hanna Kroeger, in her book, *Free Your Body of Tumors and Cysts*, said that regardless of age, they appeared very healthy.[11] "Their women at the age of eighty look as we do at forty years of age." It was revealed that the diet of this tribe "consisted of lots of apricots, vegetables, millet and other grains." (Their diet was very high in nitrilosides – B17!) It was also discovered that they "cracked the seeds of the apricots" eating the kernels.[12]

The use of laetrile in the U.S. for cancer treatment was popularized in the 1970s, but it quickly became "a subject" of bitter "controversy."[13]

In her book, *Nutrition: The Cancer Answer II*, Maureen Kennedy Salaman explained that one of the published reports from Kanematsu

Sugiura, M.D., who researched "B17" at "Memorial Sloan-Kettering Cancer Institute," stated that giving the vitamin could retard "mammary tumors in" mice. It is also able to inhibit "the formation of lung metastases," and may even halt "...the formation of new tumors." In another animal study, the vitamin was able to bring about "regression in 80 percent of animals studied" (with "spontaneous mammary tumors") and "complete regression in 40 percent..."[14] However, according to Ms. Salaman, "Sloan-Kettering announced that the results were not significant and suppressed the report," but she says that insiders "'leaked' the report to the outside world."[15]

Proponents of B17 argue that it is high in "cyanide" and therefore, dangerous, however, Ms. Salaman claims in *Nutrition: The Cancer Answer II*, that "even the FDA" has admitted that "amygdalin is 'harmless to both man and beast when used as an essential part of the metabolic approach to cancer.'"[16] As for the cyanide found in laetrile, according to website *www.alternativehealth.com*, it is broken down by the body into non-toxic substances:

> [A]n enzyme called rhodanese, which is always present in healthy tissue has the ability to break down benzaldehyde and cyanide [ingredients from Laetrile] into harmless components. Malignant cancer cells do not contain any rhodanese and therefore cannot rely on this defense mechanism.[17]

This website also noted that during the research done by the "National Cancer Institute" three decades ago, "two patients who ate almonds whilst taking amygdalin developed symptoms of cyanide poisoning."[18] (These were probably bitter almonds, rather than the sweet almonds found in most grocery stores!) Not only that but small amounts of cyanide can also be found in many berries and seeds, yet people aren't poisoned eating them! You can sometimes purchase bags of apricot kernels in natural health food stores. They are also sold on the internet.

If interested in purchasing Laetrile (B17), you can do so from "American Biologics, 1180 Walnut Ave., Chula Vista, CA 92011."[19]

Beres Drops Plus®

Dr. Josef Beres, "a Hungarian agronomist," developed mineral drops containing "iron, zinc, sodium, magnesium, manganese, potassium, copper, molybdenum, vanadium, nickel, boron, fluorine and cobalt…The drops do not exceed US RDAs."[20] Website *www.cancer-tutor.com* says that Beres tested his mineral drops "on 235 patients who had 'no chance of recovery.'[21] After giving them the drops near-ly ONE THIRD found their tumors had subsided."[22]

Breuss Total Cancer Treatment

Breuss cancer treatment involves taking a diet rich in nutrients, but in liquid form only, for a total period of 42 days. It is detailed in the book, *"The Breuss Cancer Cure"* (by "Rudolf Breuss"), which "has sold over 900,000 copies…and claims to have led to over 45,000 tes-timonials [world-wide] from cured sufferers."[23] This diet is based on the premise that you can literally "starve cancer cells…by not provid-ing any solid food proteins." The diet uses raw juices as well as teas. As described by *www.cancertutor.com*: *"Breuss juice vegetable juice," is composed of "55% red beet root, 20% carrots, 20% celery root, 3% raw potato, 2% radishes…The potato is optional except for liver cancer where it plays an important part."*[24]

I can understand why this diet would be effective, as well as very detoxifying to the body, with its use of nutrient-dense juices. (See chapter 34 of this book for information about the healing abilities imparted to the body through fasting.) The Breuss diet is a type of liq-uid fast. Cancer cells thrive on protein and sugar and this diet reduces protein intake dramatically as well as processed sugars. Many people believe that fasting will make you ill – it won't. What usually makes people ill is food. (Eating too much of the right kind or wrong kind!) Also see chapter 35 of this book for an important detoxification reg-imen. Realize that someone who is severely ill may not be able to tol-erate a juice-fast. They should always discuss a new diet plan with their physician, and they may be best doing so with a Naturopathic

Doctor, since many orthodox medicine physicians are against anything whatsoever that even hints of alternative therapy!

Burzysnski's Antineoplastons

Discussed briefly in an earlier chapter, antineoplastons were developed by Stanislaw R. Burzynski, M.D., Ph.D. In her book, *Nutrition: The Cancer Answer II,* Maureen Kennedy Salaman says that Dr. Burzynski's research revealed that "cancer patients lack a certain group of peptides in their blood."[25] He called the "peptides 'antineoplastons.'" He found a way to isolate them and use them for cancer patients, but the FDA fought him the entire way. In one particular "press release," Burzysnski reported that when he gave antineoplastons "in oral form, as opposed to intravenously, 'Some prostate cancer patients, even those who failed to respond to conventional therapy, have experienced a complete remission of their cancer in as little as five months.'"[26] Ms. Salaman further explains that when the American scientists snubbed him, Burzynski "published papers in peer-reviewed medical journals around the world," and in a recent gathering of the "International Congress of Chemotherapy...fourteen pages on antineoplastons were presented – certainly a record for what the American medical monopoly considers 'quackery.'"[27] Unfortunately (thanks to the FDA), the only place in the U.S. that you can get Burzynski's antineoplastons is Texas. "The Burzynski Research Institute" is located in "Stafford, Texas." Patients are treated at "his outpatient clinic in Houston."[28] A few insurance companies are actually beginning to cover antineoplastons, but only under very limited circumstances. Antineoplastons have been very successful alternative cancer treatments! You can reach Dr. Burzynski's Houston, Texas clinic at *www.cancermed.com.* Antineoplastons are discussed in much greater detail in chapter 13 of this book due to their tremendous success with terminal brain cancer patients! (Note that antineoplastons are not to be confused with the group of chemo drugs known as antineoplastics. They are NOT the same.)

Contortrostatin

According to website: *http://www.mnwelldir.org,* "Contortrostatin…is a protein extracted from the venom of the Southern Copperhead." Studies done at "the University of Southern California," revealed that the extract inhibited the growth of "human breast cancer cells" (transplanted into mice) up to "70%." It also kept cancer from spreading "100% of the time," and prevents "the growth of new blood vessels…"[29]

Research into this compound is described by Dr. Francis S. Markland, Ph.D., Associate Dean for Scientific Affairs and Professor of Biochemistry & Molecular Biology at the University of Southern California, Keck School of Medicine (from an article at website *www.calacademy.org):*

> Our findings indicate that contortrostatin blocks several critical steps in tumor metastasis…and is, therefore, more potent than other agents which only block a single step….In addition, contortrostatin significantly inhibits invasion of breast cancer cells…Interestingly, contortrostatin is not cytotoxic to human breast cancer cells…We found that the size of the tumor masses…in the contortrostatin-treated mice were significantly smaller than those in saline-treated mice….Even more exciting, the contortrostatin-treated group showed 65% to 85% inhibition of lung metastasis, as compared to the saline-treated group.[30]

Dr. Markland further explained that "contortrostatin also inhibits angiogenesis (the growth of new blood vessels) in breast cancer by greater than 90% using the mouse model."[30a] Thus far though, there have been no tests on humans using contortrostatin, just animal testing. Human testing may still be months or years away! The product is not promoted as a cure or treatment for humans with cancer. It is being discussed here for informational purposes only because of its enormous potential.

Another study reported by Sophia Young at *www.usc.edu/CSS F/History…,* revealed that contortrostatin effectively slowed the growth of ovarian tumors in test mice "injected with A2780 human ovarian cancer cells."[30b]

HGH – Human Growth Hormone

HGH is yet another hormone produced by our bodies in lesser amounts as we age! In their book, *What Your Doctor May Not Tell You About Immune Disorders*, Dr. Stephen Edelson and Lynn Sonberg tell us that by the time you hit 60, your body is only producing about "25 percent of the HGH secreted at age twenty," however this growth hormone does not last long in the body.[31] It is normally released from the pituitary while you are sleeping and right "after exercise." Almost immediately, the liver changes most of it to "a metabolite called insulin-like growth factor type 1 (IGF1)." If your physician wants to see if you are deficient in HGH, he or she won't measure the HGH circulating in your body, since it doesn't last very long. They will measure the amount of IGF1 that you have, since it lasts about "twenty-four to thirty-six hours."[32] Dr. Edelson and Ms. Sonberg explain that normal levels in an adult should be "200-450 ng/ml (nanograms per milliliter of blood)," and that often, "individuals with autoimmune disorders" or "chronic fatigue" syndrome have deficient levels of IGF1 and they will benefit from HGH supplements. Abnormal levels can cause "fatigue, loss of muscle and bone strength, reduced healing capacity, diminished memory…weight gain, and loss of skin tone."[33] When taken in supplement form, both authors say that HGH "Stimulates bone formation…Reduces facial wrinkles…Improves sex drive, Improves energy…Improves sleep…Enhances mood [and] Increases memory retention." HGH is available as an injectable form and "over the counter" supplements, however, you should check with your physician before taking this hormone.[34]

Insulin-induced Hypoglycemic Therapy – IHT

IHT treatment is based on the belief that "cancer cells thrive on sugar." At one time insulin was given intravenously to deliberately induce a state of hypoglycemia for about an hour (starving the cells of sugar), during which time the patient was closely monitored, however, with today's new technology, *cancertutor.com* says that this dangerous step no longer has to be done. One of the labs that uses this therapy "BioPulse [in Mexico, of course]," reports that thus far, "Every patient treated has had their tumors substantially reduced or completely eliminated."[35]

Koch Formula

Dr. William Frederick Koch developed a cure for cancer by creating a substance known as *Glyoxylide*. It was such a success that he was ultimately closed down by the cancer establishment, and he eventually left the U.S. altogether. Though he fought many battles with organized medicine, Dr. Koch was not a fraud. He earned several degrees from prestigious American colleges and even taught at two of them. Glyoxylide reportedly had the ability to enable the elimination of toxins from the body. When Dr. Koch announced that he had successfully cured several of his cancer patients, it sounded the death knoll for his career in the U.S. His peers quickly ostracized him. There is a great deal of information on Dr. Koch on the internet, and his cancer treatment has been written up in many books and journals in great detail.

Max Gerson Treatment

In *Nutrition: The Cancer Answer II*, Maureen Kennedy Salaman said that Max Gerson from Germany developed the "Gerson Treatment" which was basically a low salt, "high-potassium, no-fat, high fresh vegetable – fresh fruit diet," with "vitamin-mineral supplements and coffee enemas," as outlined in his book, "*A Cancer Therapy: Results of Fifty Cases*," written in "1958."[36] Ms. Salaman explained that

Gerson's therapy included drinking "13 glasses of fresh raw juices...and three full vegetarian meals...organically grown vegetables, fruits and whole grains."[37]

Gerson had originally started out trying to find an ideal dietary regimen for "lupus and tuberculosis" patients. Dr. Gary Null, in *The Complete Encyclopedia of Natural Healing*, said that Gerson was so successful at reversing the diseases with his diet plan, "the German physicians made him director of the clinic," and he was "something of a superstar in Europe until the 1930s."[38] At first *JAMA* was so impressed with his work, they published one of his articles, then "later attacked Gerson and called him a quack." At the "height of his career," an investigation spearheaded by "Senator Claude Pepper of Florida," asked him to present "medical documentation and patients," which he did. They were so impressed with the results, that Dr. Null says he was given a commendation.[39]

Author Conrad LeBeau, (*Hydrogen Peroxide & Ozone*), met Gerson's daughter, "Charlotte Gerson," at the "1986...National Health Federation convention in Chicago."[40] He said that the thing that impressed him the most about the lecture she gave was when she described how "they located several of the patients Dr. Gerson had treated for terminal cancer 30 years ago and found that many of them were still alive!"[41] One of Gerson's patients was "Nobel laureate Albert Schweitzer, MD," who wrote of him, "I see in him one of the most eminent medical geniuses in the history of medicine."[42]

Although I do not advocate the use of coffee enemas, according to Dr. R. W. Moss in *Cancer Therapy*, they were a popular home remedy at one time, appearing in "medical literature as early as 1917."[43] The rest of the items on the Gerson treatment are natural ingredients that are loaded with antioxidants, especially the raw juices! (He did advocate a raw liver drink that I would never recommend or use, and it was later discontinued in the diet.) Dr. Moss also said that during "1990," the "*Lancet*" did a brief "evaluation of the Gerson program" carried out by doctors at "Maudsley and Hammersmith Hospitals." Though they ended up only evaluating 7 cases, out of those "7 cases...3 (43 percent) were found to be in complete remission."[44] There is an enormous amount of information on Gerson on the internet.

MGN-3

MGN-3 is an extract taken from "three Japanese mush-rooms...Shiitake...Kawaratake...and Suehirotake...with the outer shell of rice bran." It is described as a safe, non-toxic "Immune system booster out of Tokyo, Japan." Website *www.moonbowmedia.com/health/mgn3.htm* explains that in several studies that were "first published in the International Journal of Immunotherapy, it was demonstrated that cancer patients taking MGN-3...experienced dramatic increases in their NK, or natural killer cell activity." Dr. M. Ghoneum, an "Egyptian immunology researcher," who "had been studying...MGN-3 for six years" claimed that with human cancer patients, "MGN-3 boosts NK cell growth and activity an amazing 300%."[45]

When dosages of the nutrient were studied, "a group of twenty-four individuals" were given "the highest dosage of 45 milligrams...per kilogram of body weight (roughly three grams of MGN-3 for a 150 pound person) per day, [and] natural killer cell activity had increased 800% after just one week!" This was reported by *www.drdebe.com.*, Dr. Joseph Debe's website. Then "at two months" the website explains that NK activity was compared to what it had been at the beginning of the study. After this amount of time, it was still "*27 times* greater!" This response "is reported to continue to increase after use of the product for six months," with allowance for variations in different individuals, says *drdebe.com*.[46] The website further explains that in one study with "eleven" cancer patients, "five" of them experienced "complete remission" while taking MGN-3. The patients had either "Multiple myeloma, prostate, breast, or ovarian cancers."[47] This compound is sold in the U.S. as BioBran® and can be purchased on the internet (e.g. *http://www.buy-biobran.com/index.htm*), or ordered through health food stores. You can find a great deal of information on this product at the BioBran® website: *http://www.biobran.org/index.html.*

MSM Plus Vitamin C and B12

"MSM (Methyl Sulfonyl Methane)" supplies sulfur to cells, apparently making them more "permeable." As described at *cancertutor.com,* it is popularly used in treating arthritis, because it "supports connective tissue," and decreases pain. It may "turn malignant tumors into benign tumors."[48] MSM also assists the body in balancing pH, detoxification, and "is critical to the formation of glutathione...the most plentiful antioxidant...inside the cells," says Cancer Tutor.™ [49]

A study from 1986 "showed that MSM" could prevent "mammary cancers."[50] MSM is best taken with vitamin C and B12 if you are taking it for cancer prevention and treatment. An excellent source of natural B12 is **spirulina**. Note that if you already have "plenty of sulfur in" your diet "(e.g. from eggs and onions)," *cancertutor.com* says that MSM may not prove beneficial for you. They explain that if you have allergies to sulphites, you may "also react to MSM. This is usually due to a deficiency of molybdenum and can be overcome with supplementation."[51]

Proton Beam Therapy

Proton beam therapy may offer new choices to those who are fearful of conventional radiation treatments for cancer. Though I do not personally advocate radiation therapy, I am including proton beam therapy for informational purposes only, and because this type therapy is not as hazardous as conventional radiation. Details are given in an article at OncoLink website, *www.oncolink.com*, from the Abramson Cancer Center of the University of Pennsylvania by James Metz, M.D.[52] Apparently, proton beam therapy "can be directed" so that more of the actual tumor is treated with less damage to surrounding tissues than compared to "conventional photons (x-rays)," which also means that "higher doses can safely be delivered to the tumor itself."[53] Their website article has several graphs showing very dramatic differences in side effects between conventional photon therapy and proton beam therapy, depending on the type cancer treated.

Rife Machine

During the 1930s, a scientist by the name of Royal Raymond Rife invented a very powerful microscope which had the ability to magnify organisms, but it could do so without having to destroy the objects being studied, something that science had never done before. This enabled Mr. Rife to actually study and observe living specimens. Rife used an electronic treatment to destroy viruses, thus enabling the weakened immune system to recover and bring healing to the body. According to reports, doctors using this new treatment were successfully curing hundreds of cancer patients. They were also using the therapy for treating other ailments and diseases. His work was noted in multiple prestigious medical journals, and Rife was praised by many prominent physicians of his day. However, he met with great opposition from the AMA until his work was eventually completely suppressed.

He later died under mysterious circumstances.[54] There is a great deal of information about Rife on the internet.

714X – Gaston Naessens

See chapter 15 for information on Gaston Naessens and 714X as well as the remarkable story of a young man who used 714X to cure **Hodgkins disease**. He also changed his diet and used Essiac tea, along with the 714X injections.

CHAPTER 34

TAKE THE TIME TO AVOID EVERYTHING - FASTING & DETOX

"Fasting has been proven to be the most effective means of getting the body into a natural healing process. It is also an instrument to literally reset the body's odometer and help reverse the aging process...fasting only three days a month...can increase your life span by five to seven years."

(Valerie Saxion, From her book, *How To Feel Great All The Time.)*[1]

Healing Through Fasting

Though fasting is controversial, it shouldn't be because everyone fasts at some time or another in their life and occasional fasting is a health boost! Fasting can be intentional or imposed by illness, pending surgery or other circumstances, sometimes those beyond our control. While most people are convinced that fasting several days will make them ill, what they don't realize is that it is usually too much food (even the right kind of food) that makes one ill, not fasting! While I never recommend a total fast that even excludes water, I do believe that partial fasting (half day), juice-fasting and complete food fasting (drinking water only) is very beneficial to the body if done in moderation. Not only that, but for Christians it is not merely recommended, but commanded and expected that they fast from time to time. Other religions also engage in occasional fasts as part of their belief system.

Most people look at a juice-fast as drinking ONLY juice, and a water-fast as drinking ONLY water, however, the opposite is actually true. A "water-fast" means not drinking water and a "juice-fast" means no juice. For clarification purposes, when a water or juice-fast is discussed in this chapter, it will pertain to including ONLY water or ONLY juice in the diet.

For those who want to maintain or recover optimal health, I believe the safest and healthiest fast is the juice-fast. This is a liquid fast, where no solid food is taken, but plenty of fresh raw vegetable and fruit juices are allowed.

This type of fast is very cleansing and detoxifying to the body. Dr. Don Colbert in his book, *Toxic Relief*, says that it rejuvenates and refreshes as well, and in comparison to "water-only fasting...juice-fasting...supports detoxification, alkalinizes the body and supports the liver."[2] Realize that in water-only fasts you will have a lot of "muscle loss," which is not as drastic with a juice-fast. Dr. Colbert further explains that a juice-fast will often do a more efficient job of detoxifying your liver than water-only fasting. A juice-fast will also do something that may revitalize you beyond anything else you can possibly do; it will raise the pH of your body and alkalize the tissues![3]

I have been on water-only fasts and juice-fasts. I've noticed that I actually get hungrier on a juice-fast. I believe it is because on a water-only fast, after a few days, the hunger went away. On the juice-fast it didn't, and I'm sure it's because carbs cause the body to release insulin and insulin makes you hungry. However, even juice-fasts will often begin with the first 2-3 days of water only, as suggested in the case of *The Grape Cure* diet by Johanna Brandt (discussed earlier in chapter two).

Water-only fasting is also very healthy for the body. Dr. Colbert explains that it can quickly "reduce inflammation in the body...[and] may actually cause the hardened arterial plaque of severe coronary disease to regress and possibly melt away." The same thing happens with a juice-fast, though it usually takes longer.[4]

Fasting can "bring the healing and refreshing presence of God into an individual life and into the life of a family or even a nation," says Dr. Colbert. It was after experiencing a 40 day fast that Moses, Elijah, and Jesus were greatly empowered.[5] For Christians undertaking a fast, there are many promises from the Bible that they can claim. Several are found in the Old Testament from Isaiah Chapter 58:

> Then shall thy light break forth as the morning, and thine
> health shall spring forth speedily: and thy righteousness shall
> go before thee; the glory of the Lord shall be thy reward.
> Then shalt thou call, and the Lord shall answer; thou shalt
> cry, and he shall say, Here I *am*...then shall thy light rise in

obscurity, and thy darkness be as the noonday: And the Lord shall guide thee continually, and satisfy thy soul in drought, and make fat thy bones: and thou shalt be like a watered garden, and like a spring of water, whose waters fail not. Isaiah 58: 8,9,11. (AV 1611 KJV)

Can you see that there are many blessings promised for those who undertake a scriptural fast? There are, however, reasons that God instructs people to fast. Not just for answers to prayer "[t]o make your voice to be heard on high" (Is 58:4 KJV), but God explains why he chooses fasts:

Is not this the fast that I have chosen? To loose the bands of wickedness, to undo the heavy burdens, and to let the oppressed go free, and that ye break every yoke? Is it not to deal thy bread to the hungry, and that thou bring the poor that are cast out to thy house? When thou seest the naked, that thou cover him; and that thou hide not thyself from thine own flesh? (Is: 58:6-7 KJV)

In other words, we are also to fast to loose the chains of those in bondage to sin, to help in feeding those who are hungry, and clothing the poor. Recall that at one point, when Jesus' disciples were trying to cast out demons, they failed. When they asked him why, he told them: "Howbeit this kind goeth not out but by **prayer and fasting**." (Matt: 17:21 KJV, emphasis, mine.) Meaning that there will be times in your life that praying in itself will not get answers to prayer for you. You will have to combine it with fasting to get results. Thus we see that not only is fasting great for cleansing and detoxification, for the Christian, it also has spiritual implications as well!

There are many other instances in the Bible where great answers to prayer came as a result of fasting. Esther fasted three days and saved the Jewish people from total destruction at the hands of Haman, their adversary. Daniel fasted 21 days and received an angelic visitation in answer to his prayers. Cornelius fasted in Acts 10:30 and received an angelic visitation and answer to a prayer. Many times the Jewish people fasted, not only in response to biblical commands, but in their prayers to God for assistance or deliverance in times of great distress.

Pastor Bob Rodgers of *Evangel World Prayer Center* in Louisville, Kentucky, advocates and practices fasting on a regular basis. In his very informative book, *The 21-Day Fast,* he lists many reasons for fasting: as a way of humbling ourselves, as a means of repentance and seeking the presence of God in our lives, for God's "direction" and "enlightenment," for "deliverance," financial help, "revival...salvation" of family members, for the ministry that we are in, and to obtain "mercy and grace."[6]

In the Old Testament, fasting was even part of the law given to the Hebrews. There were special feast days in the Old Testament that required everyone to fast. Fasting was an important part of their lives, emphasized by God as an important way to come before Him in humility.

According to Tony Evans, author of *Tony Evans Speaks Out On Fasting,* "[W]hen you fast, you are desperate to satisfy a need in your soul. You are desperate to make your voice heard on high...Something unique happens when we fast. God sharpens our spiritual focus so we can see things more clearly."[7]

Not only do many people experience miracles in their lives as a result of a fast, they often reap unexpected benefits as well. Writer, Arthur Wallis explains in his book, *God's Chosen Fast:*

> What of the general physical benefits? This cleansing process usually produces, after a prolonged fast, a brightness of the eye, pure breath, clear skin and a sense of physical well-being. The digestive system should become like new. A Christian worker after only a five-day fast declared, "I feel as though I've got a brand new stomach." A digestive weakness he had had for years had disappeared.[8]

When a Baptist youth pastor embarked on a 40 day fast, he did so for many reasons, including his desire for a family. He and his wife had been unable to have a child after several years of marriage. God answered his prayers, though in an unexpected way. He and his wife were not able to have a child that was biologically theirs, but they were able to adopt a beautiful baby girl!

When a dedicated Christian bible school teacher went on a partial fast to break her daughter's drug and alcohol addiction (She could not do a total fast due to blood sugar problems), God answered her fasting and prayer by breaking her daughter's addictions and at the same time, bringing salvation to another family member.

When the pastor of a Baptist Church in New England embarked on a fast to pray for his wife who had been diagnosed with cancer, God heard his prayers and honored his fast; his wife was completely healed.

When a minister's wife was diagnosed with a very painful arterial blood vessel inflammation, she was told she would die without a corticosteroid regimen. She refused the treatment much to the dismay of her friends, though her immediate family was supportive of her. She embarked on a 21 day fast and was completely healed.

As stated earlier in this book, perhaps we need to take a lesson from the animals when they are ill. When animals are sick, "they rest, drink water and fast."[9] There are many cases of chronic illnesses being cured after a period of fasting. I know of one in particular, a woman who was completely healed of lupus after a 21 day period of prayer and fasting.

According to Steve Meyerowitz in *Wheatgrass Nature's Finest Medicine*: "Fasting gives your body a chance to re-balance its own chemistry…Fasting is the great eraser, reducing all outside influences and creating a fresh start. Fasts of 3 - 50 days have achieved many miracles."[10]

When You Should NOT Fast

There are certain situations where fasting is not recommended. As described by Dr. Don Colbert in *Toxic Relief*: women who are "pregnant or nursing" should not fast, nor should you fast if you are extremely ill, "debilitated or malnourished." Individuals with mental disorders may worsen with fasting. Those with "severe liver or kidney disease" should not fast, nor if you have "cardiac arrhythmia or congestive heart failure."[11] Children should not fast unless their physician has them on a special diet that requires they avoid certain foods or certain liquids. If you are on a water or salt-restricted diet, you should not be fasting without your physician's approval. If you've just had major surgery, you should not fast, nor should you fast if you are taking chemotherapy. You need adequate nutrients for healing. If you are awaiting a transplant, you should not be fasting, unless ordered by your physician.

Dr. Colbert explains further that he tries to "wean patients off most of their medications prior to a fast," and this has to be done slowly. Of course, there are certain medications that you should take during a fast, such as if you are taking "hormone replacement therapy and thyroid medications." If you regularly take "aspirin, anti-inflammatory medications...Coumadin, diabetic medication, antidepressants, narcotics, chemotherapy medications or diuretics, you should not fast."[12] Also, Dr. Colbert recommends that if you are contemplating a long fast, always get your physician to do "blood work and a baseline EKG." A water-only fast can cause low levels of potassium, which can result in irregular heart beat and even death. This is not usually a problem with juice-fasting, because many "fresh-squeezed juices" are abundant in potassium.[13]

Any type of fast requires large amounts of water. Realize that when you increase your water consumption, you should also **add salt**, or you may end up with a dangerous sodium deficiency, which can bring on severe weakness, arrhythmias and death. You need "1/4 tsp. of salt for every **quart** of water you drink" (non refined ocean or sea salt is best).[14] See chapter 22 of this book for more details on the importance of water drinking!

Juicing to Detoxify

Cherie Calbom and Maureen Keane in their book, *Juicing For Life,* describe juices that are good for cleansing. "...[B]eet root" juice "(no more than three ounces should be consumed the first day, but this amount can be increased gradually up to six ounces), cabbage, wheatgrass, sprouts, lemon, carrot, celery, and apple."[15] Always mix beet juice with small amounts of another juice such as celery or carrot.

Ending the Fast

Whether you go on a water-only fast or a juice-fast, you need to end the fast gradually. You can not go on an extended fast, and then begin eating a regular cooked diet the same day! Your body will protest violently. Doing so has landed many unfortunate individuals in the hospital! When you are fasting, your intestines and stomach contract. How you break the fast depends on how long the fast was and the type of fast. The longer the fast you have been on, the more time you need for ending the fast. A short fast of three days will not take nearly as long to break as a 21 day or 40 day fast! If you have been on an extended water-only fast, you can begin drinking decaffeinated teas and diluted fresh juices (not full strength), then begin introducing solids slowly into your diet over a period of days. Begin with raw fruits such as bananas, whole grain breads, broth, soups, cooked cereals, such as oatmeal, or cream of wheat and cream of rice (unless you are on a totally raw diet).

If you are breaking an extended juice-fast, you have already been taking juices, so you just need to slowly start introducing solid foods again (as above), though this fast is not as delicate to break as the water-only fast. You can begin with a breakfast of raw fruit such as bananas, and a slice of whole grain bread, a broth soup for lunch with whole grain bread, and a cooked cereal such as cream of rice for supper with a sliced banana. If you have been on a 21 day or longer fast, you will need to spend several days readjusting your body to eating solids. If you have been on a fast of 7 days or more, you still have to begin slowly introducing solids into the body. (Note: if you are going to go to a total raw foods diet, you will not be eating breads, cooked soups or cooked cereals.) Do not ruin the benefits of the fast by eating junk food and highly processed sugary foods! See the next (and final) chapter of this book: *What To Do If You Are Already Ill,* for more information on detoxification and diet. Chapter 35 is not only for those who are already ill, but for those who just want to stay healthy! It is last – but not least – **the most important chapter of this book!**

CHAPTER 35

WHAT TO DO IF YOU ARE ALREADY ILL

"For I will restore health unto thee, and I will heal thee of thy wounds, saith the Lord;"

(Jeremiah 30:17 KJV)

I. Step One: Most Important – Determine Your Destiny!

You may already be struggling against an illness, or perhaps you just want to stay well. (If you have cancer, see the cancer specific chapter in this book that would apply to the type of cancer that you have, and if you have not already done so, be sure to read that immediately.)

Our physical bodies were created by a mighty King - the Creator and King of the Universe! If you are seriously ill, you should be consulting your Creator in prayer for your recovery. If you are going to consult your Creator for your healing, where do you start? Do you know who your Creator is? Do you know God? Do you know what He has said about you and about Himself? Not only did He give you life, but He gave you the right kind of food that you need for your body to sustain itself in the very best mode of operation possible!

If you want your car to perform at maximum capacity, you feed it fuel. Start putting garbage into the gas tank and the car will sputter and die, yet this is what we sometimes do to our bodies without even realizing it. Our bodies are composed not just of flesh and blood, but soul and spirit as well! You may be fighting a deadly disease and find an alternative approach in this book that could prolong or save your life, but even if you do, you are not going to live forever in the body you are now in. You will merely prolong the life God Himself has been gracious enough to give you! Eventually, someday down the road, if Jesus delays His return, you will die just like your ancestors did, just like the rest of humanity!

Jesus Himself asked, *"For what is a man profited, if he shall gain the whole world, and lose his own soul?"(Matt: 16:26)* It is your soul that makes you unique! All your dreams, aspirations, desires, loves, hates, fears, (emotions), memories, are part of what makes up your soul. It is what makes you unique! There is only ONE of you and there will never be another person to cross this earth again exactly like YOU! You truly are special and unique! However, even if you pray for healing and you are healed, unless you have accepted God's provision for your soul, you would be better off had you never been born! Once many years ago, when I told a particular person this, their response to me was, "Don't tell me about that! I don't want to hear it! Don't tell me about being bathed in the blood." You know what I can tell you about this person? They were very foolish! God told us in the Bible that one day our own words will save us or condemn us! Can you imagine standing before God one day and having that conversation thrown up in your face?

God tells us in His Word that He is a **great King**! *(Mal. 1:14)* He rules a vast domain far beyond anything you or I could possibly imagine! His throne is encompassed with splendor, honor, majesty, beauty, justice, wisdom, and glory unimaginable by mortal man! We are told in the Book of Revelations that a rainbow encircles His throne, and that out of his throne proceeds thunder, lightning and voices. This mighty Sovereign King created everything, including you and everything that you have! Angelic beings with a splendor brighter than the sun worship and bow before Him. He made you, your loved ones, your children, the world you live in and the food that you eat every day, in spite of what you may have been told about coming from a tadpole or a monkey! Darwin himself knows by now that God exists, but it is too late for him; **don't let it be too late for you**! As long as you still have breath in you, it is not too late for you!

God is totally just and totally holy. When sin entered the world through Adam and Eve's transgression, there was no way that a holy God could justify man and be just Himself, unless…and there's the catch! There was a way! Only **one way for God to do it**! Man could only be redeemed by someone who had never transgressed the laws of God – someone completely perfect, totally pure, blameless, and willing to take our place! God Himself had to pay the price for our transgression! He incarnated His only Son into the body of a young virgin, producing the God-Man, Christ Jesus, our Messiah! Jesus was born with **God's blood in Him** because He was and is God! Not Mary's blood, not Joseph's blood, but God's blood! Pure, immortal blood! You see, Jesus could never die as long as His blood coursed through his veins! He had sinless, immortal **LIFE** in His blood! He was God in the flesh. When He was crucified by the Romans, they had no idea that the only way Jesus could die was for all of His blood to be drained from His body. As long as His eternal, sinless blood kept coursing through that beating heart of His, He could not die. Only after His precious blood had been drained from His veins through the crucifixion, did He expire! You can see the awful representation of that in the movie *The Passion,* by Mel Gibson. That same blood is physical, spiritual, immortal, and pure! When you accept Jesus' sacrifice on your behalf, a spiritual "circumcision" takes place between your body and your soul. Your sins are forever cut loose from your soul. The blood of the Lamb of God is applied to your body, soul and spirit. When you die, you are free to join God in heaven, your soul forever free from the sins that Jesus Himself paid for. You are justified by the blood of the Lamb. If you never accept God's free gift of pardon, when you die, your sins are still attached to your soul. God is holy, perfect, and just. He can not allow sin into His presence. Your soul is forever consigned to hell – a place of the **lost** – a place where your sins are a permanent part of your eternal soul. Your soul never dies, neither do you! You may look different at sixty than you do at fifteen, but inside you don't feel any different. (Apart from a few aches and pains, maybe!) Ever wonder why? That is because your soul never ages. Hell is a place that you never get out of.

Maybe you think God could never forgive you, because you think you're too far gone or that you've committed the unpardonable sin. Well, what is the unpardonable sin? The only unpardonable sin I know of is rejecting Jesus as your Savior. The apostle Paul was responsible for the murders of many Christians, yet he too repented. God forgave Him and he became one of the writers of the New Testament and God blessed him remarkably. Simon Peter lied, but he repented and God forgave him too. So what have you done that is so vile that God can not forgive you? Go to the one that bled and died for you and tell HIM that what He did wasn't enough for you. Go ahead – pay for it yourself, if you like. Don't you know – that's what all those "other" religions are doing out there? They are trying to <u>pay their own way</u> without JESUS! The Buddhists think Buddha will "save" them, but Buddha did not have immortal blood and he wasn't resurrected! Neither were any of the other prophets of the world's major religions! Their bones are still in the grave awaiting the great resurrection. The only bones that were **never found** were those belonging to Jesus. That's because all those other "gods" out there are still in the GRAVE! Jesus is alive today because He is the only one that was resurrected! He had immortal blood! You need a Savior with **pure, immortal** blood! I know that I am just a sinner saved by GRACE. I know that the One who left the throne of the universe one day, paid for me with His own BLOOD. I have gladly accepted that provision. You can do it too. And if you think you don't have enough faith to do it, ask God and He will GIVE you enough faith to do it!

Are you uncertain, confused, not sure what to do? Ask Him to reveal the truth to you. Call upon Him while there is still time! You can follow every guideline in this book and help your body stay well and perhaps recover from serious illness, but it won't do a bit of good if your soul is still black as death. If you have terminal cancer, and you are not healed, you will be meeting God face-to-face in the very near future! Think about that! Are you ready? None of us are promised tomorrow, even if we are strong and healthy! This chapter will prepare you to meet God tomorrow or twenty years from now!

Below is a suggested prayer that you can pray. Pray it aloud and mean it. It isn't "magical." God knows your heart. He'll know if you're sincere or not. Sign the page and date it. Let it be a written testimony between you and God that you have accepted His provision for your sins. We are instructed in His word: *"That if thou shalt confess with thy mouth the Lord Jesus, and shalt believe in thine heart that God hath raised him from the dead, thou shalt be saved."* (Romans 10:9-10 KJV)

Jesus, I come before you with the measure of faith that you have given me. I am sorry for all the sins I have committed, and I am willing to turn from them now and put my life in your hands! Right now, the best way I know how, I confess that you died for me and paid for all my sins with your own blood. I believe that God the Father raised you from the dead and that you are alive forevermore as my advocate and Savior. Come into my life now; cleanse me with your Holy blood! I reject my own righteousness and take yours! Change me according to your power and your will! *Amen!*

Name _____ Date_____

If you signed your name after sincerely saying the above prayer, you have taken the first and most important step to getting well! Not just physical wellness, but spiritual wellness! You should be willing to tell others that you are a new Christian, confessing it with your mouth as God requires. You should also be looking for a local Bible believing church to join, be willing to follow the Lord's example in baptism, and begin growing in faith by reading your Bible every single day.

When you visit some health food stores, you will be bombarded with new age ideas and philosophies as well as Eastern religions! As a Christian, you can claim the Blood of Jesus over your mind and body to protect you from these influences!

II. Step Two: Getting Help From High Places

As a covenant child of God, you can expect God to keep His Word to you. If you are already ill, healing is promised in His Word in many places. For example, we are told in Isaiah 53:5 that Jesus *"was wounded for our transgressions, he was bruised for our iniquities: the chastisement of our peace was upon him; and with his stripes we are healed."* There are many other verses in the Bible, too numerous to list here, where God promises healing to His people. Not only that, but there are certain avenues that you can take to increase the effectiveness of your petitions before God. Combining fasting with your prayers is one very important way, and was just discussed in greater detail in Chapter 34 of this book. When you combine prayer with fasting, something supernatural happens. Don't believe it? Then read the story of Esther in the Old Testament and the story of Daniel as well. Esther prayed and fasted three days and saved a nation! Daniel prayed and fasted 21 days and was given a panoramic view of the entire future of this world! Jesus fasted 40 days before he began His powerful ministry of miracles! There are many stories in the Bible of miracles of healing, deliverance and salvation attributed to times of prayer and fasting! As Christians, we are commanded to pray and fast at certain times. Read Isaiah 58, verses 6 - 14 for all the terrific promises from God that you can claim when you fast, including the **restoration of your health!**

There are many ways that you can expect blessings from God. If you are tithing to your local church, God promises to *"...open you the windows of heaven, and pour you out a blessing, that there shall not be room enough to receive it." (Mal. 3:10)* Are you a tither?

We are also promised a blessing if we help feed and clothe the poor, for *"...he that hath mercy on the poor, happy is he* (Prov. 14:21.) and *"He that hath pity upon the poor lendeth unto the Lord; and that which he hath given will he pay him again."* (Prov. 19:17.) Have you been told by your physician that your condition is hopeless? Terminal? Read the first half of Psalm 41! If you have been helping the poor, you can claim those verses! If you haven't been helping the poor, then start doing it so that you CAN claim those verses! *"Blessed is he that considereth the poor: The Lord will deliver him in time of trouble. The Lord **will preserve him, and keep him alive**; and he shall be blessed upon the earth: and thou wilt not deliver him unto the will of his enemies. "* (Psalm 41:1-2)

Do you support your local church's missions? Have you done anything lately to help someone less fortunate than yourself? Are you a giver, or a miser?

III. Step Three: Learn the Language of Heaven

There is another avenue of gaining power in your prayer life that is sadly overlooked by many Christians in today's world. I believe it is possibly the most powerful avenue of all when it comes to getting God's attention, and that is through **PRAISE and WORSHIP**! Ask yourself this: how much time did you spend **today** worshipping God? Yesterday? This week? This month? Your entire life?

Did you know that our God is a God who desires our worship? Think about it! Why do you think you were created? What do you think your purpose is in this life and the next? I can tell you in one word – WORSHIP! You were made to worship God! Stand still right now; put your arms down at your sides, then raise up both arms toward the sky with hands and fingers straight. Your fingers point straight up toward the heavens, like arrows where God is! God desires that you lift your hands up toward heaven to exalt and worship Him! You have a voice to sing with, lungs to breathe with. You were made to worship and sing to God! Do you drive back and forth to work every day? Then you have time to worship God! Get a worship DVD and sing along with it, or sing without one! It will change your life! (I guarantee you, if everyone in your town or city would do this there would be no such thing as crime or *road rage, ever!*) Your whole body is a temple made to worship God!

What can you possibly give God that He hasn't first given YOU? Can you give Him wealth, riches, joy, purpose, strength, love, beauty, talent, power, wisdom, creativity, generosity, compassion, benevolence? There is absolutely nothing that you can give God that doesn't already belong to Him. When you contemplate just for a moment all that He has done for you (He gave you LIFE!), the enormity of it is overwhelming. There is nothing left for you to do, but to worship Him! He is worthy! He has angelic beings that stand before Him singing endless praises to Him, songs of adoration and worship, yet He still desires *your worship!* And never be led to believe that God does not care for you as an individual. Believe me, God is BIG ENOUGH to go around! He has time for you! He knows every thought you will think tomorrow before you even get up in the morning! He has numbered the hairs of your head. You are precious to Him!

Worship is the language of heaven. We are given a glimpse of God's throne room in the Book of Revelations when John is caught up into heaven in chapter four. It is a noisy place! There are thunderings, voices, lightnings, shouts, and songs of praise filling God's throne room! I am happy to say that the church I belong to has a powerful worship service, and when I visit relatives (such as a favorite sister in Texas) I attend a church there with a powerful worship service too! I can barely sing a tune, but I still like to sing.

The first time I ever went on a 21 day juice-fast, God gave me a song. I mean, He literally gave me a song! I have written poetry before, but never a song! The gist of my musical training was about 18 months of piano lessons beginning when I was twelve-years-old, so writing music was no easy task for me! I had forgotten nearly everthing I learned since then! However, you don't have to sing like a bird to sing in God's presence. He says in *Psalm 66:1: "Make a joyful noise unto God, all ye lands. Sing forth the honour of his name: make his praise glorious."* Can you make a joyful **noise**? Have you ever been in a church service where the people around you acted like they were fearful of lifting their arms during the worship and praising God audibly? They need to be educated about worship, or you might want to find a church that isn't afraid to physically worship God!

I am amazed that so many people (even those who call themselves *Christians),* can attend ball games, car races and golf outings, and they will jump up and down, stomp their feet, scream at the top of their lungs, wave their hands frantically, and shout for joy when their team scores, but get them in the worship service Sunday morning and they are blank, empty, silent, staring, spectacles of gloomy inhibition when it comes to glorifying their Creator! Suggest to them that they raise or clap their hands and shout to God and they will look at you like you just crawled out from under a dark rock for even suggesting such a thing!

There are many ways that the Bible gives us to worship God. You can worship Him through singing (the most common form of worship), through playing stringed instruments, with shouts of praise, by clapping your hands while you are singing, leaping before the Lord, and through the dance, such as David did when the Ark of God was returned to Jerusalem. Worship is noisy! Make a joyful NOISE when you come in God's presence! If you recall, David's wife, Michal, was filled with contempt when she saw him singing loudly and dancing about, and she accused him of making a fool of himself. David rebuked her, telling her he was dancing to please God, not the crowd! (II Sam. 6:20)

Throughout the entire Bible, it was very common for people to worship God by singing psalms to Him. Most of the psalms in the Old Testament were written by King David himself, and you can be certain, that he sang them out before God! David was a man after God's own heart, primarily because he was a **worshipper!**

What about you? Are you a worshipper? Do you get to church late to miss half the worship service because you don't think it's important? It is critical for you to realize, as a Christian, that God desires you to worship Him not only in the congregation of saints, but privately in your own home as well. When popular pastor, evangelist, Darlene Bishop was a guest speaker at our church, she said that God explained to her that He lives, moves, and operates within the atmosphere of WORSHIP. He BREATHES in praise and worship, like you and I inhale oxygen!

Dr. Norvel Hayes, a successful businessman, author, teacher, preacher and worshipper of God, believes that the most important time we spend in worship, is the time that we spend alone with God when no one else but God sees us. Dr. Hayes explains in his book *Worship — Your Foundation For the Victorious Life,* that God revealed to him that He has made a worship covenant with the human race:

> God said, "I will give anybody on earth who worships Me and praises My name whatever they want, because they have made Me their God...I would like for every country, city, church, home, and every individual person on earth to make a covenant with Me to worship Me."[1]

Are you seeking healing from God? Are you a woman who is trying to have a child and you are still childless? Try worshipping God! Then, bring your petition before God for a child, after you have spent daily time in worship! God always tests us to see how sincere we are. He isn't your personal vending machine. You don't just murmur a few words to Him, praise a few minutes, then – *presto* – you get your *wish*! You may spend eight months or a year worshipping him and praying before Him for a certain request before you see results. Are you being obedient to His Word? Are you tithing as He commanded (in both the Old and New Testament)? Are you doing what you can to help those Christians who are less fortunate than yourself? Are you fasting, praying and seeking God? Are you a worshipper? Are you a Christian who isn't afraid to tell someone else about Jesus?

It amazes me how many people who claim to be Christians never darken the door of their local church; never give a dime to help the needy; balk at the thought of tithing their income; would rather die than fast for one meal; watch T.V. for two or more hours a day – then claim they haven't time for prayer or for church; cringe at the thought of any sort of open expression of praise and worship to God; then come and ask **you** to pray for them because they need healing, all the while expecting God to give them a miracle and heal them when they haven't obeyed a single thing that Jesus commanded of them! Remember, God isn't demanding perfection from any of us. He knows the framework of our bodies – that we are just clay, but He also knows what we are capable of! As His creation, we are to worship God with all of our hearts and with our lives. His word tells us that *"Whoso offereth praise glorifieth me;"* (Ps. 50:23). We are also to worship Him with our thoughts. What's on your mind during your free time? As you are falling asleep at night? Do you allow your thoughts to roam uncontrollably? Do you want peace of mind? Try worshipping God with your thoughts! Exalt Him, think about Him, memorize his Words and think on them, for He promises: *"Thou wilt keep him in perfect peace, whose mind is stayed on Thee: because he trusteth in thee."(Isa 26:3.)* Keep your mind on God and <u>you won't lose it</u>!

You may argue that you have no idea HOW to worship God. Well, here is a good way to get started! Take each of the verses below and memorize one of them every day until you know them all by heart. Memorize them by SINGING them!

Sing unto him, sing psalms unto him, talk ye of all his wondrous works. (I Chron. 16:9)

Let us lift up our heart with our hands unto God in the heavens (Lamentations 3:41)

O give thanks unto the Lord; for he is good; because his mercy endureth forever. (Ps 118:1)

O clap your hands all ye people; shout unto God with the voice of triumph. (Ps 47:1)

In God we boast all the day long, and praise thy name forever...(Ps. 44:8)

Thus will I bless thee while I live: I will lift up my hands in thy name. (Ps. 63:4)

Thou art my God, and I will praise thee: thou art my God, I will exalt thee.(Ps. 118:28)

Great is the Lord, and greatly to be praised; and his greatness is unsearchable. (Ps. 145:3)

Every day will I bless thee; and I will praise thy name forever and ever. (Ps. 145:2)

Heal me, O Lord, and I shall be healed; save me, and I shall be saved; for thou art my praise. (Jer. 17:14)

...Blessed be the name of God for ever and ever: for wisdom and might are his. (Daniel 2:20)

I will praise thee: for thou hast heard me, and art become my salvation. (Ps. 118:21)

Or, if you would rather, just pick a psalm such as *Psalm 149* and memorize it. It is only nine verses, or *Psalm 150*, which is only six verses. There is even a promise from God you can claim when you are worshipping Him! It is Psalm 37:4: *Delight thyself also in the Lord; and he shall give thee the desires of thine heart.*

According to Dr. Norvel Hayes, author of *Worship – Your Foundation For the Victorious Life,* if you learn to be a worshipper of God, you will never go hungry! He explains why: "The Lord God said to me, 'Since I made Adam, there has never been one human being on earth who has ever starved to death for lack of food while they were on their knees worshipping Me and praising My name.'"[2] Think about that! It is very profound! Are you hungry or do you know someone who is? Who are they worshipping? Who is their God? Are they worshipping the true God, or idols?

God actually desires and seeks your worship! As described by Terry Law in his book: *The Power of Praise and Worship*: "It is an exciting, even an amazing fact, that **God is seeking for people to worship Him**. The very fact that God can be worshipped provides an incredible opportunity for each one of us."[3]

IV. Health & Healing From God

God sometimes heals instantly, other times, He heals gradually, but either way, He expects you to cooperate with Him in your healing! If you are praying to Him to heal you of some disease, such as cancer, you need to be doing your part! If God has healed you and you go back to eating fast-food burgers and fries every day and a very unhealthy lifestyle, don't expect to maintain your good health! You have to do your part in staying healthy! Praise God that He has more compassion on us than we sometimes have on each other! He is very forgiving, but He requires accountability and responsibility on our part. If you want healthy kids, feed them a healthy diet. Reach them with good nutrition while they are small, so it will stick when they are teenagers. I made the mistake of researching alternative health and nutrition when my child was already a teenager. Try to convince a teen to eat a nutritious diet! They already know everything, so you are wasting your time!

Our society has become a fast-food, package-crazed society, not caring, nor thinking about what we ingest. We let our tastes enslave us. God did not design all the "dead foods" that clutter our modern supermarket shelves and beckon us from the fast-food drive-throughs! Nor did He ever intend that we give these items to our children. He has already provided for us exactly what we need in the most natural, nutritious form possible! There is an old expression which says that we spend the first half of our lives acquiring wealth and the second half using our wealth to regain our health! How many of us have spent twenty or more years living on "dead foods" only to wind up complaining that we are beset with arthritis, gout, diabetes, high blood pressure, fatigue, coronary artery disease, poor circulation, and migraine headaches, yet we continue to live this way and wonder why we can't get well, feel better, or get more energy! (Note that some GOOD foods do get packaged, such as potatoes, onions, some fruits such as bags of oranges and apples, fiber breads and frozen fruits, so all "packaged" foods are not bad. Even fresh sprouts that you purchase in a health food store may be packaged, as well as frozen cubes of wheat grass juice, etc.)

Only **live** food has the **enzymes** already within it that enables you to digest it. If you take a raw vegetable like an onion with the roots still attached and put it in the ground, it will sprout and live. Cook it, then put it in the ground and it will rot. Why? Because, once cooked, you have destroyed all the life in the vegetable and it is dead! It no longer has within it the living enzymes needed for the body to digest it. Thus, your body will have to produce the enzymes to digest it — a taxing process on your entire digestive system. Not only that, cooked food moves through the bowels sluggishly, fermenting on the way. Raw food moves through the bowels much swifter, it's roughage acting as a broom to sweep out the colon along the way. Researchers are finally realizing that a diet high in fat and low in fiber (i.e. cooked vs. raw food) contributes to cancer. This is because bodily wastes that move slowly through the intestines have time to release toxins back into the body, causing illness, eventually leading to the breakdown of the immune system, auto immune disorders, and other problems.

We drown our meals with carbonated pop or water, and wonder why we can't digest our food, when what we have done, in fact, is to neutralize all the hydrochloride acid in the stomach that was intended to digest the food. It is best not to take fluids with meals. There will be exceptions to this. For example, if you are taking vitamin/mineral supplements with your meals, you will need enough fluids in order to swallow them.

V. Where To Start? Healthy Tips

There are no "quick-fixes" for optimal health, but the very first thing that you need to do is to purchase a good quality **juicer**! By the time you've gotten this far in this book, you should already have a pretty good idea which juicer you are going to purchase (if you don't already have one). Once you've done that, you are ready to begin. Below is a recipe for a tea mix that is used in the 21 day detox program described later in this chapter. This tea mix is a recipe that I blended about a year ago, because I liked the variety of herbs used. (You will end up with about seven cups of DRY ingredients once blended.) If you want a smaller amount, use half the ingredients given for ½ the recipe.

As noted earlier, be sure to discuss any new herbal tea such as this with your physician before beginning. You want to be sure you will not be ingesting anything that may be incompatible with prescription medications you are taking. You also want to be sure that you do not have a chronic disease or condition that may negate the use of herbal preparations.

Alphabet Tea

Combine the following DRY herbal ingredients in a large glass or polycarbonate jar with a reclosable, sealing lid. You will need a large jar to be able to mix and combine the contents of this tea unless you cut the amount in half for a smaller amount. Obtain these ingredients from your local herbal supplier or natural health food store. This tea should last you several weeks, depending on how many times a day you drink it. It is also part of the 21 day detox program below. (Be sure to consult with your physician about using this or any other herbal blend if you have a blood disorder, are on prescription medications, are pregnant or nursing, a transplant patient, or have any type of chronic health problems. Do not give to children without first consulting with their physician! Do not use if you have allergies to any of the ingredients.) I use a large glass jar, put the ingredients inside, close the lid and shake them all together for about five minutes to get them mixed well.

- ½ cup dried **alfalfa leaf** (omit this ingredient if you have lupus!)
- ¼ cup dried **astragalus tea** (decaffeinated)*
- ¼ cup dried **cat's claw** tea or purchase the herb in bulk (decaffeinated) (I buy the tea bags and cut them open until I have ¼ cup total)* (see note below)

- ¼ cup dried **dandelion** leaf
- ¼ cup dried **dandelion** root
- ½ cup dried **Enchinacea purpura**
- ¼ cup dried **ginkgo** leaf
- ¼ cup dried **golden ginger**
- 1 cup dried **green tea** (decaffeinated)
- ¼ cup dried **hyssop**
- ¼ cup **kelp granules** (check with your Dr. first if you have thyroid problems before using kelp!)
- ½ cup dried **milk thistle seed**
- ½ cup dried **orange peel**
- ¼ cup dried **Pau D'Arco** bark
- ¼ cup dried **peppermint**
- ½ cup dried **red clover**
- ½ cup dried **rose hips**
- ¼ cup dried **spearmint**
- ¼ cup dried **yellow dock root**

*Do not use cat's claw herb if you have an "autoimmune illness, multiple sclerosis, and tuberculosis. European practitioners avoid combining this herb with hormonal drugs, insulin or vaccines." Do not take if you are "pregnant" or breastfeeding.[4] Also, avoid astragalus during an active infectious process.[5] (Do not use any caffeinated teas. They act as diuretics in the body.) When you make the tea, you can also add herbs such as celery seed or dill to taste if desired.

When you make an 8 oz. cup of tea, you will be using two teaspoons of the *Alphabet Tea* blend. Use a stainless steel tea ball and put two teaspoons of the dried tea mixture that you blended inside the tea ball and put the tea ball into the cup. Then pour 8 oz. of boiling water over the tea ball and let it steep until it gets cool. (Or drink when still warm if you prefer warm tea.) Add a squeeze of lemon to taste if you like, and ½ tsp of royal jelly to sweeten. Put the royal jelly in the tea while it is still **hot** so that it will dissolve. (Remember, do not give honey and other bee products to children under two. Also, some individuals are allergic to bee products.) This tea is very detoxifying and rich in antioxidants.

Nutrient Supplements – Why Do We Need Them?

Most people do not get the amount of vitamins and minerals they need in their daily diet, especially in this fast-paced society in which we live. You should consider taking a potent multiple vitamin/mineral supplement daily, such as the *OLA LOA™* varieties, found in health food stores, or a mineral drink such as *Mineral Rich®,* marketed by Maureen Kennedy Salaman. You can find *Mineral Rich®* at her website *www.mksalaman.com.* It is a form of minerals in a good tasting, easily absorbable liquid. Some natural health food stores also carry *Mineral Rich®* and *OLA LOA™.*

If you are already fighting cancer, a *suggested* list of supplements is given below. As always, you should be discussing this with your physician. You may wish to incorporate some or all of these items into your diet. (They should be taken with meals unless otherwise indicated.) Though you normally would not drink large amounts of liquids with your meals, you will need to swallow enough liquid to get the supplements down.) Do NOT use pills. Always use capsules or gel-tabs whenever possible! A great deal of heat is used in compressing pills, destroying much of the nutritive value. The only exception to this would be the small chlorella pills found in some chlorella products. Also, during much of the 21 day detox program described later, you will not be taking supplements, except for your CoQ10, chlorella, topical progesterone cream (for women), apricot seeds (laetrile) and/or Haelan if you choose to use them, Graviola (if you choose to use it), milk thistle, alpha lipoic acid (if you have liver cancer), as well as any prescription medications you regularly take if the detox has been cleared with your physician. Also, during the 21 day detox, feel free to use liquid vitamin and mineral supplements daily such as *Ola Loa™* or *Mineral Rich®.* Or, if you purchase any other type of liquid vitamin-mineral preparation, these can be taken during the 21 day detox as well as the liberal use of green drinks like wheat grass juice or barley green juice. You will receive many vitamins and minerals in the juices you will be taking after day three of the fast. Regardless, I don't advise taking large amounts of supplements on an empty stomach. As explained earlier, you should always consult with your physician before beginning a new regimen such as this one, or before undertaking a detoxification program, regardless of your health status.

Suggested Supplement List

•   *Alpha lipoic acid* – 100 mg in the morning and 100 mg in the afternoon. (If you already have liver cancer or hepatitis, 200 mg. three times daily.)

•   *Apricot kernels* if you are fighting cancer – (As described by Maureen Kennedy Salaman earlier) "one kernal for every ten pounds of body weight."[6] If you weigh 120 pounds, 12 kernels daily. If you weigh 150 pounds, 15 kernels daily, etc). You may even want to consider laetrile supplements, which are discussed elsewhere in this book.

•   *Bee Pollen capsules* (if you are not allergic to bees or bee stings) 300 mg. capsules three times daily (morning, noon, and evening = total of 900 mg. daily)

•   *Beta-carotene* – if you drink several glasses daily of fresh carrot juice (and green drinks), you will be getting plenty of beta-carotene, as well as calcium. If not, you will need to supplement with both!

•   *Borage oil* – 1000 mg. daily

•   *CoQ10* – 100 mg. per day – (if you already have invasive cancer, 200 mg. twice a day for a total of 400 mg. daily) Begin with 50 mg twice a day, then gradually work up to 400 mg as noted.

•   *Chlorella* – If you already have cancer: 1 – 2 grams daily. (Take on empty stomach.)

•   Don't forget your daily dose of *vitamin D* from the sun, and you should be drinking several glasses a day of carrot and green juices to provide you with sufficient calcium, beta-carotene, and vitamin A (via the beta-carotene)

• *Flaxseed oil* – if using the liquid, take 1-2 tablespoons daily. (You will use more daily, if following the Budwig diet!)

• *Folic acid sublingual* – 400-800 **micrograms** daily.

• *Garlic* (aged garlic) such as Kyolic (if taking the liquid form, take one teaspoon morning, noon, and evening). Also, use fresh garlic liberally in your food.

• *Ginkgo biloba* – 50 mg twice daily.

• *Grapeseed extract* – 100 mg. per day. (Ok to take 50 mg twice daily)

• *Green drinks* – use liberally, such as 1-2 oz. of wheatgrass juice or 1-3 servings of barley juice, *Green Miracle*, or Kamut, or as directed on the product you choose. If you already have cancer, you may want to gradually work up to taking 6 oz. – 8 oz. of fresh wheat grass daily. If you have leukemia, you may also want to gradually work up to taking 6-8 oz. of fresh beet juice (from the root, not the green tops) daily from your juicer, but always mix a small amount of another juice with it. The 21 day detox uses wheat grass juice daily. You can take more as tolerated.

• *Green tea* – if you already have cancer, several cups of green tea daily (decaffeinated). If you can not tolerate drinking tea, use green tea (standardized) extract supplements 200 mg twice daily

• *L-Lysine* – 2 grams daily only if you already have cancer. Lysine is sometimes used to treat genital herpes outbreaks, as well as the herpes virus that causes shingles and fever blisters. It is also used for canker sores. With this amino acid, you should also be taking L-proline and L-arginine supplements. The L-proline and L-arginine can be up to one gram daily if you already have cancer. (Do not use the arginine if you have herpes! Do not take lysine if you are on antibiotics.)

• *Maitake-D-Fraction* – you may want to add this mushroom supplement to your daily diet if you are fighting cancer!

• *Milk Thistle* herbal supplement – 175 mg. daily (standardized). (However, if you have been diagnosed with liver cancer, prostate cancer, colon cancer, or hepatitis, a suggested amount is 150 mg. in the morning, afternoon and evening for a total of 450 mg. daily). Be sure it is *standardized* to contain at least 80% silymarin. Take this supplement on an empty stomach. If you work around heavy pesticides, heavy metals, with lead, cadmium, radiation, or mercury, you may want to begin supplementing with milk thistle (and alpha lipoic acid) to protect your liver! (See chapter 8.)

• *Multi-mineral* – as directed on the supplement you purchase (most of these will require that you take two to three capsules per day); or you may wish to choose a powdered nutrient drink that is mixed with water or juice, such as *Ola Loa™*. (*Ola Loa™* has great tasting vitamin and mineral drinks.) Mineral Rich® also tastes great and is in liquid form. You can find Mineral Rich® at *www.mksalaman.com*. *Ola Loa™* is in most health food stores.

• *Natural Progesterone Cream* (for **women** – see chapter 21 for directions!) This chapter will also tell you when you should **not** use this cream. Note that it is sometimes used by men.

• *Probiotics* – a formula such as HSOs, discussed in chapter five of this book or acidophilus 3-6 billion natural flora **between meals**, 2-3 times daily (Some of the green powdered drinks provide beneficial bacteria such as acidophilus).

• *Quercetin* – take as directed on the brand that you purchase.

• *Selenium* – If you already have cancer, 100 *micrograms* twice a day for a total of 200 *micrograms.* Take 100 micrograms once a day if you do not have cancer.

• *Turmeric* – 100 mg capsules 3 times per day (Do not take turmeric if you have gallstones, other gallbladder biliary problems, ulcers, or if you are on anti-coagulant medications.)[7] Discuss with your physician.

• **Multi-B vitamin** (vegetarian formula) as directed on the supplement you choose. When purchasing a B-complex capsule, try to get one that is "balanced-B" and "timed-release," for example: balanced B-100. This B-complex should have all the B-vitamins including riboflavin, biotin, thiamine, and pantothenic acid. If you choose a multi-vitamin, be sure it includes vitamin K.

• **Vitamin B-3 (Niacin)** Start with 50 mg. daily. However, if you already have cancer, you may wish to consider Dr. Hoffer's regimen earlier in this book. He used 1000 mg of niacin (and 1000 mg of vitamin C) after meals for many of his cancer patients. If so, you would start with 50 mg niacin and build up to 100 mg, then 200 mg, then 300 mg. and up to 1000 mg niacin. Discuss this first with your physician, especially if you have any type of liver cancer or liver/gallbladder disorders. You may want to seek the advice of a licensed Naturopathic Physician because some conventional medicine doctors are against any type of megavitamin therapy for cancer. If you do not choose to take the higher doses of B-3, then the balanced B-complex capsule you will be taking should already contain niacin. (Remember that niacin will give you a flush. If you take it in the form of niacinamide, it won't.) The flush opens up all your capillaries and is actually GOOD for you, but isn't particularly pleasant. If you already have cancer, you may find it difficult to tolerate, in which case, you will want niacinamide instead. Don't use the timed-release capsules. Do not take niacin if you are running a fever, it will make you feel even warmer. Also, remember that in taking larger doses of one B vitamin, it can cause deficiencies in the other B vitamins. This is another reason that your vitamin regimen (if megadose) should be regulated by your licensed Naturopathic Physician.

• **Vitamin B-12** sublingual — 500 **micrograms** daily.

• **Vitamin C** (with bioflavanoids) – At LEAST 1000 mg. morning, noon and night (total of 3000 mg per day – after meals.) If you are already diagnosed with cancer, (especially lymphoma, leukemia, or Hodgkins disease), see chapters 7 and 15 in this book, because you may want to consider taking larger doses of vitamin C! If doing so, choose a buffered vitamin C to prevent stomach upset, or use Ester C.

You may also want to consider pursuing vitamin C intravenous therapy from a Naturopathic licensed health care Physician.

• *Vitamin E* – 400 (IU) international units daily (preferably d-alpha tocopherol), and 500 mg daily of lecithin (many of these are available in gelcaps).

• *Spirulina* – If you already have cancer: 1 – 2 grams daily (Take on empty stomach.)

• DO NOT take iron supplements unless your physician already has you on them. Do not purchase multi-vitamin or mineral preparations that contain iron.

This sounds like a lot of supplements, however, you will be able to find combination supplements in some health food stores that may give you ten of these different items in one or two capsules. If you are already fighting cancer, you may want to add herbs and nutrients found in cancer specific chapters in this book, for example, Graviola if you have prostate or abdominal cancer, or Haelan fermented soy drink if you are fighting breast cancer. Haelan is always taken on an empty stomach for maximum absorption (see chapter three of this book). You may want to do a parasite cleanse first, with Dr. Clark's herbs for removing parasites (in chapter 27). You will also want to be sure that you are getting lutein and lycopene on a daily basis. There are multiple vitamin supplements in health food stores that now contain these two nutrients. Check the labels before you purchase. You may certainly want to use spirulina every day if you have mouth cancer, gymnema sylvestre if you have diabetes, and molybdenum to help prevent esophageal cancer, (especially if you have a history of smoking) or some of the many mushroom supplements mentioned in this book. Most multi-vitamin/mineral supplements will contain molybdenum. Some of the green drinks that you can purchase will have minerals, beta-carotene, calcium, quercetin, chlorella, ginkgo, B-vitamins, selenium, and probiotics, so you won't need to purchase the items separately. Some mushroom supplements contain a large variety of different mushrooms.

Liver Flush

The following is a liver tonic recipe of mine that I use occasionally for its detoxification and nutrition value. (It is also found in chapter eight.)

Juice the following RAW organic items in your juicer:

- 2 medium carrots
- 3 medium tomatoes
- Small bunch of parsley
- ¼ sweet green or red pepper (also add the seeds to the juicer)
- 1 medium beet
- 2-3 kale or collard leaves
- 6-12 spinach leaves
- 1 large celery stalk
- 1/2 small red or yellow onion
- Small bunch of cilantro
- ¼ tspn grated ginger (optional)
- ¼ tspn grated lemon peel

To the finished juice add 1 tbspn lemon juice, ½ tspn of turmeric (do not use turmeric if you have "gallstones," biliary disorders, or[8] ulcers), 1 tbspn flax oil, ¼ tspn cayenne pepper (optional, as tolerated), 1 crushed garlic clove, and one serving of a green powder such as chlorella, barley, or kamut (or 1 oz. fresh wheat grass juice if available). Add 3-4 oz. of water to dilute, only if desired. Mix well with the juice and drink. This drink is very nutritious, and detoxifying. (Be aware that some of the ingredients in this flush have blood-thinning properties.)

Raw Super Salad

This is a tasty salad that can be used once you have come off the 21 – day detox program given later in this chapter. Be aware that, as with any long fast, you must break your fast slowly, never all at once!

Combine the following fresh, raw, organic ingredients. (Use the cabbage, lettuce and spinach leaves in equal amounts as closely as possible.) Note that after you break your fast on the 21 – day detox program, the first time you use this salad, you will use a smaller amount of the cabbage, lettuce and spinach leaves. When you begin, use only a few ounces of the cabbage, romaine lettuce and spinach leaves. The first time or two that you eat it, you should eat approximately one cup of the salad, then later, two cups and finally work up to three cups.

Purple cabbage

Romaine lettuce

Spinach leaves

Small broccoli and cauliflower florets

Fresh sprouts (use liberally! Do not use alfalfa sprouts if you have lupus!)

Chopped celery

Sprig of parsley, dill & chives (fresh is best if available, rather than dried)

Diced cucumber & radishes

2 tablespoons combined sunflower seeds, pine nuts, and slivered almonds

¼ of a small chopped red or yellow onion

Tomato slices (or diced)

Chopped sweet green peppers (or red)

Small handful of pumpkin seeds

Thin slices of summer squash and carrots

½ small avocado sliced

Dressing:

2-3 tablespoons flax oil

Grated fresh ginger to taste (optional)

1 teaspoon curcumin (turmeric) do not use if you have gallbladder problems[9] or ulcers

1 tablespoon sesame seeds

1 clove garlic, diced very fine or crushed

Juice from fresh lemon and lime to taste
Sea salt to taste
Small sprinkle of kelp flakes*
¼ teaspoon grated lemon rind
Cayenne pepper (optional)
Apple cider vinegar to taste (optional), however, if using, purchase raw, unpasteurized apple cider vinegar from a reliable natural health food store.

Do not use kelp if you have thyroid problems without first checking with your physician!

Power Seed Mixture

This power seed mix can be used once you have advanced off your juice-fast. *Combine the following: (use organic products as much as possible. Do not use salted nuts or sulfured products!)* Mix all the ingredients thoroughly and refrigerate unused portion.

½ cup raisins
½ cup sunflower seeds
½ cup sesame seeds
1 cup almonds
½ cup walnuts
½ cup pecans
½ cup pine nuts
¼ cup pistachios
1 cup Brazil nuts
1 cup unsalted pumpkin seeds
½ cup red-skinned peanuts
4 dried calmyra figs, chopped
1-2 dried papaya slices
2 dried dates, chopped

(Serving size is ½ - ¾ cup.)

VI. Detoxification

Each day you should be drinking half your body weight in OUNCES of water (unless your physician has you on a special water-restricted or salt-restricted diet). For example, if you weigh 200 pounds, you need 100 ounces of water per day! If you weigh 120 pounds, you need at least 60 ounces of water per day.[10] In the 21 day detox program described below, you can count most of the juices taken on day 8 through 21 as part of your daily water quota, but you can also use water liberally and should do so unless your physician has you on a specific diet. Also feel free to drink extra servings of green tea, or green juices, if desired.

"For every 10 glasses of water...one should add to the diet about half a teaspoon of salt per day..."[11] (Based on 8 ounce glasses.) Obtain sun-dried sea salt from your local health food store for the best salt to use!

If you have diabetes or other chronic diseases, blood disorders, are pregnant or breastfeeding, or are taking prescription medications, do not attempt this detox program (or any type of fasting program) without first consulting with your physician! You should also be praying about it and seeking the Lord's leading. The first week of this program is partly based on Johanna Brandt's *The Grape Cure* diet. The first 3 days is a water-only fast; time to combine your prayers with fasting (and praise!) The only exception to this is Essiac. If you already have cancer, take 2 oz. of an Essiac tea such as *Resperin* Essiac® morning and night, every day, even during the first 7 days below. (See chapter five for more information on Essiac tea.) Be aware, of course, that the program below is going to vary with your own daily schedule. Times given are approximated. If arising earlier or later in the day, you will need to adjust the times accordingly. The chart is based on a beginning date as a Monday. Your times will be different on your days off.

If you can not get fruit in season, you can always substitute FROZEN fruit, but do not use anything canned. Be certain that the water you are using does not contain chlorine or fluoride! When drinking the juices, sip them slowly, holding them in your mouth for a few seconds before swallowing. Always use ORGANIC produce when possible! (If you are working, you will be able to mix most of the fresh juice drinks that you need either that morning or the night before work (kept in regrigerator). However, if at all possible, it is best to drink most fresh juices within ten minutes of the time that they are juiced. You never want to let fresh wheat grass juice sit overnight. Obviously, this won't always be feasible, unless you have an office setting where you are allowed to bring in your juicer. Fresh carrot juice should not be saved longer than two days in the refrigerator. For those who are already ill and unable to work, you may need to rely on family members to help with your juicing until you are stronger. Of course, anyone who is severely ill needs to consult with their physician before beginning any type of detoxification diet and fast, including this one. Many times, those who are severely ill can not tolerate raw foods only.

The sample detox program below uses a lot of beet juice, green juices and fresh fruit and vegetable juices. If you have not already done so, read the information on high-oxalate foods in chapter three of this book before beginning a detox regimen. You can avoid problems with excess oxalates simply by being sure that you are getting plenty of fluids, B-vitamins and magnesium every day.

Sample 21 - Day Detox Program

First week:

	Day 1	Day 2	Day 3	Day 4	Day 5	Day 6	Day 7
	Fast Day - Water Only (if you already have cancer, take 2 oz. Essiac tea when you first get up)	*Same as Day 1*	*Same as day 1*	*Same as day 1*	*Water, Fruit & Juices Today*	*Water, Fruit & Juices Today*	*Water, Fruit and Juices Today*
6am-6:30	*The first 10 minutes is Scripture reading, then 10 minutes of praise & worship, then 10 minutes of prayer.*	*Same as day 1*	*Same as day 1*	*Same as day 1 - except drink 8 oz. of fresh grape juice from your juicer this morning (or you can eat a large handful of fresh grapes)*	*Same as day 4*	*Same as day 4 (If you are off on weekends, you will need to adjust times accordingly)*	*Same as day 4 (If you are off on weekends, you will need to adjust times accordingly)*
6:30 AM	*Time to prepare physically for your day! This time may vary for you.*	*Same as day 1*	*Same as day 1*	*Same as day 1*	*Same as day 1*	*Same as day 1*	*Same as day 1*
7:00 AM	*This may be your work travel time. Sing to God on your way to work!*	*Same as day 1*	*Same as day 1*	*Same as day 1*	*Same as day 1*	*Same as day 1*	*Same as day 1*
8:00 AM	*Fast Day - Water Only*	*Fast Day - Water Only*	*Fast Day - Water Only*	*8 oz. of fresh grape juice from your juicer (or you can eat a large handful of fresh grapes)*	*Same as day 4*	*Same as day 4*	*Same as day 4*
9:00 AM	*Fast Day - Water Only*	*Fast Day - Water Only*	*Fast Day - Water Only*	*Remember to be taking sufficient water & salt!*	*Remember to be taking sufficient water & salt!*	*Remember to be taking sufficient water & salt!*	*Remember to be taking sufficient water & salt!*

First week: Continued

	Day 1	Day 2	Day 3	Day 4	Day 5	Day 6	Day 7
10:00 AM	*Fast Day - Water Only*	*Fast Day - Water Only*	*Fast Day - Water Only*	*8 oz. of fresh grape juice from your juicer or you can eat a large handful of fresh grapes*	*Same as day 4*	*Same as day 4*	*Same as day 4*
11:00 AM	*Fast Day - Water Only*	*Fast Day - Water Only*	*Fast Day - Water Only*	*Remember to be taking sufficient water & salt!*	*Remember to be taking sufficient water & salt!*	*Remember to be taking sufficient water & salt!*	*Remember to be taking sufficient water & salt!*
12:00 Noon	*Fast Day - Water Only*	*Fast Day - Water Only*	*Fast Day - Water Only*	*8 oz. of fresh grape juice from your juicer or you can eat a large handful of fresh grapes*	*Same as day 4*	*Same as day 4*	*Same as day 4*
1:00 PM	*Fast Day - Water Only*	*Fast Day - Water Only*	*Fast Day - Water Only*	*Remember to be taking sufficient water & salt!*	*Remember to be taking sufficient water & salt!*	*Remember to be taking sufficient water & salt!*	*Remember to be taking sufficient water & salt!*
2:00 PM	*Fast Day - Water Only*	*Fast Day - Water Only*	*Fast Day - Water Only*	*8 oz. of fresh grape juice from your juicer or you can eat a large handful of fresh grapes*	*Same as day 4*	*Same as day 4*	*Same as day 4*
3:00 PM	*Fast Day - Water Only*	*Fast Day - Water Only*	*Fast Day - Water Only*	*Remember to be taking sufficient water & salt!*	*Remember to be taking sufficient water & salt!*	*Remember to be taking sufficient water & salt!*	*Remember to be taking sufficient water & salt!*
4:00 PM	*Fast Day - Water Only*	*Fast Day - Water Only*	*Fast Day - Water Only*	*8 oz. of fresh grape juice from your juicer or you can eat a large handful of fresh grapes*	*Same as day 4*	*Same as day 4*	*Same as day 4*

First week: Continued

	Day 1	Day 2	Day 3	Day 4	Day 5	Day 6	Day 7
5:00 PM	*Fast Day - Water Only*	*Fast Day - Water Only*	*Fast Day - Water Only*	*Remember to be taking sufficient water & salt!*	*Remember to be taking sufficient water & salt!*	*Remember to be taking sufficient water & salt!*	*Remember to be taking sufficient water & salt!*
6:00 PM	*Fast Day - Water Only*	*Fast Day - Water Only*	*Fast Day - Water Only*	*8 oz. of fresh grape juice from your juicer (or you can eat a large handful of fresh grapes*	*Same as day 4*	*Same as day 4*	*Same as day 4*
6:30 PM	*Do not try to exercise on a day you are taking water-only, but do get some sunshine & fresh air!*	*Same as day 1*	*Same as day 1*	*20 minutes of sunshine (not during hottest time of day)*	*Same as day 4*	*Same as day 4*	*Same as day 4*
7:00 PM	*Fast Day - Water Only*	*Fast Day - Water Only*	*Fast Day - Water Only*	*Remember to be taking sufficient water & salt!*	*Remember to be taking sufficient water & salt!*	*Remember to be taking sufficient water & salt!*	*Remember to be taking sufficient water & salt!*
8:00 PM	*Fast Day - Water Only*	*Fast Day - Water Only*	*Fast Day - Water Only*	*8 oz. of fresh grape juice from your juicer (or you can eat a large handful of fresh grapes*	*Same as day 4*	*Same as day 4*	*Same as day 4*
9:00 PM - 9:30 PM	*Day ends - this 30 minutes should again be for Bible reading, praise & prayer! (note – if you already have cancer – take 2 oz. of Essiac tea on retiring)*	*Same as day 1*	*Same as day 1*	*Same as day 1*	*Same as day 1*	*Same as day 1*	*Same as day 1*

Second week:

	Day 8	**Day 9**	**Day 10**	**Day 11**	**Day 12**	**Day 13**	**Day 14**
	If you already have cancer, take 2 oz. of Essiac tea (such as Resperin® Essiac upon arising – do not mix it with anything else.)	*2 oz. Essiac*	*2 oz. Essiac*	*2 oz. Essiac*	*2 oz. Essiac*	*2 oz. Essiac*	*2 oz. Essiac*
6:00 - 6:30 AM	*Scripture reading, praise, then prayer for total of 30 minutes. Sip a cup of decaffeinated green tea while reading your Bible or 6 oz. of fresh-squeezed orange juice diluted with 2 oz. water. (Do not drink the green tea or juice unless you took Essiac at least an hour ago.)*	*Scripture reading & decaff green tea*	*Scripture reading & decaff green tea*	*Scripture reading & decaff green tea*	*Scripture reading & decaff green tea*	*Scripture reading & decaff green tea*	*Scripture reading & decaff green tea*
6:30 AM	*Breakfast is 1/2 banana, 4 oz. of raspberries, 4 oz. of blueberries, 1/2 kiwi & 1/2 cup of cherries (or strawberries). Put ingredients in your **blender** with water (& ice also -- only if desired) for a smoothie or slushie. (Please remove the cherry pits first or the drink will be very gritty and unpleasant!) Also add 1-2 tablespoons of flaxseed oil and 1 tsp. of bee pollen granules or open 4-6 capsules powdered bee polen and add to drink (if no allergies to bee stings or bee products).*	*Same as day 8 (note - if you have prostate cancer, use 8 oz. a day of raspberries -- If out of season, use frozen, not canned!)*	*Same as day 8*	*Same as day 8*	*Same as day 8*	*Same as day 8*	*Same as day 8*
7:30 AM	*This may be your travel time to work. If so, it is also a good time for praise music!*	*Same as day 8*	*Same as day 8*	*Same as day 8*	*Same as day 8*	*Same as day 8 unless you are off today*	*Same as day 8 unless you are off today*
8:00 AM	*1 oz. fresh wheatgrass juice combined with 1 oz. beet juice, 2 oz. celery juice and 2 oz. kale and 2 oz. broccoli juice (If fresh wheatgrass juice not available, use a tablespoon of a powdered green juice such as kamut or barley green).*	*Same as day 8*	*Same as day 8*	*Same as day 8*	*Same as day 8*	*Same as day 8*	*Same as day 8*

Second week: Continued

	Day 8	Day 9	Day 10	Day 11	Day 12	Day 13	Day 14
8:30 AM	*If you have later hours, this may be your work travel time - good time for praise music!*	*Same as day 8*	*Same as day 8*	*Same as day 8*	*Same as day 8*	*Same as day 8 unless you are off today*	*Same as day 8 unless you are off today*
9:00 AM	*Cup of Alphabet Tea - recipe is in this chapter*	*Alphabet Tea*	*Alphabet Tea*	*Alphabet Tea*	*Alphabet Tea*	*Alphabet Tea*	*Alphabet Tea*
10:00 AM	*5 oz. carrot juice with 1 oz. beet juice, 1 oz. celery juice, 1 oz. juice of raw potato*	*Same as day 8 – except use 2 oz. of the beet juice*	*Same as day 8 – except use 2 oz. of the beet juice*	*Same as day 8 – except use 2 oz. of the beet juice*	*Same as day 8 – except use 2 oz. of the beet juice*	*Same as day 8 – except use 2 oz. of the beet juice*	*Same as day 8 – except use 2 oz. of the beet juice*
11:00 AM	*8 oz. warm water mixed with 2 teaspoons of unsulfured blackstrap molasses*	*Same as day 8*	*Same as day 8*	*Same as day 8*	*Same as day 8*	*Same as day 8*	*Same as day 8*
12:00 Noon	*If you already have cancer, Lunch is the Johanna Budwig Flax Oil Mixture: 2 tablespoons of organic flaxseed oil blended well with 12 tablespoons of organic soy yogurt. Ok to add cinnamon to hide the oily taste or 1/2 cup of fruit of choice if desired - but only after the above 2 items are blended together so that the oil is not visible! If you do not already, have cancer, your noon drink can be 8 oz. fresh grape juice instead of the Budwig mix - if you prefer*	*Same as day 8 – (be sure the flax oil mixture is blended well enough that the oil is no longer visible)*	*Same as day 8*	*Same as day 8*	*Same as day 8*	*Same as day 8*	*Same as day 8*
1:00 PM	*1 oz. wheatgrass juice (if fresh not available, use a serving of one of the powdered green drinks – such as Green Miracle)*	*Same as day 8*	*Same as day 8*	*Same as day 8*	*Same as day 8*	*Same as day 8*	*Same as day 8*
2:00 PM	*Liver Flush Drink – see recipe in this chapter*	*Same as day 8*	*Same as day 8*	*Same as day 8*	*Same as day 8*	*Same as day 8*	*Same as day 8*
3:00 PM	*4 oz. fresh sprout juice, 1 oz. radish juice, 2 oz. cauliflower juice and 1 oz. beet juice mixed together*	*Same as day 8*	*Same as day 8*	*Same as day 8*	*Same as day 8*	*Same as day 8*	*Same as day 8*
4:00 PM	*6 oz. fresh grape juice mixed with 2 oz. apple juice – add 1 tsp. of fresh cinnamon*	*Same as day 8*	*Same as day 8*	*Same as day 8*	*Same as day 8*	*Same as day 8*	*Same as day 8*

Second week: Continued

	Day 8	Day 9	Day 10	Day 11	Day 12	Day 13	Day 14
5:00 PM	*This may be your work commute time – good time for praise music!*	*Same as day 8*	*Same as day 8*	*Same as day 8*	*Same as day 8*	*Same as day 8 unless you are off today*	*Same as day 8 unless you are off today*
6:00 PM	*If you already have cancer, repeat the Budwig mixture now that you had at noon – otherwise, use a green drink such as Green Miracle, fresh wheatgrass (2 oz.) or Barley Green – if using powdered mix, follow manufacturer's directions on the brand you purchase*	*Same as day 8*	*Same as day 8*	*Same as day 8*	*Same as day 8*	*Same as day 8*	*Same as day 8*
6:30 PM	*If possible, try to get your day's sunshine, but not during the hottest time of the day*	*Same as day 8*	*Same as day 8*	*Same as day 8*	*Same as day 8*	*Same as day 8*	*Same as day 8*
7:00 PM	*4 oz. pomegranate juice with 4 oz. fresh grape juice (This is one time where you can use a bottled organic pomegranate drink if fresh pomegranate not available!) Add cinnamon to taste if desired*	*Same as day 8*	*Same as day 8*	*Same as day 8*	*Same as day 8*	*Same as day 8*	*Same as day 8*
8:00 PM	*6 oz. carrot juice mixed with 2 oz. tomato juice – add juice of 1 celery stick and tablespn. flax oil*	*Same as day 8*	*Same as day 8*	*Same as day 8*	*Same as day 8*	*Same as day 8*	*Same as day 8*
8:30 PM	*Day ends approx. now - this 30 minutes should again be for Bible reading, praise & prayer!*	*Scripture reading, prayer and praise!*	*Scripture reading, prayer and praise!*	*Scripture reading, prayer and praise!*	*Scripture reading, prayer and praise!*	*Scripture reading, prayer and praise!*	*Scripture reading, prayer and praise!*
Bed time	*If you already have cancer, take 2 oz. of Essiac tea (such as Resperin Essiac®) before retiring for the day. Don't combine it with anything else.*	*2 oz. Essiac*	*2 oz. Essiac*	*2 oz. Essiac*	*2 oz. Essiac*	*2 oz. Essiac*	*2 oz. Essiac*

Third week:

	Day 15	Day 16	Day 17	Day 18	Day 19	Day 20	Day 21
	Same as day 14	*Same as day 14*	*Same as day 14*	*Same as day 14*	*Same as day 14*	*Same as day 14*	*Same as day 14*

Congratulations! You have just completed a 7 day fast, and a 14 day partial fast! If you used fresh grape juice instead of eating grapes, you have been on a 7 day <u>liquid</u> fast, the first 3 days being water only. Be certain that you are getting your quota of water and salt that you need each day as discussed earlier in this book. You can count some of the juices in day 8 through 21 as part of your water intake, but be sure that (according to your weight as discussed earlier, you are getting sufficient water & salt for the day.) As with any detox, you need plenty of water. You are flushing out your system, so you will need extra water every day during this detox program. If desired, you can even add extra water to the vegetable and fruit juices. (You will not be doing strenuous exercising during the detox program.)

VII. Now What?

Remember that detoxifying your body will make you feel worse initially. You are ridding your body of poisons that (unless you have detoxed before) have been accumulating for years! You may experience headaches and facial breakouts where poisons are being eliminated from your body. You may want to repeat the program for another 2-3 weeks, but that is up to you. You may choose a 40 day juicing only fast. What you choose will be up to you, your own strength and how you feel that the Lord is leading you. If you stay with raw foods only, good for you! You should gradually begin to introduce more and more solids into the diet, even if you stay with raw foods only! The "super salad" and "power seed mixture" should be part of your raw foods only diet, once you have advanced off the fast. If you begin adding cooked foods, do so slowly, beginning with one meal a day, such as cream of rice with fruit and toasted rye bread for breakfast, or a large baked potato for lunch or items such as hard-boiled eggs, cooked green beans and stewed tomatoes for supper. If you are using cooked foods, you may want to begin eating organic rye breads (great for high blood pressure problems) and whole wheat breads. Many people who have been on raw food only diets report having a return of their old problems when they begin incorporating cooked meals back into their diet. (One cooked item that I do support once the detox is over, and the diet has advanced somewhat is the use of hard-boiled eggs, simply because eggs are so rich in nutrients, however, this is only certified ORGANIC eggs! If not organic, they may have hormones or other unwanted chemicals in them!) Regardless of which you choose, you should stay with the prayer and praise program! Make a covenant with God to spend time every day praising Him, not just at the worship service you attend.

I don't recommend any dairy or meat products for cancer patients except for organic hard-boiled eggs, but not while on the detox program. What you decide to do is up to you. Search out the many healing verses in the Bible. Memorize them, claim them and remember that God has also promised that: *"If ye abide in me, and my words abide in you, ye shall ask what ye will, and it shall be done unto you."* (John 15:7)

God operates on faith. Your own words can determine your destiny! If you get up in the morning declaring verbally that everything will go wrong, it probably will! If you start declaring positive outcomes for each day (and for your health), God will honor your faith and move mountains for you! One of the best books I have ever read on how to put your faith into action is by Darlene Bishop, *Your Life Follows Your Words.* You can find her book at her website *www.darlenebishop.org.* She was miraculously healed of breast cancer and has a tremendous testimony.

What you choose to do with the information in this book you have just read is up to you! If you are fighting a terminal illness, pray *Psalm 119:17 every day! "Deal bountifully with thy servant, that I may live, and keep thy word,"* and declare *Psalm 118:17* BOLDLY every day: *"I shall not die, but live, and declare the works of the Lord."* Take these verses, type and print them off on your PC and tape them on your mirror so that you can memorize them and repeat them when you get up in the morning, and declare them throughout the day all day long! If you have a young child who is fighting a terminal illness, obtain some DVD praise songs and play them at your child's bedside 24 hours a day! During sleep time, turn the volume way down, if the music keeps your child awake. Remember to proclaim these same verses over your child throughout the day. You can also claim *Psalm 118:17* for them and plead the blood of Jesus over them! Sing to God and praise Him at your child's bedside, and most importantly – if they are old enough to learn, teach your children to **PRAISE THE LORD!**

Bibliography

1 "100% Science. Pure Juice." POM Wonderful Health. Online posting. 26 Dec. 2004 <http://www.pomwonderful.com/health.asp?source=google&kw= antioxidant> (used with their permission.)

2 "1999 Independent Study by Institute of Longevity Medicine." Online posting. 1 Dec. 2004 http://www.realsuccess4life.com/cgi-bin/home.cgi?6038864" Professional Networkers, Hutchinson, KS." (Used with their permission)

3 "20% of New Drugs Will Be Labeled 'Dangerous' or Withdrawn From Market JAMA Study Reports." Online posting. 30 Apr. 2004, Molocure Research, Inc. <http://www.molocure.com/adrarticle.shtml> © 2003 Molo-Cure Research, Inc. All Rights Reserved. (Used with their permission.)

4 "A Bex and a Nice Lie Down." BARISTA heartstarters for the hungry mind, Jun. 19, 2004. Online posting. 5 Jan. 2005 <http://dox.media2.org/barista/ archives/000781.html> (Used with their permission.)

5 "Abstracts of Published Studies Indicating Aloe's Potential Efficacy Against Cancer." Online posting. Life Extension Magazine, April 2002. 27 Sept. 2004. (Also see the LEF Protocol Book) <http://www.lef.org/magazine/mag2002_report _clinic_04.html> All contents © 1995-2005 Life Extension Foundation All Rights Reserved. (Used with their permission.)

6 "Agaricus Blazei Murill." Newsletter Aug. 2001, from the Wellness Directory of Minnesota™. Online posting. 18 Dec. 2004 <http://www.mnwelldir. org/docs/Newsletters/01_Aug.htm> (Used with their permission.)

7 "Agaricus." Wellness Directory of Minnesota™, Alternative Cancer Therapies, updated 10/27/04. Online posting. 28 Oct. and 20 Nov. 2004 <http:// www.mnwell.dir.org/docs/cancer1/altthrpy.htm> (Used with their permission.)

8 "Aloe Vera." Online posting. "The Alternative Cancer Treatments That Also Shrink Tumors." Cancer Tutor™ website. 17 Oct. 2004 and 28 Oct.2004 <http:// www.cancertutor.com/other/shrinktumors.html> Also see http://stopcancer.com/deathbed 1.html. (Used with their permission.)

9 "Amargo." Online posting. Raintree Nutrition's TROPICAL PLANT DATABASE. "Plant Chemicals." 24 May 2005 <http://www.rain-tree.com/amargo.htm> © Copyrighted 1996 - 2004 Raintree Nutrition, Inc., Carson City, NV. 89701 All rights reserved. This information is also found in Leslie Taylor's book, *The Healing Power of Rainforest Herbs,* Square One Publishers, Jan. 2005 (Used with their permission.)

10 "Anamu." Online posting. Raintree Nutrition's TROPICAL PLANT DATABASE. "Biological Activities & Clinical Research." 23 Nov. 2004 <http://www.rain-tree.com /anamu.htm> © Copyrighted 1996 - 2004 Raintree Nutrition, Inc., Carson City, NV. 89701 All rights reserved. This information is also found in Leslie Taylor's book, *The Healing Power of Rainforest Herbs,* Square One Publishers, Jan. 2005 (Used with their permission.)

11 "Andiroba." Online posting. Raintree Nutrition's TROPICAL PLANT DATABASE. 22 Oct. 2004 <http://www.rain-tree.com/andiroba.htm> © Copyrighted 1996 - 2004 Raintree Nutrition, Inc., Carson City, NV. 89701 All rights reserved. This information is also found in Leslie Taylor's book, *The Healing Power of Rainforest Herbs,* Square One Publishers, Jan. 2005. (Used with their permission.)

12 "Andrographis." Online posting. Herbs 2000. 17 Oct. 2004 <http://www.herbs2000.com/herbs/herbs_andrographis.htm> © 2002-2005 herbs2000.com. (Used with their permission.)

13 "Antineoplastons." Online posting. Alternatives in Cancer Therapy, from their excerpt of the book Alternatives in Cancer Therapy, by Ross, R., Ph., Pelton, Lee Overholser. 5 Dec. 2004 <http://www.curezone.com/diseases/cancer/ antineoplastons. asp> © 1996-2005 CureZone.com. (Used with their permission.)

14 "Are There Any Natural Progesterone Side Effects?" Online posting . 2 Jun. 2005 <http://www.safemenopausesolutions.com/progesteronesideeffects.html.> Copyright © Personal Wellness Network, Inc. All rights reserved. (Used with their permission.)

15 "Artemisinin." Alternative Cancer Therapies. Online posting. Wellness Directory of Minnesota. 20 Dec. 2004 <http://www.mnwelldir.org/docs/cancer/altthrpy .htm> from Dr. Lam, M.D. at website <http://www.drlam.com/A3R_brief_ in_doc_format/Artemisinin.cfm>© 2001-2004 by Michael Lam M.D. All Rights Reserved. (Used with their permission.)

16 "Aspilia." Online posting. 16 Oct. 2004 <http://www.herbs2000.com/ herbs/herbs_aspilia.htm> © 2002-2005 herbs2000.com. (Used with their permission.)

17 "Autumn Crocus." Online posting. 22 Nov. 2004 <http://www.herbs2000. com/herbs/herbs_autumn_crocus.htm>© 2002-2005 herbs2000.com. (Used with their permission.)

18 "Beres Drops." Online posting. 17 Oct. 2004. Alternative Cancer Treatment Information Center <http://www.cancertutor.com/Other/Big_List.htm> (Used with their permission.)

19 "Berry Young Juice Advantages." Online posting. 17 Oct. 2004 <http://www.aromanotes.com/87/berry-young> (Used with their permission.)

20 "Beta-Sitosterol." Online posting. 24 Oct. 2004 <www.drlam.com/opinion/beta_sitosterol.cfm> © 2001-2004 by Michael Lam M.D. All Rights Reserved

21 "Billion Dollar Drug Company Nearly Squashes Astounding Research On Natural Cancer Killer." Online posting. Health Sciences Institute, Member's Alert for Jan. 2001, Vol. 5, No. 7. 26 Apr. 2004 <http://www.hsibaltimore.com. (Used with their permission.)

22 "Bitter Melon." Online posting. Liver Cancer – Alternative Cancer Treatment Information Center. 21 Oct. 2004 <http://www.cancertutor.com/Other/Liver_Cancer.html> (Used with their permission.)

23 "Bitter Melon." Online posting. Herbs2000.com, 21 Oct. 2004 <http://www.herbs2000.com/herbs/herbs_bitter_melon.htm> © 2002-2005 herbs2000.com. (Used with their permission.)

24 "Bladder Cancer." Online posting. 17 Oct. 2004 <http://www.herbs2000.com/disorders/cancer_bladder.htm> (Used with their permission.)

25 "Bone Cancer – Another Flax Cure." Online posting. 11 Dec. 2004 <http://www.curezone.com/diseases/cancer/testimonials/Bone-cancer_another_flax_cure.asp>© 1996-2005 CureZone.com. (Used with their permission.)

26 "Bone Cancer." Online posting. 17 Oct. 2004 and 18 Dec. 2004 <http://www.herbs2000.com/disorders/cancer_bone.htm> © 2002-2005 herbs2000.com. (Used with their permission.)

27 "Bone Marrow and Stem Cell Transplants." Online posting. Overview, Bone Marrow and Stem Cell Transplants for Childhood Cancer. 21 Nov. 2004 <http://www.cancerindex.org/ccw/guide2bm.htm> (Used with their permission.)

28 "Bone Marrow Cancers (e.g. Multiple Myeloma (MM), Leukemia, etc.)" Cancer Tutor™, Alternative Cancer Treatment Information Center. Online posting. 1 Aug. 2004 <http://www.cancertutor.com/other/bone_marrow_cancer.html> (Used with their permission.)

29 "Brain Stem Gliomas." Online posting. 10 Apr. 2005 <http://www.braintumor.org/patient_info/surviving/tumor_types/othergliomas.html> Copyright 2000-2004 National Brain Tumor Foundation. (Used with their permission.)

30 "Brazilian Peppertree." Raintree Nutrition's TROPICAL PLANT DATABASE. Online posting. 1 Dec. 2004 <http://www.rain-tree.com/peppertree.htm> © Copyrighted 1996 - 2004 Raintree Nutrition, Inc., Carson City, NV. 89701 All rights reserved. This information is also found in Leslie Taylor's book, *The Healing Power of Rainforest Herbs,* Square One Publishers, Jan. 2005. (Used with their permission.)

31 "Breast Cancer – healing with herbs, vitamins and minerals." Online posting. Herbs 2000. 17 Oct. 2004 <http://www.herbs2000.com/disorders/cancer_breast.htm> © 2002-2005 herbs2000.com. (Used with their permission.)

32 "Breuss Total Cancer Treatment." Online posting. 17 Oct. 2004. Alternative Cancer Treatment Information Center – Over 200 Alternative Cancer Treatments Plus Other Information <http://www.cancertutor.com/Cancer/Breuss.html> (Used with their permission.)

33 "Broccoli and tomatoes prevent prostate cancer better than leading prescription drugs, research shows." Online posting. 03 May 2005. <http://www.news target.com/001391.html> (Used with their permission.)

34 "Bupleurum." Online posting. 25 Oct. 2004 <http://www.herbs2000.com/herbs/herbs_bupleurum.htm> © 2002-2005 herbs2000.com. (Used with their permission.)

35 "Burzynski Patient Group." "Cyrstin S." Online posting. 21 Jun. 2005 <http://burzynskipatientgroup.org/cyrstins.htm> (Used with Dr. Burzynski's permission.)

36 "Burzynski Patient Group." "Dustin K." Online posting. 21 Jun. 2005 <http://burzynskipatientgroup.org/dustink.htm> (Used with Dr. Burzynski's permission.)

37 "Burzynski Patient Group." "Jodi G." Online posting. 21 Jun. 2005 <http://burzynskipatientgroup.org/jodig.htm (Used with Dr. Burzynski's permission.)

38 "Butcher's Broom." Online posting. 22 Nov. 2004 <http://www.herbs 2000.com/herbs/herbs_butchers_broom.htm>© 2002-2005 herbs2000.com. (Used with their permission.)

39 "Cancer – Breast." "Herbs." Alternative Health Supplies (Australia), Your Health Your Choice, "Vitamins." Online Posting. 24 Oct. 2004 <http://www.alternative health.com.au/Articles/breast.htm> © 2005 Alternative Health Supplies. All Rights Reserved. (Used with their permission.)

40 "Cancer – Breast." "Quinones." Online posting. Alternative Health Supplies (Australia) Your Health Your Choice. 24 Oct. 2004 <http://www.alternative health.com.au/Articles/breast.htm>© 2005 Alternative Health Supplies. All Rights Reserved. (Used with their permission.)

41 "Cancer – Breast." Alternative Health Supplies (Australia), Your Health Your Choice, "Vitamins." Online Posting. 24 Oct. 2004 <http://www.alternative health.com.au/Articles/breast.htm>© 2005 Alternative Health Supplies. All Rights Reserved. (Used with their permission.)

42 "Cancer Adjuvant Therapy." "Ginger (Zingiber officinalis)." Life Extension. Online posting. 8 Oct. 2004. (Also see the LEF Protocol Book) <http://www.lef.org/protocols/prtcl-027b.shtml> All contents © 1995-2005 Life Extension Foundation All Rights Reserved. (Used with their permission.)

43. "Cancer Adjuvant Therapy." Online Posting. Life Extension. 8 Oct. 2004 <http://www.lef.org/protocols/prtcl-027b.html> (Also see the LEF Protocol Book) All contents © 1995-2005 Life Extension Foundation All Rights Reserved. (Used with their permission.)

44 "Cancer Adjuvant Therapy." Life Extension, Cancer Adjuvant Treatment, Online Reference for Health Concerns. Online posting. 8 Oct. 2004. (Also see the LEF Protocol Book) <http://www.lef. org /protocols/prtcl-027b.shtml> All contents © 1995-2005 Life Extension Foundation All Rights Reserved. (Used with their permission.)

45 "Cancer and Immunity." Online posting. "Immune Building Agents." "Olive Leaf." An Insider's Guide to Natural Medicine. 27 Sept. 2004 <http://www.drlam.com/A3R_brief_in_doc_format/cancer_and_immunity.cfm>© 2001-2004 by Michael Lam M.D. All Rights Reserved. (Used with their permission.)

46 "Cancer-Fighter Perillyl Alcohol Found in Tart Cherries." Online posting. FS Flavonoid Sciences. Credit: Cherry Marketing Institute Cherry Advantage Issue I. 25 May 2004 <http://www.flavonoidsciences.com/cherry-blueberry.php?page=3&title= Cancer-Fighter%20P> © 2005 Flavonoid Sciences. All Rights Reserved. (Used with their permission.)

47 "Cancer-Fighter Perillyl Alcohol Found in Tart Cherries." Online posting. 7 Mar. 2005 and 27 May, 2005 <http://www.flavonoidsciences.com/research/c3.htm>© 2005 Flavonoid Sciences. All Rights Reserved. (Used with their permission.)

48 "Cancer Types," "Skin Cancer." Online posting. 3 May 2005 <http://www.cancer-healing.com/cancer_type.php> © 2004 © Life Enthusiast Co-op. All Rights Reserved. (Used with their permission.)

49 "Cancer Types," "Lung Cancer." Online posting. 3 May 2005<http://www.cancer-healing.com/cancer_type.php>© 2004 © Life Enthusiast Co-op. All Rights Reserved. (Used with their permission.)

50 "Cansema Black Salve (Skin Cancer)." Cancer Tutor™, Alternative Cancer Treatment Information Center. Online posting. 17 Oct. 2004 <http://www.cancer-tutor. com/Cancer/Cansema.html. (Used with their permission.)

51 "Cat's Claw." Online posting. 16 Nov. 2004 <http://www.herbs2000.com/herbs/herbs_cats_claw.htm> © 2002-2005 herbs2000.com. (Used with their permission.)

52 "Caveats: Conflicting Reports on Vitamins and Minerals." June Russell's Health Facts. Online posting. "Vitamins – Antioxidants: Beta-carotene and Vitamins A and E." 14 Jan. 2005 <http://www.jrussellshealth.com/caveats_vit_min.html> (Used with their permission.)

53 "Cayenne Pepper." Alternative Cancer Therapies. Online posting. Wellness Directory of Minnesota™. 25 May. 2004 <http://mnwelldir.org/docs/cancer 1/alt-thrpy.htm. (Used with their permission.)

54 "Cervical Cancer." Online posting. 17 Oct. 2004. <http://www.herbs2000. com/disorders/cancer_cervical.htm>© 2002-2005 herbs2000.com. (Used with their permission.)

55 "Chaparral." www.curezone.com's excerpt from the book Alternatives in Cancer Therapy by Ross, Pelton, R. Ph., Lee Overholser. Online posting. 25 May 2004 <http://www.curezone.com/diseases/cancer/chaparral.asp>© 1996-2005 CureZone.com. (Used with their permission.)

56 "Chemotherapy: A Dull Weapon! Kyle Slavik A Success Story," from website OPTIONS – Revolutionary Ideas on the War on Cancer. Online posting. 5 Dec. 2004 <http://www.karlloren.com/biopsy/p60.htm> © Vibrant Life. All Rights Reserved. (Used with Mr. Loren's permission.)

57 "Chicory Root." Over 200 Alternative Cancer Treatments Plus Other Information – Cancer Tutor™ website. Online posting. 11 Dec. 2004 <http;//www. cancertutor.com/Other/Big_List.htm> (Used with their permission.)

58 "Chinese asparagus." Earthnotes Herb Library. Online posting 21 Jan. 2005 <http://earthnotes.tripod.com/asparagus.htm# aspother> © 2000 by Ernestina Parziale CH (Used with Ms. Parziale's permission.)

59 "Chronic Fatigue: Chronic Fatigue Syndrome, Gastritis, Gastric Ulcer…" Corporate Overview, Molo-Cure Research, Inc. Online posting. 31 Dec. 2004 <http:// www.molocure.com/about.shtml> © 2003 Molo-Cure Research, Inc. All Rights Reserved. (Used with their permission.)

60 "Chuchuhuasi, Chuchuhuasi Or 'tree of life' Venezuela." Information online from http://www.rain-tree.com/chuchuhuasi.htm. 17 Oct. 2004 <http://www.life-enthusiast.com/excula/ingredients/ing_Chuchuhuasi.htm> © Copyrighted 1996 - 2004 Raintree Nutrition, Inc., Carson City, NV. 89701 All rights reserved. This information is also found in Leslie Taylor's book, *The Healing Power of Rainforest Herbs,* Square One Publishers, Jan. 2005. (Used with Ms.Taylor's permission.)

61 "Cilantro: A Common Spice/Herb That Can Save Your Life." Online posting. Wellness Directory of Minnesota™. 18 Dec. 2004 <http://www.mnwell.dir. org/ docs/detox/cilantro.htm> (Used with their permission.)

62 "Clodronate." Online posting. Cancer Tutor™, Alternative Cancer Treatment Information Center. 17 Oct. 2004 <http://www.cancertutor.com/Other /Big_List.htm> (Used with their permission.)

63 "Colorectal Cancer." Online posting. Herbs2000.com. 17 Oct. 2004 <http://www.herbs2000.com/disorders/cancer_colorectal.htm> © 2002-2005 herbs2000.com. (Used with their permission.)

64 "Comfrey Plant." Cancer Tutor™ website. Online posting. 17 Oct. 2004 <http://www.cancertutor.com/Other/Big_List.htm> (Used with their permission.)

65 "Comparison of Glutathione in Fresh vs. Cooked Foods (in milligrams per 3 ½ oz (100 g) serving)." Online posting. Reprinted with permission of www.nutritionadvisor.com, President Steven P. Petrosino, Ph.D, 6 May, 2005 <http://www.nutritionadvisor.com/glutatione_foods.php> © 2004 Nutritionadvisor, LLC (Used with their permission.)

66 "Compound from rare plant shows promise in treating breast cancer." Charlottesville, VA. Feb. 1, 2005. Contact Bob Beard reb8e@virginia.edu. Online posting. 1 Feb. 2005 <http://www.eurekalert.org/pub_releases/2005-02/uovh-cfr013 105.php> (Used with their permission.)

67 "Congestive Heart Failure," "Co-enzyme Q10. This is Very Important." Online posting 2005, Mar. 21 <http://www.doctoryourself.com/congestive.html> Copyright 2003 and prior years by Andrew W. Saul. From the book *DOCTOR YOURSELF,* available from Andrew Saul, Number 8 Van Buren Street, Holley, New York 14470 USA   (From his website – used with Dr. Saul's permission.)

68 "Contortrostatin," and "C-Statin." Alternative Cancer Therapies.Wellness Directory of Minnesota™. Online posting. 20 Dec. 2004 <http://www.mnwelldir .org/docs/cancer1/altthrpy.htm> (Used with their permission.)

69 "Cot Death & Vaccines." Online Posting, NVIC. 19 Jun. 2005 <http://www.whale.to/m/quotes17.html> (Used with their permission.)

70 "Cranberry Juice." Online Posting. Cancer Tutor™. 17 Oct. 2004 <http://www.cancer tutor.com/Other/Big_list.htm> (Used with their permission.)

71 "Curcumin/Tumeric." Online posting. Cancer Tutor™. 17 Oct. and 30 Nov. 2004 <http://www.cancertutor.com/Other/Big_List.htm> (Used with their permission.)

72 "Dandelion Plant (herb – NOT just the root)." Online posting. Cancer Tutor™. 17 Oct. 2004 <http://www.cancertutor.com/OtherBig_List.htm> (Used with their permission.)

73 "DHEA protects against prostate cancer." Online posting. 3 May 2005 <www.yourhealthbase.com/prostate_cancer.htm> © 1999-2004 by Hans R. Larsen. (Used with their permission.)

74 "DIM (diindolylmethane)," Online posting. Cancer Tutor™, 14 Apr. 2005 <http://www.cancertutor.com/OtherBig_List.htm> (Used with their permission.)

75 "D-limonene," and "Perillyl Alcohol." Online posting. Cancer Tutor™. 17 Oct. 2004 <http://www.cancertutor.com/Other/Big_List.htm> (Used with their permission.)

76 "D-limonene." Cancer Tutor™, Online posting. 3 Dec. 2004 <http://www.cancertutor.com/ Other/Big_List.htm> (Used with their permission.)

77 "Doctors Discover Lapacho." Online posting. Red-Purple Lapacho (also known as Pau D' Arco or Taheebo). 21 Oct. 2004 <http://www.oralchelation.com/taheebo /lapacho2.htm> (Used with Mr. Loren's permission.)

78 "Dr. Budwig's Diet & Cancer Healing Protocol," at website *Healing Cancer Naturally.* The quote is from Dr. Johanna Budwig in *Flax Oil as a True Aid.* Online posting. 17 Jan. 2005 <http://www.healingcancernaturally.com/budwig_proto-col .html> © 2004 & 2005 Healingcancernaturally.com. All Rights Reserved. (Used with their permission.)

79 "Dr. Budwig's Diet & Cancer Healing Protocol." From website Healing Cancer Naturally. Online posting 17 Jan. 2005<http://www.healingcancernatural-ly. com/budwig_protocol.html> from Dr. Budwig in "Der Toddes Tumors, Band II." (The Death of the Tumor, Vol. II) transcribing an interview broadcast by the Siddeutscher Rundfunk Stuttgart (South German Radio Station) on 11 Sept. 1967. © 2004 & 2005 Healingcancernaturally.com. All Rights Reserved. (Used with their permission.)

80 "Drug Firms and Doctors: The Offers Pour In." Online Posting. 30 Apr. 2004, Molocure Research, Inc. <http://www.molocure.com/bostonglobe.shtml> © 2003 Mole-Cure Research, Inc. All Rights Reserved. (Used with their permission.)

81 "Drug giant accused of false claims." Psych Drug Truth. NBC NEWS. Online posting. 5 Jan. 2005 http://www.prozactruth.com/article_drug_giant_accused. htm> (Used with their permission.)

82 "Dyer's Woad (Isatis Indigotica Fortune)." Online posting. Prostate Problem – Enlargement of the Prostate – Prostate Cancer – Bladder Infection...3 Dec. 2004 <http://www.nutrition2000.com/ prostatepchope.htm> (Used with their permis-sion.)

83 "Effects of Estrogen Dominance." Diagnose-Me: Condition: Progesterone Low or Estrogen Dominance. Online posting. 24 Dec. 2004 <http://www. diag-nose-me.com/cond/C8779.html> (Used with their permission.)

84 "Ellagic Acid." Online Posting. 10 Apr. 2005 <http://www.cancer-prevention.net> (Used with their permission.)

85 "Ellagic Acid." Online Posting. Wellness Directory of Minnesota™, Alternative Cancer Therapies. The Information on H. Pylori is from Dr. Glen Halvorson's book, *Chemo-preventive Properties of Phytochemicals.* 28 Oct. 2004<http://www.mnwell dir.org/docs/ cancer1/altthrpy.htm> (Used with their permission.)

86 "Emmanuel Revici." Online posting. 17 Oct. 2004 <http://www.cancer tutor.com/Other/Big_List.htm> (Used with their permission.)

87 "Endometrial Cancer." Online posting. 17 Oct. 2004 <http://www.herbs 2000.com/disorders/cancer_endometrial.htm>© 2002-2005 herbs2000.com (Used with their permission.)

88 "Espinheira Santa." Online posting. 16 Oct. 2004 <http://www.herbs2000. com/herbs/herbs_espinheirasanta.htm>>© 2002-2005 herbs2000.com. (Used with their permission.)

89 "Essential Fatty Acids." Online posting. 23 Jan. 2005 <http://www. absolute-lythepurest.com/other%20parts/essentialfattyacids.html> © 2003 Thymely Solutions, Inc. All Rights Reserved (Used with their permission.)

90 "Estrogen Information Summary." National Institute of Neurological Disorders and Stroke, "Estrogen." Online posting. 27 May, 2005 <http://www.ninds.nih. gov/funding/research/parkinsonsweb/drug_summaries /estrogen.htm>

91 "Everyone Gets Rich When You Get Sick." Wellness Directory of Minnesota™, "Newsletter Aug. 2001." Online posting. 18 Dec. 2004 <http://www. mnwelldir.org/docs/Newsletters01_Aug.htm> (Used with their per-mission.)

92 "Ewing's sarcoma in children." CancerBACUP Helping people live with can-cer. Online posting. 19 Jan. 2005 <http://www.cancer bacup.org.nk/Cancertype/ Childrenscancers/Typesofchildrenscancers/Ew...> © CancerBACUP 2003. (Used with their permission.)

93 "Exula Health Products." Online posting. 28 Dec. 2004 <http://www.life-enthusiast.com/exsula/exsula_main.htm> and <www.lifeenthusiast.com/exsula/pr_ iridesca.htm> © 2003 Life Enthusiast Co-op. All Rights Reserved (Used with their permission.)

94 "FAQs." ExToxNet Recommendation 14 Background. Online posting. 24 Oct. 2004 <http://extoxnet.orst.edu/faqs/dietcancer/ web14/fourteenphyto.html> (Used with their permission.)

95 "FDA Opens Baycol Probe." Agency Feeling the Heat After Vioxx Withdrawal, NEWS. Online posting. Copyright © 2003-2004 ConsumerAffairs.com, 26 Dec. 2004 <http://www.consumeraffairs.com/news04/vioxx_baycol_fda.html> (Used with the permission.)

96 "Food as Medicine: Other Phytochemicals. How Other Phytochemicals Help Protect Against Cancer." Online posting. The Cancer Project. 18 May 2004 http://www.cancerproject.org/medicine/phytochemicals.html (Used with their permission.)

97 "Food sources of Lysine." From the "Lysine Amino Acid Information page." Zest for Life Supplements webpage. Available: http://www.anyvitamins.com/lysine-info.htm (accessed 2005, Jan. 26) (Used with their permission.)

98 Online posting 26 Jan. 2005 <http://www.anyvitamins.com/glutamic-acid-info.htm> © 1999-2003 Sallamander Concepts (Used with their permission.)

99 "Foods that Harm, Foods That Heal – Tasty Ways to Keep the Doctor Away." Reader's Digest, from the book, April 2004. The book was *Foods That Harm, Foods That Heal* (1st edition) in Mar. 2004. Used with permission of Global Books & Home Entertainment, The Reader's Digest Association, Inc.

100 "Geraniol." Online posting. "Health Conditions Starting with C and herbal remedies used to treat them." 16 Oct. 2004 <http://earthnotes.tripod.com/ckbk_c.htm> (Used with Ms. Parziale's permission.)

101 "Gill-Over-The-Ground." The Backyard Herbalist, Ernestina Parziale CH, "Health Conditions Starting with C and herbal remedies used to treat them." Online posting. 16 Oct. 2004 <http://earthnotes.tripod.com/ckbk_c.htm> © 1998-2005 Ernestina Parziale. (Used with Ms. Parziale's permission.)

102 "Ginseng and Cancer: A follow-up." Perspectives Research and Creative Activities, Spring 2004, Southern Illinois University Carbondale. Online posting. 19 Dec. 2004 <http://www.siu.edu/~perspect/04_sp/ginseng.html> © 2004 Board of Trustees, Southern Illinois University. (Used with their permission.)

103 "Glandulars." Cancer Tutor™, Alternative Cancer Treatment Information Center. 17 Oct. 2004 <http://www.cancertutor.com/other/Big_List.htm> (Used with their permission.)

104 "Grape Vitis Vinifera." Online posting. 7 June 2004 <http://www.herbs 2000.com/herbs/_grape.htm>© 2002-2005 herbs2000.com (Used with their permission.)

105 "Grape." Online posting. 23 Jun. 2004 <http://www.herbs2000.com/herbs/herbs_grape.htm> © 2002-2005 herbs2000.com (Used with their permission.)

106 "Grapes Inhibit Cancer Growth." Online Posting. From CNN interactive, Jan 10, 1997. 18 May 2004 <http://www.cnn.com/HEALTH/ 9701/10/grapes.Cancer/index.html>© 2001 Cable News Network. All Rights Reserved. (Used by permission of CNN.com.)

107 "Graviola." Online posting. Alternative Cancer Therapies. 25 May 2004 <http://www.mnwelldir.org/docs/cancer1/altthrpy2.htm> (Used with their permission.)

108 "Green tea could prevent cancer of the esophagus." News & Analysis Science & Nutrition 25/05/2004. Online posting. 28 Oct. 2004 <http://www.food navigator.com/news/news-NG.asp?id=52331> Industry & Science News 2000/2005 NOVIS – All Rights Reserved (Used with their permission.)

109 "Green Tea Fights Killer Disease." Online posting. FoodNavigator.com, News & Analysis Science & Nutrition, 2/4/2004. 28 Oct. 2004 <http://www. foodnavigator.com/news/news-NG.asp?id=51104> Industry & Science News 2000/2005 NOVIS – All Rights Reserved (Used with their permission.)

110 "Grocery warning: curry sauces contain dangerous levels of food coloring chemicals." News Target Network, News and Commentary on Today's Top Stories. Monday, Jan. 23, 2005 commentary. Online posting.4 Jan. 2005 <http://www.news target.com/001027.html> New Target Network © 2004, 2005 All Rights Reserved (Used with their permission.)

111 "Guacatonga." Raintree Nutrition's TROPICAL PLANT DATABASE. Online posting. 22 Oct.2004 <http://www.rain-tree.com/guacatonga.htm> © Copyrighted 1996 - 2004 Raintree Nutrition, Inc., Carson City, NV. 89701 All rights reserved. This information is also found in Leslie Taylor's book, *The Healing Power of Rainforest Herbs,* Square One Publishers, Jan. 2005. Used with Ms. Taylor's permission.

112 "Headway on Natural Chemotherapy for Prostate Cancer." News & Analysis Research, 20/04/2004, "Natural Treatments for Prostate Cancer are Fast Gaining Scientific Evidence for their efficacy in human patients." Online posting. 28 Oct. 2004 <http://www.nutraingredients.com/news/news-NG.asp?id=51500> Industry & Science News 2000/2005 NOVIS – All Rights Reserved (Used with their permission.)

113 "Healing Cancer." Excerpt From a book by Robert Barefoot, Death by Diet. Online posting. 3 Jan. 2005 <http://www.cancer-healing.com/net_alkalize _diet.php> (Used with their permission.)

114 "Healing Colon Cancer with RAW Food: A personal account." Online Posting. Holistic Health: Testimonials of Amazing Health Recovery. 23 May 2004 <http://www.shirleys-wellness-café.com/cancer.htm> © 1996-2005 All Rights Reserved (Used with their permission.)

115 "Health Information." Online posting. Jones Biomedicals & Laboratory, Inc. 29 Jan. 2005 <http://members.aol.com/jonbio/nutrition.htm> (Used with their permission.)

116 Healing With Vitamins, by The Editors of *Prevention* Health Books (City, State, n.g.), Rodale, Inc., 1996 (Used with their permission.)

117 "Herbs and Supplements: Goldenseal." HPN – Healing People Network – safety issues. Online posting. 5 Dec. 2004 <http://www.healingpeople.com/index.php ?option=com_staticfile=encyclopedia/pg0001> Healing People Network, L.P. An Alliance Health Company, all rights reserved (Used with their permission.)

118 "Herbs." Cancer – Breast, Your Health Your Choice, Alternative Health Supplies (Australia). Online posting. 24 Oct. 2004 <http://www.alternativehealth.com.au/Articles/breast.htm> © 2005 Alternative Health Supplies. All Rights Reserved. (Used with their permission.)

119 "High dietary boron linked to reduced risk for prostate cancer." From Reuters Health Information. Available: http://www.oncolink.com/resources/article.cfm?c=3&s=8&ss=23&id=1188&month=04&year=2001. Oncolink Cancer News (accessed 2005, June 2) Copyright © 1994-2005 © Trustees of the University of Pennsylvania. Copyright © 2005 Reuters Limited. All rights reserved. Reprinted with their permission. Reuters shall not be liable for any errors or delays in the content, or for any actions taken in reliance thereon.

120 "Hodgkin Lymphoma and Non-Hodgkin Lymphoma." Cancer Types, Classification. Online posting. 28 Dec. 2004 <http://www.cancer-healing.com/cancer_type.php> © 2004 Life Enthusiast Co-op. All Rights Reserved (Used with their permission.)

121 "Hoelen." Online posting. 22 Jan. 2005 <http://www.herbs2000.com/herbs/herbs_hoelen.htm> © 2002-2005 herbs2000.com (Used with their permission.)

122 "Horseradish." Online posting. Herbs 2000.com. 5 Dec. 2004 <http://www.herbs2000.com/herbs/herbs_horseradish.htm> © 2002-2005 herbs2000.com (Used with their permission.)

123 "How Shark Cartilage Works On Cancer." Online posting.16 Nov. 2004 <http://www.nutritionfarm.com/GLOSSARY/REPORTS/sharkrept.htm> © 1996-2005 The Nutrition Farm® All Rights Reserved. Used by permission from their website.

124 "Hoxsey Formula." Wellness Directory of Minnesota™. Alternative Cancer Therapies. Online posting. 28 Oct. 2004 <http://www.mnwelldir.org/docs /cancer1/altthrpy2.htm> (Used with their permission.)

125 "HRT Comes With Serious Risks and Side Effects." Online posting. 9 Nov. 2004 <http://www.safemenopausesolutions.com/hrt.html> Copyright © Personal Wellness Network, Inc., All rights reserved. (Used with their permission.)

126 "HSI Members Battle Prostate Cancer with Herbal Complex From the Amazon." Health Archives. HSI Health Sciences Institute, 2/1/2002. Online posting. 21 Oct. 2004 <http://www.hsibaltimore.com/misc/hsi_0202c.shtml> © 1997-2005 by Institute of Health Sciences, LLC. (Used with their permission.)

127 "ICHT (Intra-Cellular Hyperthermia Therapy." Integrated Medical Specialists. Online posting. 12 Dec. 2004 <http://www.heatkillscancer.com/cancer _heat.html>(Used with their permission.)

128 "Independent Lab Verifies Cancer-Fighting Agents In Cherries." Online posting. FS Flavonoid Sciences. Credit: Cherry Marketing Institute Cherry Advantage Issue I. 25 May 2004 <http://www.flavonoidsciences.com/cherry-blueberry.php? page=3 &title=Cancer-Fighter%20P> © Flavonoid Sciences All Rights Reserved. Used by permission of FS Flavonoid Sciences website owners.

129 "Insulin-induced Hypoglycemic Therapy (IHT)." Online posting. 11 Dec. 2004 <http://www.cancertutor.com/Other/Big_List.htm> (Used with their permission.)

130 "IPT Fact sheet." Online posting. 12 Dec. 2004 <http://iptq.com/fact_ sheet.htm> (Used with their permission.)

131 "Is the Budwig Protocol 'just flaxseed oil and cottage cheese'"? Online posting. 17 Jan. 2005 <http://www.healingcancernaturally.com/budwig_protocol.html> © 2004 & 2005 www.healingcancernaturally.com. All Rights Reserved. (Used with their permission.)

132 "Johanna Brandt / Fred Wortman Grape Cure For Cancer." Cancer Tutor™, Alternative Cancer Treatment Information Center. Online posting. 1 Aug. 2004 <http://www.cancertutor.com/Cancer/GrapeCure.html> (Used with their permission.)

133 "Johanna Budwig Revisited." Wellness Directory of Minnesota™. Online posting. 20 Dec. 2004 <http://www.mnwelldir.org/docs/cancer1budwig.htm> (Used with their permission.)

134 "Kidney Cancer (Renal Cell Carcinoma)." Online posting. 17 Oct. 2004 <http://www.herbs2000.com/disorders/cancer_kidney.htm>© 2002-2005 herbs2000.com (Used with their permission.)

135 "Kiwi Fruit." The World's Healthiest Foods: Feeling Great, George Mateljan Foundation. Online posting. 17 Dec. 2004 <http://www.whfoods.com /gen-pagephp?tname=foodspice&dbid=41> © 2002-2005 The George Mateljan Foundation. (Used with their permission.)

136 "Lactose Intake May Increase Ovarian Cancer Risk in Postmenopausal Women." HSI, Health Sciences Institute. Online posting. 30 Dec. 2004 http://www.hsibaltimore.com/ealerts/ea200412/ea20041214.html> © 1997-2005 by Institute of Health Sciences, LLC. (Used with their permission.) Also rec'd this as an email alert on 12/14/04 from HSI/Research@healthiernews.com.

137 "Laetrile." Alternative Health Supplies (Australia). Your Health™, Your Choice®, "Review of Laetrile (Vitamin B17). Online posting. 5 Jan. 2005 <http://www.alternativehealth.com.au/articles/laetril.htm>© 2005 Alternative Health Supplies. All Rights Reserved. (Used with their permission.)

138 "Let the Buyer Beware." Online posting. Red-Purple Lapacho (also known as Pau D' Arco or Taheebo). 21 Oct. 2004 <http://www.oralchelation.com/taheebo/lapacho2.htm> © 2003 by Vibrant Life. All Rights Reserved. (Used with Karl Loren's permission.)

139 "Light Therapy Tackles Cancer." Online posting. 31 May, 2005 <http://news.bbc.co.uk/1/hi/health/1871474.stm> permission granted from BBC News at bbcnews.com, © BBC.

140 "Liver Cancer." Online posting. Liver Cancer – Healing with Herbs, Vitamins and Minerals. 17 Oct. 2004 <http://www.herbs2000.com/disorders /cancer_liver.htm>© 2002-2005 herbs2000.com (Used with their permission.)

141 "Lorenzo's oil for adrenolenkodystrophy and adrenomyeloneuropathy." "Evidence based thinking about health care." Online posting. "Lorenzo's oil for AMN and ALD." <http://www.jr2.ox.ac.uk/bandolier/booth/neurol/lorenz.html> ©1994-2005. (Used with their permission.)

142 "Lung Cancer." Online posting. 17 Oct. 2004 <http://www.herbs2000.com/disorders/cancer_lung.htm>© 2002-2005 herbs2000.com (Used with their permission.)

143 "Lycium Berries (Wolf Berries)." Online posting. 18 Dec. 2004 <http://www.spectrumwellbeing.co.uk/lycium.htm> © Martin Dowling 2002/2003/2004 2005 (Used with their permission.)

144 "Lyprinol." Online posting. 6 May, 2005 <http://www.primohealth.com /PILyprinol.a.html> (Used with their permission.)

145 "Macela." Raintree Nutrition's TROPICAL PLANT DATABASE. Online posting. "Biological Activities and Clinical Research." 22 Oct. 2004 <http://www.rain-tree.com/macela.htm> © 1996 - 2004 Raintree Nutrition, Inc., Carson City, NV. 89701 All rights reserved. This information is also found in Leslie Taylor's book, *The Healing Power of Rainforest Herbs,* Square One Publishers, Jan. 2005 (Used with Ms. Taylor's permission.)

146 "Maitake." Herbs 2000.com. Online posting. 22 Nov. and 29 Dec. 2004 <http://www.herbs2000.com/herbs/herbs_maitake.htm>© 2002-2005 herbs2000.com. (Used with their permission.)

147 "Mammograms Worthless Over Breast Exam Alone." Online posting. Karl Loren's website. 24 May, 2005 <http://www.karlloren.com/biopsy/p88.htm> With permission from Mr. Loren.

148"Mangosteen Treatment for Cancer." Online Posting. 17 Oct. 2004 <http://www.cancertutor.com/Cancer/Mangosteen.html> (Used with their permission.) (note that they give their source for this article is given as: "'Antiproliferation, antioxidation and induction of apoptosis by Garcinia mangostana (mangosteen) on SKBR3 human breast cancer cell line,' by Moongkarndi P, Kosem N, Kaslungka S, Luanratana O, Pongpan N, Neungton N.")

149 "Medical Conditions." Cancer Prevention website. "Botanicals." Copyright 1998 – 2005 by L. Vicky Crouse, N.D. and James S. Reiley, N.D. (ISSN 1527-0661), Online posting. 2 Feb. 2005 <http://www.naturalopinion.com> (Used with their permission.)

150 "Melatonin." Melatonin for Sleep Disorders and antioxidant protection. Online posting. 30 Nov. 2004 <http://www.health-n-energy.com/melatin.htm> (Used with their permission.)

151 "Melatonin: Supplements, What Works." Online posting. 30 Nov. 2004 <http://www.healthyroads.com/mylibrary/data/pelletier/chapter3/p_melatonin.asp> © 2001 Healthyroads. All rights reserved (Used with their permission.)

152 "Migraine." Online posting. 24 Dec. 2004 <http://www.mcvitamins.com/ migraine.htm> (Used with their permission.)

153 "Milk and Dairy." The Food Web. "Milk and Dairy Products." Online posting. 12 Nov. 2004 <http://www.anarac.com/milk_and_dairy.htm> (Used with their permission.)

154 "Milk Thistle (Carduus marianus or Silybum marianum)." Online posting. Dietary Supplement Information Bureau™, nhi, 13 Jan. 2005 <http://content. nhiondemand.com/dse/consumer/monoAll-style.asp? objID=100072&ctype=...> (Used with their permission.)

155 "Milk Thistle." Side Effects and Cautions. Online posting. Herbs2000.com. 29 Dec. 2004 <http://www.herbs2000.com/herbs/herbs_thistle_ milk.htm>© 2002-2005 herbs2000.com (Used with their permission.)

156 "MSM Plus Vitamin C and B12 Cancer Treatment." Online posting. 1 Dec. 2004 <http://www.cancertutor.com/Cancer/MSM.html> (Used with their permission.) (This study was done by "Dr. McCabe, Dr. P. O'Dwyer, Dr. B. Sickle-Antanello, Dr. E. Woltering, Dr. H. Abou-Issa and Dr. A. James, published in the Archives of Surgery, 12/1986.")

157 "Mullaca." Online posting. "Plant Chemicals." TROPICAL PLANT DATABASE of Raintree Nutrition. 21 Oct. 2004 <http://www.rain-tree.com/mullaca.htm> © Copyrighted 1996 - 2004 Raintree Nutrition, Inc., Carson City, NV. 89701 All rights reserved. This information is also found in Leslie Taylor's book, *The Healing Power of Rainforest Herbs,* Square One Publishers, Jan. 2005 (Used with Ms. Taylor's permission)

158 "Mushrooms - Shiitake - Lentinula edodes." Online posting. (1 Aug. 2004) <http://www2.mcdaniel.edu/ Biology/botf99/herbnew/phytomedicine/tomushrooms. html> (Used with their permission.)

159 "Myeloma Cancer." Online posting. Discount Vitamins & 4 Herbs Health News. 1 Aug. 2004 Available: http://www.discount-vitamins-herbs.net/healthnews30 .htm#121 p. 4 (accessed 2004, Aug. 1) (Used with their permission.) Note that Discount-Vitamins gives their reference for this article as: "Bharti AC, Donato N,Singh S, Aggarwal BB. 'Curcumin (diferuloylmethane) down-regulates the constitutive activation of nuclear factor-kappa B and Ikappa Balpha kinase in human multiple myeloma cells, leading to suppression of proliferation and induction of apoptosis.' From *Blood.* 2003 Feb 1;101(3):1053-62."

160 "Natural Progesterone," With permission: AltMedDex® System: Klasco RK (Ed): AltMedDex® System: Thomson Micromedex, Greenwood Village, Colorado (2005, Jan. 24)

161 "Natural Progesterone," "Other Possible Side Effects." With permission: AltMedDex® System: Klasco RK (Ed): AltMedDex® System: Thomson Micromedex, Greenwood Village, Colorado (2005, Jan. 24)

162 "Newsletter Aug. 2001." The Wellness Directory of Minnesota™. Online posting. 18 Dec. 2004 <http://www.mnwelldir.org/docs/Newsletters/01_Aug.htm> (Used with their permission.)

163 "NINDS Adrenoleukodystrophy Information Page," from the National Institute of Neurological Disorders and Stroke. Online posting. 14 May 2005 <http://www.ninds.nih.gov/disorders/adrenoleukodystrophy/adrenoleukodystro-phy.htm>

164 "Non-Hodgkin's Lymphoma – oncology channel." Online posting. This information reprinted with permission © Healthcommunities.com, Inc., 2005. All rights reserved. 13 Dec. 2004 <http://www.oncology/channel.com/nonhodgkins>

165 "Oat Beta Glucan." Effective Natural Cancer Treatments. Online posting. 1 Dec. 2004 <http://www.cancer-treatments.net/cancer.html> (Used with their permission.)

166 "'Off-The-Shelf' Cancer Cure?" Online posting. HSI, Health Archives, 6/1/2001, Health Sciences Institute. 30 Dec. 2004 <http://www.hsibaltimore.com/ea 2001/ea_010301.html> © 1997-2005 by Institute of Health Sciences, LLC. (Used with their permission.)

167 "Oil of Oregano." Online posting. 1 Dec. 2004 <http://www.cancertutor. com/OtherBig_List.htm> (Used with their permission.)

168 "ORAC Values of Fruits & Vegetables." Online posting. 22 Dec. 2004 <http://www.youngagain.com/orac.html> © 1999-2005 Young Again Nutrients. All rights reserved (Used with their permission.)

169 "Ovarian Cancer." Online posting. Website labtestsonline.org. 27 Apr. 2005 <http://www.labtestsonline.org/understanding/conditions/ovarian-2.html. (Used with their permission.) Lab Tests Online is a non-commercial web site published by the American Association for Clinical Chemistry. For up-to-date information on clinical lab tests, visit their website above. © 2001-2005 American Association for Clinical Chemistry.

170 "Pancreatic Cancer: Story of Maribel C. Lim." Cancer Central (Aug. 2003), Manila, Philippines. Online posting. 17 Oct.2004 <http://www.cancer-central.com/ pancreas-cancer/pancreas-caer-3.htm> © 2003 Green & Gold Int'l Exports (Used with their permission.)

171 "Parsley." Online posting. 28 Oct. 2004 <http://www.herbs2000.com/ herbs/herbs_parsley.htm>© 2002-2005 herbs2000.com (Used with their permission.)

172 "Pau D' Arco {Teehebo} Ancient Herb, Modern Miracle." In-depth Pau D'arco Article by Dr. Mowry. Online posting. 10 Dec. 2004 <http://www.oral chelation.com/taheebo/research/page1.htm> © 2003 Vibrant Life. All rights reserved (Used with permission of Mr. Karl Loren.)

173 "Pau d' arco and Cancer." Herbal Remedies for Immunity, Cancer, Lapacho, Natural Herbal Remedies for Cancer. Online posting. 21 Oct. 2004 <http:// www.holistic-online.com/cancer/Cancer_lapacho_herb-rem.htm> © 1998-2005 ICBS, Inc. All rights reserved (Used with their permission.)

174 "PawPaw Alternative Cancer Treatment." Online posting. 14 Dec. 2004 <http://alternativecancer.us/pawpaw.htm> (Used with their permission.)

175 "Phyllanthus." Online posting. 9 April 2005 <http://www.herbs2000.com/ herbs/herbs_phyllanthus.htm>© 2002-2005 herbs2000.com (Used with their permission.)

176 "Pituitary Tumors." National Institute of Neurological Disorders and Stroke. Online posting. 17 May 2005 <http://www.ninds.nih.gov/disorders/pituitary _tumors/pituitary_tumors.htm>

177 "Poly-MVA New hope for cancer patients. New hope for brain cancer patients," online posting, 7 Jul. 2005 <http://www.mnwelldir. org/docs/cancer1/poly.htm> (Used with their permission).

178 "Polysaccharide Kureha (PSK)." Online posting. Herbs2000.com.25 Oct. 2004 (Used with their permission). <http://www.herbs2000.com/miss/psk.htm> © 2002-2005 herbs2000.com (Used with their permission.)

179 "Pomegranate extract blocks skin tumors in mice." New York, Reuters Health. From OncoLink Cancer News, *Reuters Health Information*. Available: http://www.oncolink .com/resources/article.cfm?c=3&s=8&ss=23&id=11481&month = 01&year=2005, posting date Jan 20, 2005 (accessed 2005, June 2) Copyright © 1994-2005 © Trustees of the University of Pennsylvania. From *Reuters Health Information*, Copyright © 2005 Reuters Limited. All rights reserved. Reprinted with their permission. Reuters shall not be liable for any errors or delays in the content, or for any actions taken in reliance thereon.

180 "Preserving the living and the dead." New Agriculturist on-line – Reporting Agriculture for the 21st Century. "Spice Preservatives." Online posting. 20 Dec. 2004 <http://www.new-agri.co.uk/02-1/focuson/focuson8.html> (Used with their permission.)

181 "Prostate Cancer." Herbs 2000. Online posting. 17 Oct. 2004 <http://www.herbs2000.com/disorders/cancer_prostate.htm>© 2002-2005 herbs2000.com (Used with their permission.)

182 "Provera Side Effects, and Drug Interactions – Medroxyprogesterone Acetate – RxList Mon…" Side Effects. Online posting. 24 Jan. 2005 <http://www.rxlist.com/cgi/generic/medrox_ad.htm> © 2005 by RxList, Inc. (Used with their permission.)

183 "Prozac: What is the Truth behind it? The Prozac Truth Exposed on this Web Site." Online posting. 5 Jan. 2005 <http://www.prozactruth.com> (Used with their permission.)

184 "Psoralea." Online posting. 30 Nov. 2004 and 25 Oct. 2004 <http://www.herbs2000.com/herbs/herbs_psoralea.htm>© 2002-2005 herbs2000.com (Used with their permission.)

185 "Raw Dairy Sales Illegal in Manhattan." HSI Health Sciences Institute. "The Milkman Cometh." Online posting. 30 Dec. 2004 <http://www.hsialert.com/ ealerts/ea200412/ea20041222.html> © 1997-2005 by Institute of Health Sciences, LLC. Also received this as an email on 12-22-04 from HSIResearch@healthiernews.com. (Used with their permission.)

186 "Recent Scientific Advances in Rare Diseases Research," Report on the Rare Diseases Research Activities at the National Institutes of Health FY 2003," "Beta-Sitosterolemia," Online posting. 2 Jul. 2005. <http://rarediseases.info.nih.gov/html/reports/fy2003/ nhlbi.html>

187 "Red Beet." Leukemia, from "Herbal Formulas for Leukemia." Online posting. 1 Aug. 2004 <http://www.herbsfirst.com/ailmentsdescriptions/leukemiapg.html> (note that this information is now under the article "Leukemia," at website http://herballegacy.com/id118.htm, which is linked to herbfirst.com) (Used with their permission.) their website says that this was taken from the book *School of Natural Healing* by John R. Christopher, 1976, Christopher Publications, P O Box 412, Springville, UT. 84663.

188 "Red Clover (Trifolium praetense)." Online Posting. Cancer Tutor™ Alternative Cancer Treatment Information Center. 17 Oct. 2004 <http://www.cancertutor.com/Other/Big_List.htm> (Used with their permission.)

189 "Rhodiola Rosea." New Page 5. Online posting. Planet Herbs. 21 Oct. 2004 <http://www.planetherbs.com/articles/rhodiolia%20rosea/htm> © PlanetHerbs Online 01/04/04 (Used with their permission.)

190 "Rhodiola Rosea." Online posting. Planet Herbs. 21 Oct. 2004 <http://www.planetherbs.com/articles/rhodiolia%20rosea/htm> © PlanetHerbs Online 01/04/04 - (Used with their permission.) from their reference: Artic Root (Rhodiola Rosea): The Powerful New Ginseng Alternative by Carl Germano, R.D., C.N.S., L.D.N., and Zakir Ramazanov, Ph.D., published by Kensington Health Books.

191 "Royal Jelly (a bee product)." Online posting. Alternative Cancer Treatment Information Center. 21 Nov. 2004 <http://www.cancertutor. com/Other/Big_List.htm> (Used with their permission.)

192 "Royal Rife Machine." Online posting. 17 Oct. 2004 <http://www.cancer tutor.com/Other/Big_List.htm> (Used with their permission.)

193 "Saliva vs. Serum or Plasma Testing For Progesterone." Special Report from the John R. Lee, M.D. Medical Letter, Saliva Hormone Testing. Online posting. 24 Dec. 2004 <http://www.johnleemd.com/store/saliva_serum.html> © Hormones, Etc. (Used with their permission.)

194 "Sarcoma." Online posting. Cancer-healing.com website. "Cancer Types." 3 May 2005 <http://www.cancer-healing.com/cancer_type.php> © 2004 Life Enthusiast Co-op, All rights reserved (Used with their permission.)

195 "Schisandra Berries More Than a Liver Aid," From the January 2001 issue of Nutrition Science News, NewHope.com. Online posting. "Protects the Liver." 25 Nov. 2004 <http://www.newhope.com/nutritionsciencenews/NSN_backs/Jan_01 /schisandra.cfm> Copyright © 2004, Penton Media, Inc. (Used with their permission.)

196 "Seven Essentials." Healthy-Living.org. Online posting. 21 Dec. 2004 <http://www.healthy-living.org/html/essential_seven.html> © 2002-2004 Healthy-Living.org. All rights reserved (Used with their permission.)

197 "Shark Cartilage." Enerex.ca. Online posting. 30 Jun. 2004 <http://www. enerex.ca/articles/shark_cartilage.htm> © 1997-2005 Enerex Botanicals Ltd., All rights reserved (Used with their permission.)

198 "Sheep Sorrel." Online posting. Cancer and Immunity, Immune Building Agents, Dr.Lam.com. 21 Nov. 2004 <http://www.drlam.com/A3R_brief_in_doc_ format/cancer_and_immunity.cfm>© 2001-2004 by Michael Lam M.D. All Rights Reserved (Used with Dr. Lam's permission.)

199 "Shiitake Mushroom (Lentinula edodes)." Online posting. 7 May, 2005 <http://www.stoneycreekmushrooms.com/about.htm> (Used with their permission.)

200 "Simarouba." Online posting. "Simarouba glauca, amara Simarouba – Simarouba glauca," TROPICAL PLANT DATABASE of Raintree Nutrition. "Biological Activities & Clinical Research." 22 Oct. 2004 <http://www.rain-tree.com/simarouba .htm> © 1996 - 2004 Raintree Nutrition, Inc., Carson City, NV. 89701 All rights reserved. This information is also found in Leslie Taylor's book, *The Healing Power of Rainforest Herbs,* Square One Publishers, Jan. 2005 (Used with Ms. Taylor's permission.)

201 "Snow Fungus." Online posting. 20 Nov. 2004 <http://www.herbs2000. com/herbs/herbs_snow_fungus.htm> © 2002-2005 herbs2000.com (Used with their permission.)

202 "Stomach Cancer." Online posting. 17 Oct. 2004 <http://www.herbs2000. com/disorders/cancer_stomach.htm> © 2002-2005 herbs2000.com. (Used with their permission.)

203 "Suma." Raintree Nutrition Tropical Plant Database. Online posting. 22 Oct. 2004 <http://www.rain-tree.com/suma.htm> © 1996 - 2004 Raintree Nutrition, Inc., Carson City, NV. 89701 All rights reserved. This information is also found in Leslie Taylor's book, *The Healing Power of Rainforest Herbs,* Square One Publishers, Jan. 2005 (Used with Ms. Taylor's permission.)

204 "Sun exposure prevents prostate cancer." yourhealthbase.com. Online posting. 3 May 2005 <http://www.yourhealthbase.com/cancer_prostate.htm> © 1994-2005 by Hans R. Larsen (Used with their permission.)

205 "Sweet Wormwood (herb)." Online posting. The Cancer Tutor™, Alternative Cancer Treatment Information Center. 17 Oct. 2004 <http://www. cancertutor.com/Other/Big_List.htm> (Used with their permission.)

206 *Taber's Cyclopedic Medical Dictionary.* 20th Edition, Philadelphia, PA: F.A. Davis Co., © 2005. (Used with their permission.)

207 "Tetrahydrocannabinol (THC – medical marijuana)." Cancer Tutor™, Alternative Cancer Treatment Information Center. Online posting. 17 Oct. 2004 <http://www.cancertutor.com/Other/Big_List.htm> (Used with their permission.)

208 "The Benefits of Beta Glucan and MSM Supplements from a Terminal Cancer Survivor's perspective." Why Beta Glucan for Immune System Response? Online posting. 17 Oct. 2004 <http://www.aboutbetaglucan.com> © 2002-2004 Aboutbetaglucan.com. All rights reserved (Used with their permission.)

209 "The Cure That Killed The Patient." Karl Loren's website. From "Chemotherapy: A Dull Weapon." Online posting. 5 Dec. 2004 <http://www.karl loren.com/biopsy/p60htm (Used with Mr. Loren's permission.)

210 "The Effect of Ukrain on Cancer." Online posting. 13 Oct. 2004 <http://www.ukrin.com/standardtexte/Standardbrief_2_eng.htm> © Ukrainian Anti-Cancer Institute 1997-2005. (Used with their permission.)

211 "The Health Effects of Chlorine in our Water." Online posting. 15 Jan. 2005 <http://www.wizardofeyez.com/chlorine.html> ©: 9/8/2001, A.D., with the Freedom against the Egypt-Calendar: G. M. Swartwout© (Used with their permission.)

212 The Healing Power of Vitamins, Minerals, and Herbs. Reader's Digest, Pleasantville, N.Y. Reader's Digest Assoc., Inc., 1998, 1999, 2000. Quoted with permission of Global Books & Home Entertainment, The Reader's Digest Association, Inc.

213 "The Latest Research on Selenium and Prostate Cancer." Online posting. American Federation for Aging Research, Prostate Cancer Information Center. 26 Oct. 2004 <http://www.infoaging.org/d-prost-17—r-selenium.htm> © 2000-05 American Federation for Aging Research. All rights reserved (Used with their permission.)

214 "Tian Xian." Cancer Alternative Treatments. Online posting. Tian Xian liquid. 17 Oct. 2004 <http://www.tianxian.com> © 2004 Green & Gold Int'l. Exports. All rights reserved. (Used with their permission.)

215 "Transfer Factor." Cancer Tutor™ website, Online posting. 1 Dec. 2004 <http://www.cancertutor.com/Other/Big_ List.htm> (Used with their permission.)

216 "Treatment: Hydrazine Sulfate." Online posting. 20 Jan. 2005 <http://www. diagnoseme.com/treat/T396383.html> (Used with their permission.)

217 "Triptolide." Alternative Cancer Therapies. The Wellness Directory of Minnesota™. Online posting. 21 Oct. 2004 <http://www.mnwelldir.org/docs/cancer1/ altthrpy3.htm> (Used with their permission.)

218 "Tumor Types: Non Gliomas." Online posting. 10 Apr. 2005 <http://www.braintumors.org/patient_info/surviving/tumor_types/nongliomas.htm l> © 2000-2004 National Brain Tumor Foundation. (Used with their permission.)

219 "Tumor Types: Other Brain-Related Conditions." Online posting. 10 Apr. 2005 <http://www.braintumors.org/patient_info/surviving/tumor_types/other-brain.html> © 2000-2004 National Brain Tumor Foundation. (Used with their permission.)

220 "Turmeric Curcuma longa syn C. domestica." 29 Jan. 2005 <http://www .herbs2000.com/herbs/herbs_turmeric.htm>© 2002-2005 herbs2000.com. (Used with their permission.)

221 "Turmeric May Be Effective Adjunct Cancer Therapy." Discount Vitamins & Herbs – Health News. Online posting. 17 Nov. 2004 <http://www. discount-vitamins-net/health-news30.htm> (Note that the reference the website gives for their article is: "The annual meeting of the American Association for Cancer Research, San Francisco, California. April 9, 2002.") © 2001-2005 Discount Herbs & Vitamins, Inc. All rights reserved. (Used with their permission.)

222 "Vassourinha." Online posting. Raintree Nutrition's TROPICAL PLANT DATABASE. "Plant Chemicals." 21 Oct. 2004 <http://www.rain-tree.com/vassourinha .htm> © 1996 - 2004 Raintree Nutrition, Inc., Carson City, NV. 89701 All rights reserved. This information is also found in Leslie Taylor's book, *The Healing Power of Rainforest Herbs,* Square One Publishers, Jan. 2005 (Used with Ms. Taylor's permission.)

223 "Vitamin A may prevent prostate cancer." yourhealthbase.com. Online posting. 3 May 2005 <http://www.yourhealthbase.com/cancer_prostate.htm> © 1994-2005 by Hans R. Larsen (Used with their permission.)

224 "Vitamin A and Carotenoids." Facts About Dietary Supplements, National Institutes of Health Office of Dietary Supplements. Online posting. 14 Jan. 2005 <http://ods.od.nih.gov/factsheets/cc/vita.html> (Used with their permission.)

225 "Vitamin D supplements to protect against MS," 03/01/2005. NUTRAingredients.com/ Europe. Online posting. 23 Jun. 2005 <http://www.nutraingredients.com/news/news-ng.asp?n=56996-vitamin-d-supplements> (Used with their permission.) NOVIS Industry & Science News © 2001/2005 – NOVIS – All rights reserved

226 "We have the formula!" Alternative Cancer Therapies. Wellness Directory of Minnesota™. Online posting. 20 Dec. 2004. <http://www.mnwelldir. org/docs/cancer1 /altthrpy.htm> (Used with their permission.)

227 "What are the reasons to have a hysterectomy?" "When is a hysterectomy necessary?" Online posting. 9 Nov. 2004 <http://www.safemenopausesolutions.com /hysterectomy.html> Copy © Personal Wellness Network, Inc. All rights reserved (Used with their permission.)

228 "What is graft-versus-host disease? (If you are having a transplant from a donor)." Online posting. CancerBACUP Helping people live with cancer. 21 Nov. 2004 <http://www.cancerBACUP.org.uk/ Treatments/stemcellbonemarrow transplants/ Generalinfo...> © CancerBACUP 2003 (Used with their permission.)

229 "What is Leukodystrophy?" National Institute of Neurological Disorders and Stroke, NINDS Leukodystrophy Information Page, Online posting. 2 Jul. 2005 <http://www.ninds.nih.gov/disorders/ leukodystrophy/leukodystrophy.html>

230 "What is the health risk of too many carotenoids?" Facts About Dietary Supplements, "Vitamin A and Carotenoids, National Institutes of Health Office of Dietary Supplements. Online posting. 14 Jan. 2005 <http://ods.od.nih.gov/fact-sheets/cc /vita.html> (Used with their permission.)

231 "Wheatgrass Treatment For Cancer." Cancer Tutor™ website. Online posting. 12 Dec. 2004 <http://www.cancertutor.com/Cancer/Wheatgrass.html> (Used with their permission.)

232 "Wormwood." Alternative Cancer Therapies. Dr. Lam, M.D. at http://www.drlam.com/A3R_brief_in_doc_format/Artemisinin.cfm; © 2001-2004 by Michael Lam M.D. All Rights Reserved. Note that quotes are from the Wellness Directory of Minnesota's™ website, online posting. 20 Dec. 2004 <http://www.mnwell dir.org/docs/cancer1/altthrpy.htm> (Used with their permission.)

233 "Xi Shu." Online posting. 28 Oct. 2004 <http://www.herbs2000.com/ herbs/herbs_xi_shu.htm>© 2002-2005 herbs2000.com (Used with their permission.)

234 Anderson, Nina, "120 and Healthy! It's Common in the Republic of Georgia." Online posting. Many Hands Feature Articles at the Alternative Medical Journal of New England. 17 Oct. 2004 <http://www.manyhands.com/articles/georgia.html> © 1996-2003 Many Hands Magazine. All rights reserved (Used with permission from www.manyhands.com.)

235 Antol, Marie N. *Healing Teas*: How to Prepare and Use Teas to Maximize Your Health, (City, State, n.g.) Avery Publishing, Penguin Group (USA), Inc., 1996.

236 Atkins, Robert, M.D. "Nutritional Doctor Quotes." From *Whale* website. Online posting. 28 May, 2005 <http://www.whale.to/m/quotes2.html> (Used with their permission.)

237 Baker, M. L. "Drug Makers Support Clinical Trial Disclosure." June 18, 2004. BARISTA headstarters for the hungry mind. June 19, 2004, "A Bex and a Nice Lie Down." Online posting. 5 Jan. 2005 <http://www.dox.media2.org/barista/archives/000781.html> (Used with their permission.)

238 Balch, James F., M.D. From *The Super Anti-Oxidants –Why They Will Change the Face of Healthcare in the 21st Century*, copyright © 1998 by James F. Balch. Reprinted by the permission of the publisher, M. Evans & Company, New York

239 Balch, Phyllia A., C.N.C. and James F, M.D., *Prescription for Nutritional Healing*. New York: Avery Publishing, 2000.

240 Baroody, Theodore A., N.D., D.C., Ph.D. Nutrition, C.N.C. *Alkalize or Die – Superior Health Through Proper Alkaline-Acid Balance*. Waynesville, N.C: Holographic Health Press, 1991. (Used with Dr. Baroody's approval.)

241 Batmanghelidj, F., M.D. *Your Body's Many Cries For Water*. Vienna, VA: Global Health Solutions, Inc. 1992, 1995, 1997. (Used with permission of Mr. Bob Butts.)

242 Becker, Sue. "Bulk Up On Fiber." Online posting. 8 Jun. 2005 <http://www/breadbeckers.com/bulkuponfiber.html> Copyright 2003, The Bread Beckers, Inc. © (Used with their permission.)

243 Berkson, Bert, M.D., Ph.D. From *The Alpha Lipoic Acid Breakthrough: The Superb Antioxidant That May Slow Aging, Repair Liver Damage, and Reduce the Risk of Cancer, Heart Disease, and Diabetes*. Copyright © 1998 by Bert Berkson. Used by permission of Prima Publishing, Division of Random House, Inc.

244 Best, Billy and Sue Best. "The Boy Who Ran Away From Chemotherapy, Billy's Story." Online posting. 7 Jan 2005 <http://www.grand-strand.com/suebest /boywho.htm> © 2004 Grandstrand Information Technologies. (Used by permission of Sue Best.)

245 Bharti, A.C., et al. "Turmeric May Be Effective Adjunct Cancer Therapy." Discount Vitamins and Herbs Health News (from "The Annual Meeting of the American Assoc. for Cancer Research, San Francisco, CA.) April 9, 2002. Online posting. 1 Aug. 2004 <http://www.discount-vitamins-herbs.net/health-news30htm> (Used with their permission.)

246 Billingsley, J. "Red Wine May Protect Against Breast Cancer – Phytochemicals Appear to Block Estrogen Formation." Online posting. HealthDay. 18 May 2004 <http://www.healthday.com/view.cfm?id=516350> © 2005 Scout News, LLC. All rights reserved. (Used with their permission.)

247 Blauer, Stephen. *The Juicing Book: A Complete Guide to the Juicing of Fruits and Vegetables for Maximum Health.* (City, State, n.g.) Avery Publishing, 1989.

248 Blaylock, Russell. L., M.D. *Natural Strategies For Cancer Patients.* New York: Twin Streams, Kensington Publishing Corp., © 2003, All rights reserved. Reprinted by arrangement with Kensington Publishing Corp. www.kensington-books.com.

249 Borek, C., Ph.D. "Beta Glucan Boosts Immunity," Beta Glucan vs. Cancer," and "Beta Glucan the Supplement." Online posting. 17 Oct. 2004 <http://www.newhope.com/ nutritionsciencenews/NSN_backs/Jan_01/betaglu-can.cfm> Copyright © 2004 Penton Media, Inc. (Used with their permission.)

250 Brandt, Johanna. *The Grape Cure.* Yonkers, New York: Ehret Literature Publishing Co., Inc., P O Box 24, Dobbs Ferry, N.Y., 10522, 1971. Their website is at www.arnold ehret.org. (Used with permission of Ehret Literature Publishing Co.)

251 Brandt, Johanna., N.D. *How to Conquer Cancer Naturally.* Joshua Tree, Ca: Tree of Life Publications, 1989. (Used with their permission.)

252 Broadhurst, C. Leigh, Ph.D. *Health and Healing with Bee Products.* Vancouver, Canada: with permission from Alive Publishing Group, Inc., Canada.www.alive.com <http://www.alive.com> 2000.

253 Brown, Anthony J., M.D., Reuters Health, New York, posting date May 23, 2005. "Pomegranate juice shows promise as treatment for recurrent prostate cancer." Available: http://www.oncolink.com/resources /article.cfm? =3&s=8&ss=23&id=11913&month= 058&year=2005 OncoLink Cancer News, Copyright © 1994-2005 © Trustees of the University of Pennsylvania. Copyright © 2005 Reuters Limited. All rights reserved. Reprinted with their permission. Reuters shall not be liable for any errors or delays in the content, or for any actions taken in reliance thereon. (accessed 2005, June 2)

254 Brown, Arlin J. "Comprehensive Cancer Therapy." Online posting. The Cancer Homepage. 18 May 2004 <http://www.curezone.com/diseases/cancer/can-cer _arlin_therapy.html>© 1996-2005 CureZone.com (Used with their permission.)

255 Charles Brusch, M.D. "Alternative Medical Doctor Quotes," from *Whale* website. 9 Jun. 2005 <http://www.whale.to/m/quotes6.html> (Used with their permission.)

256 Budwig, Johanna, Dr. "The Budwig Diet Quotes," from *Whale* website. 28, Jun. 2005 <http://www.whale.to/a/budwig_q.html> (Used with their permission.)

257 Calbom, Cheri and Maureen Keane. *Juicing For Life*. (City, State, n.g.) Avery, member of Penguin Putnam, Inc., 1992, Trillium Health Products.

258 Carper, Jean. *The Food Pharmacy: Dramatic New Evidence That Food Is our Best Medicine.* New York: Bantam Books, 1988. Reprinted with Ms. Carper's permission.

259 Carper, Jean. *Miracle Cures: Dramatic New Scientific Discoveries Revealing the Healing Powers of Herbs, Vitamins, and Other Natural Remedies* New York: Harper Collins, 1997. Reprinted with Ms. Carper's permission.

260 Cassani, Margareta-Erminia. "MGN-3: Mushroom Extract Boosts Immune System, Kills Diseased Cells." Moonbow Media, MGN-3 Disease Killing Mushrooms. Online posting. 6 Jan. 2005 <http://www.moonbowmedia.com/health/mgn3.htm> © Magareta-Erminia Cassani, 2000-2004 All rights reserved (Used with their permission.)

261 Cathcart, Robert F., M.D. "Vitamin C – Orthomed.com," "Polio Cure Systematically Suppressed." Online Posting. 28 May, 2005 <http://www.orthomed.com> © 2005 & prior years, Robert F. Cathcart, M.D. (Used with their permission.)

262 Challem, Jack. *All About Carotenoids Beta-Carotene, Lutein & Lycopene.* Garden City Park, N.Y: Avery Publishing, 1999, permission granted from Mr. Challem for all quotes.

263 Cheraskin, E., M.D., D.M.D. *Vitamin C Who Needs It?* Birmingham, AL: Arlington Press & Co., 1993. (Used with their permission.)

264 Chowka, Peter, "Suzanne Somers' Use of Mistletoe," "Actress Suzanne Somers chooses an alternative therapy to treat her breast cancer © By Peter Chowka (April 1, 2001), <http://store.yahoo.com/annieappleseedproject/suzso-museofm.html> (accessed 2005, Jul. 4) Used with their permission.

265 Clark, Hulda Regehr, Ph.D., N.D. *The Cure For All Cancers: Including over 100 Case Histories of Persons Cured,* Chula Vista, CA: New Century Press, 1993. (Reprinted with permission from New Century Press.)

266 Clark S.S., Zhoung L, Filiult, D, Perman S, Ren Z, Gould, M, Yang,"Anti-leukemia effect of perillyl alcohol in Ber/Abl-transformed cells indirectly inhibits signaling through Mek in a Ras- and Raf-independent fashion," Online posting. NCBI, PubMed, Clin Cancer Res. 2003 Oct. 1:9(12):4494-504, 1 Jul. 2005 <http://www.ncbi.nlm.nih.gov/ entrez/query.fcgi? cmd=Retrieve&db= pubmed&dopt=Abstract&list_uids=14555523& query_hl=38>

267 Colbert, Don, M.D. *Walking in Divine Health*. Lake Mary, FL: Siloam, A Strang Co., 1999. Used with permission of Siloam, A Strang Company.

268 Colbert, Don, M.D. *Toxic Relief.* Lake Mary, FL: Siloam, A Strang Co., 2001, 2003. Used with permission of Siloam, A Strang Company.

269 Colbert, Don, M.D. *What You Don't Know May Be Killing You.* Lake Mary, FL: Siloam, A Strang Co., 2000. Used with permission of Siloam, A Strang Company.

270 Connor, John G. "Cancer Prevention and Diet." Online posting. 21 May 2005 <http://www.compassionateacupuncture.com/cancer.htm> copyright © 2005 John G. Connor. (Used with their permission.)

271 Costello, M. "Essiac Quotes." Online posting. 28 Jun. 2005 *<http://www.whale.to/c/ quotes.html>* (Used with their permission.)

272 Debe, J.A., D.C., D.A.C.B.N., C.C.S.P., C.C.N. "MGN-3 – New Super Immune Stimulator." Online posting. 1 Aug. 2004 <http://www.drdebe.com/MGN.htm> Copyright © Nov. 9, 1998 by Joseph A. Debe. (Used with their permission.)

273 Deoul, Kathleen. "Cancer Cover-Up The Neal Deoul Story." Frequently Asked Questions from cancer-coverup.com. Online posting. 26 Dec. 2004 <http://www.cancer-coverup. com/faqs/is-this-treatment-safe.htm> (Used with their permission.)

274 Dubin, Reese. From *Miracle Food Cures From The Bible* by Reese Dubin, copyright © 1999 by Prentice Hall. Used by permission of Avery Publishing, an imprint of Penguin Group (USA) Inc.

275 Duke, James A., Ph.D. *The Green Pharmacy, The Ultimate Compendium of Natural Remedies from the World's Foremost Authority on Healing Herbs*, New York: St. Martin's Paperbacks, 1998, published in arrangement with Rodale Press, Inc., 1997. (Used with their permission.)

276 Duke, James A., Ph.D., with Michael Castleman. *The Green Pharmacy-Anti-Aging Prescriptions Herbs, Foods, and Natural Formulas to Keep You Young,* (City, State, n.g.) Rodale Press, Inc., 2001. (Used with their permission.)

277 Edelson, Stephen.B., M.D. and Lynn Sonberg. *WHAT YOUR DOCTOR MAY NOT TELL YOU ABOUT IMMUNE DISORDERS: The Revolutionary Drug-free Treatments for Thyroid Disease, Lupus, MS, IBD, Chronic Fatigue, Rheumatoid Arthritis, and Other Diseases,* New York: Warner Books, A Lynn Sonberg Book, 2003. From *What Your Doctor May Not Tell You About ™: Autoimmune Disorders*

by Stephen Edelson, M.D., Copyright © 2003 by Stephen Edelson and Lynn Sonberg. By permission of Warner Books, Inc.

278 Eftekhar, J. L. *Heal Yourself. Globe Digests™*. Boca Raton, FL and New York: Globe Communications Corp., 1995. Reproduced with permission of Globe Digests.

279 Elkins, Rita, M.H. *Healing from the Hive Bee Pollen Royal Jelly Propolis AND Honey*. Pleasant Grove, UT: Woodland Publishing, 1996. (Used with their permission.)

280 Elkins, Rita, M.H. *Cat's Claw (Uno de Gato),* Pleasant Grove, UT: Woodland Publishing, Inc.,1995. (Used with their permission.)

281 Elkins, Rita, M.H. *Powerful Protector Against Breast and Prostate Cancers D-Glucarate™,* Pleasant Grove, UT: Woodland Publishing, Inc., 1999. (Used with their permission.)

282 Elkins, Rita, M.H. *Natural Alternatives to HRT: Overcome Osteoporosis, Heart Disease and Other Menopausal Conditions Without Risky Synthetic Hormone Replacement.* Orem, UT: Woodland Publishing, 2003. (Used with their permission.)

283 Elkins, Rita, M.H. *Noni (Morinda citrifolia),* Pleasant Grove, UT: Woodland Publishing, 1997. (Used with their permission.)

284 Elkins, Rita. *Chinese Red Yeast Rice.* Pleasant Grove, UT: Woodland Publishing, 1998. (Used with their permission.)

285 Ellison, S., M.Sc. "Beyond Vioxx." From "Details on the Vioxx Recall, Possible Vioxx Side Effects, Vioxx Lawsuit, Information and Alternative Natural Treatments..." Online Posting. 9 Nov. 2004 <http://www.safemenopausesolutions.com/vioxx.html> Copyright © Personal Wellness Network, Inc. All rights reserved (Used with their permission.)

286 Evans, Tony. *Tony Evans Speaks Out on Fasting.* Chicago: Moody Publishers, 2000. (Used with their permission.)

287 Forgionne, G. A., Ph.D. "Nutritional Therapy for Primary Peritoneal Cancer: A Case Study." From the CancerLynx website. Online posting. 14 Dec. 2004 <http://www. cancerlynx.com/peritonealcase.html> Copyright CancerLynx 1999-2005 (Used with their permission.)

288 Fox, Marilyn. "Multiple Sclerosis Testimonials," Online posting. 22 Mar. 2005 <http://www.watercure2.org> (Used with permission of Mr. Bob Butts.)

289 Gale, K. Reuters Health. "Herbal COX-2 Inhibitor Induces Prostate Cancer Cell Apoptosis." 29 Jul. 2003, Online Posting. Oncolink – Abramson Cancer Center of the Univ. of Pennsylvania. "Prostate Cancer." Copyright 1994-2004 © Trustees of the University of PA. 4 Jan. 2005 <http://www.oncolink.com/resources/article.cfm?c=3&s =8&ss=23&id=9953&month=07&year=2003> Copyright © 2005 Reuters Limited. All rights reserved. Reprinted with their permission. Reuters shall not be liable for any errors or delays in the content, or for any actions taken in reliance thereon. Also see <http:// www.oncolink.com/custom_tags/print_article. cfm?Page=2&id=9953&Section=Reut...>

290 Gardiner, Eric. *How I conquered Cancer – A Naturopathic Alternative.* Houston, TX: Emerald Ink Publishing, 1997. (Used by permission of Emerald Ink Publishing)

291 Gittleman, Ann Louise, M.S. *Natural Healing For Parasites.* New York: Healing Wisdom Publications, 1995. (Used with permission of Ms. Gittleman.)

292 Gordon, Serena. "Vitamin K Might Prevent Liver Cancer – Wards disease Off in Women with Cirrhosis." Online posting. 25 Nov. 2004 <http://www.health-day.com/view. cfm?id=520187> (Used with their permission.)

293 Gottlieb, Bill. *Alternative Cures – The Most Effective Natural Home Remedies for 160 Health Problems.* (City, State, n.g.) Rodale, Inc., 2000 (Used with Rodale's permission.)

294 Greenberg, Alan, M.D. "Cancer Quotes." Online posting. 19 Jun. 2005 < *http://www. whale.to/cancer/quotes.html>* (Used with their permission.)

295 Griffith, H. Winter, M.D. VITAMINS, HERBS, MINERALS & SUPPLEMENTS, THE COMPLETE GUIDE. Rev. Edition. (City, State, n.g.) Fisher Books, Member of Perseus Books Group, 1988, 1998. (Used with their permission.)

296 Gupta, Chris, "The FDA versus Folic Acid." Share the Wealth, July 14, 2003. Online posting. 20 Nov. 2004 <http://www.newmediaexplorer.org/chris/2003/07/14/the _fda_versus_folic_acid.htm> (Used with Mr. Gupta's permission.)

297 Gupta, Chris, "The FDA versus Folic Acid – Share The Wealth." "It's time to revolt." Online posting. 20 Nov. 2004 <http://www.newmediaexplorer.org/chris/2003/07/14/ the_fda_versus_folic_acid.htm> (Used with Mr. Gupta's permission.)

298 Gursche, Siegfried. *Fantastic Flax, A Powerful Defense Against Cancer, Heart Disease and Digestive Disorders.* Burnaby BC V5J 5B9: Vancouver, Canada: 2003, with permission from Alive Publishing Group, Inc. Canada. www.alive.com <http://www.alive. com>

299 Gursche, Siegfried. *Good Fats and Oils, Why We Need Them and How to Use Them in the Kitchen,* 2000, with Permission from Alive Publishing Group, Inc., www.alive.com <http://www.alive.com>

300 Guttersen, C., R.D., Ph.D. "Take Two Carrots and Call Me In the Morning." Online Posting. Foodservice – Diet and Breast Cancer. 11 May 2004 <http://www.calolive.org/ foodservice/findings/findings2002q3html> Copyright © 2005 California Olive Industry. All rights reserved (Used with permission of the California Olive Industry's website.)

301 "Gymnema Sylvestre for Diabetes," Brain Wave Entrainment Technology. Online posting, 3 Jan. 2005 <http://intelegen.com/nutrients/gymnema _sylvestre_for_diabetes.htm> p. 1 © Vitamin Research Products, Inc., 2001, used with Intelegen's permission.

302 Hawken, C.M. *Green Foods "Phyto Foods" for Super Health.* Pleasant Grove, UT: Woodland Publishing, 1998. (Used with their permission.)

303 Hayes, Norvel. *Worship Your Foundation For The Victorious Life.* (Tulsa: Harrison House Publishers, copyright 1997.) (Used with their permission.)

304 Hayes, Norvel. *Worship Breaking Through to His Presence and Power.* (Tulsa: Harrison House Publishers, copyright 1993.) (Used with their permission.)

305 Heinerman, John. *Healing Power of Herbs.* Boca Raton, FL: *Globe Digests™*, Globe Communications Corp., 1995. Reproduced with permission of Globe Digests.

306 Heinerman, John. *HEINERMAN'S ENCYCLOPEDIA OF HEALING JUICES*, New York: Reward Books by Penguin Putnam, Inc., 1994.

307 Hirneise, Lothar. "Lothar Hirneise's Cancer Research." Online posting. 17 Jan. 2005 <http://www.healingcancernaturally.com/lotharhirneise.html> © 2004 & 2005 www.healingcancernaturally.com. All rights reserved. (Used with their permission.)

308 Hoffer, Abram, M.D., Ph.D., FRCP(C). "Clinical Procedures in Treating Terminally Ill Cancer Patients with Vitamin C." Supportive Vitamin C Therapy for Cancer Patients. Online posting. 1 Aug. 2004 <http://www.doctoryourself.com/hoffer_cancer_2.html> Used with permission from Dr. Hoffer and the website as well.

309 Hoffer, Abram, M.D., Ph.D., FRCP(C). "Hoffer's Home Page – Orthomolecular Treatment of Cancer." Online posting. 28 May, 2005 <http://www.islandnet.com/~hoffer/ (Used with Dr. Hoffer's permission.)

310 Hoffer, Abram, M.D., F.R.C.P.(C), with Linus Pauling, Ph.D. *Healing Cancer – Complementary Vitamin & Drug Treatments,* Toronto, Ontario Canada: CCNM Presss, Inc., 2004 (Used by permission of Bob Hilderley at CCNM Press as well as Dr. Abram Hoffer.)

311 Howell, Mike and Sandra Goodman, Ph.D. This quote was taken from "An Interview with Udo Erasmus." Positive Health Magazine, Integrated Magazine for the 21st century, Issue 12/May/June 1996. Online posting. 23 Jan. 2005 <http://www.positivehealth.com/ articles.asp?I=818> Content © Positive Health Publications Ltd. 1994-2005. All rights reserved. (Used with their permission.)

312 Hunsberger, Mae Eydie with C. Loeffler. *How I Conquered Cancer Naturally*. Garden City Park, N.Y.: Avery Publishing Group, Inc., 1992.

313 Jaehnig, K.C. "Ginseng Root May Help Slow Growth of Cancer Cells." Online posting. 9 May, 2005 <http://news.siu.edu/news/January05/011105kj4109.htm> © 2003, Board of Trustees, Southern Illinois University. (Used with their permission.)

314 Keegan, Lynn, Ph.D., R.N. *Healing Nutrition*. Albany, N.Y: From *Healing Nutrition* 2nd Edition by KEEGAN. © 2002. Reprinted with permission of Delmar Learning, a division of Thomson Learning: www.thomsonrights.com. Fax 800 730-2215.

315 Kradjian, Robert M., M.D. "The Milk Letter: A Message To My Patients," from Dr. Robert M. Kradjian, M.D. *Breast Surgery,* Chief Div. of General Surgery, Seton Medical Centre #302 – 1800 Sullivan Ave., Daly City, CA 94015 USA. Online posting. 26 Jan. 2005 <http://www.notmilk.com/Kradjian.html> © notmilk.com (Used with their permission.)

316 Kramer, Thomas, A.M., M.D. "Understanding Clinical Trials in Context." 10/02/03, from Medscape General Medicine™, Medscape from WebMD. Online posting. 7 Jan. 2005 <http://www.medscape.com/viewarticle/462046_3> "Support and Sponsorship." Reprinted with permission from *Medscape General Medicine 5 (4), 2003,* http://www.medscape.com/viewarticle/462046 © 2003, Medscape.

317 Kroeger, Hanna, Ms.D. *Free Your Body of Tumors and Cysts*. (City, State, n.g.) Hanna Kroeger Publications, 1997. (Used by permission from family of Ms. H. Kroeger.)

318 Kroeger. Hanna. *Parasites The Enemy Within*. (City, State, n.g.) Hanna Kroeger Publications, 1991. (Used by permission from family of Ms. H. Kroeger.)

319 Krystosik, James D.C. *Nature's Prescription for Over 60 Diseases – Grape Seed and Pine Bark Extract*. (The prior title of this book was: *Pycnogenols-Pine Bark (OPC's) Grape Seed (OPC's) "Superstar Antioxidants."* Garrettsville, OH: Good New Press, 1995. (Use approved by Dr. James Krystosik, D.C.)

320 Laino, Charlene. MSNBC, "Chinese Folk Remedy Fights Cancer Plant Compound Sparks Chain Reaction That Kills Tumor Cells." HerbTime, The Natural Health Center. Online posting. 1 Nov. 2004 <http://www.herbtime.com/InformationPages/ChineseFolk RemedyFightsCancer.htm> Copyright © 1998-2005 by Herbtime. Used with permission of herbtime.com.

321 Lam, Michael, M.D. "Medicinal Mushrooms." "Cancer and Immunity." Online posting. 27 Sept. 2004 <http://www.drlam.com/A3R_brief_in_doc_format/cancer_ and_immunity.cfm, © 2001-2004 by Michael Lam M.D. All Rights Reserved. Used with Dr. Lam's permission.

322 Lang, Susan,"Onions Anti-cancer Effects." R.H. Liu, M.D., Ph.D. Online posting. Cornell News for release Oct. 7, 2004, contact Susan S. Lang. 29 Dec. 2004 <http://www.news .cornell.edu/releases/Oct04/onions.cancer. ssl.html> (Used with permission of news.cornell.edu)

323 Law, Terry. *THE POWER OF PRAISE AND WORSHIP*. Tulsa, OK: Victory House Publishers, 1985. (Used with their permission.)

324 LeBeau, Conrad. *Hydrogen Peroxide & Ozone*. 13th Edition. West Allis, WI: Vital Health Publications, 2001. Used with their permission.

325 Lee, Deborah. *JUICING: Your Liquid Nutritional Supplement*. Pleasant Grove, UT: Woodland Publishing, 1998. (Used with their permission.)

326 Lee, John R., M.D., et al. What Your Doctor May Not Tell You About Breast Cancer *How Hormone Balance Can Help Save Your Life:* New York: From WHAT YOUR DOCTOR MAY NOT TELL YOU ABOUT BREAST CANCER by Dr. John Lee, M.D., Virginia Hopkins, M.A. and David T. Zava, Ph.D., Warner Books, Inc., 2002. Copyright © 2002 by John R. Lee, M. D., Virginia Hopkins, M.A., and David T. Zava, Ph.D., by permission of Warner Books, Inc.

327 Lee, John R., M.D. with Virginia Hopkins. WHAT YOUR DOCTOR MAY NOT TELL YOU ABOUT™ MENOPAUSE *The Breakthrough Book on Natural Progesterone.* New York: Warner Books, Inc., 1996. From WHAT YOUR DOCTOR MAY NOT TELL YOU ABOUT MENOPAUSE by Dr. John Lee, M.D. Copyright © 1996 by John R. Lee, M.D. and Virginia Hopkins. By permission of Warner Books, Inc.

328 Ley, Beth.M., Ph.D. *BILBERRY & LUTEIN: the Vision Enhancers Protect Against Cataracts, Macular Degeneration, Glaucoma, Retinopathy & Other Health Problems,* B. L. Publications, 2001. (Used with their permission.)

329 Lieberman, Shari. Ph.D. and Ken Balbal, C.N. *Maitake Mushroom AND D-Fraction.* Pleasant Grove, UT: Woodland Publishing, 2001 (Used with their permission.)

330 P.F. Lin. "Antitumor effect of actinidia chinensis polysaccharide on murine tumor," Institute of Molecular Medicine, Zhejiang College of Traditional Chinese Medicine, Hangzhou, Online posting. Zhonghua Zhong Liu Za Zhi. 1988 Nov;10(6):441-4, <http://www.ncbi.nlm.nih.gov/entrez/query.fcgi?cmd=Retrieve&db=pubmed&dopt=Abstract&list_uids=2855056&query_hl=33>, p. 1 (accessed 2005, Jul. 1)

331 K. Lockwood, S. Moesgaard, and K. Folkers, "Partial and complete regression of breast cancer in patients in relation to dosage of coenzyme Q10," PubMed, NCBI, Biochem Biophys Res Commun. 1994 Mar 30;199(3):1504-8, p. 1. Online posting. 1 Jul. 2005 <http://www.ncbi.nlm.nih.gov/entrez/query.fcgi?cmd=Retriev&db=pubmed&dopt=Abstract&list_uids=7808519&query_hl=32>

332 K. Lockwood, S. Moesgaard, T. Yamamoto, and K. Folkers, "Progress on therapy of breast cancer with vitamin Q10 and the regression of metastases," PubMed, NCBI, Biochem Biophys Res Commun. 1995 Jul 6;212(1):172-7, p. 1, Online posting. 25 Nov. 2004<http://www.ncbi.nlm.nih.gov/entrez/query.fcgi?cmd=Retrieve&db=pubmed&dopt=Abstract&list_uids=7612003

333 Lynes, Barry. *Helping The Cancer Victim.* Queensville, Ontario: Marcus Books, 1990. (Used with permission from Marcus Books.)

334 Mae, Eydie with C. Loeffler. *How I Conquered Cancer Naturally.* Garden City Park, N.Y.: Avery Publishing Group, Inc., 1992.

335 Malkmus, George, Rev. "From Death to Life – A Miraculous Recovery." Rita Myers. Back to the Garden – Teaching Health From a Biblical Perspective. Hallelujah Acres - Publisher: Rev. George H. Malkmus, Fall 2004, Issue #29. (Used with permission from Rev. G. Malkmus.)

336 Malkmus, Rev. George. "How to Eliminate Sickness Seminar." "Hallelujah Acres Brings You Back to the Garden: the biblical natural diet." Online posting. 25 May 2004 <http://www.hacres.com/seminars.asp.> (Used with permission of Rev. Malkmus.)

337 Markland, Francis S., Ph.D. "A Snake Venom Protein with Unique Anti-tumor and Anti-angiogenic Activities." Online posting. 5 Feb. 2005 http://www.calacademy.org/ education/bioforum2000-2001/venoms/markland-sum.../ © 2005 California Academy of Sciences. (Used with their permission.)

338 Martarelli D, Martarelli B, Pediconi D, Nabissi MI, Perfumi M, Pompei P. "Hypericum perforatum methanolic extract inhibits growth of human prostatic carcinoma cell line orthotopically implanted in nude mice." *Cancer Letters* 210 (1): 27-33, Jul 82004, from Positive Health Magazine. Inegrated Medicine for the 21st Century. Online posting. 23 Jun. 2005 <http://www.positivehealth.com/research.asp?i=3318> Content © Positive Health Publications Ltd., 1994-2005. All rights reserved. (Used with their permission.)

339 Mercola, Joseph, M.D. "Sunlight Actually Prevents Cancer." Online Posting. 12 Nov. 2004 http://www.mercola.com/2002/apr/3/sun_prevents_cancer.htm © 2005 Dr. Joseph Mercola. All rights reserved. (Used with permission from Dr. Mercola.)

340 Mercola, Joseph, M.D. "Chlorella: A Natural Wonder Food, Anti-Cancer Properties of Chlorella." Online posting. "How Much Chlorella Should A Person Take If They Have Cancer." 25 Nov. 2004 <http://www.mercola.com/chlorella/anti_cancer.htm> © 2005 Dr. Joseph Mercola. All rights reserved. (Used with permission of Dr.Mercola.)

341 Mercola, Joseph, M.D. "The Benefits of Probiotics 9/29/04." Online posting. 31 Dec. 2004 <http://www.mercola.com/2004/sept/29/probiotics_benefits.htm> © 2005 Dr. Joseph Mercola. All rights reserved. (Used with permission of Dr. Mercola.)

342 Metz, James, M.D. "Reduced Normal Tissue Toxicity With Proton Therapy." Online posting April 28, 2002. OncoLink website, The Abramson Cancer Center of the University of Pennsylvania, 1 Jun. 2005, <http://www.oncolink.com/treat-ment/ article.cfm?c=9&s=70&id=211> Copyright © 1994-2005 © Trustees of the University of Pennsylvania. (Used with their permission.)

343 Meyerowitz, Steve. "Benefits of Wheatgrass." Online posting - International Specialty Supply. 1 Aug., 2004 <http://www.sproutnet.com/Press/benefits_of_wheatgrass.htm> Used with Mr. Meyerowitz's permission.)

344 Meyerowitz, Steve. *Sprouts, The Miracle Food, The Complete Guide to Sprouting.* (City, State, n.g.) Sproutman Publications, 1983, 1998. (Used with Mr. Meyerowitz's permission.)

345 Meyerowitz, Steve. *Water The Ultimate Cure: Discover Why Water is the Most Important Ingredient in Your Diet and Find Out Which Water is Right for You.* Great Barrington, MA: Distributed by: Book Publishing Company, Summertown, TN., © 2000, 2001. (Used with Mr. Meyerowitz's permission.)

346 Meyerowitz, Steve. *Wheat Grass Nature's Finest Medicine: The Complete Guide to Using Grass Foods & Juices to Revitalize Your Health.* Great Barrington, MA: Sproutman Publications, 1999. (Used with Mr. Meyerowitz's permission.)

347 Mindell, Earl L., R.Ph., Ph.D. with V.L. Hopkins. *Dr. Earl Mindell's What You Should Know About The Super Antioxidant Miracle.* New York: the McGraw-Hill Companies, 1996. Reproduced with permission of the McGraw-Hill Companies

348 Mindell, Earl, R.Ph., Ph.D. *EARL MINDELL'S FOOD AS MEDICINE: WHAT YOU CAN EAT TO HELP PREVENT EVERYTHING FROM COLDS TO HEART DISEASE TO CANCER,* New York: Reprinted with permission of Simon & Schuster Adult Publishing Group From EARL MINDELL'S FOOD AS MEDI-CINE, by Earl Mindell, R.Ph., Ph.D, © by Earl Mindell, R.Ph., Ph.D., and Carol Colman.

349 Mindell, Earl, R.Ph., Ph.D. *EARL MINDELL'S HERB BIBLE,* New York: Reprinted with permission of Simon & Schuster Adult Publishing Group, from EARL MINDELL'S HERB BIBLE by Earl Mindell, R.Ph., Ph.D., © 1992 by Earl Mindell, R.Ph., Ph.D., and Carol Colman.

350 Mindell, Earl, R.Ph., Ph.D. *EARL MINDELL'S SOY MIRACLE.* New York: Reprinted with permission of Simon & Schuster Adult Publishing Group, from EARL MINDELL'S SOY MIRACLE © 1995 by Earl Mindell

351 Miners, S.E. "Hope For Cancer Sufferers." Online posting. "An 'Official Miracle.'" 7 Jan. 2005 <http://www.1001herbs.com/webarticles/essiac/essiac-extras.html> ©Copyright 2005 100lherbs.com. All rights reserved. Established April 1998. (Used with their permission.)

352 Mirkin, Gabe., M.D. "Breast Milk Prevents Childhood Diabetes?" Online posting. 12 Nov. 2004 <http://www.drmirkin.com/diabetes/D216.htm> Copyright © 2003 www.drmirkin.com. (Used with their permission.)

353 Mitchell. Terri, "Resveratrol Powerful Protection Against Prostate Cancer." Online Posting. From Life Extension Magazine Report. 18 May 2004. (Also see the LEF Protocol Book) <http://www.lef.org/magazine/mag2004/apr2004_report_resver_01.html> All contents © 1995-2005 Life Extension Foundation All Rights Reserved. (Used with their permission.)

354 Morse, Robert, N.D. *THE DETOX MIRACLE SOURCEBOOK*, Prescott, AZ: Hohm Press, 2004. (Used with permission of Hohm Press.)

355 Moss, Ralph W., Ph.D. *CANCER THERAPY: THE INDEPENDENT CONSUMER'S GUIDE to Non-Toxic Treatment & Prevention.* New York: Equinox Press, 1992. (Used with their permission through A. Beattie.) Moss, Ralph W., Ph.D. *The Cancer Industry.* Brooklyn: Equinox Press, 2002. (Used with their permission through A. Beattie.)

356 Moss, Ralph W., Ph.D. *THE CANCER INDUSTRY*, Brooklyn: Equinox Press, 2002. (Used with their permission through A. Beattie.)

357 Moss, Ralph W., Ph.D. "Intriguing New Anticancer Compound From East Europe." Online posting. From The Cancer Chronicles #27, © June 1995 by Ralph W. Moss, Ph.D. 13 Oct. 2004 <http://www.ralphmoss.com/html/ukrain.shtml> (Used with their permission through A. Beattie.)

358 Moss, Ralph W., Ph.D. *Antioxidants against Cancer.* State College PA: Equinox Press, Inc., 2000. (Used with their permission through A. Beattie.)

359 Moss, Ralph,W., Ph.D. "A Reply to Dr. Klausner: Natural Products Should be Tested First Against Cancer," from The Cancer Chronicles #29 © Sept. 1995 by Ralph W. Moss, Ph.D. "Landmark Study." Ralph Moss on Cancer – Expert Guidance for Crucial Decisions. Online posting. 2 Feb. 2005 <http://www.ralph-moss.com/html/try.shtml> (Used with their permission through A. Beattie.)

360 Mowrey, D., Ph.D. Rainforest Remedies, "Undiscovered Riches," Important Herbs from South American Rainforests. Online posting. "Lapacho." 21 Oct. 2004 <http://www.rain-tree.com/article4.htm> © 1996 - 2004 Raintree Nutrition, Inc., Carson City, NV. 89701 All rights reserved. This information is also found in Leslie Taylor's book, *The Healing Power of Rainforest Herbs,* Square One Publishers, Jan. 2005. Used with Ms. Taylor's permission.

361 Mowrey, Daniel B., Ph.D. *The Scientific Validation of Herbal Medicine.* HOW TO REMEDY AND PREVENT DISEASE WITH HERBS, VITAMINS, MINERALS, AND OTHER NUTRIENTS, New York: McGraw-Hill Companies, 1986. Reproduced with permission of McGraw-Hill Companies

362 Murray, Dr. Michael T. "Question of the Week." Online posting. 25 Nov. 2004 <http://www.doctormurray.com/Qarchive/ip6.htm> Used with their permission.

363 Murray, Frank. *Remifemin: Herbal Relief for Menopausal Symptoms.* New York: McGraw-Hill Companies, 1996. Reproduced with permission of the McGraw-Hill Companies.

364 Nolfi, Kristine, M.D. *RAW FOOD TREATMENT OF CANCER.* Translated from the book, "Raw Food Treatment of Cancer," Copyright © 1995 by TEACH Services, Inc. Published by TEACH Services, Inc., 254 Donovan Rd., Brushton, N.Y. 12916, 518/358-3494. Used with their permission.

365 Norton, Amy, "Bee Products Fight Tumors in Mice Study Shows." From *Reuters Health Information.* New York, Dec. 16, 2004. Reuters content is the intellectual property of Reuters Limited. Reprinted with their permission. Reuters shall not be liable for any errors or delays in content, or for any actions taken in reliance thereon. "News," from cancerpage.com. Online posting. 19 Dec. 2004 <http://www.cancerpage.com/news/ article.asp?id=7827> cancerpage.com 2000-2005. All rights reserved.

366 Null, Gary., Ph.D. *THE COMPLETE ENCYCLOPEDIA OF NATURAL HEALING: A comprehensive A-Z listing of common and chronic illnesses and their proven natural treatments,* New York, N.Y. © 2000, 2001, 2002, Kensington Publishing Corp. All rights reserved. Reprinted by arrangement with Kensington Publishing Corp., *www.kensingtonbooks.com.*

367 O'Brien, James E. *The Miracle of Garlic & Vinegar and other Exciting Natural Wonders.* Globe Mini Mags®. Boca Raton, FL: Globe Communications Corp., 1991. Reproduced with permission of Globe Digests.

368 Olsen, Cynthia, with contributions by Jim Chan and Christopher Gussa. *ESSIAC A Native Herbal Cancer Remedy.* Reprinted with permission from *Essiac: A Native Herbal Cancer Remedy* by Cynthia Olsen, Lotus Press, P O Box 325, Twin Lakes, WI. 53181. ©1996 All Rights Reserved. (Used with their permission.)

369 Oski, Frank A., M.D. *Don't Drink Your Milk!* NEW FRIGHTENING MEDICAL FACTS ABOUT THE WORLD'S MOST OVERRATED NUTRIENT. Brushton, N.Y: Teach Services, Inc., 1996. Translated from the book, *Don't Drink Your Milk!* Copyright © 1996 by TEACH Services, Inc., 254 Donovan Road, Brushton, N.Y. 12916 518/358-3494. (Used with their permission.)

370 Patton, D. "Vitamin E has protective role in bladder cancer." Online posting. News & Analysis Science and Nutrition 30/03/2004. 28 Oct. 2004 <http://www.food navigator.com/news/news-NG.asp?id=9537> © 2000/2005 – NOVIS – All rights reserved (Used with their permission.)

371 Phillips, Gavin. "The Cancer Racket – The Hoxsey Remedies." Online posting. 24 May, 2005 < http://www.getipm.com/personal/cancer-racket.htm> (Used with their permission.)

372 Pressinger, R., M.Ed., and Wayne Sinclair. Allergy, Asthma & Immunology. "About Neuroblastoma." Causes of Neuroblastoma Research New Warnings About Where You Live. "Neuroblastoma and Chlordane." (CANCER, 59:1853-1859, 1987.) Online posting. 10 Dec. 2004 <http://www.chem-tox.com/neuroblastoma/default.htm> (Used with their permission.)

373 Quinn, Dick.*LEFT FOR DEAD*. Minneapolis, MN: Quinn Publishing Co., 1992. (Used with their permission.)

374 Rajkapoor,B., et al. "Antitumor Activity of Elephantopus scaber Linn Against Dalton's Ascitic Lymphoma." Online posting. IJPS – The *Indian Journal of Pharmaceutical Sciences*. The Indian Pharmaceutical Assoc (IPA). 19 Jan. 2004 <http://www.indian pharma.org/journal/index.php/2002/1jan%20-%feb/antitumoractivity.html> Permission to quote granted by Rao V.S.V. Vadlamudi, Ph.D., Editor, *Indian Journal of Pharmaceutical Sciences,* Indian Pharmaceutical Assn.

375 Rivers, Charmaine. *Manna from Heaven - Healing Foods From The Bible.* Boca Raton, FL. And New York: *Globe Digests*™. American Media Mini Mags., Inc., 2002. Reproduced with permission of Globe Digests.

376 Rodgers, Bob. *The 21 Day Fast: 21 Days that will revolutionize your life!* Louisville, KY: Bob Rodgers Ministries, 2001. Reprinted with permission of Dr. Bob Rodgers.

377 Rollins, Catherine P. "Estrogen Dominance Linked to Cancer." Online posting. "Synthetic HRT and Cancer." 24 Dec. 2004 <http://www.natural-progesterone-advisory-network.com/estrogen-dominance-linked-to-cancer.htm> Copyright © 2005 Making Plans Pty Ltd. All Rights Reserved. (Used with their permission.)

378 Rollins, Catherine P. "Is Natural Progesterone Safe?" Online posting. 9 Nov. 2004 <http://www.natural-progesterone-advisory-network.com/is-natural-progesterone-safe.htm> Copyright © 2005 Making Plans Pty Ltd. All Rights Reserved. (Used with their permission.)

379 Rollins, Catherine P." Can Progesterone Help Alleviate Autoimmune Disorders Like Hashimoto's Disease, Grave's Disease, Multiple Sclerosis or Lupus?" "Estrogens." Online posting. 24 Dec. 2004 <http://www.natural-progesterone-advisory-network.com/News/article040622-3> Copyright © 2002-04,Making Plans Pty Ltd, All Rights Reserved. (Used with their permission.)

380 Rubin, Jordan S., N.M.D., Ph.D. *THE MAKER'S DIET.* Lake Mary FL: Siloam Publishing, 2004. Used with permission of Siloam, a Srang Company.

381 Ryan, Caroline. BBC News. "Sunshine Prevents Cancer." From website The Greatest Herbs on Earth™. Online posting. 12 Nov. 2004http://www.greatestherbsonearth.com/ articles/sunshine_prevents_cancer.htm. Copyright 2000-2005 Greatest Herbs On Earth © All rights reserved (Used with their permission.)

382 Sage, Donna., M.S.S.A. "Haelan Reverses Cancer Cell Growth." Online Posting. From Well Being Journal Special Edition: Healing Cancer Naturally. 17 Oct. 2004 http://www.wellbeingjournal.com/haelan.htm (c) 2000 Well Being Journal. All rights reserved. Used with permission of wellbeing journal and Donna Sage M.S.S.A.

383 Sahelian, Ray, M.D. "Ashwagandha: by Ray Sahelian, M.D., Ashwagandha Benefits." Online posting. 17 Jan. 2005 <http://www.raysahelian.com/ashwagandha.html> © Copyright 2005 All Rights Reserved RaySahelian.com (Used with their permission.)

384 Sahelian, Ray, M.D. "Gymnema." Gymnema and diabetes – gynnema and blood sugar. Online posting. 3 Jan. 2005 <http://www.raysahelian.com/gymnema.html> © Copyright 2005 All Rights Reserved RaySahelian.com (Used with their permission.)

385 Sahelian, Ray. *SAW PALMETTO NATURE'S PROSTATE HEALER*, New York: Kensington Publishing, 1998, also see www.raysahelian.com/saw.html (Used with Dr. Sahelian's permission and permission of Kensington Publishng.)

386 Salaman, Maureen Kennedy, *FOODS That Heal.* Menlo Park, CA: Statford Publishing, 1989. (Reprinted with Ms. Salaman's permission.)

387 Salaman, Maureen Kennedy. *NUTRITION: THE CANCER ANSWER II,.* Menlo Park, Ca: Statford Publishing, 1995, 2002. (Reprinted with Ms. Salaman's permission.)

388 Salaman, Maureen Kennedy. *ALL YOUR HEALTH QUESTIONS ANSWERED NATURALLY*, MKS, Inc., 1998. (Reprinted with Ms. Salaman's permission.)

389 Salaman, Maureen Kennedy. *How to RENEW YOU*, Menlo Park, CA: MKS, Inc., 2003. (Reprinted with Ms. Salaman's permission.)

390 Saxion, Valerie. *HOW TO Feel Great ALL THE TIME A LIFELONG PLAN for UNLIMITED ENERGY and RADIANT GOOD HEALTH,* Little Rock, Arkansas: Lions Head Publishing, 2002. (Reprinted with Ms. Saxion's permission.)

391 Schulick, Paul. *Ginger Common Spice & Wonder Drug.* Revised Edition. Brattleboro, VT: Herbal Free Press, Ltd., 1994. (Used with their permission.)

392 Schwartz, J., Shklar, G., Reid, S., Trickler, D., "Prevention of experimental oral cancer by extracts of Spirulina-Dunaliella algae," Online posting. Nutr Cancer. 1988;11(2):127-34, Department of Oral Medicine and Oral Patholody, Harvard School of Dental Medicine Boston. 1 Jul. 2005 <http://www.ncbi.nlm.nih.gov/entrez/query.fcgi?cmd=Retriev&db =pubmed &dopt=Abstract&list_uids=3129701&query_hl=35>, p. 1(accessed 2005, Jul. 1)

393 Scott, C., and Lust, John, Naturopath. *Crude Black Molasses, A Natural "Wonder Food."* New York, N.Y., Benedict Lust Publications, 1980, 1992. (Used with their permission.)

394 Shealy, C. Norman, M.D., Ph.D. *Natural Progesterone Cream: Safe and Natural Hormone Replacement,* New York: Mc-Graw Hill Companies, 1999. Reproduced with permission of the McGraw-Hill Companies.

395 Shogren, E. "FDA kept suicide findings secret." Los Angeles Times, published on 4/6/4, Psyche Drug Truth. Online posting 5 Jan. 2005 <http://www.prozactruth.com /article_fda_secret_findings.htm> (Used with their permission.)

396 Shulze, Dick, N.D. "Herbal Naturopathy Quotes," "Politics." Online posting. 21 Jun. 2005 <http://www.whale.to/a /herbal_q.html> (Used with their permission.)

397 Sinatra, Stephen, M.D., F.A.C.C. *THE COENZYME Q10 PHENOMENON: The breakthrough nutrient that helps combat heart disease, cancer, aging and more,* New York: the McGraw-Hill Companies, 1998. Reproduced with permission of the McGraw-Hill Companies.

398 Sinatra, Stephen.T., M.D., F.A.C.C. *Coenzyme Q10 and the Heart*: New York: the McGraw-Hill Companies, 1999. Reproduced with permission of the McGraw-Hill Companies.

399 Skousen, Max B. *ALOE VERA HANDBOOK: The Ancient Egyptian Medicine Plant*. (City, State, n.g.) Aloe Vera Research Institute, 1992 (Used with their permission.)

400 Smith, E.D. "Effects of Homogenization and Pasteurization of Milk." Online posting. 5 Dec. 2004 <http://www.karloren.com/aajonus/p1.htm> from Karl Loren's website. (Used with permission from Mr. Loren.)

401 Srinivas, G., Anto, R.J., Srinivas, P., Vidhyalakshmi, S., Senan, V.P., Karunagaran, D. Div. Of Cancer Biology, Rajiv Gandhi Centre for Biotechnology, Poojapura, Thiruvananthapuram 695 014, Kerala, India. Pub Med, "Emodin induces apoptosis of human cervical cancer cells through poly (ADP-ribose) polymerase cleavage and activation of caspase-9." Online posting. 27 Sept. 2004. <http://www.ncbi.nlm.nih.gov/ entrez/query.fcgi?cmd=Retrieve& db=PubMed &list_uids=12892828" Eur J Pharmacol. 2003 JVL 25;473(2-3):117-25 p. 1

402 Stengler, Mark, N.D., From *The Natural Physician's Healing Therapies: Proven Remedies that Medical Doctors Don't Know,* by Mark Stengler, N.D., copyright © 2001 by Mark Stengler. Used by permission of Avery Publishing, an imprint of Penguin Group (USA) Inc.

403 Stone, Irwin, Ph.D. From "Nutritional Doctor Quotes." From *Whale* website. Online posting. <http://www.whale.to/w/quotes4.html> 9 Jun. 2005. (Used with their permission.)

404 Strand, Ray D., M.D. with Donna K. Wallace. *DEATH BY PRESCRIPTION: THE SHOCKING TRUTH BEHIND AN OVERMEDICATED NATION*. Nashville, TN: Thomas Nelson Publishers®, 2003. (Used with their permission.)

405 Strand, Ray., M.D. *WHAT YOUR DOCTOR DOESN'T KNOW ABOUT NUTRITIONAL MEDICINE MAY BE KILLING YOU,* Nashville: Thomas Nelson Publishers®, 2002. (Used with their permission.)

406 Tenney, D. *Medicinal Mushrooms: Cancer Fighters and Immunity Enhancers*. Pleasant Grove, UT: Woodland Publishing, 1997. (Used with their permission.)

407 Tenney, L., M.H. *HEALTH HANDBOOK,* Pleasant Grove, UT: Woodland Publishing, 1996. (Used with their permission.)

408 Editors of Bottom Line Publications. *The World's Greatest Treasury of HEALTH SECRETS*. Greenwich, CT: Boardroom, Inc., 2000. (Used with their permission.)

409 Tietze, Harald W. *Papaya The Healing Fruit*. Vancouver, Canada: Alive Books, Alive Natural Health Guides, 2000 (from Andrea Ehring, author of Das Krebsheilmittel Der Aborigines: (Papaya: The Cancer Healing Remedy of the Aborigines.) With permission from Alive Publishing Group, Inc. Canada. www.alive.com, <http://www.alive.com>

410 Udall, K. Gilbert. *Cordyceps Sinensis: Immune and Stamina Booster*, Pleasant Grove, UT: Woodland Publishing, 2000. (Used with their permission.)

411 Vyas, J. J. and V. K. Jain. "Ukrain Treatment in Carcinoma of the Esophagus (Case Report). 13 Oct. 2004 <http://www.ukrin.com/Ukrainbook1/195final.htm> (Used with their permission.)

412 Wade, Carlson. *Carlson Wade's New FACT BOOK ON Bee Pollen and Your Health*. New York, the McGraw Hill Companies, 1978, 1992. Reproduced with permission of the McGraw-Hill Companies.

413 Walker, M., D.P.M. "Medical Journalist Report of Innovative Biologies," from the Townsend Letter For Doctors & Patients – Feb/Mar 2001, Homeostatic Soil Organisms for One's Primal Defense." Online posting. 31 Dec. 2004 <http://www.vital-nutrients.com /drwalker_on_hsos_1.htm> Copyright 1999-2005 by Ron Pellegrini. All rights reserved.

414 Wallis, Arthur. *GOD'S CHOSEN FAST: A Spiritual and Practical Guide to Fasting*, Ft. Washington, PA: Christian Literature Crusade, copyright © 1968, published by CLC Publications, Fort Washington, PA, Used by permission.

415 Ward, B. "Garlic." Optimal Diet Healthy Eating Website, "Letters to Friends," Glorious Garlic 04 Oct. 2003. Taken from "Healing Foods of the Bible," by Bernard Ward. Online Posting. 29 Dec. 2004 <http://homodiet.Netfirms.com/otherssay/ letters/garlic.htm> (Used with their permission.)

416 Warner, Glen, from "Alternative Medical Doctor Quotes." From *Whale* website. Online posting. 9 Jun. 2005 <http;//www.whale.to/m/quotes6.html> (Used with their permission.)

417 Warner, Jennifer, "Substance In Peppers Kills Cancer Cells," WebMD Medical News, "Capsaicin (Hot Pepper Substance) Kills Cancer Cells," Sept. 3, 2002, retrieved 4 Jul. 2005 from <http://store.yahoo.com/annieappleseedproject/caphotpepsub.html> (Used with their permission.)

418 White, Linda B., M.D., Steven Foster and the staff of Herbs for Health. *THE HERBAL DRUGSTORE: THE BEST NATURAL ALTERNATIVES TO OVER-THE-COUNTER AND PRESCRIPTION MEDICINES,* (City, State, n.g.) Rodale, Inc., 2000. (Used with their permission.)

419 Wigmore, Ann. *THE HIPPOCRATES DIET and HEALTH PROGRAM,* (City, State, n.g.) Avery Publishing, 1984.

420 Wigmore, Ann. *The Sprouting Book: HOW TO GROW AND USE SPROUTS TO MAXIMIZE YOUR HEALTH AND VITALITY,* Wayne, N.J: Avery Publishing Group, Inc., 1986

421 Wigmore, Ann. *The Wheatgrass Book: HOW TO GROW AND USE WHEAT-GRASS TO MAXIMIZE YOUR HEALTH AND VITALITY,* (City, State, n.g.) Avery Publishing, member of Penguin Putnam, Inc., and The Hippocrates Health Institute, Inc., 1985.

422 Willner, Robert, M.D., Ph.D. "Dr. Johanna Budwig Diet Cancer, Arthritis, Multiple Sclerosis, Psoriasis, Eczema, Acne…Flaxseed oil and cottage cheese." 29 Jun. 2004 <http://www.alternativehealth.co.nz/cancer/budwig.htm> (Used with their permission.)

423 Willner, Robert, M.D., Ph.D. From *Whale* website. "Doctor Robert Willner, M.D., Ph.D." Online posting. 9 Jun. 2005 <http://www.whale.to/c/willner.html> (Used with their permission.)

424 Winters, Jason. "Sir Jason Winters Story – About Sir Jason Winters." Online posting. 6 Jan. 2005 <http://www.sirjasonwinters.com/story.htm> Copyright © 1997-2005 Tri-Sun International. Used with permission.

425 Wood, R. "Mushrooms Detoxify." Kitchen Coaching, Healing With Food, Food as Medicine, Mushrooms Detoxify web article, online posting. 17 Oct. 2004 <http://www .rwood.com/Articles/Mushrooms_Detoxify.htm> © 2002-2004 Rebecca Wood. (Used with their permission.)

426 Wright, Lloyd. "Milk Thistle Ancient Blessing." Triumph Over Hepatitis C website. Online posting. 8 Apr. 2005 <http://www.hepatitisCfree.com/milk_thistle_book.htm> (Used with their permission.)

427 Yeager, Selene, et al. *Doctors Book of FOOD REMEDIES: The Newest Discoveries in the Power of Food to Cure and Prevent Health Problems – From Aging and Diabetes to Ulcers and Yeast Infections,* (City, State, n.g.): Rodale, Inc., 1998. (Used with their permission.)

428 Yiamouyiannis, John. "Fluoride Toxicity, Immune System and Aging." Online posting. 9 Nov. 2004 <http://www.health-science.com/fluoride_ toxicity.html> © 1995-2004 Health & Science Research Institute, USA. (Used with their permission.)

429 Young, Gary D. "New Discovery on the Chinese Wolfberry." Special Health Advisory on Immunity and Anti-Aging. Online posting. 17 Oct. 2004 <http://www.aroma-essence.com/research-reports/chinese-wolfberry.html> Copyright © 1996-2004 aroma-essence.com and its licensors. All rights reserved. (Used with their permission.)

430 Young, Robert.O., Ph.D., and Shelley Redford Young. *The pH MIRACLE Balance Your Diet, Reclaim Your Health.* New York: Warner Books, Inc. 2002, from *Ph Miracle, The,* by Robert Young, Ph.D., Copyright © 2002 by Robert Young, Ph.D. By permission of Warner Books, Inc.

431 Young, S. "Contortrostatin: Evaluation of Its Effect on Ovarian Tumor Growth." California State Science Fair, 2002 Project Summary, Project Number S1435. Online posting. 5 Feb. 2005 <http://www.usc.edu/CSSF/History/2002/Projects/S1435.pdf> (Used with their permission.)

432 Zentaro, N. "With Tian Xian Liquid, I shall Never Surrender to Liver Cancer." Tian Xian. Online Posting. 17 Oct. 2004 <http://www.tianxian.com/testimonials/liver_ cancer.asp>(Used with their permission.)

433 Ziff, Samuel., Ziff, Michael F., D.D.S. *Dentistry Without Mercury.* Orlando, FL: Bio=Probe, Inc., 1985. (Used with Dr. Ziff's permission.)

NOTES

Chapter 1

[1] R. Moss, Ph.D., *The Cancer Industry.* Brooklyn, N.Y.: Equinox Press, 2002, p. 42

[2] M. Kennedy Salaman. *Nutrition: The Cancer Answer II,* Menlo Park, CA:MKS., Inc., Statford Publishing, 1995, 2002, p. 28

[2a] R. Willner, M.D., Ph.D. From *Whale* website. "Dr. Robert Willner, M.D., Ph.D." Available: http://www.whale.to/c/willner.html (accessed 2005, Jun. 6)

[2b] Moss, p. 17

[3] Ibid., p. 12

[4] Moss, p. 5

[5] Ibid., p. 412

[6] B. Lynes. *Helping The Cancer Victim*, Queensville, Ontario: Marcus Books,1990, p. 24

[7] Ibid., p. 45

[8] R. Willner, M.D., Ph.D. From *Whale* website. "Dr. Robert Willner, M.D., Ph.D." Available: http://www.whale.to/c/willner.html (accessed 2005, Jun. 6)

[8a] A. Hoffer, M.D., F.R.C.P.(C), with L. Pauling, Ph.D. *Healing Cancer – Complementary Vitamin & Drug Treatment,* Toronto, Ontario Canada: CCNM Press, Inc., 2004, p. 13-14

[8b] Ibid., p. 170

[9] Lynes, p. 3-4.

[10] Ibid., p. 4

[11] A. Hoffer, M.D., F.R.C.P.(C) with L. *Pauling. Healing Cancer – Complimentary Vitamin & Drug Treatment,* Toronto, Ontario, Canada: CCNM Press, 2004, p. 130

[12] "Newsletter Aug. 2001," Wellness Directory of Minnesota™, Available: http://www.mnwelldir.org/docs/Newsletters/01_Aug.htm (accessed 2004, Dec. 18)

[13] J. R. Lee, M.D., David Zava, Ph.D., and Virginia Hopkins. New York: Warner Books, Inc., 2002, p. 6 – From *What Your Doctor May Not Tell You About™: Breast Cancer* by John R.Lee, M.D., copyright © 2002 by John R. Lee, M. D., Virginia Hopkins, M.A., and David T. Zava, Ph.D., by permission of Warner Books, Inc.

[14] Lynes, p.6 (quoting Dr. Robert Jones from the *Seattle Times*)

[15] "The Cure That Killed the Patient," from Karl Loren's website, "Chemotherapy: A Dull Weapon," Available: http://www.karlloren.com/biopsy/p60.htm (accessed 2004, Dec. 5)

[16] Ibid.

[17] Molo-Cure Research, Inc., *20% of New Drugs Will Be Labeled "Dangerous" or Withdrawn from Market JAMA Study Reports,* Available: http://www.molocure.com/adrarticle.shtml, p. 1 (accessed 2004, April 30).

[18] Ibid.

[19] Health Sciences Institute, Member's Alert for Jan 2001, Vol. 5, No. 7, "Billion-dollar drug company nearly squashes astounding research on natural cancer killer." Available: http://www.hsibaltimore.com (accessed 2004, Apr. 26)

[20] Molo-Cure Research, Inc., *The Boston Globe - "Drug Firms and doctors: the offers pour in."* Available: http://www.molocure.com/bostonglobe.shtml, p. 1 (accessed 2004, April 30)

[21] Ibid.

[22] Ibid.

23 Ibid., p. 36-37

24 "Cancer Cover-Up The Neal Deoul Story," by Kathleen Deoul, Frequently Asked Questions, Available: http://www.cancer-coverup.com/faqs/is-this-treatment-safe.htm, (accessed 2004, Dec. 26) Quoted with their permission.

25 "FDA Opens Baycol Probe," Agency Feeling the Heat After Vioxx Withdrawal, NEWS – Available http://www.consumeraffairs.com/news04/vioxx_baycol_fda.html, p. 1, Copyright © 2003-2004 ConsumerAffairs.Com, Inc. (Accessed 2004, Dec. 26)

26 Strand, et al., p. 58

27 Ibid., p. 73

28 S. Ellison, M.Sc., "Beyond Vioxx," 2004, p. 2 - from "Details on the Vioxx recall, possible Vioxx side effects, Vioxx lawsuit, information and alternative natural treatments...," Available: http://www.safemenopausesolutions.com/vioxx.html., p. 2 (accessed 2004, Nov. 9) Copyright © Personal Wellness Network, Inc. All rights reserved.

29 Ibid.

30 "Cot Death & Vaccines," available: http://www.whale.to/m/quotes17.html, (accessed 2005, June 19)

31 "Newsletter Aug 2001," Wellness Directory of Minnesota™, available: http://www.mnwell dir.org/docs/Newsletters/01_Aug.htm, (accessed 2004, Dec. 18)

32 "Everyone gets rich when you get sick," Wellness Directory of Minnesota™, "Newsletter Aug. 2001," Available: http://www.mnwelldir.org/docs/Newsletters/01_Aug.htm (accessed 2004, Dec. 18)

33 M. Kennedy Salaman. *Nutrition: The Cancer Answer II*, Menlo Park, California: Statford Publishing, 1995, p. 8

Chapter 2

1 M. Kennedy Salaman. *Nutrition: The Cancer Answer II,* Statford Publishing 1995, from her note at the beginning of the book - 2002 edition.

2 J. Brandt. *The Grape Cure,* Yonkers, New York, 1971, p. 19-20. Ehret Literature Publishing Co., Inc., P O Box 24, Dobbs Ferry, N. Y. 10522 website address is: www.arnoldehret.org.

2a Ibid.

3 Ibid., p. 20-21

4 Ibid., p. 21-22

5 Ibid., p. 42

6 J. Brandt. *The Grape Cure,* Yonkers, New York, 1971, p. 43. Ehret Literature Publishing Co., Inc., P O Box 24, Dobbs Ferry, N. Y. 10522 website address is: www.arnold-ehret.org.

7 Ibid., p. 43

8 Ibid., p. 44

9 Brandt, p. 48

10 Ibid., p. 51

11 Ibid., p. 54-55

12 Brandt, p. 60

13 Ibid., p. 147

13a R. Dubin. P. 214. From *Miracle Food Cures From The Bible* by Reese Dubin, copyright © 1999 by Prentice Hall. Used by permission of Avery Publishing, an imprint of Penguin Group (USA) Inc.

[14] J. F. Balch, M.D. From *The Super Anti-Oxidants: Why They Will Change the Face of Healthcare in the 21st Century,* copyright © 1998 by James F. Balch. Reprinted by permission of the publisher, M. Evans & Company, New York, p. 113

[15] Ibid., p. 113

[16] Dubin, p. 213

[17] Ibid., p. 212

[18] Ibid., p. 211

[19] Ibid., p. 211-212

[20] Dubin, p. 215-216

[21] Ibid., p. 216

[22] Ibid.

[23] J. Carper. *The Food Pharmacy - Dramatic New Evidence That Food Is Your Best Medicine,* New York: Bantam Books, 1988, p. 212

[24] E. Mindell, R.Ph., Ph.D. *Earl Mindell's Food as Medicine,* New York: p. 23. Reprinted with permission of Simon & Schuster Adult Publishing Group, from *Earl Mindell's Food As Medicine,* by Earl Mindell R.Ph., Ph.D © 1994 by Earl Mindell, R.Ph., Ph.D. and Carol Colman

[25] Ibid., p. 127

[26] J. Brandt., N.D. *How to Conquer Cancer Naturally*, Joshua Tree, CA: Tree of Life Publications, 1989, p. 92

[27] Ibid., p. 94

[28] T. A. Baroody, N.D., D.C., Ph.D. Nutrition, C.N.C., *Alkalize or Die*, Waynesville, N.C.: Holographic Health Press,1991, p. 15, 45

[29] Ibid., p. 15

[30] J. G. Connor, M.Ac, LAc, "Cancer Prevention and Diet," "Useful Fruit," Available: http://www.compassionateacupuncture.com/cancer.htm (accessed 2005, May 21) copyright © 2005 John G. Connor, M.Ac, Lac.

[31] T. Mitchell. "Resveratrol Powerful Protection Against Prostate Cancer," from Life Extension™ Magazine Report, Available: http://www.lef.org/magazine/mag2004/apr2004_report_resver _ 01.html, (accessed 2004, May 18) Also see the LEF Protocol Book!

[32] Ibid.

[33] "Study: Grapes Inhibit Cancer Growth," from CNN interactive, Jan 10, 1997, L. Ciampa contributed to this report. Available: http://www.cnn.com/HEALTH/9701/10/grapes. Cancer/index.html., p. 1 (accessed 2004, May 18)

[34] "Food as Medicine: Other Phytochemicals. How Other Phytochemicals Help Protect Against Cancer," The Cancer Project, Available: http://www.cancerproject.org/medi-cine/Phytochemicals,html, p 2 (accessed 2004, May 18)

[35] J. F. Balch, M.D. From *The Super Anti-Oxidants: Why They Will Change the Face of Healthcare in the 21st Century,* copyright © 1998, by James F. Balch. Reprinted by the permission of the publisher, M. Evans & Company, New York, p. 115

Chapter 3

[1] R. Atkins. "Nutritional Doctor Quotes." From *Whale* website. Available: http://www.whale. to/m/quotes2.html (accessed 2005, May 28)

[2] C. Guttersen, R.D., Ph.D. Foodservice - *Diet and Breast Cancer* - "Take Two Carrots and Call Me in the Morning," Available: http://wwwcalolive.org/foodservice/findings/find-ings_2002q3html, p. 1 (accessed 2004, May 11)

[2a] E. Mae with C. Loeffler. *How I Conquered Cancer Naturally*, Garden City Park, N.Y.: Avery Publishing Group, Inc., 1992, p. 38-39

[3] Ibid., p. 39

[4] Ibid., p. 103

[5] Ibid., p. 131

[6] K. Nolfi, M.D. *Raw Food Treatment Of Cancer,* Brushton, N.Y.: TEACH Services, Inc., 1995, p. 2-3, Translated from the book, "Raw Food Treatment Of Cancer," Copyright © 1995 by TEACH Services, Inc. published by: TEACH Services, Inc., 254 Donovan Rd. Brushton, New York 12916, 518/358-3494

[7] Ibid., p. 2

[8] Ibid., p. 31

[9] Ibid., p. 32

[10] Ibid., p. 34-35

[11] G. Malkmus, Rev. Back to the Garden - Teaching Health from a Biblical Perspective – Rita Myers, *From Death to Life A Miraculous Recovery,* Hallelujah Acres - Rev. George H. Malkmus, Publisher, Fall 2004, Issue #29, p. 1, 19

[12] S. Meyerowitz. *Wheat Grass Nature's Finest Medicine.*, Great Barrington, MA: Sproutman Publications, 1999, p. 93, 94

[13] "Kiwi Fruit," The World's Healthiest Foods: Feeling Great, George Mateljan Foundation, Whfoods.com. Available: http://www.whfoods.com/genpagephp?tname=foodspice&dbid=41 p. 2-3, (accessed 2004, dec. 17)

[14] Ibid.

[15] S. Sinatra, M.D., F.A.C.C. *The Coenzyme Q10 Phenomenon*, New York: the McGraw-Hill Companies, 1998, p. 82-83. Reproduced with permission of the McGraw-Hill Companies

[16] Ibid., p. 83

[17] R.W. Moss, Ph.D. *Antioxidants against Cancer*, State College, PA.: Equinox Press, Inc., 2000, 2002, p. 71-72

[18] Ibid., p. 76

[19] Ibid., p. 77

[20] Moss, p. 81

[20a] "DIM (diindolylmethane)," Available: www.cancertutor.com/OtherBig_list.htm, (accessed 15 Apr 2005)

[21] Moss, p. 73

[22] Ibid., p. 74

[23] M. Kennedy Salaman. *Nutrition: The Cancer Answer II,* Menlo Park, CA: Statford Publishing, 1995, p. 235

[24] Ibid., p. 235-236

[25] Ibid., p. 236

[26] Ibid.

[27] Ibid.

[27a] "Exsula Health Products," Available: http://www.life-enthusiast.com/exsula/exsula_main.htm, and www.life-enthusiast.com/exsula/pr_iridesca.htm (accessed 2004, Dec. 28)

[27b] "Cancer - Breast," Alternative Health Supplies (Australia) *Your Health Your Choice,* "Vitamins," Available: http://www.alternativehealth.com.au/Articles/breast.htm, p. 5-6, (accessed 2004, Oct. 24)

[28] A. Hoffer, M.D., F.R.C.P.(C), with L. Pauling, Ph.D. *Healing Cancer – Complementary Vitamin & Drug Treatments,* Toronto, Ontario, Canada: CCNM Press, 2004, p. 46

[28a] "Cancer - Breast," Alternative Health Supplies (Australia) *Your Health Your Choice,* "Vitamins," Available: http://www.alternativehealth.com.au/Articles/breast.htm, p. 5-6, (accessed 2004, Oct. 24)

[29] Ibid., p. 6

[30] Ibid., p. 6

[31] Ibid., p. 6

[32] "Billion-dollar drug company nearly squashes astounding research on natural cancer killer," Health Sciences Institute, Members Alert for January 2001, Vol. 5, No. 7, Available: http://www.hsibaltimore.com (accessed 2004, April 26)

[33] Ibid., p. 1

[34] Ibid., p. 3

[35] S. Yeager & the Editors of Prevention Health Books. *Doctors Book of FOOD REMEDIES,* (City, State n.g.): Rodale, Inc, 1998, p. 392, 393

[36] Ibid.

[37] Ibid., p. 429

[38] Ibid.

[39] M. Kennedy Salaman. *How to Renew You,* Menlo Park, CA., MKS, Inc., 2003, p. 131

[40] Ibid., p. 132

[41] *Cranberry Juice,* Available: http://www.cancertutor.com/Other/Big_List.htm, p. 13 (accessed 2004, Oct. 17)

[42] D. Colbert, M.D. *Walking in Divine Health,* Lake Mary, Fl.: Siloam, 1999, p. 57

[43] Ibid.

[44] Ibid.

[45] Ibid.

[46] H. W. Tietze. *Papaya The Healing Fruit,* with permission from Alive Publishing Group, Inc. Canada. www.alive.com <http://www.alive.com> 2000, p. 8-9

[47] Ibid.

[48] "Mangosteen Treatment for Cancer," The Cancer Tutor™ Alternative Cancer Treatment Information Center, Available://http://www.cancertutor.com/Cancer/Mangosteen.html, p. 2, 3 (accessed 2004, Oct. 17) Note that they give their souce as: "Antiproliferation, antioxidation and induction of apoptosis by Garcinia mangostana (mangosteen) on SKBR3 human breast cancer cell line,' by Moongkarndi P, Kosem N, Kaslungka S, Luanratana O, Pongpan N, Neungton N."

[49] S. Yeager, p. 125-126

[50] Ibid., p. 126

[51] Ibid.

[52] "Cancer - Breast," Alternative Health Supplies (Australia) *Your Health Your Choice,* "Vegetables," Available: http://www.alternativehealth.com.au/Articles/breast.htm, p.8 (accessed 2004, Oct. 24)

[53] S. Lieberman, Ph.D., and K. Babal, C.N. *Maitake Mushroom AND D-Fraction*, Pleasant Grove, UT: Woodland Publishing, 2001, p. 16

[53a] "Maitake," from website Herbs2000.com, Available: http://www.herbs2000.com/herbs/herbs_maitake, htm, p. 2 (accessed 2004, Dec. 29)

[54] C. Borek, Ph.D., "Beta Glucan Boosts Immunity," "Beta Glucan vs. Cancer," and "Beta-Glucan the Supplement." Available: http://www.newhope.com/nutritionsciencenews/NSN_backs/ Jan_01/betaglucan.cfm, p. 1-2 (accessed 2004, Oct 17) (Dr. Borek is a research professor at Tufts University School of Medicine in Boston) Copyright © 2004 Penton Media, Inc.

[55] Ibid., p. 2

[56] "Cancer - Breast," Alternative Health Supplies (Australia) *Your Health Your Choice,* Available: http://www.alternativehealth.com.au/Articles/breast.htm p. 3 (accessed 2004, Oct. 24)

[57] Ibid.

[57a] "Kiwi Fruit," The World's Healthiest Foods: Feeling Great, George Mateljan Foundation, Whfoods.com. Available: http://www.whfoods.com/genpagephp?tname=foodspice&dbid=41 p. 2-3, (Accessed 2004, dec. 17)

[58] D. Colbert, M.D. *Walking in Divine Health*, Lake Mark, Fl.: Siloam, 1999, p. 49-50

[59] Ibid.

[60] Donna Sage, M.S.S.A., "*Haelan Reverses Cancer Cell Growth*," from *Well Being Journal Special Edition: Healing Cancer Naturally*, Available: http://www.wellbeingjournal.com/haelan.htm, p. 1, 6 (accessed 2004, Oct. 17)

[61] Ibid., p. 3-4

[62] Ibid., p. 4

[63] Sage, p. 4-5

[64] Ibid., p. 11-12

[65] Sage., p 12-13

[66] Ibid., p. 12

[67] Sage, p. 12

[68] Ibid., p. 13

[69] "Cancer Adjuvant Therapy," LifeExtension, Available: http://www.lef.org/protocols/prtcl-027b.html (accessed 2004, Oct. 8) Also see the LEF Protocol Book!

[70] "Andrographis," herbs2000.com, Available: http://www.herbs2000.com/herbs/herbs_andrographis.htm, p 1-2 (accessed 2004, Oct. 17)

[71] Ibid.

[72] Ibid., p. 2

[73] R. Elkins, M.H. *Cat's Claw (Uno de Gato),* Pleasant Grove, UT: Woodland Publishing Inc., 1995, p. 24, 27

[74] Ibid.

[75] "Cat's Claw," herbs2000.com, Available: http://www.herbs2000.com/herbs/herbs_cats_claw.htm, p. 2-3 (accessed 2004, Nov 16)

[76] "Dandelion Plant (herb - NOT just the root)", Available: http://www.cancertutor.com/Other Big_List.htm, p. 14, (accessed 2004, Oct. 17)

[77] Ibid.

[78] "Garlic," Optimal Diet Healthy Eating website "Letters to Friends," *Glorious Garlic* 04 Oct, 2003, from "Healing Foods of the Bible" by Bernard Ward. Available http://homodiet.Netfirms.com/otherssay/letters/garlic.htm (accessed 2004, Dec. 29)

[79] J. Carper. *The Food Pharmacy - Dramatic New Evidence That Food Is Your Best Medicine,* New York: Bantam Books, 1988-1989, p. 203

[80] "Breast Cancer - healing with herbs, vitamins and minerals," herbs 2000.com, Available: http://www.herbs2000.com/disorders/cancer_breast.htm, p.2 (accessed 2004, Oct 17)

[81] Ibid.

[82] "Milk Thistle," "Side Effects And Cautions" - Herbs2000.com website - Available: http://www. herbs2000.com/herbs/herbs_thistle_milk.htm, p. 4 (accessed 2004, Dec. 29)

[83] R.L. Blaylock, M.D. *Natural Strategies For Cancer Patients*, New York: Twin Streams Kensington Publishing Corp., © 2003, p. 171. All right reserved. Reprinted by arrangement with Kensington Publishing Corp. www.kensingtonbooks.com.

[84] "Cancer - Breast," "Quinones," Alternative Health Supplies (Australia) *Your Health Your Choice*, Available: http://www.alternativehealth.com.au/Articles/breast.htm p. 5 (accessed 2004, Oct.24)

[85] Ibid., "Herbs," p. 7

[86] J. A. Duke, Ph.D. *The Green Pharmacy*, New York: St. Martin's Paperbacks, 1998, (Published in arrangement with Rodale Press, Inc.,) p. 481-482

[87] "Rhodiola Rosea," New Page 5, Available: http://www.planetherbs.com/articles/rhodiolia%20rosea/htm, p. 1-2 (accessed 2004, Oct. 21)

[88] Ibid.

[89] "Cancer - Breast," "Herbs," Alternative Health Supplies (Australia) *Your Health Your Choice*, Available: http://www.alternativehealth.com.au/Articles/breast.htm p. 7 (accessed 2004, Oct. 24)

[90] Duke, p. 378-379

[91] "Breast Cancer - healing with herbs, vitamins and minerals," herbs 2000.com, Available: http://www.herbs2000.com/disorders/cancer_breast.htm, p.2 (accessed 2004, Oct 17)

[92] Ibid., p. 2

[92a] Mark Stengler, N.D., p 445 *The Natural Physician's Healing Therapies* by Mark Stengler, N.D copyright © 2001 by Mark Stengler. Used by permission of Avery Publishing, an imprint of Penguin Group (USA) Inc.

[93] "Sweet Wormwood (herb)," The Cancer Tutor™, Alternative Cancer Treatment Information Center, Available: http://www.cancertutor.com/Other/Big_List.htm, p. 36 (accessed 2004, Oct. 17)

[94] Ibid.

[95] Ibid.

[96] R. Elkins, M.H. *D-Glucarate, Powerful Protector Against Breast and Prostate Cancers,* Pleasant Grove, UT: Woodland Publishing, Inc., 1999, p. 6

[97] Ibid., p. 13, 18

[98] Ibid.

[99] "How Shark Cartilage Works On Cancer," Available: http://www.nutritionfarm.com GLOSSARY/REPORTS/sharkrept.htm, p. 1 (accessed 2004, Nov. 16)

[100] Ibid.

[101] Ibid.

[102] "Clodronate," The Cancer Tutor™, Alternative Cancer Treatment Information Center, Available: http://www.cancertutor.com/Other/Big_List.htm, p. 11 (accessed 2004, Oct. 17) (Also see http://www.mnwelldir.org/docs/cancer1/altthrpy.htm.)

[103] R.W. Moss, Ph.D. *Cancer Therapy - The Independent Consumer's Guide To Non-Toxic Treatment & Prevention*, Equinox Press, 1992, p. 407, 408

[104] "The Effect of Ukrain on Cancer," Available: http://www.ukrin.com/standardtexte/Standard brief_2_eng.htm, p. 1 (accessed 2004, Oct. 13)

[105] Ibid., p. 2

[106] Ibid., p. 3

[107] M. Kennedy Salaman. *Nutrition: The Cancer Answer II,* Menlo Park, CA.: Statford Publishing, 1995, p. 238

[108] F. Batmanghelidj, M.D. *Your Body's Many Cries For Water,* Vienna, VA: Global Health Solutions, Inc., 1992, 1995, 1997, p. 161

Chapter 4

[1] R.D. Strand with D.K. Wallace. *What Your Doctor Doesn't Know About Nutritional Medicine May Be Killing You,* Nashville: Thomas Nelson Publishers, 2002, p. 111

[2] "Billion dollar drug company nearly squashes astounding research on natural cancer killer," Health Sciences Institute January Newsletter, Members Alert for January 2001 Vol. 5, No. 7, Available: http://www.hsibaltimore.com (accessed 2004, April 26)

[3] A. Hoffer, Ph.D., M.D., FRCP(C). "Hoffer's Home Page – Orthomolecular Treatment of Cancer," Available: http://www.islandnet.com/~hoffer/ p. 3 (accessed 2005, May 28)

[4] T. Mitchell. "Resveratrol - Powerful Protection Against Prostate Cancer." Available: http://www.lef.org/magazine/mag2004/apr2004_report_resver_01.htm, p. 1, Life Extension website, (accessed 2004, May 18) Also see the LEF Protocol Book!

[5] R. Elkins, M.H. *D-Glucarate, Powerful Protector Against Breast and Prostate Cancers,* Pleasant Grove, Utah: Woodland Publishing, 1999, p. 23

[6] J. Challem. *All About Carotenoids Beta-carotene, Lutein & Lycopene*, Garden City Park, N.Y. Avery Publishing, 1999, p. 27, 28, Quotes reprinted with Mr. Challem's permission.

[7] Challem, p. 27, 28

[8] Elkins., p. 24

[9] K. Gale, *Reuters Health,* "Herbal COX-2 inhibitor induces prostate cancer cell apoptosis," posting date July 29, 2003, OncoLink Cancer News from *Reuters Health Information –* Abramson Cancer Center of the University of Pennsylvania, "Prostate Cancer." Available: http://www.oncolink.com/resources/article.cfm?c=3&s=8&ss=23&id=9953&month=07 &year=2003. Copyright © 2005 Reuters Limited. All rights reserved. Reuters shall not be liable for any errors or delays in the content, or for any actions taken in reliance thereon. Reprinted with their permission. Also see http://www.oncolink.com/custom_tags/print_article.cfm?Page=2&id=9953&Section=Re ut...Copyright © 1994-2004 Trustees of the University of Pennsylvania, (accessed 2005, Jan 4)

[10] "High dietary boron linked to reduced risk for prostate cancer." From Reuters Health Information. Available: http://www.oncolink.com/resources/article.cfm?c=3&s=8&ss=23&id=1188&month=04&year=2001. Oncolink Cancer News (accessed 2005, June 2) Copyright © 2005 Reuters Limited. All rights reserved. Reprinted with their permission. Reuters shall not be liable for any errors or delays in the content, or for any actions taken in reliance thereon. OncoLinkCopyright © 1994-2005 © Trustees of the University of Pennsylvania

[11] Ibid.

[12] Ibid.

[13] Elkins, p. 6

[14] Ibid., p. 6, 7, 16

[15] Elkins, p. 10

[16] Ibid., p. 18

[17] Cancer-Fighter Perillyl Alcohol Found in Tart Cherries," FS Flavonoid Sciences. Available: http://www.flavonoidsciences.com/cherryblueberry.php?page=3&title=Cancer-Fighter%20P p. 1 (accessed 2004, May 25) Credit: Cherry Marketing Institute Cherry Advantage Issue I

[18] Ibid.

[19] Ibid., p. 1

[20] "Independent Lab Verifies Cancer-Fighting Agents In Cherries." Available: http://www.flavonoidsciences.com/cherry-blueberry.php?page=3&title=Cancer-Fighter%20P...p. 1 (accessed 2004, May 25) Credit: Cherry Marketing Institute Cherry Advantage Issue I

[20a] "DHEA protects against prostate cancer." Available: http:///www.yourhealthbase.com/prostate_cancer.htm (accessed 2005, May 3)

[21] E. Gardiner. *How I Conquered Cancer - A Naturopathic Alternative,* Houston, TX: Emerald Ink Publishing, 1997, p. 36, reprinted with their permission

[22] Ibid., p. 38

[23] Ibid., p. 38

[24] Ibid., p. 69

[25] "Ellagic Acid," Wellness Directory of Minnesota™, Alternative Cancer Therapies, Available: http://www.mnwelldir.org/docs/cancer1/altthrpy.htm, p. 1 (accessed 2004, Oct. 28)

[26] Ibid.

[27] "Ellagic Acid," Wellness Directory of Minnesota™, Alternative Cancer Therapies, (This website says that their information about H.pylori is from Dr. Glen Halvorson's Book, *Chemo-preventive Properties of Phytochemicals)* Available: http://www.mnwelldir.org/docs/cancer1/altthrpy.htm, p. 2-3 (accessed 2004, Oct. 28)

[28] M. Stengler, N.D. p 187. *The Natural Physician's Healing Therapies* by Mark Stengler, N.D. copyright © 2001 by Mark Stengler. Used by permission of Avery Publishing, an imprint of Penguin Group (USA) Inc.

[29] "Cancer Adjuvant Therapy," "Ginger (Zingiber officinalis)," LifeExtension, Available: http://www.lef.org/protocols/prtcl-027b.shtml, (accessed 2004, Oct 8) Also see the LEF Protocol Book!

[30] Ginseng and Cancer: A Follow-up," Perspectives Research and Creative Activities, Spring 2004, Southern Illinois University Carbondale, Available: http://www.siu.edu/~perspect/04_sp/ginseng.html, p 1 (accessed 2004, Dec. 19) © 2003, Board of Trustees, Southern Illinois University

[31] K. C. Jaehnig, "Ginseng Root May Help Slow Growth of Cancer Cells," Available: http://news.siu.edu/news/January05/011105kj4109.htm, (accessed 2005, May 9) © 2003, Board of Trustees, Southern Illinois University

[31a] Ibid.

[31b] Ibid.

[32] Laura Murphy. From an email to me on 2005, May 10

[33] "Headway on natural chemotherapy for prostate cancer," Nutraingredients.com, News & Analysis Research, 20/04/2004 "Natural treatments for prostate cancer are fast gaining scientific evidence for their efficacy in human patients," Available: http://www.nutraingredients.com/news/news-NG.asp?id=51500, p. 1 (accessed 2004, Oct. 28)

[34] "Foods That Harm, Foods That Heal - Tasty ways to keep the doctor away," *Reader's Digest*, from the book, (April 2004), p. 97-98 The book itself was published (1st edition) in Mar. 2004.

[35] *The World's Greatest Treasury of Health Secrets*, From the Editors of Bottom Line Publications, Greenwich, CT.: Boardroom, Inc., 2000, p. 217

[36] Ibid., p. 217

[37] J.F. Balch, M.D. From *The Super Anti-Oxidants: Why They Will Change the Face of Healthcare in the 21st Century,* copyright © 1998 by James F. Balch. Reprinted by permission of the publisher, M. Evans & Company, New York, p. 129

[38] Ibid., p. 130

[39] Ibid., p. 132-133

[40] Balch, M.D., p. 129

[41] J. Carper. *The Food Pharmacy - Dramatic New Evidence That Food Is Your Best Medicine,* New York: Bantam Books, 1988, p. 297-298

[42] "Prostate Cancer," herbs2000.com, "Available: http://www.herbs2000.com/disorders/cancer_prostate.htm, p. 2 (accessed 2004, Oct. 17)

[43] "Broccoli and tomatoes prevent prostate cancer better than leading prescription drugs, research shows," Sun. May 01, 2005, newstarget.com. Available: http://www.newstarget.com/001391.html (accessed 2005, May 3)

[44] R. Sahelian, M.D. *Saw Palmetto Nature's Prostate Healer*, New York: Kensington Publishing, 1998, p. 71-85. Also see Dr. Sahelian's website at www.raysahelian.com/saw.html

[45] Ibid.

[46] "Prostate Cancer," herbs2000.com, p. 2

[47] S. Lieberman, Ph.D., and K. Babal, C.N. *Maitake Mushroom AND D-Fraction*, Pleasant Grove, Utah: Woodland Publishing, 2001, p. 18

[48] Ibid.

[49] "Maitake," herbs2000.com, Available: http://www.herbs2000.com/herbs/herbs_maitake.htm, p. 1 (accessed 2004, Nov. 22)

[50] "Maitake," herbs2000.com

[51] Ibid.

51aA. J. Brown, M.D., Reuters Health, New York, posting date May 23, 2005. "Pomegranate juice shows promise as treatment for recurrent prostate cancer." Available: http://www.oncolink.com/resources/article.cfm?=3&s=8&ss=23&id=11913&month=058&year=2005 Copyright © 2005 Reuters Limited. All rights reserved. Reprinted with their permission. Reuters shall not be liable for any errors or delays in the content, or for any actions taken in reliance thereon. OncoLink Cancer News is Copyright © 1994-2005 © Trustees of the University of Pennsylvania, (accessed 2005, June 2)

51b Ibid.

51c Ibid.

52 Elkins, *D-Glucarate*, p. 24

53 M. K. Salaman. *Nutrition: The Cancer Answer II*, Menlo Park, CA.: Statford Publishing, 2002 (this edition), p. 263

54 Ibid., p. 264

55 Salaman, p. 355

56 Ibid., p. 354

57 Ibid., p. 356, 358

58 T. Mitchell. "Resveratrol - Powerful Protection Against Prostate Cancer," Available: http://www.lef.org/magazine/mag2004/apr2004_report_resver_01.htm, p. 1, Life Extension website, (accessed 2004, May 18) Also see the LEF Protocol Book!

59 Ibid.

60 T. Mitchell

61 Ibid.

62 R. Sahelian, M.D. *Saw Palmetto Nature's Prostate Healer*, New York: Kensington Publishing, 1998, p. 96, also see www.raysahelian.com/saw.html

63 J. Carper. *Miracle Cures: Dramatic New Scientific Discoveries Revealing the Healing Powers of Herbs, Vitamins, and Other Natural Remedies* New York: Harper Collins 1997, p. 193

64 Ibid., p. 193

64a Martarelli D, Martarelli B, Pediconi D, Nabissi MI, Perfumi M, Pompei P. "Hypericum perforatum methanolic extract inhibits growth of human prostatic carcinoma cell line orthotopically implanted in nude mice." *Cancer Letters* 210 (1): 27-33, Jul 8 2004, from Positive Health Magazine. Inegrated Medicine for the 21st Century. Available: http://www.positivehealth.com/research.asp?i=3318 (accessed 2005, Jun. 23)

64b "Sun exposure prevents prostate cancer," Available: http://www.yourhealthbase.com/cancer_prostate.htm, (accessed 2005, May 3)

65 "Turmeric May Be Effective Adjunct Cancer Therapy," Discount Vitamins & Herbs - Health News. Available: http://www.discount-vitamins-herbs.net/health-news30.htm, p. 2-3 (accessed 2004, Nov. 17) Note that the reference the website gives for their article is: "The annual meeting of the American Association for Cancer Research, San Francisco, California. April 9, 2002."

66 "Prostate Cancer," herbs2000.com, Available: http://www.herbs2000.com/disorders/cancer_prostate.htm, p. 2 (accessed 2004, Oct. 17)

66a Mark Stengler, N.D., p 445 *The Natural Physician's Healing Therapies* by Mark Stengler, N.D copyright © 2001 by Mark Stengler. Used by permission of Avery Publishing, an imprint of Penguin Group (USA) Inc.

67 "The latest research on selenium and prostate cancer," American Federation for Aging Research - Prostate Cancer Information Center. Available: http://www.infoaging.org/d-prost-17—r-selenium.htm, p. 1 (accessed 2004, Oct. 26)

68 D. Patton, "Vitamin E has protective role in bladder cancer," FoodNavigator.com, News & Analysis Science & Nutrition. Available: http://www.foodnavigator.com/news/news-Ngasp?id=9537 (accessed 2004, Oct. 28)

69 Ibid.

70 "Red Clover (Trifolium pratense)," Cancer Tutor™, Alternative Cancer Treatment Information Center, Available: http://wwwcancertutor.com/Other/Big_List.htm, p. 32, (accessed 2004, Oct 17

71 Ibid.

72 "Prostate Cancer," herbs2000.com, Available: http://www.herbs2000.com/disorders/cancer_prostate.htm, p. 2 (accessed 2004, Oct. 17)

73 "Polysaccharide Kureha (PSK)," Herbs 2000, Available: http://www.herbs2000.com/miss/psk.htm, p. 1 (accessed 2004, Oct. 25)

74 "The Effect of Ukrain on Cancer," Available: http://www.ukrin.com/standardtexte/Standardbrief_2_eng.htm, p. 1 (accessed 2004, Oct. 13)

75 Ibid., p. 2

76 F. Batmanghelidj, M.D. *Your Body's Many Cries For Water,* Vienna, VA: Global Health Solutions, Inc., 1992, 1995, 1997, p. 161

Chapter 5

1 R. D. Strand, M.D., with Donna K. Wallace. *What Your Doctor Doesn't Know About Nutritional Medicine May Be Killing You,* Thomas Nelson Publishers, 2002 p. 163

2 "Healing Colon Cancer with RAW Food: A personal account," Holistic Health: Testimonials of Amazing Health Recovery. Available: http://www.shirleys-wellness-café.com/cancer.htm, p. 1 (accessed 2004, May 23)

3 Rev. George Malkmus, "How to Eliminate Sickness Seminar," Hallelujah Acres Brings you back to the Garden: the biblical natural diet. Available: http://www.hacres.com/seminars.asp, p. 1 (accessed 2004, May 25)

4 Ibid.

5 Ibid., p. 2

5a R. Willner, M.D., Ph.D. "Dr. Johanna Budwig Diet – Cancer, Arthritis, Multiple Sclerosis, Psoriasis, Eczema, Acne…Flaxseed oil and cottage cheese," The Cancer Homepage, Available: http://www.alternativehealth.co.nz/cancer/budwig.htm, from Ed McCabe (p85, "Oxygen Therapies") discussing his view on the role of essential fatty acids, p. 10 (accessed 2004, June 29)

5b "Dr. Budwig's Diet & Cancer Healing Protocol," website: Healing Cancer Naturally. Available: http://www.healingcancernaturally.com/budwig_protocol.html, from Dr. Budwig in "Der Tod des Tumors, Band II" (The Death of the Tumor, Vol. II) transcribing an interview broadcast by the Siddeutscher Rundfunk Stuttgart (South German Radio Station) on 11 Sep 1967, (accessed website 2005, Jan 17)

6 "Dr. Budwig's Diet & Cancer Healing Protocol," website: Healing Cancer Naturally, Available: http://www.healingcancernaturally.com/budwig_protocol.html, (accessed 2005, Jan 17)

6a R. Elkins, M.H. *D-Glucarate, Powerful Protector Against Breast and Prostate Cancers*, Pleasant Grove, UT: Woodland Publishing, 1999, p. 21-22

6b A. Hoffer, M.D., Ph.D., F.R.C.P. (C) "Hoffer's Home Page – Orthomolecular Treatment of Cancer," (accessed 2005, Jun. 11)

7 J. S. Rubin, N.M.D., Ph.D. *The Maker's Diet,* Lake Mary, FL.: Siloam, 2004, p. 26

7a Ibid.

8 Rubin, p. 26-27, 29

9 Ibid., p. 36

10 Ibid., p. 195

11 "Wormwood," Alternative Cancer Therapies, According to Dr. Lam MD at http://www.drlam.com/A3R_brief_in_doc_format/Artemisinin.cfm, quotes are from the Wellness Directory of Minnesota™ website, Available: http://www.mnwelldir.org/docs/cancer1/altthrpy.htm, (accessed 2004, Dec. 20)

11a "Colorectal Cancer," herbs2000.com. Available: http://www.2000herbs.com/disorder-scancer_colorectal.htm p. 2 (accessed 2004, Oct. 17)

12 "Graviola," Alternative Cancer Therapies. Available: http://www.mnwelldir.org/docs/cancer1/altthrpy2.htm, p. 1 (accessed 2004, May 25)

13 Ibid.

14 Ibid.

15 Ibid.

16 "Billion-dollar drug company nearly squashes astounding research on natural cancer killer," Health Sciences Institute January Newsletter, Members Alert for January 2001 - Vol. 5, No. 7. Available: http://www.hsibaltimore.com (accessed 2004, April 26)

17 Ibid., p. 2

18 Ibid., p. 2, 3

19 Ibid., p. 3

20 "Billion-dollar drug company…" p. 3

21 Ibid.

22 Ibid., p. 4

23 Ibid.

24 Ibid., p. 5

25 R. Dubin. p. 62. From *Miracle Food Cures From The Bible* by Reese Dubin, copyright © 1999 by Prentice Hall. Used by permission of Avery Publishing, an imprint of Penguin Group (USA) Inc.

26 Ibid.

27 Ibid., p. 62, 63

28 Dubin, p. 63

29 Ibid., p. 64

30 Dubin, p. 65

31 C. Olsen, with contributions by Dr. Jim Chan & Christopher Gussa, *Essiac A Native Herbal Cancer Remedy*, p.13. Reprinted with permission from *Essiac: A Native Herbal Cancer Remedy* by Cynthia Olsen, Lotus Press, PO Box 325, Twin Lakes, WI 53181. © 1996 All Rights Reserved.

32 Ibid., p. 15

33 Ibid., p. 16

34 Dubin., p. 71, 72

[35] Ibid., p. 73

[36] Ibid., p. 73

[37] Olsen, p.18

[38] Ibid., p. 19

[38a] C. Brusch, M.D. From *Whale* website. "Alternative Medical Doctor Quotes." Available: http://www.whale.to/m/quotes6.html (accessed 2005, Jun. 9)

[38b] Olsen, p. 20

[39] Ibid.

[40] Ibid., p. 21

[41] Dubin, p. 69, 84

[42] Ibid., p. 87

[43] Dubin. p, 78, 79

[44] Ibid., p. 316

[45] "Cancer Adjuvant Therapy," LifeExtension, Available: http://www.lef.org/protocols/prtcl027b.shtml., p. 1 (accessed 2004, Oct 8) Also see the LEF Protocol Book!

[46] Ibid.

[47] "Colorectal Cancer," Herbs2000.com, *Healing with herbs, vitamins and minerals*, Available: http://www.herbs2000.com/disorders/cancer_liver.htm, p. 1 (accessed 2004, Oct. 17)

[47a] Cancer Adjuvant Therapy," LifeExtension, Available: http://www.lef.org/protocols/prtcl027b.shtml (accessed 2004, Oct. 8) Also see the LEF Protocol Book!

[48] Ibid.

[49] "'Off-The-Shelf' Cancer Cure?" HSI, Health Archives, Health Sciences Institute, 6/1/2001, Available: http://www.hsibaltimore.com/ea2001/ea_010601.html (accessed 2004, Dec. 30)

[50] Nina Anderson. "120 and Healthy! It's Common in the Republic of Georgia," Many Hands Feature Articles, at the Alternative Medicine Journal of New England, Available: http://www.manyhands.com/articles/georgia.html, p. 1 (accessed 2004, Oct. 17)

[51] Ibid.

[52] Ibid., p. 2 (the website gives their souce of this information as: Professor Dr. Zakir Ramazanov, Ph.D. and excerpted from the book, *The Secrets of Staying Young*)

[53] "Suma," Raintree Nutrition, TROPICAL PLANT DATABASE, p. 1,2,3 Available: http://www.raintree.com/suma.htm, (accessed 2004, Oct. 22) This information is also found in Leslie Taylor's book, *The Healing Power of Rainforest Herbs,* Square One Publishers, Jan. 2005

[54] Ibid., p. 6

[55] "Colorectal Cancer," herbs2000.com, Available: http://www.herbs2000.com/disorders/cancer_colorectal.htm p. 1, 2 (accessed 2004, Oct. 17)

[56] Mark Stengler, N.D., p 445 *The Natural Physician's Healing Therapies* by Mark Stengler, N.D copyright © 2001 by Mark Stengler. Used by permission of Avery Publishing, an imprint of Penguin Group (USA) Inc.

[57] B. Gottlieb. *Alternative Cures*, (City, State, n.g.) Rodale, 2000, p. 170

[57a] "Cat's Claw," herbs2000.com, Available: http://www.herbs2000.com/herbs/herbs_cats_claw.htm, p. 2-3 (accessed 2004, Nov 16)

58 "Colorectal Cancer,"herbs2000.com, Available:
    http://www.herbs2000.com/disorders/cancer_colorectal_htm p. 3 (accessed 2004, Oct 17)

59 M. Kennedy Salaman. *All Your Health Questions Answered Naturally*, MKS, Inc., 1998, (City, State, n.g.) p. 211

60 Stengler, p. 355

61 "Colorectal Cancer," herbs2000.com, *Colorectal Cancer*. Available:
    http://www.herbs2000.com/disorders/cancer_ colorectal.htm, p. 2 (accessed 2004, Oct. 17)

61a Susan S. Lang, "Onions anti-cancer effects," Cornell News, for release Oct. 7, 2004, (contact Susan S. Lang). R.H. Liu, M.D., Ph.D. Available:
    http://www.news.cornell.edu/releases/Oct04/onions.cancer.ssl.html p. 1-2 (accessed 2004, Dec. 29)

61b Ibid.

62 S. Sinatra, M.D., F.A.C.C. *The Coenzyme Q10 Phenomenon*, New York: the McGraw Hill Companies, 1998, p. 82-83. Reproduced with permission of the McGraw-Hill Companies

63 Ibid.

64 Ibid., p. 83

65 Ibid.

66 Strand, M.D. et. al., p. 145

66aIbid.

67 R. W. Moss, Ph.D. *Antioxidants against Cancer,* State College, PA.: Equinox Press, Inc. p. 73

68 Ibid., p. 74

69 C. Gupta, "The FDA versus Folic Acid," *Share the Wealth*, July 14, 2003. Available:
    http://www.newmediaexplorer.org/chris/2003/07/14/the_fda_versus_folic_acid.htm, p. 1 (accessed 2004, Nov. 20)

70 Ibid., p. 1

71 Ibid.

72 R. W. Moss. *Antioxidants against Cancer*, State College, PA., Equinox Press, Inc. p. 82

73 Ibid., p. 83-84

74 Ibid.

75 Ibid.

76 Ibid.

77 J. Heinerman. *Heinerman's New Encyclopedia of Fruits & Vegetables*, Reward Books, 1995, p. 75

78 "Stomach Cancer," herbs2000.com. Available: http://www.herbs2000.com/disorders/cancer_stomach.htm, p. 2, (accessed 2004, Oct. 17)

79 "Colorectal Cancer" herbs2000.com, Available:
    http://www.herbs2000.com/disorders/cancer_colorectal.htm, p. 2 (accessed 2004, Oct. 17)

80 Shari Lieberman, Ph.D. and Ken Babal, C.N., *Maitake Mushroom AND D-Fraction,* Pleasant Grove, UT: Woodland Publishing, 2001, p. 28-29

81 "Polysaccharide Kureha (PSK)," herbs2000.com. Available:
    http://www.herbs2000.com/miss/psk.htm, p. 1 (accessed 2004, Oct. 25)

82 Lieberman, et al., p. 11

83 "Colorectal Cancer," herbs2000.com. Available:
    http://www.herbs2000.com/disorders/cancer_colorectal.htm, p. 2 (accessed 2004, Oct. 17)

[84] Deanne Tenney, *Medicinal Mushrooms*, Pleasant Grove, UT:Woodland Publishing, 1997, p. 11-12

[85] Ibid.

[86] "Stomach Cancer," herbs2000.com. Available: http://www.herbs2000.com/disorders/cancer_stomach..htm, p. 2 (accessed 2004, Oct. 17)

[87] Tenney, p. 12

[88] S. Yeager & the Editors of Prevention Health Books. *Doctors Book of FOOD REMEDIES*, (city, state, n.g.): Rodale, Inc., 1998, p. 429

[89] Ibid., p. 429

[90] "Beta-Sitosterol," DrLam.com. Available: www.drlam.com/opinion/beta_sitosterol.cfm, 1-3, (accessed 2004, Oct. 24)

[91] Ibid.

[92] "Recent Scientific Advances in Rare Diseases Research," Report on the Rare Diseases Research Activities at the National Institutes of Health FY 2003," "Beta-Sitosterolemia,"Available: http://rarediseases.info.nih.gov/html/reports/fy2003/nhlbi.html, (accessed 2005, Jul 2)

[93] "What is Leukodystrophy?" National Institute of Neurological Disorders and Stroke, NINDS Leukodystrophy Information Page, Available: *http*://www.ninds.nih.gov/disorders/leukodystrophy/leukodystrophy.htm, (accessed 2005, Jul. 2)

[94] "Colorectal Cancer," herbs2000.com. Available: http://www.herbs2000.com/disorders/cancer_colorectal.htm, p. 3 (accessed 2004, Oct. 17)

[94a] Ibid.

[94b] Ibid.

[95] M. Kennedy Salaman. *Nutrition: The Cancer Answer II*, Menlo Park, CA: Statford Publishing, MKS, Inc. 2002, p. 348

[95a] Ibid., p. 348

[96] Ibid., p. 349

[97] Donna Sage, M.S.S.A., *Haelan Reverses Cancer Cell Growth*, from *Well Being Journal Special Edition: Healing Cancer Naturally*. Available: http://www.wellbeingjournal.com/haelan.htm, p. 1, 6 (2004, Oct. 17)

[97a] Ibid.

[98] S. Meyerowitz. *Wheat Grass Nature's Finest Medicine*, Great Barrington, Mass: Sproutman Publications, 1999, p. 98-101

[99] "The Effect of Ukrain on Cancer." Available: http://www.ukrin.com/standardtexte/Standardbrief_2_eng.htm, p. 1 (accessed 2004, Oct. 13)

[100] Ibid., p. 1

[101] Ibid.

[102] Ibid., p. 1, 2

[103] Ibid.

[104] "Colorectal Cancer," herbs2000.com. Available: http://www.herbs2000.com/disorders/cancer_ colorectal.htm, p. 3 (accessed 2004, Oct. 17)

[105] F. Batmanghelidg, M.D. *Your Body's Many Cries For Water*, Vienna, VA: Global Health Solutions, 1992, 1995, 1997, p. 161

Chapter 6

[1] B. Berkson, M.D., Ph.D. From *The Alpha Lipoic Acid Breakthrough,* copyright © 1998 by Burt Berkson. Used by permission of Prima Publishing, a division of Random House, Inc., p. 75

[2] J. Challem. *All About Carotenoids Beta-carotene, Lutein & Lycopene*, Garden City Park, N.Y.: Avery Publishing Group 1999, p. 27, reprinted with Mr. Challem's permission

[3] E. Mindell, R.Ph., Ph.D. *Earl Mindell's Food as Medicine,* New York. P. 219. Reprinted with permission of Simon & Schuster Adult Publishing Group, from EARL MINDELL'S FOOD AS MEDICINE, by Earl Mindell, R.Ph., Ph.D. © 1994 by Earl Mindell, R.Ph., Ph.D., and Carol Colman.

[4] S. Yeager and the Editors of Prevention Health Books. (City, State n.g.) *Doctor's Book Of Food Remedies,* Rodale, Inc., 1998, p. 503

[5] Ibid.

[6] J. Carper. *The Food Pharmacy,* New York: Bantam Books, 1988, p. 147

[7] "Cancer-Fighter Perillyl Alcohol Found in Tart Cherries." FS Flavonoid Sciences website. Available: http://www.flavonoidsciences.com/cherryblueberry.php?page=3&title=Cancer-Fighter%20P p. 1 (accessed 2004, May 25) Credit: Cherry Marketing Institute Cherry Advantage Issue I

[8] Ibid., p. 1

[9] R. Blaylock, M.D. *Natural Strategies For Cancer Patients,* New York: Twin Streams, Kensington Publishing Corp., © 2003, p. 260. All rights reserved. Reprinted by arrangement with Kensington Publishing Corp. www.kensingtonbooks.com.

[10] Ibid.

[10a] S. Becker. "Bulk Up On Fiber." Available at http://www.breadbeckers.com/bulkupon-fiber.htm (accessed 8 June, 2005) Copyright 2003 The Bread Beckers, Inc.©

[10b] "Ellagic Acid," "Cancer Weakness #7 – Use Free Radical Scavengers (That are Cancer Killers)." Available: http://www.cancer-prevention.net (Accessed 10 Apr. 2005)

[10c] Ibid.

[11] M. Stengler, N.D. p. 187. *The Natural Physician's Healing Therapies* by Mark Stengler, N.D. copyright © 2001 by Mark Stengler. Used by permission of Avery Publishing, an imprint of Penguin Group (USA) Inc.

[12] R.W. Moss, Ph.D. *Antioxidants against Cancer*, State College, PA.: Equinox Press, Inc., 2000, p. 37

[13] Ibid.

[13a] "Agaricus," Wellness Directory of Minnesota™, Alternative Cancer Therapies, updated 10-27-04. Available: http://www.mnwelldir.org/docs/cancer1/altthrpy.htm, p. 1-3 (accessed 2004, Nov. 20)

[13b] Ibid.

[14] Ibid.

[15] Ibid.

[16] "Polysaccharide Kureha (PSK)," herbs2000.com. Available: http:///www.herbs2000.miss/psk.htm, p. 1 (accessed 2004, Oct. 25)

[16a] Ibid.

[17] "Agaricus," Wellness Directory of Minnesota™, Alternative Cancer Therapies, updated 10-27-04. Available: http://www.mnwelldir.org/docs/cancer1/altthrpy.htm, p. 1-3 (accessed 2004, Nov. 20)

[18] J. Lee, M.D. with Virginia Hopkins. *What Your Doctor May Not Tell You About Menopause - The Breakthrough Book On Natural Progesterone*, New York: Warner Books, Inc. 1996, p. 46-47, From *What Your Doctor May Not Tell You About Menopause* by Dr. John Lee, M.D., Copyright © 1996 by John R. Lee, M.D. and Virginia Hopkins. By permission of Warner Books, Inc.

[19] Ibid., p. 47, 226

[20] *Healing with Vitamins* (by the Editors of *Prevention* Health Books), (City, State, n.g.) Rodale, Inc., p. 136-137

[21] R. Blaylock, M.D. *Natural Strategies For Cancer Patients,* New York: Twin Streams Kensington Publishing Corp., © 2003, p. 10-11. All rights reserved. Reprinted by arrangement with Kensington Publishing Corp. www.kensingtonbooks.com

[22] H. Winter Griffith, M.D. *Vitamins Herbs, Minerals & Supplements, The Complete Guide,* Rev. Edition, (City, State, n.g.) Fisher Books, Member of Perseus Books Group, 1988, 1998, p. 49

[23] "Cervical Cancer." Herbs2000.com. Available: http://www.herbs2000.com/disorders/cancer_cervical.htm, p. 2 (accessed 2004, Oct. 17)

[24] Ibid., p. 3

[25] *The Healing Power of Vitamins, Minerals, and Herbs*, Reader's Digest, Pleasantville, N.Y. Reader's Digest Assoc., Inc., p. 352, 353. Quoted with permission of Global Books & Home Entertainment, The Reader's Digest Association, Inc.

[25a] Ibid.

[25b] "Andiroba," Raintree Nutrition, TROPICAL PLANT DATABASE. Available: http://www.raintree.com/andiroba.htm p. 1,3,4 (accessed 2004, Oct. 22) This information is also found in Leslie Taylor's book, *The Healing Power of Rainforest Herbs,* Square One Publishers, Jan. 2005

[25c] Ibid.

[26] Ibid.

[27] "Endometrial Cancer." Herbs2000.com. Available: http://www.herbs2000.com/disorders/cancer_endometrial.htm, p. 1 (accessed 2004, Oct. 17)

[28] Ibid., p. 1-2

[29] "Cat's Claw." Herbs2000.com. Available: http://www.herbs2000.com/herbs/herbs_cats_claw.htm, p. 3 (accessed 2005, Jan 11)

[30] J. G. Connor, M.Ac, Lac, "Cancer Prevention and Diet." "Herbal Nutritional Support." Available: http://www.compassionateacupuncture.com/cancer.htm (accessed 2005, May 21)

[30a] G. Srinivas, R.J. Anto, P. Srinivas, S. Vidhyalakshmi, V.P. Senan, D. Karunagaran. Div. Of Cancer Biology, Rajiv Gandhi Centre for Biotechnology, Poojapura, Thiruvananthapuram 695 014, Kerala, India. Pub Med, "Emodin induces apoptosis of human cervical cancer cells through poly (ADP-ribose) polymerase cleavage and activation of caspase-9." Available: http://www.ncbi.nlm.nih.gov/entrez/query.fcgi?cmd=Retrieve&db=PubMed&list_uids=12892828, Eur J Pharmacol. 2003 JVL 25;473(2-3):117-25 p. 1, (accessed 2004, Sept. 27)

[31] S. E. Miners, "Hope for Cancer Sufferers," 1001herbs.com, "An 'Official Miracle.'" Available: http://www.1001herbs.com/webarticles/essiac/essiac-extras.html, p. 2 (accessed 2005, Jan. 7)

[32] Ibid., p. 2

[33] Ibid., p. 3

[34] "Espinheira Santa," Herbs2000.com. Available:
http://www.herbs2000.com/herbs/herbs_espinheirasanta.htm, p. 1,2 (accessed 2004, Oct. 16)

[35] "Endometrial Cancer," Herbs2000.com. Available: http://www.herbs2000.com/disorders/cancer_endometrial.htm, p. 2 (accessed 2004, Oct. 25)

[36] Ibid., p. 2

[36a] "Snow Fungus," Herbs2000.com. Available:
http://www.herbs2000.com/herbs/herbs_snow_fungus.htm, p. 1 (accessed 2004, Nov. 20)

[37] Ibid.

[38] Ibid., p. 1

[38a] "Cervical Cancer," Herbs2000.com. Available:
http://www.herbs2000.com/disorders/cancer_cervical.htm, p. 2 (accessed 2004, Oct. 17)

[39] Ibid.

[39a] "Turmeric Curcuma longa syn. C. domestica," Herbs2000.com. Available:
http://www.herbs2000.com/herbs/herbs_turmeric.htm, p. 3 (accessed 2005, Jan 29)

[40] Blaylock, p. 177

[41] Ibid., p. 178-180, 185, 258

[42] R. Dubin. From *Miracle Food Cures From The Bible* by Reese Dubin, copyright © 1999 by Prentice Hall. Used by permission of Avery Publishing, an imprint of Penguin Group (USA) Inc., p. 164-165

[43] Ibid., p. 165

[44] Ibid.

[45] Dubin, p. 165

[46] Ibid., p. 166

[47] Ibid., p. 167

[48] Dubin, p. 168, 169

[49] Ibid.

[50] J. L. Eftekhar, *Heal Yourself, Globe Digests™*, Boca Raton, FL., and New York: Globe Communications Corp., 1995, pg. 22

[51] "Shark Cartilage," Enerex.ca. Available:
http://www.enerex.ca/articles/shark_cartilage.htm, p. 2 (accessed 2004, Jun. 30)

[51a] G. A. Forgionne, Ph.D., "Nutritional Therapy for Primary Peritoneal Cancer: A Case Study," from the *CancerLynx* website July 8, 2002 article. Available: http://www.cancerlynx.com/peritonealcase.html, p. 1-3 (accessed 2004, Dec. 14)

[52] "Endometrial Cancer," Herbs2000.com, Available: http://www.herbs2000.com/herbs/herbs_espinheirasanta.htm, p. 2 (accessed 2004, Oct. 16)

[53] Ibid.

[54] S. Yeager and the Editors of *Prevention* Health Books. *Doctors Book of FOOD REMEDIES,* (City, State, n.g.) Rodale, Inc. 1998, p. 108

[55] J. A. Duke, Ph.D., with M. Castleman. *The Green Pharmacy anti-aging Prescriptions*, (City, State, n.g.), Rodale Press, Inc., 2001. P. 87

[56] Salaman, p. 199

[57] R. Morse, N.D. *The Detox Miracle Sourcebook*, Prescott, AZ.: Hohm Press, 2004, p. 154

Chapter 7

[1] M. Kennedy Salaman. *All Your Health Questions Answered Naturally*, MKS, Inc. 1998, (Distributed by Bay to Bay Distribution, Inc. Mountain View, CA.) p. 657

[2] Taber's Cyclopedic Medical Dictionary, Philadelphia: F.A. Davis Co., © 2005, 20th Edition, p. 1414

[3] "Bone Marrow and Stem Cell Transplants," Overview, Bone Marrow and Stem Cell Transplants for Childhood Cancer. Available: http://www.cancerindex.org/ccw/guide2bm.htm, p. 1 (accessed 2004, Nov. 21)

[4] "What is graft-versus-host disease? (if you are having a transplant from a donor),"CANCERBACUP Helping people live with cancer, Available: //www.cancerbacup.org.uk/Treatments/Stemcellbonemarrowtransplants/Generalinfo…, p. 1 (accessed 2004, Nov.21)

[5] Taber's, p. 1283-1284

[6] M. Kennedy Salaman. *Nutrition: The Cancer Answer II*, Menlo Park, CA: Statford Publishing, 2002 edition, p. 279-280

[7] Ibid..

[8] Ibid., p. 280

[9] Ibid., p. 280, 281

[10] Ibid., p. 279

[11] Ibid.

[12] R. F. Cathcart M.D., "Vitamin C – Orthomed.com.," "Polio Cure Systematically Suppressed,"Available: http://www.orthomed.com (accessed 2005, May 28)

[13] A. Hoffer, M.D., F.R.C.P.(C), with Linus Pauling, Ph.D. *Healing Cancer – Complementary Vitamin & Drug Treatments,* Toronto Ontario, Canada: 2004, p. 35

[14] Ibid., p. 37

[15] Ibid., p. 42

[16] Hoffer, et al., p. 61

[17] R. W. Moss, Ph.D. *Antioxidants against Cancer*, State College, PA.: Equinox Press, Inc., 2000, 2002, p. 59

[18] M. Kennedy Salaman. *All Your Health Questions Answered Naturally*, MKS, Inc., 1998, p. 655

[19] Ibid.

[20] Ibid., p. 658

[21] "Vitamin A may prevent prostate cancer," yourhealthbase.com. Available: http://www.yourhealthbase.com/cancer_prostate.htm (accessed 2005, May 3)

[22] Hoffer, et al., p. 59

[23] "Bone Cancer." Herbs2000.com. Available: http://www.herbs2000.com/disorders/cancer_bone.htm p. 2 (accessed 2004, Oct. 17)

[24] Ibid., p. 2

[25] "Red Beet," Leukemia, from "Herbal Formulas for Leukemia." Available: http://www.herbsfirst.com/ailments descriptions/Leukemiapg.html, p. 1 (accessed 2004, Aug. 1) herbsfirst is now linked with http://herballegacy.com/id118.htm and this information is under the "Leukemia" article at herballegacy.com (accessed 2005, May 6) Permission to quote obtained from The Shool of Natural Healing, taken from the book *The School of Natural Healing* by John R. Christopher, 1976, Christopher Publications, P O Box 412, Springville, UT 84663.

26 S. Meyerowitz, "Benefits of Wheatgrass," International Specialty Supply. Available: http://www.sproutnet.com/Press/benefits_of_wheatgrass.htm p. 1, 2, (accessed 2004, Aug. 1)

27 Ibid., p. 2

28 Moss, p. 70

29 Ibid.

30 Ibid., p. 92, 93

31 Ibid.,

32 Ibid., p. 92, 93

32a Salaman, p. 659-660

33 H. Winter Griffith, M.D. *Vitamins, Herbs, Minerals & Supplements - The Complete Guide,* (City, State, n.g.): Perseus (Fisher Books), 1988, 1998, p. 49

34 M. Kennedy Salaman. *All Your Health Questions Answered Naturally*, (Distributed by Bay to Bay Distrib., Inc. Mountain View, CA.) MKS, Inc., 1998, p. 653, 654

34a R. Blaylock, M.D. *Natural Strategies for Cancer Patients,* New York: Twin Streams, Kensington Publishing Corp., © 2003, p. 143-144. All rights reserved. Reprinted by arrangement with Kensington Publishing Corp. www.kensingtonbooks.com

35 Ibid.

36 Ibid., p. 144

37 Blaylock, p. 144

37aIbid., p. 170-172

38 Ibid.

39 "Grape." Herbs2000.com. Available: http://www.herbs2000.com/herbs/herbs_grape.htm., p. 3 (accessed 2004, Jun 23)

40 Ibid.

41 Ibid., p. 3

42 "Mangosteen Treatment For Cancer," Cancer Tutor™, Alternative Cancer Treatment Information Center. Available: http://www.cancertutor.com/Cancer/Mangosteen.html, p. 1, 2 (accessed 2004, Oct. 17) (Note that they give their source as: "'Antiproliferation, antioxidation and induction of apoptosis by Garcinia mangostana (mangosteen) on SKBR3 human breast cancer cell line,' by Moongkarndi P, Kosem N, Kaslungka S, Luanratana O, Pongpan N, Neungton N."

42a Ibid.

43 "Health Information, "Jones Biomedicals & Laboratory, Inc. Available: http://members.aol.com/jonbio/nutrition.htm (accessed 2005, Jan 29)

44 S. Lieberman, Ph.D., and K. Babal, C.N., *Maitake Mushroom AND D-Fraction*, Pleasant Grove, UT.: Woodland Publishing, 2001, p. 27

45 Ibid.

46 Ibid.

47 "Maitake," Herbs2000.com. Available: http://www.herbs2000.com/herbs/herbs_maitake.htm, p. 1 (Accessed 2004, Nov. 22)

48 "Shiitake Mushroom (Lentinula edodes)." Available: http://www.stoneycreekmushrooms.com/about.htm (accessed 2005, May 7)

48a Ibid.

49 Salaman. p. 657-658

49a J. F. Balch, M.D. From *The Super Antioxidants: Why They Will Change the Face of Healthcare in the 21st Century,* copyright © 1998, by James F. Balch. Reprinted by the permission of the publisher M. Evans & Company, New York, p. 120

49b Salaman, p. 211

50 "Royal Jelly (a bee product)," Cancer Tutor™, Alternative Cancer Treatment Information Center. Available: http://www.cancertutor.com/Other/Big_List.htm, p. 33 (accessed 2004, Nov. 21)

51 P.A. Balch, C.N.C. et al., Prescription For Nutritional Healing, New York: Avery Publishing, 2000, p. 253

51a J. Carper. *The Food Pharmacy*, New York: Bantam Books, 1988, p. 282, 283

52 Ibid.

52a S.S. Clark, L. Zhoung, D. Filiault, S. Perman, Z. Ren, M. Gould and X. Yang, "Antileukemia effect of perillyl alcohol in Ber/Abl-transformed cells indirectly inhibits signaling through Mek in a Ras- and Raf-independent fashion," Online posting, NCBI, PubMed, Clin Cancer Res. 2003 Oct. 1:9(12):4494-504, Available: http://www.ncbi.nlm.nih.gov/entrez/query.fcgi?cmd=Retrieve&db=pubmed&dopt=Abstract&list_uids=14555523&query_hl=38, p. 1 (accessed 2005, Jul. 1)

53 R. W. Moss, Ph.D. *Cancer Therapy - The Independent Consumer's Guide to Non-Toxic Treatment and Prevention*, New York: Equinox Press, 1992, p. 203

54 Ibid., p. 204

55 Ibid., p. 127

56 "Sheep Sorrel," Cancer and Immunity, Immune Building Agents, DrLam.com. Available at http://www.drlam.com/A3R_brief_in_doc_format/cancer_and_immunity.cfm, p. 4 (accessed 2004, Nov. 21)

57 "Artemisinin," Alternative Cancer Therapies. Available: http://www.mnwelldir.org/docs/cancer1/altthrpy,htm, Wellness Directory of Minnesota™, from Dr. Lam, M.D. at http://www.drlam.com/A3R_brief_in_doc_forat/Artemisinin.cfm, (accessed 2004, Dec. 20)

58 Ibid.

58a Ibid.

59 "Bone Cancer." Herbs2000.com. Available: http://www.herbs2000.com/disorders/cancer_bone.htm p. 2 (accessed 2004, Oct. 17)

59a "Autumn Crocus." Herbs2000.com. Available: http://www.herbs2000.com/herbs/herbs_autumn_crocus.htm, p.1 (accessed 2004, Nov. 22)

60 "Butcher's Broom." Herbs2000.com. Available: http://www.herbs2000.com/herbs/herbs_butchers_broom.htm. p. 2 (accessed 2004, Nov. 22)

61 R. Elkins, M.H. *Cat's Claw (Uno de Gato),* Pleasant Grove, UT: Woodland Publishing, Inc., 1995, p. 24

62 Ibid., p. 24-25

62a "Cat's Claw," "Side Effects and Cautions," Herbs2000.com. Available: http://www.herbs2000.com/herbs/herbs_cats_claw.htm, p. 3 (accessed 2004, Dec. 21)

63 L. Tenney, M.H. *Health Handbook*, Pleasant Grove, UT: Woodland Publishing, 1996, p. 165

64 Blaylock, p. 170-171

[65] Ibid.

[66] "Green tea fights killer disease," FoodNavigator.com, News & Analysis Science & Nutrition, 2/4/2004. Available: http://www.foodnavigator.com/news/newsNG.asp?id=51104, p. 1 (accessed 2004, Oct. 28)

[67] "Cancer Adjuvant Therapy." Life Extension. Available: http://www.lef.org/protocols/prtcl027b.shtml (accessed 2004, October 8) Also see the LEF Protocol Book!

[68] "Liver Cancer." Herbs2000.com, "Liver Cancer - healing with herbs, vitamins and minerals," Available: http://www.herbs2000.com/disorders/cancer_liver.htm p. 1 (accessed 2004, Oct. 17)

[69] G. Null. *The Complete Encyclopedia of Natural Healing.* New York, N.Y. Kensington Publishing Corp. © 2000, 2001, 2002, p. 85. All rights reserved. Reprinted by arrangement with Kensington Publishing Corp., *www.kensingtonbooks.com.*

[70] D. Mowrey, Ph.D, "Rainforest Remedies, Undiscovered Riches, Important Herbs From South American Rainforests," "Lapacho." Available: http://www.raintree.com/article4.htm, p. 1(accessed 2004, Oct. 21) This information is also found in Leslie Taylor's book, *The Healing Power of Rainforest Herbs,* Square One Publishers, Jan. 2005

[71] "Pau d'arco and Cancer," "Herbal Remedies For Immunity," Cancer, Lapacho, Natural Herbal Remedies for Cancer, Holisticonline.com. Available: http://www.holisticonline.com/cancer/Cancer_lapacho_herb-rem.htm, p. 1, 2 (2004, Oct. 21)

[71a] Ibid.

[72] Ibid.

[73] "Doctors Discover Lapacho," Red-Purple Lapacho, (also known as Pau D'Arco or Taheebo). Available: http://www.oralchelation.com/taheebo/lapacho2.htm, p. 1-2 (accessed 2004, Oct 21)

[74] "Let the Buyer Beware," Red-Purple Lapacho, (also known as Pau D'Arco or Taheebo), Available: http://www.oralchelation.com/taheebo/lapacho2.htm, p. 1-4 (accessed 2004, Oct 21)

[75] S. Yeager and the Editors of Prevention Health Books. *Doctor's Book of Food Remedies,* (City, State, n.g.), Rodale, Inc., 1998, p. 497

[76] R.W. Moss, Ph.D. *Cancer Therapy - The Independent Consumer's Guide To Non-Toxic Treatment & Prevention*, New York: Equinox Press, 1992, p. 256

[77] Ibid.

[78] R.W. Moss, Ph.D. *Cancer Therapy - The Independent Consumer's Guide To Non-Toxic Treatment & Prevention*, New York: Equinox Press, 1992, p. 257-258

[79] "Myeloma Cancer," Discount Vitamins & 4herbs Health News. 1 Aug. 2004. Available: http://www.discount-vitamins-herbs.net/health-news30.htm#121. (accessed 1 Aug. 2004) (This article was later re-named "Component of Turmeric Stops the Spread of Myeloma Cancer," and was listed as #118 on the website, rather than #121) Note that the reference discount-vitamin gives for this article at their website is: "Bharti AC, Donato N, Singh S, Aggarwal BB, 'Curcumin (diferuloylmethane) down-regulates the constitutive activation of nuclear factor-kappa B and Ikappa Balpha kinase in human multiple myeloma cells leading to suppression of proliferation and induction of apoptosis.' Blood 2003 Feb 1;101(3):1053-62.)"

[80] "Turmeric Curcuma longa syn. C. domestica," Herbs2000.com. Available: http://www.herbs2000.com/herbs/herbs_turmeric.htm, p. 3 (accessed 2005, Jan 29)

[81] S. Yeager and the Editors of Prevention Health Books. *Doctors Book of FOOD REMEDIES*, Rodale, Inc., 1998, p. 496-497

[82] AC Bharti, N. Donato, S. Singh, BB Aggarwal, "Turmeric May Be Effective Adjunct Cancer Therapy," - Discount Vitamins & Herbs Health News, (from "The annual meeting of the American Association for Cancer Research, San Francisco, California. April 9, 2002.") Available: http://www.discount-vitamins-herbs.net/healthnews30.htm, p. 4 (accessed 2004, Aug. 1)

[82a] "Kiwi Fruit," The World's Healthiest Foods: Feeling Great, George Mateljan Foundation, Whfoods.com. Available: http://www.whfoods.com/genpagephp?tname=foodspice&dbid=41 p. 2-3, (Accessed 2004, dec. 17)

[83] Beta-Sitosterol," DrLam.com. Available: www.drlam.com/opinion/beta-sitosterol.cfm, p. 1-2 (accessed 2004, Oct. 24)

[84] Ibid.

[85] J. F. Balch, M.D. From *The Super Anti-Oxidants: Why They Will Change the Face of Healthcare in the 21st Century,* copyright © 1998, by James F. Balch. Reprinted by the permission of the publisher, M. Evans & Company, New York, p. 147, 279

[86] Ibid., p. 148

[87] Ibid.

[88] Ibid., p. 144-147

[89] "Mullaca," Raintree Nutrition, "Plant Chemicals," TROPICAL PLANT DATABASE. Available: http://www.com/mullaca.htm, p. 1-2 (accessed 2004, Oct. 21) This information is also found in Leslie Taylor's book, *The Healing Power of Rainforest Herbs,* Square One Publishers, Jan. 2005

[90] Ibid., p. 2-3

[90a] Ibid.

[91] Ibid., p. 3

[92] Ibid., p. 4, 5

[92a] "Simarouba," Raintree Nutrition, Simarouba glauca, amara Simarouba - Simaroubaglauca TROPICAL PLANT DATABASE, "Biological Activities And Clinical Research." Available: http://www.rain-tree.com/simarouba.htm 1-3 (Accessed 2004, Oct. 22) This information is also found in Leslie Taylor's book, *The Healing Power of Rainforest Herbs,* Square One Publishers, Jan. 2005

[93] Ibid.

[94] Ibid., p. 4

[95] "Anamu," Raintree Nutrition, ANAMU - Petiveria alliacea - ANAMU, TROPICAL PLANT DATABASE, "Biological Activities And Clinical Research." Available: http://www.rain-tree-com/anamu.htm, p. 1-3 (accessed 2004, Nov. 23) This information is also found in Leslie Taylor's book, *The Healing Power of Rainforest Herbs,* Square One Publishers, Jan. 2005

[96] Ibid.

[97] Ibid., p. 5-6

[97a] "Amargo," Raintree Nutrition, TROPICAL PLANT DATABASE, "Plant chemicals." Available: http://www.rain-tree.com/amargo.htm, p.3 (accessed 2005, May 24) This information is also found in Leslie Taylor's book, *The Healing Power of Rainforest Herbs*, Square One Publishers, Jan. 2005.

[98] "Vassourinha," Raintree Nutrition, Vassourinha - Scoparis dulcis, TROPICAL PLANT DATABASE, "Plant Chemicals." Available: http://www.raintree.com/vassourinha.htm, p. 1-2 (accessed 2004, Oct.21) This information is also found in Leslie Taylor's book, *The Healing Power of Rainforest Herbs,* Square One Publishers, Jan. 2005

[99] "HSI members battle prostate cancer with herbal complex from the Amazon," Health Archives, HSI, Health Sciences Institute, 2/1/2002. Available: http://www.hsibaltimore.com/misc/hsi_0202c.shtml p.2,3 (accessed 2004, Oct. 21)

[100] "Andrographis." Herbs2000.com. Available: http://www.herbs2000.com/herbs/herbs_andrographis.htm, p. 1 (accessed2004, Oct. 17)

[101] Ibid., p. 1, 2

[102] Ibid., p. 2

[103] Ibid.

[104] "Bitter Melon," Liver Cancer - Alternative Treatments, Cancer Tutor™, Alternative Cancer Treatment Information Center. Available: http://www.cancertutor.com/Other/Liver_Cancer.Html (accessed 2004, Oct. 21)

[104a] "Bitter Melon." Available: http://www.herbs2000.com/herbs/herbs_bitter_melon.htm (accessed 2004, Oct. 21)

[105] D. B. Mowrey, Ph.D. *The Scientific Validation of Herbal Medicine. How To Remedy and Prevent Disease With Herbs, Vitamins, Minerals, And Other Nutrients,* New York: McGraw-Hill Companies, 1986, p. 61, reproduced with permission of McGraw-Hill Companies

[105a] "Dyer's Woad (Isatis Indigotica Fortune)," Prostate Problem - Enlargement of the Prostate-Prostate Cancer - Bladder Infection...Available: http://www.nutrition2000.com/prostatepchope.htm, p. 3 (accessed 2004, Dec. 3)

[106] "Bone Cancer." Herbs2000.com. Available: http://www.herbs2000.com/disorders/cancer_bone.htm, p. 2 (accessed 2004, Oct. 17)

[107] R. Dubin. From *Miracle Food Cures From The Bible* by Reese Dubin, copyright © 1999 by Prentice Hall. Used by permission of Avery Publishing, an imprint of Penguin Group (USA) Inc., p 160

[107a] R. W. Moss, Ph.D, "Intriguing New Anticancer Compound From East Europe," From The Cancer Chronicles #27, © June 1995 by Ralph W. Moss, Ph.D. Available: http://www.ralph moss.com/ukrain.html, p. 1, 2 (accessed 2004, Oct 13)

[107b] Ibid.

[108] Ibid.

[109] "Xi Shu," Herbs2000.com. Available: http://www.herbs2000.com/herbs/herbs_xi_shu.htm, p.2 (accessed 2004, Oct. 28)

[110] M. Kennedy Salaman. *All Your Health Questions Answered Naturally*, MKS, Inc., 1998, p. 653-654

[111] Blaylock, p. 242

Chapter 8

[1] B. Berkson, M.D., Ph.D. From *The Alpha Lipoic Acid Breakthrough,* copyright © 1998 by Burt Berkson. Used by permission of Prima Publishing, a division of Random House, Inc., p. 70

[2] J. Carper. *Miracle Cures*, New York: Harper Collins, 1997, p. 136-137

2aIbid., p. 137, 138

2bIbid.

3 Ibid., p. 137,138

4 Ibid., p. 138

5 Carper, p. 139

6 Ibid., p. 139

7 Ibid., p. 140

8 J. A. Duke, Ph.D., with Michael Castleman, *The Green Pharmacy anti-aging Prescriptions,* (City, State, n.g.) Rodale, 2001, p. 187

9 Ibid.

10 R. L. Blaylock, M.D. *Natural Strategies For Cancer Patients*, New York: Twin Streams Kensington Publishing Corp., © 2003, p.171. All rights reserved. Reprinted by arrangement with Kensington Publishing Corp. www.kensingtonbooks.com

11 M. Stengler, N.D. *The Natural Physician's Healing Therapies* by Mark Stengler, N.D. copyright © 2001 by Mark Stengler. Used by permission of Avery Publishing, an imprint of Penguin Group (USA) Inc., p. 330-331

12 Ibid., p. 331

13 Ibid.

14 Ibid., p. 333

15 J. F. Balch, M.D. From *The Super Anti-Oxidants*: *Why They Will Change the Face of Healthcare in the 21st Century,* copyright © 1998, by James F. Balch. Reprinted with permission of the publisher, M. Evans & Company, p. 52

16 Ibid.

17 Ibid.

18 *The Healing Power of Vitamins, Minerals, and Herbs*, Pleasantville, N.Y., The Reader's Digest Assoc., Inc., 1999, 2000, p. 331. Quoted with permission of Global Books & Home Entertainment, The Reader's Digest Association, Inc.

19 Ibid.

20 Ibid.

21 Ibid.

22 "Milk Thistle (Carduus marianus or Silybum marianum)," Dietary Supplement Information Bureau™, nhi. Available: http://content.nhiondemand.com/dse/consumer/monoAll-style.asp?objID=100072&ctype=...p. 1 (accessed 2005, Jan 13)

23 M. Kennedy Salaman. *All Your Health Questions Answered Naturally.* (City, State, n.g.) MKS, Inc., 1998, p. 669

24 J. A. Duke, Ph.D., with Michael Castleman, *The Green Pharmacy anti-aging Prescriptions,* Rodale, 2001, p. 186

24a Lloyd Wright. "Milk Thistle Ancient Blessing," Triumph Over Hepatitis C website. Available: http://www.hepatitisCfree.com/milk_thistle_book.htm (accessed 2005, Apr. 8)

24b Carper., p. 140-141

25 Salaman, p. 669

26 "Abstracts of Published Studies Indicating Aloe's Potential Efficacy Against Cancer," Life Extension. LE Magazine April 2002, Available: http://www.lef.org/magazine/mag2002report_clinic_04.html (accessed 2004, Sept. 27), p 1. Also see the LEF Protocol Book!

[27] B. Berkson, M.D., Ph.D. From *The Alpha Lipoic Acid Breakthrough*, copyright © 1998 by Burt Berkson. Used by permission of Prima Publishing, a division of Random House, Inc., p. 11, 14

[28] Berkson, p. 102, 103

[28a] "Kiwi Fruit," The World's Healthiest Foods: Feeling Great, George Mateljan Foundation, Whfoods.com. Available: http://www.whfoods.com/genpagephp?tname=foodspice&dbid=41 p. 2-3, (Accessed 2004, dec. 17)

[29] "Liver Cancer." Herbs2000.com. Available: http://www.herbs2000.com/disorders/cancer_liver.htm, (accessed 2004, Oct. 17)

[30] J. Heinerman. *Heinerman's Encyclopedia of Healing Juices*, New York: Reward Books, 1994 by Penguin Putnam, Inc, p. 36-39

[31] S. Yeager & the Editors of Prevention Health Books, *Doctor's Book of Food Remedies,* (City, State, n.g.) Rodale, Inc., 1998, p. 429

[32] "Liver Cancer." Herbs2000.com. Available: http://www.herbs2000.com/disorders/cancer_liver. htm, p. 1-2 (accessed 2004, Oct. 17)

[32a] K. Lockwood, S. Moesgaard, and K. Folkers, "Partial and complete regression of breast cancer in patients in relation to dosage of coenzyme Q10," PubMed, NCBI, Biochem Biophys Res Commun. 1994 Mar 30; 199(3):1504-8, p. 1. Available: http://www.ncbi.nlm.nih.gov/entrez/query.fcgi?cmd=Retriev&db=pubmed&dopt=Abstract&list_uids=7808519&query_hl=32 (accessed 2005, Jul. 1)

[33] K. Lockwood, S. Moesgaard, T. Yamamoto, and K. Folkers, "Progress on therapy of breast cancer with vitamin Q10 and the regression of metastases," PubMed, NCBI, Biochem Biophys Res Commun. 1995 Jul 6; 212(1):172-7, p. 1. Available: http://www.ncbi.nlm.nih.gov/entrez/query.fcgi?cmd=Retrieve&db=pubmed&dopt=Abstract&list_uids=7612003&query_hl=30 (accessed 2004, Nov. 25)

[33a] J. G. Connor, M.Ac., LAc "Cancer Prevention and Diet." "Herbs and Nutritional Support." Available: http://www.compassionate/acupuncture.com/cancer.htm (accessed 2005, May 21)

[34] M. N. Antol. *Healing Teas*, Avery, 1996, p. 95

[35] "Liver Cancer," Herbs2000.com, Available: http://www.herbs2000.com/disorders/cancer_liver.htm, p. 1 (accessed 2004, Oct. 17)

[36] Ibid.

[37] E. L. Mindell, R.Ph. with V. L. Hopkins. *Dr. Earl Mindell's What You Should Know About The Super Antioxidant Miracle,* New York: the McGraw-Hill Companies, 1996, p. 50. Reproduced with permission of the McGraw-Hill Companies.

[38] Ibid., p. 53-54

[39] Ibid., p. 52-53

[40] "Liver Cancer." Herbs2000.com. Available: http://www.herbs2000.com/disorders/cancer_liver.htm, p. 2 (accessed 2004, Oct. 17)

[41] Ibid.

[42] Ibid.

[43] C. M. Hawken. *Green Foods, "Phyto-Foods" for Super Health,* Pleasant Grove, UT: Woodland Publishing, 1998, p 13-14

[44] Ibid., p. 15-16

[45] Dr. J. Mercola, "Chlorella: A Natural Wonder Food - Anti Cancer Properties of Chlorella," "How Much Chlorella Should a Person Take If They Have Cancer?" Available: http://www.mercola.com/chlorella/anti_cancer.htm, p. 2 (accessed 2004, Nov. 25)

[46] A. Wigmore. *The Wheatgrass Book,* 1985 (City, State, n.g.) Avery Publishing and The Hippocrates Health Institute, p.10

[47] Ibid., p. 22

[48] M. Kennedy Salaman. *All Your Health Questions Answered Naturally.* (City, State, n.g.) MKS, Inc., 1998, p. 188

[49] "Question of the Week," Dr. Michael T. Murray online of the *Question of the Week,* Available: http://www.doctormurray.com/Qarchive/ip6.htm, p. 1 (accessed 2004, Nov. 25)

[50] Heinerman, p. 258-259

[51] Yeager, p. 392-393

[52] Ibid.

[53] Ibid.

[54] Ibid., p. 393

[55] S. Lieberman, Ph.D., and Ken Babal, C.N. *Maitake Mushroom AND D-Fraction,* Pleasant Grove, UT: Woodland Publishing, 2001, p. 13

[56] Ibid., p. 12

[57] "Maitake," Herbs2000.com. Available: http://www.herbs2000.com/herbs/herbs_maitake.htm, p. 1 (accessed 2004, Nov. 22)

[58] "Liver Cancer," Herbs2000.com. Available: http://www.herbs2000.com/disorders/cancer_liver.htm, p.2 (accessed 2004, Oct. 17)

[59] Ibid., p. 2

[60] "Agaricus," Wellness Directory of Minnesota™, Alternative Cancer Therapies. Available: http://www.mnwelldir.org/docs/cancer1/altthrpy.htm, p. 1,2,3 (accessed 2004, Oct. 8)

[61] R. H. Liu, Cornell News "Onions anti-cancer effects," Oct. 7, 2004, contact Susan S. Lang, Available: http://www.news.cornell.edu/releases/Oct04/onions.cancer.ssl.html (accessed 2004, Dec. 29)

[61a] Ibid.

[62] Salaman, p. 667

[63] Ibid.

[64] Ibid., p. 667-669

[64a] "Phyllanthus," Herbs2000.com. Available: http://www.herbs2000.com/herbs/herbs_phyl-lanthus.htm, p. 1 (accessed 2005, April 9)

[64b] Ibid.

[65] "Liver Cancer." Herbs2000.com. Available: http://www.herbs2000.com/disorders/cancer_liver.htm, p.3 (accessed 2004, Oct. 17)

[66] J. F. Balch, M.D. From *The Super Anti-Oxidants: Why They Will Change The Face of Healthcare in the 21st Century,* copyright © 1998, by James F. Balch. Reprinted by the permission of the publisher, M. Evans & Company, New York, p. 210, 213

[66a] H. Winter Griffith, M.D. *Vitamins Herbs, Minerals & Supplements The Complete Guide,* Revised Edition, (City, State, n.g.) Perseus (Fisher Books), 1988, 1998, p. 108

[67] M. Kennedy Salaman. *Nutrition: The Cancer Answer II,* Menlo Park, CA: Statford Publishing, MKS, Inc.,2002, p. 349

[68] "Liver Cancer." Herbs2000.com. Available: http://www.herbs2000.com/disorders/cancer_liver.htm, p. 2 (2004, Oct. 17)

[68a] Ibid.

[69] N. Zentaro, "With Tian Xian Liquid, I shall Never Surrender to Liver Cancer," "Liver Cancer: Stories of Liver Cancer Survivors, Tian Xian," Nishimura Zentaro. Available: http://www.tianxian.com/testimonials/liver_cancer.asp?u=MV-A..., p.1 (accessed 2004, Oct. 17)

69a Ibid.

70 Serena Gordon, "Vitamin K Might Prevent Liver Cancer - Wards disease off in women
with cirrhosis," HealthDay.com. Available:
http://www.healthday.com/view.cfm?id=520187, p. 1-2, (accessed 2004, Nov. 25)

70a Ibid.

70b "Kiwi Fruit," The World's Healthiest Foods: Feeling Great, George Mateljan
Foundation, Whfoods.com. Available:
http://www.whfoods.com/genpagephp?tname=
foodspice&dbid=41 p. 2-3, (Accessed 2004, dec. 17)

71 R.W. Moss, Ph.D. *Cancer Therapy The Independent Consumer's Guide to Non-Toxic Treatment and Prevention,* Equinox Press, 1992, p. 142

72 "Liver Cancer," p. 2

72a "Bupleurum," Herbs2000.com. Available: http://www.herbs2000.com/herbs
/herbs_bupleurum.htm, p.1 (accessed 2004, Oct. 25)

73 Ibid.

74 "Bone Cancer." Herbs2000.com. Available: http://www.herbs2000.com/disorders/
cancer_bone.htm, p. 2 (Accessed 2004, Dec. 18)

74a J. A. Duke, Ph.D., with Michael Castleman, *The Green Pharmacy Anti-aging
Prescriptions,* Rodale, 2001, Ibid., p. 191

75 Ibid., p. 188-189

76 M. N. Antol. *Healing Teas,* 1996, (City, State, n.g.) Avery, p. 122-123

77 Duke et. al, p. 189

78 Ibid.

79 "Macela," Raintree Nutrition, *TROPICAL PLANT DATABASE.* Available:
http://www.rain-
tree.com/macela.htm, "Biological Activities and Clinical Research," p. 1-3
(accessed
2004, October 22) Per Raintree website, part of the information on this herb was
from *The Healing Power of Rainforest Herbs* by Leslie Taylor, copyrighted ©
2004.

79a Ibid., p. 2, 3

80 Ibid.

81 Duke, et al., p. 191

82 "Herbs," Cancer - Breast, *Your Health Your Choice,* Alternative Health Supplies
(Australia) Available: http://www.alternativehealth.com.au/Articles/breast.htm
p. 7 (accessed 2004, Oct. 24)

83 Duke, et al., p. 189

84 "Schisandra Berries More Than a Liver Aid," from The January 2001 issue of
Nutrition Science News, NewHope.com, "Protects The Liver." Available:
http://www.newhope.com/nutritionsciencenews/NSN_backs/Jan_01/schisan
dra.cfm, p. 1-2 (accessed 2004, Nov. 25) Copyright © 2004, Penton Media, Inc.

84a "Liver Cancer," p. 2

85 Ibid.

86 Ibid., p. 2

87 Duke et. al, p. 190-191

88 Mark Stengler, N.D., p 445 *The Natural Physician's Healing Therapies* by Mark
Stengler, N.D copyright © 2001 by Mark Stengler. Used by permission of Avery
Publishing, an imprint of Penguin Group (USA) Inc.

[89] Duke et al., p. 190-191

[90] "Turmeric *Curcuma longa syn. C. domestica*," Herbs2000.com. Available: http://www.herbs.2000.com/herbs/herbs_turmeric.htm, p. 3 (accessed 2005, Feb. 11)

Chapter 9

[1] M. Howell and S. Goodman, Ph.D. "An Interview with Udo Erasmus," <u>Positive Health</u> Magazine, Integrated magazine for the 21st century, Issue 12 - May/June 1996. Available: http://www.positivehealth.com/articles.asp?I=818 (accessed 2005, Jan. 23)

[2] "Cancer Types," "Lung Cancer." Available: http://www.cancer-healing.com/cancer_type.php (accessed 2005, May 3)

[2a] "Lung Cancer," Herbs2000.com. Available: http://www.herbs2000.com/disorders/cancer_lung.htm, p 3 (accessed 2004, Oct. 17)

[3] J. Heinerman, *Heinerman's Encyclopedia of Healing Juices*, New York: Reward Books, Penguin Putnam, Inc., 1994, p. 37

[4] J. Heinerman. *Heinerman's New Encyclopedia of Fruits & Vegetables,* New York: Reward Books, Penguin Putnam, Inc., 1995, p. 39

[5] R. W. Moss, Ph.D. *Cancer Therapy The Independent Consumer's Guide to Non-Toxic Treatment & Prevention,* New York: Equinox Press, 1992, p. 236

[6] Ibid.

[7] "Caveats: Conflicting Reports on Vitamins and Minerals," June Russell's Health Facts, "Vitamins - Antioxidants: Beta-carotene and Vitamins A and E -" Available: http://www.jrussellshealth.com/caveats_vit_min.html, p. 1 (accessed 2005, Jan 14)

[8] Ibid., p. 1

[9] R. W. Moss, Ph.D. *Antioxidants against Cancer*, State College, PA, 2000, 2002, p. 32, 33

[10] Ibid.

[11] "Vitamin A and Carotenoids," Facts About Dietary Supplements, National Institutes of Health Office of Dietary Supplements. Available: http://ods.od.nih.gov/factsheets/cc/vita.html, p. 18 (accessed 2005, Jan 14)

[12] Ibid., p. 75

[13] Ibid.

[14] "Lung Cancer," Herbs2000.com. Available: http://www.herbs2000.com/disorders/cancer_lung.htm, p. 3 (accessed 2004, Oct. 17)

[15] "What is the health risk of too many carotenoids?" Facts About Dietary Supplements, "Vitamin A and Carotenoids," National Institutes of Health, Office of Dietary Supplements, Available: http://ods.od.nih.gov/factsheets/cc/vita.html, p. 17 (accessed 2005, Jan 14)

[15a] C.M. Hawken. *Green Foods - "Phyto-Foods" for Super Health,* Pleasant Grove, UT: Wood-land Publishing, 1998, p. 9

[16] S. Yeager & the Editors of Prevention Health Books. *Doctors Book of FOOD REMEDIES,* (City, State, n.g.) Rodale, Inc., p. 429

[16a] Ibid.

[16b] R. W. Moss. *Antioxidants against Cancer*, State College, PA: Equinox Press, Inc., 2000, 2002, p. 69

[17] Ibid.

[17a] "Congestive Heart Failure," "Co-Enzyme Q10. This is very important." Available: http://www.doctoryourself.com/congestive.html (accessed 2005, Mar. 21) Copyright 2003 and prior years by Andrew W. Saul. From the book *DOCTOR YOURSELF*, available from Andrew Saul, Number 8 Van Buren Street, Holley, New York 14470 USA

[17b] Stephen T. Sinatra, M.D., F.A.C.C. *The Coenzyme Q10 Phenomenon,* New York: the McGraw-Hill Companies, 1998, p. 82-84. Reproduced with permission of the McGraw-Hill Companies

[18] Ibid.

[18a] Ibid., p. 5, 6

[19] Ibid.

[20] Sinatra, p. 6, 7

[21] Ibid., p. 66, 67

[22] S.T. Sinatra, M.D., F.A.C.C. *Coenzyme Q10 and the Heart,* New York: the McGraw-Hill Companies,1999, p. 11. Reproduced with permission of the McGraw Hill Companies

[23] James F. Balch, M.D. From *The Super Antioxidants: Why They Will Change The Face of Healthcare in the 21st Century,* copyright © 1998, by James F. Balch. Reprinted by permission of the publisher, M. Evans & Company, New York, p. 140-141

[24] R. W. Moss, Ph.D. *Cancer Therapy The Independent Consumer's Guide to Non-Toxic Treatment & Prevention,* New York: Equinox Press, 1992, p. 305

[24a] R. W. Moss, Ph,.D. *Antioxidants against Cancer,* New York: Equinox Press, Inc., 2000, 2002, p. 73,74

[25] Ibid.

[26] J. A. Duke, Ph.D. with M. Castleman. *The Green Pharmacy anti-aging Prescriptions,* (City, State, n.g.) Rodale, Inc., 2001, p. 94

[27] Ibid.

[28] R. W. Moss, Ph.D. *Cancer Therapy: The Independent Consumer's Guide to Non-Toxic Treatment & Prevention,* New York: Equinox Press, 1992, p. 423-426

[29] R. W. Moss, Ph.D. *Antioxidants against Cancer,* State College, PA: Equinox Press, Inc., 2000, 2002, p 36-38

[30] James F. Balch, M.D. From *The Super Antioxidants: Why They Will Change The Face Of Healthcare In The 21st Century,* copyright © 1998, by James F. Balch. Reprinted by the permission of the publisher, M. Evans & Company, New York, p. 132-133

[30a] Hoffer, Abram, M.D., Ph.D., F.R.C.P. (C) "Hoffer's Home Page – Orthomolecular Treatment of Cancer." Available: http://www.islandnet.com/~hoffer/ p. 1-2 (accessed 2005, May 28)

[30b] Ibid., p. 11

[31] Balch, p. 93-95

[32] B. Berkson, M.D., Ph.D., From *The Alpha Lipoic Acid Breakthrough* copyright © 1998 by Burt Berkson. Used by permission of Prima Publishing, a division of Random House, Inc., p. 18

[33] *Healing with Vitamins,* from the Editors of Prevention Health Books, (City, State, n.g.) Rodale, Inc., 1996, p. 136-137

[34] E. Cheraskin, M.D., D.M.D. *Vitamin C Who Needs It?* Birmingham, AL: Arlington Press & Co., 1993, p.159

[35] E. Mindell, R.Ph, with Virginia Hopkins. *Dr. Earl Mindell's What You Should Know About The Super Antioxidant Miracle,* New York, the McGraw-Hill Companies, 1996, p. 39. Reproduced with permission of the McGraw-Hill Companies.

[36] Ibid., p. 40-41

[37] James F Balch, M.D. From *The Super Antioxidants: Why They Will Change The Face of Healthcare in the 21st Century,* copyright © 1998, by James F. Balch. Reprinted by the permission of the publisher, M. Evans & Company, New York, p. 95

38 Ibid., p. 96

38a Ibid., p. 98-100

39 Ibid.

39a "Comparison of Glutathione in Fresh vs. Cooked Foods (in milligrams per 3 ½ oz (100 g) serving)." Available from nutrition advisor website, President, Dr. Steven P. Petrosino, Ph.D. http://www.nutritionadvisor.com/glutathione_foods.php (accessed 2005, May 6) Reprinted with their permission.

40 Ibid.

41 Ibid.

41a R. W. Moss, Ph.D. *Antioxidants against Cancer*, State College PA: Equinox Press, Inc., 2000 p. 76-78

42 Ibid.

43 Moss, *Antioxidants against Cancer*, p. 78

44 H. W. Griffith, M.D. *VITAMINS Herbs, Minerals & Supplements The Complete Guide*, (City, State n.g.) Perseus (Fisher Books), 1988, 1998, p. 108

45 "Lung Cancer," Herbs2000.com. Available: http://www.herbs2000.com, p. 3 (accessed 2004, Oct. 17)

46 "Emanuel Revici," The Cancer Tutor™. Available: http://www.cancertutor.com/Other/Big_List.htm, p. 16 (accessed 2004, Oct. 17)

47 "Melatonin: Supplements, What Works," Healthyroads.com. Available: http://www.healthy-roads.com/mylibrary/data/pelletier/chapter3/p_melatonin.asp, p. 1 (accessed 2004, Nov. 30)

48 Ibid.

49 "Melatonin," Melatonin for Sleep Disorders and a powerful antioxidant. Available: http://www.health-n-energy.com/melatin.htm, p. 2 (accessed 2004, Nov. 30)

50 Ibid.

51 Moss, *Antioxidants against Cancer*, p. 89, 91

51a "Melatonin: Supplements, What Works," www.healthyroads.com, p. 2

52 Ibid.

52a "Cancer-Fighter Perillyl Alcohol Found in Tart Cherries." "Independent Lab Verifies Cancer-Fighting Agents in Cherries." Available: http://www.flavonoidsciences.com/research/c3.htm, (accessed 2005, May 27)

53 "Lung Cancer." Herbs2000.com. Available: http://www.herbs2000.com/disorders/cancer_lung.htm p. 1 (accessed 2004, Oct. 17)

53a "Aspilia," Herbs2000.com. Available: http://www.herbs2000.com/herbs/herbs_aspilia.htm, p. 1-2, (accessed 2004, Oct. 16)

54 Moss, *Cancer Therapy The Independent Consumer's Guide to Non-Toxic Treatment & Prevention,* p. 130

55 Ibid., p. 130,131

56 "Lung Cancer," Herbs2000.com. Available: http://www.herbs2000.com/disorders/cancer_lung.htm p. 1-2 (accessed 2004, Oct. 17)

57 Ibid., p. 2

58 "Cat's Claw," "Side Effects and Cautions." Available: http://www.herbs2000.com/herbs/herbs_cats_claw.htm, p. 3 (accessed 2005, Jan 11)

59 "Lung Cancer," Herbs2000.com., p. 2

59a "Espinheira Santa," Herbs2000.com. Available: http://www.herbs2000.com/herbs/herbs_espinheirasanta.htm, p. 1-2 (accessed 2004, Oct. 16)

[60] Ibid.

[61] Moss, p. 158

[61a] Ibid.

[62] Ibid., p. 158, 159

[63] "Lung Cancer," Herbs2000.com, p. 3

[64] Ibid., p. 2

[65] "Parsley," Herbs2000.com. Available: http://www.herbs2000.com/herbs/herbs_parsley.htm, p. 2 (accessed 2004, Oct.28)

[66] "Psoralea," Herbs2000.com. Available: http://www.herbs2000.com/herbs/herbs_psoralea.htm, p. 1-2 (accessed 2004, Nov. 30)

[67] "Lung Cancer," herbs2000.com, p. 3

[67a] "Rhodiola Rosea," New Page 5. Available: http://www.planetherbs.com/articles/rhodiolia%20rosea.htm, p. 1,2 (accessed 2004, Oct. 21)

[68] Ibid.

[69] Moss, p. 256

[70] J. Carper. *The Food Pharmacy*, New York: Bantam Books, 1988, p. 266

[71] Ibid.

[72] "Tian Xian," Cancer Alternative Treatments - Tian Xian Liquid. Available: http://www.tianxian.com/p. 1 (accessed 2004, Oct. 17)

[73] Ibid.

[74] "Curcumin /Turmeric." Available at http://www.cancertutor.com?Other/Big_List.htm, p. 13, (accessed 2004, Nov. 30)

[75] "Lung Cancer," Herbs2000.com. Available: http://www.herbs2000.com/disorders/cancer_lung.htm, p. 2 (accessed 2004, Oct. 17)

[75a] Mark Stengler, N.D., p. 445 *The Natural Physician's Healing Therapies* by Mark Stengler, N.D copyright © 2001 by Mark Stengler. Used by permission of Avery Publishing, an imprint of Penguin Group (USA) Inc.

[76] C. Borek, Ph.D., *Beta Glucan Boosts Immunity*, Beta Glucan vs. Cancer and Beta Glucan the Supplement. Available: http://www.newhope.com/nutritionsciencenews/NSN_backs/Jan_01/betaglucan.cfm, p. 2 (accessed 2004, Oct 17) (Dr. Borek "is a research professor at Tufts University School of Medicine in Boston"), Copyright © 2004, Penton Media, Inc.

[77] Ibid.

[77a] "Oat Beta Glucan," Effective Natural Cancer Treatments. Available: http://www.cancer-treatments.net/cancer.html, p. 1 (Accessed 2004, Dec. 1)

[78] R. Elkins, M.H. *D-Glucarate™, Powerful Protector Against Breast and Prostate Cancers,* Woodland Publishing, Inc., 1999, p. 6

[79] Ibid., p. 6, 7, 16

[80] Ibid., p. 10

[81] Elkins, p. 11

[82] Ibid., p. 14, 16

[83] Ibid., p. 18

[84] R. Elkins, M.H. *Noni (Morinda citrifolia) Prize Herb of Tahiti and the South Pacific,* Pleasant Grove, UT: Woodland Publishing, 1997, p. 20-22

[85] "The Effect of Ukrain on Cancer." Available: http://www.ukrin.com/standardtexte/Standard brief_2_eng.htm, p. 1 (accessed 2004, Oct. 13)

[86] Ibid., p. 2

[87] Ibid., p. 2, 3

[88] "Lung Cancer," herbs2000.com, Available:
http://www.herbs2000.com/disorders/cancer_lung.htm, p. 2 (accessed 2004, Oct. 17)

[89] D. Colbert, M.D. *Walking in Divine Health,* Lake Mary, FL: Siloam, 1999, p. 28-29

[90] M. K. Salaman. *Nutrition: The Cancer Answer II,* Menlo Park, CA: Statford Publishing, 1995, p. 257

[91] Ibid.

Chapter 10

[1] C. Gupta, "The FDA Versus Folic Acid - Share The Wealth." "It's time to revolt." Available:
http://www.newmediaexplorer.org/chris/2003/07/14/the_fda_versus_folic_acid.htm, p. 1 (accessed 2004, Nov. 20)

[2] J. Challem. *All About Carotenoids Beta-Carotene, Lutein & Lycopene,* Garden City Park, N.Y: Avery Publishing Group, 1999, p. 24, quotes reprinted with Mr. Challem's permission.

[3] R. W. Moss, Ph.D. *Antioxidants against Cancer*, Equinox Press, Inc., 2000, p. 25

[4] Ibid., p. 32

[5] Ibid., p. 29

[6] Health Archives, HSI, Health Sciences Institute 2/1/2002, "HSI members battle prostate cancer with herbal complex from the Amazon." Available:
http://www.hsibaltimore.com/misc/hsi_0202 _c.shtml, p. 3 (accessed 2004, Oct. 21)

[7] "Brazilian Peppertree," TROPICAL PLANT DATABASE, Raintree Nutrition. Available:
http://www.rain-tree.com/peppertree.htm, p. 1, 5 (accessed 2004, Dec. 1) This information is also found in Leslie Taylor's book, *The Healing Power of Rainforest Herbs,* Square One Publishers, Jan. 2005

[8] R. W. Moss, Ph.D. *Cancer Therapy The Independent Consumer's Guide To non-Toxic Treatment & Prevention,* New York: Equinox Press, 1992, p. 305

[9] J. F. Balch, M.D. From *The Super Anti-Oxidants*: *Why They Will Change the Face of Healthcare in the 21st Century*, copyright © 1998, by James F. Balch. Reprinted by the permission of the publisher, M. Evans & Company, New York, p. 162-163

[10] Ibid.

[10a] Ibid.

[11] "Cancer Adjuvant Therapy," LifeExtension website. Available: http://www.lef.org/protocols/prtcl-027b shtml (accessed 2004, Oct. 8) Also see the LEF Protocol Book!

[11a] Ibid.

[12] "Green tea could prevent cancer of the esophagus," FoodNavigator.com, News & Analysis Science & Nutrition25/05/2004. Available: http://www.foodnavigator.com/news/news-NG.asp?id=52331, p. 1 (accessed 2004, Oct. 28)

[12a] Ibid.

[12b] Ibid.

[13] Moss, *Antioxidants against Cancer*, p. 37

[13a] Moss, *Cancer Therapy: The Independent Consumer's Guide to Non-Toxic Treatment & Prevention,* p. 107

[14] Ibid.

[15] "Mullaca," Raintree Nutrition, TROPICAL PLANT DATABASE, "Plant Chemicals." Available: http://www.rain-tree.com/mullaca.htm, p. 1-2 (accessed 2004, Oct. 21) This information is also found in Leslie Taylor's book, *The Healing Power of Rainforest Herbs,* Square One Publishers, Jan. 2005

[16] "Mullaca," Raintree Nutrition, p. 2, 3

[17] Ibid., p. 4, 5

[18] J. Carper. *The Food Pharmacy.* New York: Bantam Books, 1088, 1989, p. 249, 250

[18a] R. W. Moss, Ph.D. *Cancer Therapy The Independent Consumer's Guide To Non-Toxic Treatment & Prevention,* New York: Equinox Press, 1992, p. 41-42

[19] Ibid.

[20] R.W. Moss, Ph.D. *Antioxidants against Cancer,* State College, PA: Equinox Press, 2002, p. 83

[21] Ibid.

[22] Ibid.

[22a] J. Schwartz, G.Shklar, S. Reid, D. Trickler, "Prevention of experimental oral cancer by extracts of Spirulina-Dunaliella algae," Nutr Cancer. 1988;11(2):127-34, Department of Oral Medicine and Oral Patholody, Harvard School of Dental Medicine Boston, Available: http://www.ncbi.nlm.nih.gov/entrez/query.fcgi?cmd=Retriev&db=pubmed&dopt=Ab stract &list_uids=3129701&query_hl=35, p. 1(accessed 2005, Jul. 1)

[23] Simarouba," Raintree Nutrition, TROPICAL PLANT DATABASE, "Biological Activities and Clinical Research." Available: http://www.rain-tree.com/simarouba.htm, p. 1-5 (accessed 2004, Oct. 22) This information is also found in Leslie Taylor's book, *The Healing Power of Rainforest Herbs,* Square One Publishers, Jan. 2005

[24] Ibid.

[25] "Transfer Factor." Available: http://www.cancertutor.com/Other/Big_List.htm, p. 1 (accessed 2004, Dec. 1)

[26] Ibid.

[27] "1999 Independent Study by Institute of Longevity Medicine." Available: http://www.realsuccess4life.com/cgi-bin/home.cgi?6038864, p. 1 "Professional Networkers, Hutchinson, KS," (accessed 2004, Dec. 1)

[28] J.J. Vyas and V.K. Jain, "Ukrain Treatment in Carcinoma of the Esophagus (Case Report)," Available: http://www.ukrin.com/Ukrainbook1/195final.htm, p. 1 (accessed2004, Oct. 13)

[29] Ibid., p. 2

[30] Ibid.

[31] Vyas et al, p. 2

[32] Ibid., p. 2

[33] Moss, *Cancer Therapy,* p. 54

Chapter 11

[1] M. Kennedy Salaman. *All Your Health Questions Answered Naturally,* (City, State, n.g.) MKS, Inc., 1998, p. 204

[2] G. Null, Ph.D. *The Complete Encyclopedia of Natural Healing*, New York, N.Y: Kensington Publishing Corp. 3rd edition, © 2000, 2001, 2002, p. 475-476. All rights reserved. Reprinted by arrangement with Kensington Publishing Corp., *www.kens-ingtonbooks.com.*

[3] R. W. Moss, Ph.D. *Cancer Therapy - The Independent Consumer's Guide To Non-Toxic Treatment & Prevention*, New York: Equinox Press, 1992, p. 187-188

[4] Ibid.

[5] Ibid., p. 187-188

[6] Null, p. 473

[7] Ibid.

[8] Ibid.

[9] A. Hoffer, M.D., FRCP(C), with Linus Pauling, Ph.D. *Healing Cancer – Complementary Vitamin & Drug Treatments,* Toronto, Ontario, Canada: CCNM Press, 2004, p. 93

[10] A. Hoffer, Ph.D., M.D., Ph.D., FRCP(C). "Hoffer's Home Page – Orthomolecular Treatment of Cancer," Available: http://www.islandnet.com/~hoffer/ p. 3 (accessed 2005, May 28)

[11] Ibid.

[12] D-limonene," and "Perillyl Alcohol." Available: http://www.cancertutor.com/Other/Big_List.htm, p. 15, 30 (accessed 2004, Oct. 17)

[13] Ibid.

[14] J.Carper. *The Food Pharmacy*, New York: Bantam Books, 1988, 1989, p. 215

[15] Ibid.

[16] S. T. Sinatra, M.D., F.A.C.C. *The Coenzyme Q10 Phenomenon*, New York: the McGraw-Hill Companies, 1998 p. 15. Reproduced with permission of the McGraw-Hill Companies

[17] Ibid., p. 83-85

[18] Carper, *The Food Pharmacy*, p. 189

[19] Ibid.

[20] "FAQs" ExToxNet Recommendation 14 Background. Available: http://extoxnet.orst.edu/faqs/dietcancer/web14/fourteenphyto.html, p. 2 (accessed 2004, Oct. 24)

[21] M. K. Salaman. *All Your Health Questions Answered Naturally,* (City, State, n.g.) MKS, Inc., p. 207

[22] Ibid.

[23] Ibid.

[24] R. L. Blaylock, M.D. *Natural Strategies For Cancer Patients,* New York: Twin Streams, Kensington Publishing Corp., © 2003, p. 2. All rights reserved. Reprinted by arrangement with Kensington Publishing Corp., www.kensingtonbooks.com

[25] Ibid.

[26] Ibid.

[27] Salaman, *All Your Health Questions Answered Naturally*, p. 206

[28] Ibid.

[29] Ibid., p. 205

[30] Ibid.

[31] Ibid., p. 206

[32] "Light Therapy Tackles Cancer." Available: http://news.bbc.co.uk/1/hi/health/1871474.htm (accessed 2005, May 31) Reprinted with permission from BBC News at bbcnews.com © BBC

[33] Ibid.

[34] Ibid.

[35] "Light Therapy Tackles Cancer," bbbnews.com

[36] Ibid.

[37] Ibid.

[38] R. Sahelian, M.D. *Saw Palmetto Nature's Prostate Healer,* New York: Kensington Books, Kensington Publishing Corp., 1998, p. 96, also see www.raysahelian.com/saw.html © 1998, All rights reserved. Reprinted by arrangement with Kensington Publishing Corp., www.Kensingtonbooks.com

[38a] Mark Stengler, N.D., p 445 *The Natural Physician's Healing Therapies* by Mark Stengler, N.D copyright © 2001 by Mark Stengler. Used by permission of Avery Publishing, an imprint of Penguin Group (USA) Inc.

[39] Salaman, *All Your Health Questions Answered Naturally,* p. 206

[40] "Pancreatic Cancer: Story of Maribel C. Lim," Cancer Central, (August 2003), Manila, Philippines, Available: http://www.cancer-central.com/pancreas-cancer/pancreas-cancer-3.Htm, p. 1, 2 (accessed 2004, Oct. 17)

[41] "The Effect of Ukrain on Cancer." Available: http://www.ukrin.com/standardtexte/Standardbrief_2_eng.htm p.1 (accessed 2004, Oct 13)

[42] Ibid., p .3

[43] Ibid., p. 3, 4

Chapter 12

[1] R. D. Strand, M.D. *What Your Doctor Doesn't Know About Nutritional Medicine May Be Killing You,* Nashville, TN: Thomas Nelson Publishers®, 2002, p. 83

[2] "Kidney Cancer (Renal Cell Carcinoma)." Herbs2000.com. Available: herbs2000.com/disorders/cancer_kidney.htm, p. 1 (accessed 2004, Oct. 17)

[3] "Bladder Cancer." Herbs2000.com. Available: herbs2000.com/disorders/cancer_bladder.htm p. 1-2, (accessed 2004, Oct. 17)

[4] "Cancer Adjuvant Therapy," LifeExtension, Cancer Adjuvant Treatment - Page 3 of 11: Online Reference for Health Concerns, Available: http://www.lef.org/protocols/prtcl-027b.shtml, p. 3 (accessed 2004, Oct. 8) Also see the LEF Protocol Book!

[5] "Herbs and Supplements: Goldenseal," HPN - Healing People Network - safety issues, Available: http://www.healingpeople.com/index.php?option=com_staticfile=encyclopedia/pg/0001, p. 1 (accessed 2004, Dec. 5)

[6] Ibid.

[7] "Liver Cancer," Herbs2000.com. Available: http://www.herbs2000.com/disorders/cancer_liver_htm, p. 1 (accessed 2004, Oct. 17)

[8] R. W. Moss, Ph.D. *The Cancer Industry*, Brooklyn, N.Y: Equinox Press, 1999, 2002, p. 293-294

[9] Ibid., p. 317, 320

[10] "Kidney Cancer (Renal Cell Carcinoma)," Herbs2000.com. Available: herbs2000.com/disorders/cancer_kidney.htm, p. 1 (accessed 2004, Oct. 17)

[10a] "Cat's Claw," Side Effects and Cautions. Available: http://www.herbs2000.com/herbs/herbs_cats_claw.htm, p. 3 (accessed 2005, Jan 11)

[11] "The Health Effects of Chlorine in our Water." Available: http://www.wizardofeyez.com/chlorine.html, (accessed 2005, Jan 15)

[12] R.W. Moss, Ph.D. *Cancer Therapy - The Independent Consumer's Guide To Non-Toxic Treatment & Prevention,* New York: Equinox Press, 1992, p. 220

[13] Siegfried Gursche. *Good Fats and Oils, Why We Need them and How to Use Them in the Kitchen,* with permission from Alive Publishing Group, Inc. Canada. www.alive.com, <http://www.alive.com> 2000, p. 28-31, 41

[14] J. Carper. *The Food Pharmacy*, New York: Bantam Books, 1988, 1989, p. 204

[15] Ibid., p. 200, 203

[16] "Grape Vitis Vinifera." Herbs 2000.com. Available:
http://www.herbs2000.com/herbs_grape.htm, p. 2 (accessed 2004, June 7)

[17] Ibid.

[18] "Bladder Cancer," Herbs2000.com. Available:
herbs2000.com/disorders/cancer_bladder.htm, p. 2 (accessed 2004, Oct. 17)

[19] "Mushrooms - Shiitake - Lentinula edodes," 2. Available:
http://www2.mcdaniel.edu/Biology/botf99/herbnew/phytomedicine/tomushrooms.html
(accessed 2004, Aug 1)

[20] Ibid., p. 2, 3

[20a] "Bladder Cancer," Herbs2000.com. Available:
herbs2000.com/disorders/cancer_bladder.htm, p. 2 (accessed 2004, Oct. 17)

[20b] "Rhodiola Rosea," Available: http://www.planetherbs.com/articles/rhodiolia%20roseahtm,
p 1, 2 (accessed 2004, Oct. 21) Their reference: *Arctic Root (Rhodiola Rosea): The
Powerful New Ginseng Alternative* by Carl Germano, R.D., C.N.S., L.D.N., and Zakir
Ramazanov, Ph.D, published by Kensington Health Books

[21] Ibid., p. 2

[22] R. Sahelian, M.D. *Saw Palmetto Nature's Prostate Healer,* New York: Kensington Books,
Kensington Publishing Corp., 1998, p. 96, also see www.raysahelian.com/saw.html ©
1998, All rights reserved. Reprinted by arrangement with Kensington Publishing Corp.,
www.Kensingtonbooks.com

[23] "Baikal Scullcap (Scutellaria Baicalensis)," Prostate & Health - Prostate Protocol.
Available: http://www.nutrition2000.com/prostate_and_health/pancreatic-cancer-infor-
mation.asp, p. 2, 3 (accessed 2004, Dec. 3)

[24] "The Effect of Ukrain on Cancer," Ukrin.com. Available: http://www.ukrin.com/standard-
texte/Standardbrief_2_eng.htm, p. 1 (accessed 2004, Oct. 13)

[25] Ibid., p. 2

[26] Ibid., p. 4

[27] M. Kennedy Salaman. *Foods That Heal*, Menlo Park, CA: Statford Publishing, 1989, p.
128

[28] Ibid., p. 128

[29] Ibid., p. 128-129

[30] "Bladder Cancer," Herbs2000.com, p. 3

[31] "Kidney Cancer (Renal Cell Carcinoma)." Herbs2000.com. Available: herbs2000.com/dis-
orders/cancer_kidney.htm, p. 2 (accessed 2004, Oct. 17)

[32] D. Patton, "Vitamin E has protective role in bladder cancer," FoodNavigator.com, News &
Analysis Science & Nutrition, 03/30/2004. Available:
http://www.foodnavigator.com/news/news- NG.asp?id=9537, p. 1 (accessed 2004, Oct.
28)

[33] H. Winter Griffith, M.D. *Vitamins Herbs, Minerals & Supplements - The Complete Guide*,
(City, State, n.g.), Perseus (Fisher Books), 1988, 1998, p. 45

[34] E. L. Mindell, R.Ph. with V. L. Hopkins. *Dr. Earl Mindell's What You Should Know About
the Super Antioxidant Miracle,* New York: the McGraw-Hill Companies, 1996, p. 14.
Reproduced with permission of the the McGraw-Hill Companies

[35] R.W. Moss, Ph.D. *Antioxidants against Cancer*, State College, PA: Equinox Press, Inc.,
2000, 2002, p. 11

[36] Ibid., p. 11-12

[37] Ibid.

[38] Moss, *Antioxidants against Cancer*, p. 12

[39] Ibid., p. 13

[40] Ibid.

[41] "Bladder Cancer," Herbs2000.com. Available: http://www.herbs2000.com/disorders/cancer_bladder.htm, p. 3 (accessed 2004, Oct 17)

[42] S. Meyerowitz. *Wheat Grass Nature's Finest Medicine.*, Great Barrington, MA: Sproutman Publications, 1999, p. 95

Chapter 13

[1] A. Greenberg, M.D. "Cancer Quotes," Available: *http://www.whale.to/cancer/quotes.html* (accessed 2005, Jun. 19)

[1a] "Burzynski Patient Group," "Dustin K." Available: http://burzynskipatientgroup.org/dustink.htm (accessed 21 Jun. 2005)

[1b] "Burzynski Patient Group," "Crystin S." Available: http://burzynskipatientgroup.org/cyrstins. htm

[1c] "Burzynski Patient Group," "Jodi G." Available: http://burzynskipatientgroup.org/jodig.htm, (accessed 2005, June 21)

[2] "Antineoplastons," Alternatives In Cancer Therapy website, from their except of the book *Alternatives in Cancer Therapy,* by Ross, R. Ph. Pelton, Lee Overholser. Available: http://www.curezone.com/diseases/cancer/antineoplastons.asp, p. 1, 2, 4

[2a] Ibid.

[3] Ibid..

[4] Ibid., p. 4

[4a] "Antineoplastons," p. 4

[5] Ibid..

[6] Ibid..

[7] R.W. Moss., Ph.D. *The Cancer Industry*, Brooklyn, N.Y: Equinox Press, 1999, 2000, p. 320, 321

[8] "Antineoplastons," Alternatives In Cancer Therapy website, from their except of the book *Alternatives in Cancer Therapy,* by Ross, R. Ph. Pelton, Lee Overholser, the web article is: *Antineoplastons,* Available: http://www.curezone.com/diseases/cancer/antineoplastons.asp, p. 5 (accessed 2004, Dec. 5)

[8a] "Wormwood," Alternative Cancer Therapies, According to Dr. Lam MD at http://www.drlam.com/A3R_brief_in_doc_format/Artemisinin.cfm, quotes are from the Wellness Directory of Minnesota™ website. Available: http://www.mnwelldir.org/docs/cancer1/altthrpy.htm, (accessed 2004, Dec. 20)

[8b] Ibid.

[9] Ibid..

[9a] R. Pressinger, M.Ed. and Wayne Sinclair, M.D., Allergy, Asthma & Immunology, "About Neuroblastoma," Causes of Neuroblastoma Research: New Warnings about Where You Live, "Neuroblastoma and Chlordane," (CANCER, 59:1853-1859, 1987), Available: http://www.chemtox.com/neuroblastoma/default.htm, p. 1-2 (accessed 2004, Dec. 10)

[10] Ibid.

[11] Ibid.

11a "Chemotherapy: A Dull Weapon! Kyle Slavik A Success Story," From website OPTIONS - *Revolutionary Ideas in the War on Cancer.* Available: http://www.karlloren.com/biopsy/htm, p. 1 (accessed 2004, Dec. 5)

12 Ibid.

13 Ibid.

14 Ibid., p. 2

15 "Cayenne Pepper," Alternative Cancer Therapies. Available: http://www.mnwelldir.org/docs/cancer1/altthrpy.htm, Wellness Directory of Minnesota™, p. 1 (accessed 2004, May 25)

16 Ibid., p. 1

17 R.W. Moss, Ph.D. *Cancer Therapy - The Independent Consumer's Guide To Non-Toxic Treatment & Prevention,* New York: Equinox Press, 1992, p. 137

18 Ibid., p. 138

19 R. Willner, M.D., Ph.D. "Dr. Johanna Budwig Diet – Cancer, Arthritis, Multiple Sclerosis, Psoriasis, Eczema, Acne…Flaxseed oil and cottage cheese," The Cancer Homepage, Available: http://www.alternativehealth.co.nz/cancer/budwig.htm, from Ed McCabe (p 85, "Oxygen Therapies") discussing his view on the role of essential fatty acids, p. 2, 9, (accessed 2004, June 29)

20 "Dr. Budwig's Diet & Cancer Healing Protocol," website: Healing Cancer Naturally, Available: http://www.healingcancernaturally.com/budwig_protocol.html, (accessed 2005, Jan 17)

21 Willner, p. 8-9

22 Ibid., p. 1, 3, 8

23 "Is the Budwig Protocol 'just flaxseed oil and cottage cheese'"? website: Healing Cancer Naturally. Available: http://www.healingcancernaturally.com/budwig_protocol.html, (accessed 2005, Jan 17)

24 "Dr. Budwig's Diet & Cancer Healing Protocol," website: Healing Cancer Naturally, Available: http://www.healingcancernaturally.com/budwig_protocol.html, quote is from Dr. Johanna Budwig in <u>Flax Oil as a True Aid,</u> (accessed 2005, Jan 17)

25 Willner, p. 10

26 Ibid.

27 "Dr. Budwig's Diet & Cancer Healing Protocol," website Healing Cancer Naturally. Available: http://www.healingcancernaturally.com/budwig_protocol.html, from Dr. Budwig in "Der Tod des Tumors, Band II" (The Death of the Tumor, Vol. II) transcribing an interview broadcast by the Siddeutscher Rundfunk Stuttgart (South German Radio Station) on 11 Sep 1967, (accessed website: 2005, Jan 17)

28 Willner, p. 8

29 Ibid., p. 5

30 R. L. Blaylock, M.D. *Natural Strategies For Cancer Patients*, New York: Twin Streams, Kensington Publishing Corp., © 2003, p. 143-144. All rights reserved. Reprinted by arrangement with Kensington Publishing Corp. www.kensingtonbooks.com

31 Ibid., p. 144

32 "Cancer Adjuvant Therapy," LifeExtension, *Cancer Adjuvant Therapy*. Available: http://www.lef.org/protocols/prtcl- 027b.shtml (2004, Oct 8) Also see the LEF Protocol Book!

33 Ibid.

34 "Liver Cancer," Herbs2000.com. Available: http://www.herbs2000.com/disorders/cancer_liver.htm, p. 1 (accessed 2004, Oct. 17)

34a J. L. Eftekhar. *Heal Yourself, Globe Digests™,* New York, N.Y. (and Boca Raton, FL.) Globe Communications Corp., 1995, p. 19-20

35 Ibid.

36 R.W. Moss, Ph.D. *Cancer Therapy - The Independent Consumer's Guide To Non-Toxic Treatment & Prevention,* New York: Equinox Press, 1992, p. 195-196

36a "Tetrahydrocannabinol (THC -medical marijuana)," Cancer Tutor™, Alternative Cancer Treatment Information Center Available: http://www.cancertutor.com/Other/Big_List.htm, p. 36-37, (accessed 2004, Oct. 17)

37 Ibid.

38 Ibid., p. 37

39 R.W. Moss, Ph.D. *Antioxidants against Cancer*, State College, PA: Equinox Press, Inc., 2000, 2002, p. 89

40 "Mullaca," Raintree Nutrition, TROPICAL PLANT DATABASE, Available: http://www.raintree.com/mullaca.htm, p. 1-2 (accessed 2004, Oct. 21) This information is also found in Leslie Taylor's book, *The Healing Power of Rainforest Herbs,* Square One Publishers, Jan. 2005

40a "Brain Stem Gliomas." Available: http://www.braintumor.org/patient_info/surviving/tumor_types/othergliomas.html (accessed 2005, Apr. 10) copyright 2000-2004 National Brain Tumor Foundation.

40b Ibid.

40c "Tumor Types: Non Gliomas." Available: http://www.braintumor.org/patient_info/surviving/tumor_types/nongliomas.html (accessed 2005, Apr. 10) copyright 2000-2004 National Brain Tumor Foundation.

40d "Tumor Types: Other Brain-Related Conditions." Available: http://www.braintumor.org/patient_ info/ surviving/ tumor_types/otherbrain.html (accessed 2005, Apr. 10) copyright 2000-2004 National Brain Tumor Foundation

41 "Mullaca," Raintree Nutrition, p. 2, 3

42 Ibid., p. 4, 5

43 S. Lieberman, Ph.D. and K. Babal, C.N. *Maitake Mushroom AND D-Fraction,* Pleasant Grove, UT: Woodland Publishing, 2001, p. 14

43a "Pituitary Tumors," National Institute of Neurological Disorders and Stroke. Available: http://www.ninds.nih.gov/disorders/pituitary_tumors/pituitary_tumors.htm (accessed 2005, May 17)

43b Ibid.

43c Ibid.

44 Ibid.

44a "Poly-MVA New hope for cancer patients. New hope for brain cancer patients," Available: http://www.mnwelldir.org/docs/cancer1/poly.htm, (accessed 2005, Jul. 7)

45 R. W. Moss, Ph.D. *Cancer Therapy: The Independent Consumer's Guide to Non-Toxic Treatment & Prevention,* New York: Equinox Press, 1992, p. 170

45a "Pau d'arco {Teehebo} Ancient Herb, Modern Miracle," In-depth Pau D'arco Article by Dr. Mowry, Available: http://www.oralchelation.com/taheebo/research/page1.htm, p. 1, (accessed 2004, Dec. 10)

46 Ibid.

47 R. W. Moss, Ph.D. "Intriguing New Anticancer Compound From East Europe," From The Cancer Chronicles #27 © June 1995 by Ralph W. Moss, Ph.D., Available: http://www.ralphmoss.com/html/Ukrain.shtml, p. 1 (accessed 2004, Oct 13)

48 "The Effect of Ukrain on Cancer," Ukrin.com. Available: http://www.ukrin.com/standard-texte/Standardbrief_2_eng.htm, p. 1-3 (accessed 2004, Oct. 13)

49 Ibid.

50 Ibid., p. 2, 3

51 Ibid., p. 1

51a "Vassourinha," Raintree Nutrition, TROPICAL PLANT DATABASE, Plant Chemicals. Available: http://www.rain-tree.com/vassourinha.htm, p. 1, 3-5 (accessed 2004, Oct. 21) This information is also found in Leslie Taylor's book, *The Healing Power of Rainforest Herbs,* Square One Publishers, Jan. 2005

52 Ibid.

52a "Anamu," Raintree Nutrition, TROPICAL PLANT DATABASE, Biological Activities and Clinical Research. Available: http://www.rain-tree.com/anamu.htm, p. 1, 3-6 (accessed 2004, Nov. 23) This information is also found in Leslie Taylor's book, *The Healing Power of Rainforest Herbs,* Square One Publishers, Jan. 2005

53 Ibid.

Chapter 14

1 B. Berkson, M.D., Ph.D. From *The Alpha Lipoic Acid Breakthrough,* copyright © 1998 by Burt Berkson. Used by permission of Prima Publishing, a division of Random House, Inc., 1998, p. vii

2 "Cancer Types," "Skin Cancer." Available: http://www.cancer-healing.com/cancer_type.php (accessed 2005, May 3)

2a Ibid.

2b Ibid.

3 M.K. Salaman. *All Your Health Questions Answered Naturally*, (City, State, n.g.) MKS, Inc., 1998, p. 223

4 Ibid., p. 224

5 R. W. Moss, Ph.D. *Cancer Therapy: The Independent Consumer's Guide To Non-Toxic Treatment & Prevention,* New York: Equinox Press, 1992, p. 291

5a C. Borek, Ph.D., "Beta Glucan Boosts Immunity," "Beta Glucan vs. Cancer" and "Beta Glucan the Supplement." Available: http://www.newhope.com/nutritionsciencenews/NSN_backs/Jan_01/betaglucan.cfm, p. 1-2 (accessed 2004, Oct 17) Copyright © 2004, Penton Media, Inc.

5b Ibid.

6 Ibid.

7 "Oat Beta Glucan," Effective Natural Cancer Treatments. Available: http://www.cancer-treatments.net/cancer.html., p.1 (accessed 2004, Dec. 1)

8 "Cansema Black Topical Salve (Skin Cancer)," Cancer Tutor™, Alternative Cancer Treatment Information Center. Available: http://www.cancertutor.com/Cancer/Cansema, html, p. 1, 9 (accessed 2004, Oct. 17)

9 "Gill-Over-The-Ground," The Backyard Herbalist, Ernestina Parziale CH, "Health Conditions Starting with C and herbal remedies used to treat them." Available: http://earthnotes.tripod. com/ckbk_c.htm, p. 2 (accessed 2004, Oct. 16)

10 "Chaparral," www.curezone.com's except from the book *Alternatives in Cancer Therapy* by Ross, R.Ph., Pelton, Lee Overholser. Available: www.curezone.com/diseases/cancer/chaparral.asp, p. 1 (accessed 2004, May 25)

11 Ibid.

[12] Ibid., p. 1

[13] Ibid., p. 1

[14] Curezone.com., p. 2

[15] Ibid.

[16] Ibid.

[17] Ibid.

[18] R. D. Strand, M.D., with Donna K. Wallace. *Death by Prescription*, Nashville, TN: Thomas Nelson Publishers, 2003, p. 167-168

[19] Ibid., p. 94-95

[20] "Cancer Cover-Up The Neal Deoul Story," by Kathleen Deoul, *Frequently Asked Questions*, Available: http://www.cancer-coverup.com/faqs/is-this-treatment-safe.htm, (accessed 2004, Dec. 26) Quoted with their permission.

[20a] Warner, Jennifer, "Substance In Peppers Kills Cancer Cells," WebMD Medical News, "Capsaicin (Hot Pepper Substance) Kills Cancer Cells," Sept. 3, 2002, Available: http://store.yahoo.com/annieappleseedproject/caphotpepsub.html, (accessed 4 Jul. 2005) Used with permission from annieappleseedproject.

[21] Cancer Tutor™, Alternative Cancer Treatment Information Center, "Cansema Black Topical Salve (Skin Cancer)" Available: http://www.cancertutor.com/Cancer/Cansema, html, p. 1, 9 (2004, Oct. 17)

[22] Ibid.

[23] Ibid.

[24] "Comfrey plant," from www.cancertutor.com website Available: http://www.cancertutor.com/Other/Big_List.htm p. 12 (accessed 2004, Oct 17)

[25] "Espinheira Santa." Herbs2000.com. Available: http://www.herbs2000.com/herbs/herbs_espinheirasanta.Htm , p. 1 (accessed 2004, Oct. 16)

[26] Ibid., p. 1, 2

[27] M.K. Salaman. *All Your Health Questions Answered Naturally,* MKS, Inc., 1998 p. 226

[28] Ibid., p. 225, 226

[29] Ibid., p. 225

[30] R. W. Moss, Ph.D. *Cancer Therapy - the Independent Consumer's Guide To Non-Toxic Treatment & Prevention,* Equinox Press, 1992, p. 163

[30a] The Reader's Digest Assoc., Inc. *The Healing Power of Vitamins, Minerals, and Herbs,* 1999, 2000, p. 331. Quoted with permission of Global Books & Home Entertainment, The Reader's Digest Association, Inc.

[31] Ibid.

[32] "Pomegranate extract blocks skin tumors in mice." New York, Reuters Health. From OncoLink Cancer News, *Reuters Health Information.* Available: http://www.oncolink.com/resources//article.cfm?c=3&s=8&ss=23&id=11481&month=01&year=2005, posting date Jan. 20, 2005 (accessed 2005, June 2) Copyright © 1994-2005 © Trustees of the University of Pennsylvania. From *Reuters Health Information,* Copyright © 2005 Reuters Limited. All rights reserved. Reprinted with their permission. Reuters shall not be liable for any errors or delays in the content, or for any actions taken in reliance thereon.

[33] Ibid.

[34] Salaman, *All Your Health Questions Answered Naturally*, p. 224

[35] R. W. Moss, Ph.D. *Antioxidants against Cancer*, State College, PA: Equinox Press, Inc., 2002, p. 77-78

[36] M. Kennedy Salaman. *Nutrition: The Cancer Answer II*, MKS, Inc./Statford Publishing, 2002, p. 349

[37] D. Sage, M.S.S.A., "Haelan Reverses Cancer Cell Growth," "Precancerous Skin Condition," Healing Cancer Naturally, - Haelan, From Well Being Journal Special Edition: Healing Cancer Naturally, Available: http://www.wellbeingjournal.com/haelan.htm, p. 9-10 (accessed 2004, Oct. 17)

[38] "Vassourinha," Raintree Nutrition, TROPICAL PLANT DATABASE, Database Entry: Vassourinha - Scoparia dulcis Vassourinha, Available: http://www.raintree.com/vassourinha.htm, p. 2 (accessed 2004, Oct. 21) This information is also found in Leslie Taylor's book, *The Healing Power of Rainforest Herbs,* Square One Publishers, Jan. 2005

[39] Ibid., p. 4, 5

[40] S. Meyerowitz. *Wheat Grass Nature's Finest Medicine*, Great Barrington, MA: Sproutman Publications, 1999, p. 103, 104

Chapter 15

[1] Costello, M. "Essiac Quotes." Available: *http://www.whale.to/c/quotes.html* (accessed 28, Jun. 2005)

[2] "Sarcoma," Available: http://www.cancer-healing.com/cancer_type.php, "Cancer Types" (accessed 2005, May 3)

[2a] "Non-Hodgkin's Lymphoma - oncology channel." Available: http://www.oncologychannel.com/nonhodgkins, p. 1. This information reprinted with permission © Healthcommunities.com, Inc., 2005. All rights reserved. (accessed 2004, Dec. 13)

[3] "Hodgkin Lymphoma and Non-Hodgkin Lymphoma," Cancer Types, Classification, Available: http://www.cancer-healing.com/cancer_type.php, (accessed 2004, Dec. 28)

[4] Ibid..

[5] M. Kennedy Salaman. *Nutrition: The Cancer Answer II*, Menlo Park, CA.: Statford Publishing, 2002 edition, p. 279-280

[6] Ibid..

[7] "Andrographis," herbs2000.com. Available: http://www.herbs2000.com/herbs/herbs_andrographis.htm, p. 1-2 (accessed 2004, Oct. 17)

[8] Ibid., p. 2

[9] "Ashwagandha: by Ray Sahelian, M.D., Ashwagandha Benefits." Available: http://www.raysahelian.com/ashwagandha.html, p. 3 (accessed 2005, Jan 17

[10] B. Rajkapoor, B. Jayakar and R. Anandian Vinayaka, "Antitumour Activity of Elephantopus scaber Linn Against Dalton's Ascitic Lymphoma," The *Indian Journal of Pharmaceutical Sciences,* The Indian Pharmaceutical Association (IPA), 2002, Jan – Feb. Available: http://www.indianpharma.org/journal/index.php/2002/1jan%20%20feb/antitumouractivity, (accessed 2005, Jan 19) Accepted 4 October 2001 Revised 10 September 2001 Received 13 February 2001. Quoted with permission by Rao V.S.V. Vadlamudi, Ph.D., Editor, Indian Journal of Pharmaceutical Sciences, Indian Pharmaceutical Assn.

[11] "The benefits of Beta Glucan and MSM supplements from a terminal cancer survivor's perspective," Why Beta Glucan for Immune System Response? About betaglucan.com. Available: http://www.aboutbetaglucan.com, p. 1 (accessed 2004, Oct 17)

[12] Ibid.

[13] Ibid.

14 "Oat Beta Glucan," Effective Natural Cancer Treatments, Available: http://www.cancer-treatments.net/cancer.html, p. 1 (accessed 2004, Dec. 1)

15 Ibid.

16 Dr. J. Mercola, "Chlorella: A Natural Wonder Food, Anti Cancer Properties of Chlorella," "How Much Chlorella Should a Person Take If They Have Cancer?" Available: http://www.mercola.com/chlorella/anti_cancer.htm, p. 2 (accessed 2004, Nov. 25)

17 "Dr. Budwig's Diet and Cancer Healing Protocol," website - Healing Cancer Naturally. Available: http://www.healingcancernaturally.com/budwig_protocol.html, (accessed 2005, Jan. 17)

18 "Bone Cancer - Another Flax Cure." Available: http://www.curezone.com/diseases/cancer/testimonials/Bone_cancer_another_flax_cure.asp, p. 1 (accessed 2004, Dec. 11)

19 Ibid.

20 Ibid.

21 Ibid., p. 52

22 "Geraniol," website: earthnotes.tripod.com, "Health Conditions Starting with C and herbal remedies used to treat them." Available: http://earthnotes.tripod.com/ckbk_c.htm, p. 2, (accessed 2004, Oct. 16)

23 J. A. Duke with Michael Castleman. *The Green Pharmacy Anti-Aging Prescriptions*, (City, State, n.g.) Rodale, Inc., 2001, p. 93

24 "Cancer Adjuvant Therapy," Life Extension. Available: http://www.lef.org/protocols/prtcl027b.shtml, (accessed 2004, Oct 8) Also see the LEF Protocol Book!

25 "Ewing's sarcoma in children," CANCERBACUP Helping people live with cancer. Available: http://www.cancerbacup.org.uk/Cancertype/Childrenscancers/Typesofchildrenscancers/Ew...p. 1 (accessed 2005, Jan 19)

26 "Guacatonga," Raintree Nutrition, TROPICAL PLANT DATABASE. Available: http://www.rain-tree.com/guacatonga.htm, p 1, 2-3 (accessed 2004, Oct. 22) This information is also found in Leslie Taylor's book, *The Healing Power of Rainforest Herb*, Square One Publishers, Jan. 2005

27 Ibid., p. 2, 3, 7

28 "Andiroba," Raintree Nutrition, TROPICAL PLANT DATABASE. Available: http://www.rain-tree.com/andiroba.htm p. 1, 3, 4 (accessed 2004, Oct. 22) This information is also found in Leslie Taylor's book, *The Healing Power of Rainforest Herb*, Square One Publishers, Jan. 2005

29 R. W. Moss, Ph.D. *The Cancer Industry*, Brooklyn, N.Y: Equinox Press, 1999, 2002, p. 492

30 Ibid.

31 B. Best, S. Best, "The Boy Who Ran Away From Chemotherapy, Billy's Story." Available: http://www.grand-strand.com/suebest/boywho.htm, (accessed 2005, Jan. 7)

32 Ibid.

33 Ibid.

34 Ibid.

35 R.W. Moss, Ph.D., p. 187, 189

36 Ibid., p. 190

37 Ibid.

38 Ibid.

[39] Ibid., p. 192, 193

[40] Moss, p. 192, 193

[41] Ibid., 195-200

[42] Moss., p. 209, 210

[43] "Treatment: Hydrazine Sulfate." Available: http://www.diagnose-me.com/treat/T396383.html, (accessed 2005, Jan 20)

[44] Ibid.

[45] G. Null, Ph.D. *The Complete Encyclopedia of Natural Healing*, New York, N.Y. © 2000, 2001, 2002 Kensington Publishing Corp. p. 85. All rights reserved. Reprinted by arrangement with Kensington Publishing Corp., *www.kensingtonbooks.com.*

[46] "ICHT (Intra-Cellular Hyperthermia Therapy," Integrated Medical Specialists. Available: http://www.heatkillscancer.com/cancer_heat.html, p. 1-2 (accessed 2004, Dec. 12)

[47] "IPT Fact Sheet." Available: http://iptq.com/fact_sheet.htm, p. 1 (accessed 2004, Dec. 12)

[48] "Psoralea," herbs2000.com. Available: http://www.herbs2000.com/herbs/herbs_psoralea.htm, p. 1 (accessed 2004, Oct. 25)

[49] R. Dubin. p 161, From *Miracle Food Cures From The Bible* by Reese Dubin, copyright © 1999 by Prentice Hall. Used by permission of Avery Publishing, an imprint of Penguin Group (USA) Inc.

[50] "Glandulars," Cancer Tutor™, Alternative Cancer Treatment Information Center. Available: http://www.cancertutor.com/Other/Big_List.htm, p. 19 (accessed 2004, Oct 17

[51] Ibid.

[52] A. Hoffer, M.D., Ph.D., "Clinical Procedures in Treating Terminally Ill Cancer Patients with Vitamin C," Supportive Vitamin C Therapy for Cancer Patients, DoctorYourself.Com. Available: http://www.doctoryourself.com/hoffer_cancer_2.html, p. 1,8 (accessed 2004, Aug 1)

[53] Ibid.

[54] Ibid.

[55] Ibid., p. 8-9

[56] A. Hoffer, M.D., Ph.D., FRCP(C), "Hoffer's Home Page – Orthomolecular Treatment of Cancer." Available: http://www.islandnet.com/~hoffer/, p. 2 (accessed 2005, May 28)

[57] Ibid., p. 11

[58] S. Meyerowitz. *Wheat Grass Nature's Finest Medicine*, Great Barrington, MA: Sproutman Publications, p. 107-108

Chapter 16

[1] D. Shulze, N.D. "Herbal Naturopathy Quotes," "Politics." Available: http://www.whale.to/a/herbal_q.html (accessed 2005, Jun.21)

[2] A. Wigmore. *The Wheatgrass Book*, From the Foreword by Brian Clement of Boston, MA, Nov. 1984, (City, State, n.g.) Avery, member of Penguin Putnam, Inc., 1985, p. x

[3] Ibid.

[4] G. A. Forgionne, Ph.D., "Nutritional Therapy for Primary Peritoneal Cancer: A Case Study," from the *CancerLynx* website July 8, 2002 article. Available: http://www.cancerlynx.com/peritonealcase.html, p. 1-3 (accessed 2004, Dec. 14)

[5] Forgionne, p. 4

[5a] Ibid., p. 6, 7

[6] Ibid.

6a "Ovarian Cancer." From labtestsonline.org website. Available: http://www.labtestsonline.org/understanding/conditions/ovarian-2.html (accessed 2005, Apr. 27) Labtestsonline is a non-commercial website published by the American Association for Clinical Chemistry. For up-to-date information on clinical lab tests, visit the website at www.labtestsonline.org

6b Ibid.

6c Ibid.

7 Wigmore, p. 47

8 "Wheatgrass Treatment For Cancer," Cancer Tutor™ website, Available: http://www.cancertutor.com/Cancer/Wheatgrass.html., (accessed 2004, Dec. 12)

9 A. Wigmore. *The Hippocrates Diet and Health Program*, (City, State, n.g.) Avery, 1984, p. 49

9a S. Meyerowitz. *Wheat Grass Nature's Finest Medicine.*, Great Barrington, MA: Sproutman Publications, 1999, p. 31, 32

9b Ibid.

10 Ibid.

11 Ibid., p. 34

12 Meyerowitz, p. 93, 94

13 Ibid., p. 95

14 Ibid., p. 98, 101

15 Meyerowitz, p. 103, 104

16 Ibid., p. 108

17 A. Wigmore. *The Hippocrates Diet and Health Program*, (City, State, n.g.) Avery, 1984, p. 95-96

18 S. Blauer. *The Juicing Book*, (City, State, n.g.) Avery, 1989, p. 12-13

19 Ibid.

20 E. Mindell, R.Ph., Ph.D., *Earl Mindell's Soy Miracle*, New York, p. 106. E. Mindell, R.Ph., Ph.D. *Earl Mindell's Soy Miracle,* New York, p. 106. Reprinted with permission from Simon & Schuster Adult Publishing Group, from EARL MINDELL'S SOY MIRACLE by Earl Mindell, R.Ph., Ph.D. © 1995 by Earl Mindell, R.Ph.,Ph.D, and Carol Colman.

21 Ibid., p. 106-107

22 J. E. O'Brien. *The Miracle of Garlic & Vinegar and other Exciting Natural Wonders*, Globe Mini Mags®, Boca Raton, FL: Globe Communications Corp., 1991, p. 62

23 Ibid., p. 62

24 Ibid.

25 M. Stengler, N.D. *The Natural Physician's Healing Therapies* by Mark Stengler, N.D. copyright © 2001 by Mark Stengler. Used by permission of Avery Publishing, an imprint of Penguin Group (USA) Inc., p. 426

25a Ibid., p. 426-427

25b Ibid.

26 Stengler, p. 426-427

26a Ibid., p. 428, 429

27 Ibid.

28 C.M. Hawken. *Green Foods "Phyto-Foods" for Super Health* Pleasant Grove, UT: Woodland Publishing, 1998, p. 11-12

29 Stengler, p. 428, 429

[30] R. Dubin. p. 128-130 From *Miracle Food Cures From The Bible* by Reese Dubin, copyright © 1999 by Prentice Hall. Used by permission of Avery Publishing, an imprint of Penguin Group (USA) Inc.

[31] Ibid., p. 128

[32] Dubin, p. 128-129

[33] Ibid., p. 130, 133

[34] Hawken, p. 13

[35] Ibid., p. 13-15

[36] Hawken, p. 14

[37] Ibid., p. 20-21

[38] Ibid., p. 6

[39] Ibid., p. 19, 20

[40] A. Wigmore. *The Sprouting Book,* Wayne, N. J.: Avery Publishing Group, Inc., 1986, p. 4

[41] Ibid., p. 7-9

[42] Ibid., p. 10, 11

[43] Ibid., p. 11

Chapter 17

[1] Budwig, Johanna, Dr. "The Budwig Diet Quotes." Available: http://www.whale.to/a/budwig_q.html, (accessed 2005 Jun. 28)

[2] M. Kennedy Salaman. *Nutrition: The Cancer Answer II,* Menlo Park, CA: Statford Publishing, 1995, 2002, p. 123

[3] Ibid., p. 123

[4] Ibid., p. 122

[5] Salaman, p. 123

[6] S. Gursche. From the book *Fantastic Flax, A Powerful Defense Against Cancer, Heart Disease and Digestive Disorders*: with permission from Alive Publishing Group, Inc., Canada. www.alive.com, <http://www.alive.com> p. 13

[7] Ibid., p. 6

[8] Gursche, p. 8

[9] Ibid., p. 8, 9

[9a] Ibid., p. 12

[10] Ibid.

[10a] Gursche, p. 13-19

[11] Ibid.

[11a] Gursche, p. 20, 21

[12] Ibid.

[12a] Ibid.

[13] Gursche, p. 20, 21

[13a] Ibid., p. 20, 22, 26

[14] Ibid.

[15] M. Stengler, N.D., p. 187. *The Natural Physician's Healing Therapies* by Mark Stengler, N.D. copyright © 2001 by Mark Stengler. Used by permission of Avery Publishing, an imprint of Penguin Group (USA) Inc.

[16] Ibid., p. 187-188

[17] Ibid.

[17a] M. Kennedy Salaman. *All Your Health Questions Answered Naturally,* (City, State, n.g.) MKS., Inc., 1998, p 378

[18] Ibid.

[19] R. Dubin. From *Miracle Food Cures From The Bible* by Reese Dubin, copyright © 1999 by Prentice Hall. Used by permission of Avery Publishing, an imprint of Penguin Group (USA) Inc., p. 138

[20] Ibid., p. 138

[20a] Ibid., p. 139

[21] Ibid.

[22] E. Mindell, R.Ph., Ph.D., *Earl Mindell's Food as Medicine*, New York, p. 20, 192. Reprinted with permission of Simon & Schuster Adult Publishing Group from EARL MINDELL'S FOOD AS MEDICINE by Earl Mindell, R.Ph., Ph.D. ©1994 by Earl Mindell R.Ph., Ph.D and Carol Colman.

[23] S. Meyerowitz. *Sprouts, The Miracle Food, The Complete Guide to Sprouting,* Sproutman Publications, 1983-1998, p. 160

[24] S. Yeager and the Editors of *Prevention* Health Books, (City, State, n.g.) *Doctors Book of FOOD REMEDIES,* Rodale, 1998, p. 221-222

[25] Ibid.

[25a] Gursche, Siegfried. *Good Fats and Oils*, with permission from Alive Publishing Group, Inc., Canada. www.alive.com p. 16-21

[26] Ibid.

[27] Ibid., p. 19

[27a] Ibid., p. 28-38

[27b] Gursche, p. 28-38

[28] Ibid.

[29] "Dr. Budwig's Diet & Cancer Healing Protocol," website: Healing Cancer Naturally. Available: http://www.healingcancernaturally.com/budwig_protocol.html, (accessed 2005, Jan. 17)

[30] R. Blaylock, M.D. *Natural Strategies for Cancer Patients*, New York: Twin Streams, Kensington Publishing Corp., © 2003, p. 142-144, All rights reserved. Reprinted by arrangement with Kensington Publishing Corp. www.kensingtonbooks.com

[31] *The Healing Power of Vitamins, Minerals, and Herbs*, Pleasantville, N.Y./Montreal: *Reader's Digest*, Reader's Digest Assn., 1999, p. 290-291. Quoted with permission of Global Books & Home Entertainment, The Reader's Digest Association, Inc.

[32] "Johanna Budwig Revisited," Wellness Directory of Minnesota™ website. Available: http://www.mnwelldir.org/docs/cancer1/budwig.htm, p. 1 (accessed 2004, Dec. 20)

[33] Kelley, p. 1

[34] Ibid.

[35] R. Willner, M.D., Ph.D. The Cancer Homepage. "Dr. Johanna Budwig Diet Cancer, Arthritis, Multiple Sclerosis, Psoriasis, Eczema, Acne...Flaxseed oil and cottage cheese." Available: http://www.alternativehealth.co.nz/cancer/budwig.htm, p. 7 (accessed 2004, Jun. 29)

[36] Ibid., p. 1-2

[37] Ibid., p. 2

[38] R. Willner, M.D., Ph.D. The Cancer Homepage. "Dr. Johanna Budwig Diet Cancer, Arthritis, Multiple Sclerosis, Psoriasis, Eczema, Acne...Flaxseed oil and cottage cheese." Available: http://www.alternativehealth.co.nz/cancer/budwig.html, p. 9, from Ed McCabe (p85, "Oxygen Therapies") discussing his view on the role of essential fatty acids, (accessed 2004, Jun. 29)

[39] Ibid., p. 10-11

[40] Willner, p. 11

[41] "Bone Cancer - Another Flax Cure." Available: http://www.curezone.com/diseases/cancer/testimonials/Bone_cancer_another_flax_cure.asp, p. 1 (accessed 2004, Dec. 11)

[41a] Willner, p. 3

[42] Ibid.

[43] S. Yeager and the Editors of Prevention Health Books. *Doctor's Book of Food Remedies,* (City, State, n.g.) Rodale, Inc. 1998, p. 44

[44] R. W. Moss, Ph.D. *Cancer Therapy: The Independent Consumer's Guide To Non-Toxic Treatment & Prevention,* New York: Equinox Press, 1992

[45] "Lyprinol." Available: http://www.primohealth.com/PILyprinol.a.html (accessed 2005, May 6)

Chapter 18

[1] From the AV1611 *King James Holy Bible* - Genesis 1:29

[2] P.F. Lin. "Antitumor effect of actinidia chinensis polysaccharide on murine tumor," Institute of Molecular Medicine, Zhejiang College of Traditional Chinese Medicine, Hangzhou, Online posting. Zhonghua Zhong Liu Za Zhi. 1988 Nov;10(6):441-4, Available: http://www.ncbi.nlm.nih.gov/entrez/query.fcgi?cmd=Retrieve&db=pubmeddopt=Abstract&list_uids=2855056&query_hl=33, p. 1 (accessed 2005, Jul. 1)

[2a] Ibid.

[3] "Kiwi Fruit," The World's Healthiest Foods: Feeling Great, George Mateljan Foundation, Whfoods.com. Available: http://www.whfoods.com/genpagephp?tname=foodspice&dbid=41 p. 2-3, (Accessed 2004, dec. 17)

[3a] Ibid.

[4] Ibid.

[4a] Ibid.

[5] M. B. Skousen. *The Ancient Egyptian Medicine Plant, Aloe Vera Hand Book,* (City, State, n.g.) Aloe Vera Research Institute, 1992, p. 10-14 Ibid., p. 12

[6] Charlene Laino, MSNBC, "Chinese Folk Remedy Fights Cancer - Plant Compound Sparks Chain Reaction That Kills Tumor Cells," HerbTime The Natural Health Center. Available: http://www.herbtime.com/InformationPages/ChineseFolkRemedyFightsCancer.htm, p. 1 (accessed 2004, Nov. 1)

[7] "Ashwagandha," Herbs2000.com. Available: http://www.herbs2000.com/herbs/herbs_ashwagandha,htm, p 1-2 (accessed 2004, Oct. 16)

[8] R. Sahelian, M.D., "Ashwagandha." Available: http://www.raysahelian.com/ashwagandha.html, (accessed 2005, Jan 17, p. 3

[9] Ibid., p. 3, Life Sci.2003 Nov 21;74(1):125-32)

[10] "Ashwagandha," Herbs2000.com p. 2

[10a] "Aspilia," herbs2000.com. Available: http://www.herbs2000.com/herbs/herbs_aspilia.htm, p. 1-2, (accessed 2004, Oct. 16)

[11] E. Mindell, R.Ph., Ph.D. *Earl Mindell's Soy Miracle,*" New York, p. 123. E. Mindell, R.Ph., Ph.D. New York, p. 106. Reprinted with permission from Simon & Schuster Adult Publishing Group, from EARL MINDELL'S SOY MIRACLE by Earl Mindell, R.Ph., Ph.D. © 1995 by Earl Mindell, R.Ph., Ph.D, and Carol Colman.

11a "Bladder Cancer." Herbs2000.com. Available: herbs2000.com/disorders/cancer_bladder.htm p. 1-2, (accessed 2004, Oct. 17)

11b M. Stengler, N.D., p.75, *The Natural Physician's Healing Therapies* by Mark Stengler, N.D. copyright © 2001 by Mark Stengler. Used by permission of Avery Publishing, an imprint of Penguin Group (USA) Inc.

12 Ibid.

13 B. Gottlieb. *Alternative Cures - The Most Effective Natural Home Remedies for 160 Health Problems,* (City, State, n.g.) Rodale 2000, p. 167

13a "Bupleurum," Herbs2000.com. Available:
http://www.herbs2000.com/herbs/herbs_bupleurum. htm,p. 1, 2 (accessed 2004, Oct. 25)

14 Ibid.

15 "Bone Cancer," Herbs2000.com. Available: http://www.herbs2000.com/disorders/cancer_bone. htm, p. 2 (accessed 2004, Dec. 18)

15a M. Nadine Antol. *Healing Teas*, (City, State, n.g.) Avery, 1996, p. 112, 113

16 Ibid.

17 "Chicory Root." Available: http://www.cancertutor.com/OtherBig_List.htm, p. 11 (accessed 2004, Dec. 11)

17a "Chinese Asparagus," Earthnotes Herb Library. Available:
http://earthnotes.tripod.com/asparagus.htm#aspother, (accessed 2005, Jan. 21)

18 Ibid.

19 "Cilantro: A Common Spice/Herb That Can Save your Life."Available:
http://www.mnwell.dir.org/docs/detox/cilantro.htm, p. 1-2 (accessed 2004, Dec. 18)

20 Ibid.

21 K. Gilbert Udall. *Immune and Stamina Booster Cordyceps Sinensis,* Pleasant Grove, UT: Woodland Publishing, 2000, p. 25-27.

21a E. Mindell, R.Ph., Ph.D. *Earl Mindell's Herb Bible,* New York, p. 77. Reprinted with permission of Simon & Schuster Adult Publishing Group from EARL MINDELL'S HERB BIBLE by Earl Mindell, R.Ph., Ph.D, © 1992 by Earl Mindell R.Ph., Ph.D. and Carol Colman.

22 Ibid.

23 Website www.cancertutor.com, "Curcumin /Turmeric." Available at http://www.cancertutor.com/Other/Big_List.htm, p. 13 (accessed 2004, Oct. 17)

24 "Grocery warning: curry sauces contain dangerous levels of food coloring chemicals," News Target Network, News and Commentary on Today's Top Stories, Monday, Jan 03, 2005 commentary: available: http://www.newstarget.com/001027.html, p. 1 (accessed 2005, Jan 4)

24a Mark Stengler, N.D., p 445, *The Natural Physician's Healing Therapies* by Mark Stengler, N.D copyright © 2001 by Mark Stengler. Used by permission of Avery Publishing, an imprint of Penguin Group (USA) Inc.

24b Antol, p. 122-123

24c Ibid.

25 "D-limonene," Cancertutor.com. Available:
http://www.cancertutor.com/Other/Big_List_htm, p. 15, (accessed 2004, Dec. 3)

25a D. B. Mowrey, Ph.D. *The Scientific Validation of Herbal Medicine*, New York: McGraw-Hill Companies, 1986, reproduced with permission of McGraw-Hill Companies, p. 118-119

26 Ibid.

27 Dr. J. Heinerman. *Healing Power of Herbs,* Boca Raton, FL: *Globe Digests™,* Globe Communications Corp., 1995, p. 34, 35

27a "Compound from rare plant shows promise in treating breast cancer," Charlottesville, Va., Feb. 1, 2005. Available: http://www.eurekalert.org/pub_releases/2005-02/uovh-cfr013105.php (accessed 2005, Feb. 1)

28 Antol, p. 143

29 E. Mindell, R.Ph., Ph.D. *Earl Mindell's Herb Bible,* New York, p.104-105. Reprinted with permission of Simon & Schuster Adult Publishing Group from EARL MINDELL'S HERB BIBLE by Earl Mindell, R.Ph., Ph.D, © 1992 by Earl Mindell R.Ph., Ph.D. and Carol Colman

30 Ibid., p. 106

31 R. W. Moss, Ph.D. *Cancer Therapy - The Independent Consumer's Guide to Non-Toxic Treatment & Prevention,* New York: Equinox Press, 1992, p Moss, p. 155

32 E. Mindell, R.Ph., Ph.D. *Earl Mindell's Herb Bible,* p. 107, 108 Reprinted with permission of Simon & Schuster Adult Publishing Group from EARL MINDELL'S HERB BIBLE by Earl Mindell, R.Ph., Ph.D, © 1992 by Earl Mindell R.Ph., Ph.D. and Carol Colman.

33 Ibid.

34 Ibid., p. 108

35 E. Mindell, R.Ph., Ph.D. *Earl Mindell's Herb Bible,* p 102, 103

36 R. Sahelian, M.D. "Gymnema," Gymnema and diabetes, gymnema and blood sugar. Available: http://www.raysahelian.com/gymnema.html, p. 1-2 (accessed 2005, Jan. 3)

37 Ibid., p. 1-2

38 Ibid., p. 3

39 Ibid.

39a "Gymnema Sylvestre for Diabetes," Brain Wave Entrainment Technology, Available: http://intelegen.com/nutrients/gymnema_sylvestre_for_diabetes.htm, p. 1 © Vitamin Research Products, Inc., 2001, (accessed 2005, Jan 3)

39b Ibid., p. 1-2

40 Moss, p. 160-161

41 "Medical Conditions," Cancer Prevention website, "Botanicals." Available: http://www.naturalopinion.com. Copyright 1998 - 2005 by L. Vicky Crouse, N.D. and James S. Reiley, N.D...(ISSN 1527-0661), (accessed 2005, Feb. 2)

42 Moss, p. 162, 163

43 Ibid.

44 Gavin Phillips. "The Cancer Racket...The Hoxsey Remedies." Available: http://www.getipm.com/personal/cancer-racket.htm., p. 4-6 (accessed 2005, May 24)

44a Chowka, Peter, "Suzanne Somers' Use of Mistletoe," "Actress Suzanne Somers chooses an alternative therapy to treat her breast cancer © By Peter Chowka (April 1, 2001), Available: http://store.yahoo.com/annieappleseedproject/suzsomuseofm.html, (accessed 2005, Jul. 4) Used with their permission.

45 Antol, p. 162, 163

46 Ibid.

47 Ibid., p. 163

48 "Cancer and Immunity," DrLam.com, "Immune Building Agents," "Olive Leaf," An Insider's Guide to Natural Medicine. Available: http://www.drlam.com/A3R_brief_in_doc_format/cancer_and_immunity.cfm., (accessed 2004, sept. 27)

49 Ibid.

[50] Antol, p. 175, 177

[51] "Parsley," Herbs2000.com. Available:
http://www.herbs2000.com/herbs/herbs_parsley.htm, p. 2 (accessed 2004, Oct. 28)

[51a] Dr. J. Heinerman. *Healing Power of Herbs*, Boca Raton, FL: *Globe Digests™*, Globe
Communications Corp., 1995, p. 79-80

[52] Ibid.

[53] Ibid., p. 80

[54] L. B. White, M.D., S. Foster and the staff of Herbs for Health. *The Herbal Drugstore -
The Best Natural Alternatives to Over-the-Counter and Prescription Medicines!*
(City, State,n.g.) Rodale, Inc., 2000, p, 51, 60, 442

[55] Ibid.

[56] Ibid., p. 164

[56a] Antol, p.188-190

[57] Ibid.

[57a] "Triptolide," Alternative Cancer Therapies, Wellness Directory of Minnesota™.
Available: http://www.mnwelldir.org/docs/cancer1/altthrpy3.htm,p. 1 (accessed 2004,
Oct. 21)

[58] Ibid.

[59] "Aspilia," herbs2000.com. Available:
http://www.herbs2000.com/herbs/herbs_aspilia.htm, p. 2 (accessed 2004, Oct. 16)

[60] Ibid.

[60a] D. Gary Young, "New Discovery on the Chinese Wolfberry," Special Health Advisory
on Immunity and Anti-Aging, Aroma-Essence.com. Available: http://www.aro-
maessence.com/research-reports/chinese-wolfberry.html, p. 12 (accessed 2004, Oct.
17)

[61] Ibid.

[62] Ibid., p. 2

[63] Ibid.

[64] "*Berry Young Juice* Advantages." Available: http://www.aromanotes.com/87/berry-
young/ p. 1-2, (accessed 2004, Oct. 17)

[65] "Lycium Berries (Wolf Berries)," Available: http://www.spectrumwellbeing.co.uk/lyci-
um.htm, p. 1 (accessed 2004, Dec. 18)

[66] "Xi Shu," Herbs2000.com. Available:
http://www.herbs2000.com/herbs/herbs_xi_shu.htm, p. 2 (accessed 2004, Oct. 28)

[67] Ibid.

Chapter 19

[1] S.T. Sinatra, M.D. *Coenzyme Q10 and the Heart*, New York: the McGraw-Hill
Companies, 1999, p. 10. Reproduced with permission of the McGraw-Hill
Companies

[2] Ibid., p. 10

[3] Ibid., p. 11, 12

[4] Ibid., p. 30

[5] R.D. Strand, M.D., with D. K. Wallace. Nashville, TN: *What Your Doctor Doesn't Know
About Nutritional Medicine May Be Killing You,* Thomas Nelson Publishers, 2002, p.
81

[6] L. Keegan, Ph.D., R.N., Albany, N.Y: p. 97. From *Healing Nutrition* 2nd Edition by KEE-GAN, © 2002. Reprinted with permission of Delmar Learning, a division of Thomson Learning: www.thomsonrights.com. Fax 800 730-2215.

[6a] Ibid.

[7] Ibid.

[8] Ibid., p. 10

[9] S.T. Sinatra, M.D. *Coenzyme Q10 and the Heart*, New York: the McGraw-Hill Companies, 1999, p. 35. Reproduced with permission of the McGraw-Hill Companies

[10] Ibid.

[11] Ibid., p. 24

[12] Ibid., p. 25-27

[13] Sinatra, p. 11

[14] Ibid.

[15] Ibid., p. 49

[16] J. F. Balch, M.D. From *The Super Anti-Oxidants Why They Will Change The Face of Healthcare in the 21st Century,* copyright © 1998, by James F. Balch. Reprinted by the permission of the publisher, M. Evans & Company, New York, p. 136, 137, 142

[17] Ibid., p. 136, 137, 142

[17a] Strand, p. 67

[18] Ibid., p. 67-68

[19] R.W. Moss. *Antioxidants against Cancer*, State College, PA: Equinox Press, Inc., 2000, 2002, p. 69

[20] H. Winter Griffith, M.D. *VITAMINS Herbs, Minerals & Supplements The Complete Guide,* Revised Edition, (City, State n.g.) Perseus (Fisher Books), 1988, 1998, p. 154

[20a] "Kiwi Fruit," The World's Healthiest Foods: Feeling Great, George Mateljan Foundation, Whfoods.com. Available: http://www.whfoods.com/genpagephp?tname=foodspice&dbid=41 p. 2-3, (Accessed 2004, dec. 17)

[21] M. Stengler, N.D. p. 108 *The Natural Physician's Healing Therapies* by Mark Stengler, N.D. copyright © 2001 by Mark Stengler. Used by permission of Avery Publishing, an imprint of Penguin Group (USA) Inc.

[22] Ibid., p. 56-57

[22a] Stengler, p. 56-57

[22b] J. D. Krystosik, D.C. *Nature's Prescription for Over 60 Diseases – Grape Seed and Pine Bark Extract. (The prior title of this book was Pycnogenols-Pine Bark (OPC's) Grape Seed (OPC's) "Super Antioxidants."* Garrettsville, OH., Good News Press, 1995, p. 6

[23] Ibid.

[24] Ibid., p. 1

[24a] Krystosik., p. 1, 2

[25] Ibid.

[26] Ibid., p. 3, 16

[27] Ibid., p. 16, 17

[28] Krystosik, p. 34

[29] Ibid., p. 15-16

[30] R. Elkins, M.H. *Cat's Claw (Uno de Gato),* Pleasant Grove, UT: Woodland Publishing, Inc., 1995, p. 17

[31] Ibid., p. 24

[32] "Cat's Claw," "Side Effects and Cautions," herbs2000.com. Available: http://www.herbs2000.com/herbs/herbs_cats_claw.htm., p. 3 (accessed 2004, Dec. 21)

[33] J. F. Balch, M.D. From *The Super Anti-Oxidants: Why They Will Change the Face of Healthcare in the 21st Century,* copyright © 1998, by James F. Balch. Reprinted by the permission of the publisher, M. Evans & Company, New York, p. 115

[33a] "100% Science. Pure Juice," POM Wonderful Health. Available: http://www.pomwonderful.com/health.asp?source=google&kw=antioxidant, p. 1 (accessed 2004, Dec. 26)

[34] Ibid.

[35] Balch, p. 120

[36] M. Kennedy Salaman, Menlo Park, CA: *How To Renew You,* MKS, Inc. p. 138

[37] R. W Moss., Ph.D. *Antioxidants against Cancer,* Equinox Press, Inc., 2000, 2002, p. 15

[38] "Seven Essentials," Healthy-Living.org. Available: http://www.healthyliving.org/html/essential_seven.html, (accessed 2004, Dec. 21)

[39] "ORAC Values Of Fruits & Vegetables." Available: http://www.youngagain.com/orac.html, (Accessed 2004, Dec. 22)

[40] B. Berkson, M.D., Ph.D. From *The Alpha Lipoic Acid Breakthrough* copyright © 1998 by Burt Berkson. Used by permission of Prima Publishing, a division of Random House, Inc., (Quote from the cover of the book)

[41] Moss, *Antioxidants against Cancer,* p. 67

[42] Ibid., p. 67

[43] B. Berkson, M.D., Ph.D., p. 11, 13, XV

[44] Ibid., p. 14

[44a] Ibid., p. 102, 103

[45] Ibid.

[46] Moss, *Antioxidants against Cancer,* p. 61, 62

[47] Ibid., p. 62

[48] Editors of Prevention Health Books, *Prevention's Healing with Vitamins,* (City, State, n.g.) Rodale, 1996, p. 371

[48a] S. Gursche. From the book *Fantastic Flax, A Powerful Defense Against Cancer, Heart Disease and Digestive Disorders*: with permission from Alive Publishing Group, Inc., Canada. www.alive.com, <http://www.alive.com> p. 20, 22, 26

[49] "Cancer Fighting Foods and Spices," The Cancer Cure Foundation. Available: http://www.cancure.org/cancer_fighting_foods.htm, (accessed 2005, Jan 3)

[50] Moss, *"Antioxidants against Cancer,* p. 62

[51] Ibid.

[52] Moss, p. 63

[53] Beth M. Ley, Ph.D. *Bilberry & Lutein the Vision Enhancers,* BL Publications, 2001, p. 16-20

[54] M. Kennedy Salaman. *All Your Health Questions Answered Naturally*, (City, State, n.g.) MKS, Inc., 1998, p. 766

[55] Ibid., p. 769

[56] "NINDS Adrenoleukodystrophy Information page." National Institute of Neurological Disorders & Stroke. Available: http://www.ninds.nih.gov/disorders/adrenoleukodystrophy/adrenoleukodystrophy.htm (accessed 2005, May 14)

[57] Ibid.

[58] "Lorenzo's oil for adrenoleukodystrophy and adrenomyeloneuropathy," Bandolier, "Evidence based thinking about health care," "Lorenzo's oil for AMN and ALD." Available: http://www.jr2.ox.ac.uk/bandolier/booth/neurol/lorenz.html, (accessed 2005, Jan 22), © 1994-2005

[59] Ibid.

[60] Salaman, *All Your Health Questions Answered Naturally,* p. 784-785

[61] Ibid., p. 784-785, 787

[62] H. Winter Griffith, M.D. *Vitamins Herbs, Minerals & Supplements The Complete Guide,* Revised Edition, (City, State, n.g.) Perseus (Fisher Books), 1988, 1998, p. 40

[63] Salaman, p. 784-785, 787

[64] Ibid., p. 397-398

[65] D. Colbert, M.D. *Walking in Divine Health*, Siloam, 1999, p. 49-50

Chapter 20

[1] B. Berkson, M.D., Ph.D. From *The Alpha Lipoic Acid Breakthrough,* copyright © 1998 by Burt Berkson. Used by permission of Prima Publishing, a division of Random House, Inc., p. 69

[1a] J. Challem. *All About Carotenoids Beta-carotene, Lutein & Lycopene*, Avery's FAQs Series, Garden City Park, N.Y: Avery Publishing Group 1999, p. 7, 8, quotes reprinted with Mr. Challem's permission.

[2] Ibid.

[3] Ibid., p. 19

[3a] Challem, p. 19, 20

[4] Ibid.

[5] Ibid., p. 24

[6] Ibid., p. 22, 34, 36, 38, 39

[7] Ibid., p. 39-40

[8] H.Winter Griffith, M.D. *VITAMINS Herbs, Minerals & Supplements The Complete Guide*, Revised Edition, (City, State, n.g.) Perseus (Fisher Books), 1988, 1998, p. 28

[9] Ibid., p. 28-29

[10] H. W. Tietze. *Papaya The Healing Fruit*, with permission from Alive Publishing Group, Inc. Canada. www.alive.com http://www.alive.com 2000, p. 16

[10a] Ibid., p. 16

[11] Ibid.

[12] Ibid., p. 17 (From Andrea Ehring, author of *Das Krebsheilmittel Der Aborigines: (Papaya: The Cancer Healing Remedy of the Aborigines.)*

[13] Ibid., p. 14, 19

[14] Tietze, p. 5, 8, 9, 19

[14a] Ibid., p. 21, 26

[15] Ibid.

[16] S.Yeager and the Editors of *Prevention* Health Books. *Doctor's Book Of Food Remedies,* Rodale, Inc., 1998, p. 538, 539

[17] Ibid., p. 539

[18] Ibid., p. 20

[18a] "Paw Paw Alternative Cancer Treatment." Available: http://alternativecancer.us/pawpaw.htm p. 1 (accessed 2004, Dec. 14)

[19] Ibid.

[20] Ibid., p. 2, 5-6

[21] Ibid., p. 6, 8

[22] Yeager, et al., p. 539

[23] Ibid., p. 416-417

[24] C. Rivers. *Manna from Heaven - Healing Foods From The Bible,* Boca Raton, FL. and New York, N.Y. *Globe Digests*™, American Media Mini Mags, Inc., 2002, p. 52-53

[24a] Challem, p. 67-69

[25] Ibid.

[26] Ibid., p. 69

[27] Ibid., p. 70

[27a] Rivers, p. 23-24

[28] Ibid., p. 27

[28a] Yeager, p. 33, 35-36

[29] Ibid., p. 45-46

[30] Ibid., p. 59-60

[31] Yeager, p. 94-95

[31a] Ibid., p. 98, 101

[31b] Ibid.

[32] Ibid.

[32a] Yeager, p. 129-131

[32b] Ibid.

[33] Ibid.

[33a] R. Elkins, M.H. *Chinese Red Yeast Rice*, Pleasant Grove, UT: Woodland Publishing, 1998, p. 5, 17

[34] Ibid.

[35] "Food sources of Lysine." From the "Lysine Amino Acid Information page." Zest for Life Supplements webpage. Available: http: //www.anyvitamins.com/lysine-info.htm (accessed 2005, Jan. 26)

[36] E. Cheraskin, M.D., D.M.D. *Vitamin C Who Needs It?* Birmingham, AL: Arlington Press & Company, 1993, p. 159, 160

[37] "Essential Fatty Acids." Available: http://www.absolutelythepurest.com/other%20parts/essentialfattyacids.html, p. 1, (accessed 2005, Jan 23)

[38] Ibid., p. 1

[39] R. W. Moss, Ph.D. *Cancer Therapy - The Independent Consumer's Guide To Non-Toxic Treatment & Prevention,* New York: Equinox Press, 1992, p. 217-218

[40] Ibid.

[41] Ibid., p. 218

[42] Ibid., p. 219-220

Chapter 21

[1] J. R. Lee, M.D., David Zava, Ph.D., and Virginia Hopkins. *What Your Doctor May Not Tell You About Breast Cancer - How Hormone Balance Can Help Save Your Life*, New York: Warner Books, Inc., 2002, p. 182 - From *What Your Doctor May Not Tell You About ™: Breast Cancer* by John R. Lee, M.D., copyright © 2002 by John R. Lee, M. D., Virginia Hopkins, M.A., and David T. Zava, Ph.D., by permission of Warner Books, Inc.

[1a] J. R. Lee, M.D. with Virginia Hopkins. *What Your Doctor May Not Tell You About Menopause The Breakthrough Book on Natural Progesterone*, New York: Warner Books, Inc., 1996, p. 34-35, 37. From *What Your Doctor May Not Tell You About Menopause* by John Lee, M.D., Copyright © 1996 by John R. Lee, M.D., and Virginia Hopkins. By Permission of Warner Books, Inc.

[1b] Ibid.

[2] Ibid.

[3] Ibid., p. 35

[4] "Problems Associated with Early Puberty - Cancer Alternatives." Available: http://www.alkalizeforhealth.net/earlymenarchy.htm, p. 1 (accessed 2004, Dec. 16)

[5] Lee, et al., *What Your Doctor May Not Tell You About Breast Cancer,* p. 136

[6] Ibid., p. 136

[6a] Lee, et al., *What Your Doctor May Not Tell You About Menopause*, p. 36-37,

[6b] Ibid.

[7] Ibid.

[8] Lee, et al., *What Your Doctor May Not Tell You About Breast Cancer*, p. 105

[9] Ibid., p. 99-101

[10] "Effects of Estrogen Dominance," Diagnose-Me Condition: "Progesterone Low or Estrogen Dominance," Available: http://www.diagnoseme.com/cond/C8779.html, p. 1 (accessed 2004, Dec. 24)

[11] Lee, et al., *What Your Doctor May Not Tell You About Breast Cancer* p. 99-101

[12] Lee, et al., *What Your Doctor May Not Tell You About Menopause*, p. 25, 26

[13] Ibid., p. 34

[14] R.D. Strand, M.D., with Donna K. Wallace. *What Your Doctor Doesn't Know About Nutritional Medicine May Be Killing You*, Nashville, TN., Thomas Nelson Publishers®, 2002, p. 115

[15] Catherine P. Rollins, "Estrogen Dominance Linked to Cancer," "Synthetic HRT and Cancer." Available: http://www.natural-progesterone-advisory-network.com/estrogen-dominance-linked-to-cancer.htm (accessed 2004, Dec. 24) Copyright © 2005 Making Plans Pty Ltd. All Rights Reserved.

[16] Ibid.

[16a] Lee, et al., *What Your Doctor May Not Tell You About Breast Cancer*, p. 141-142

[17] Ibid.

[18] C. Norman Shealy, M.D., Ph.D. *Natural Progesterone Cream*, New York: McGraw-Hill Companies, 1999, p. 31, reproduced with permission of the McGraw-Hill Companies.

[19] Lee, et al., *What Your Doctor May Not Tell You About Breast Cancer*, p. 142

[20] "Estrogen Information Summary." From the National Institute of Neurological Disorders and Stroke, "Estrogen." Available: http://www.ninds.nih.gov/funding/research/parkinsonsweb/drug_ summaries/estrogen.htm (accessed 2005, May 27)

[21] Lee, et al., *What Your Doctor May Not Tell You About Breast Cancer*, p. 143

[22] Ibid., p. 143-152

23 Ibid.

24 Ibid.

25 Ibid.

26 "What are the reasons to have a hysterectomy?" "When is a hysterectomy necessary?" SafeMenopauseSolutions.com. Available: http://www.safemenopausesolutions.com/hysterectomy.html, p. 2, (accessed 2004, Nov. 9) Copyright © Personal Wellness Network, Inc. All rights reserved.

27 Lee, et al., *What Your Doctor May Not Tell You About Breast Cancer,* Warner Books, 2002, p. 153 - From *What Your Doctor May Not Tell You About ™: Breast Cancer* by John R. Lee, M.D., copyright © 2002 by John R. Lee, M. D., Virginia Hopkins, M.A., and David T. Zava, Ph.D., by permission of Warner Books, Inc.

28 Ibid., p. 159

29 "Provera Side Effects, and Drug Interactions - Medroxyprogesterone Acetate - RxList Mon…" Side Effects. Available: http://www.rxlist.com/cgi/generic/medrox_ad.htm, p. 1-4 (accessed 2005, Jan 24)

29a Lee, et al., *What Your Doctor May Not Tell You About Breast Cancer*, p. 105

30 Ibid.

31 "HRT Comes With Serious Risks and Side Effects," SafeMenopauseSolutions.com. Available: http://www.safemenopausesolutions.com/hrt.html, p. 2 (accessed 2004, Nov. 9) Copyright © Personal Wellness Network, Inc. All rights reserved.

32 Ibid., p. 3

33 C. Norman Shealy, M.D., Ph.D. *Natural Progesterone Cream*, New York: McGraw-Hill Companies, 1999, p. 12, reproduced with permission of the McGraw-Hill Companies.

34 Ibid.

35 "Natural Progesterone," "Other Possible Side Effects." With permission: AltMedDex® System: Klasco RK (Ed): AltMedDex® System: Thomson Micromedex, Greenwood Village, Colorado (2005, Jan. 24)

36 Ibid.

37 Ibid.

38 "Are There Any Natural Progesterone Side Effects?" Available: http://www.safe-menopausesolutions.com/progesteronesideeffects.html. (accessed 2005, Jun. 3) © Personal Wellness Network, Inc. All rights reserved.

39 Lee, et al., *What Your Doctor May Not Tell You About Breast Cancer*, p. 158-159

40 M. Kennedy Salaman. *How To Renew You*, Menlo Park, CA: MKS, Inc., 2003, p. 116

41 Ibid., p. 116

42 Lee, et al., *What Your Doctor May Not Tell You About Menopause,* p. 272

43 "Effects of Estrogen Dominance," Diagnose-Me: Condition: Progesterone Low or Estrogen Dominance. Available: http:www.diagnose-me.com/cond/C8779.html., (accessed 2004, Dec. 24)

44 Ibid.

45 Lee, et al., *What You Doctor May Not Tell You About Menopause*, Ibid., p. 269-271

46 Ibid., p. 271-272

47 Lee, et al., *What Your Doctor May Not Tell You About Menopause*, p. 44

48 Ibid.

49 Lee, et al., *What Your Doctor May Not Tell You About Menopause*, p. 102

50 Ibid., p. 259

[51] Lee, et al., *What Your Doctor May Not Tell You About Menopause*, p. 161

[52] Ibid., p. 272-277

[53] Ibid., p. 278

[53a] Ibid.

[54] Ibid.

[55] Ibid., p. 277-278

[55a] Migraine." Available: http://www.mcvitamins.com/migraine.htm, (accessed 2004, Dec. 24)

[56] "Ibid.

[57] "Saliva vs. Serum or Plasma Testing For Progesterone," Special Report from the John R. Lee, M.D. Medical Letter, Saliva Hormone Testing, Available: http://www.johnleemd.com/store/saliva_serum.html, p.2 (accessed 2004, Dec. 24)

[57a] Ibid.

[58] Ibid.

[58a] Ibid.

[58b] Ibid.

[59] Ibid.

[59a] "Saliva vs. Serum…"

[60] Ibid.

[61] Lee, et al., *What Your Doctor May Not Tell You About Menopause*, p.69

[61a] "Saliva vs. Serum…"

[61b] Ibid.

[62] Ibid.

[63] Ibid.

[64] Lee, et al., *What Your Doctor May Not Tell You About Breast Cancer,* p.7

[65] Ibid., p. 8

[66] Ibid., p. 25

[67] Ibid., p. 16

[67a] Lee, et al., *What Your Doctor May Not Tell You About Menopause*, p. 289

[68] Ibid.

[69] C. P. Rollins, "Is Natural Progesterone Safe?" Available: www.natural-progesterone-advisory-network.com/is-natural-progesterone-safe.htm, (accessed 2004, Nov. 9) Copyright © 2005 Making Plans Pty Ltd. All Rights Reserved.

[69a] Lee, et al., *What Your Doctor May Not Tell You About Breast Cancer*, p. 18

[70] Ibid.

[71] Ibid., p. 166

[71a] Lee, et al., *What Your Doctor May Not Tell You About Breast Cancer,* p. 166

[72] Ibid.

[73] C. P. Rollins, "Can Progesterone Help Alleviate Autoimmune Disorders Like Hashimoto's Disease, Graves Disease, Multiple Sclerosis or Lupus?' "Estrogens." Available: http://www.natural-progesterone-advisory-network.com/News/article040622-3.htm, Copyright © 2002-04, Making Plans Pty Ltd., p. 1 (accessed 2004, Dec. 24)

[74] R. Elkins, M.H. *Natural Alternatives to HRT,* Orem, UT: Woodland Publishing, 2003, p.23-24

[75] Lee, et al., *What Your Doctor May Not Tell You About Menopause*, p. 253

[76] Ibid., p. 155

[77] Ibid., p. 158

[78] Ibid., p. 159, 160

[79] Elkins, p. 28

[80] Ibid.

[81] F. Murray. *Remifemin: Herbal Relief for Menopausal Symptoms,* New York: McGraw-Hill Companies, 1996, p. 22-23. Reproduced with permission of McGraw-Hill Companies.

[82] Ibid.

[83] Salaman, p. 121

[84] Ibid., p. 123

[85] Ibid., p. 90

[86] Elkins, p. 30

[87] Elkins, p. 30-34

[88] Ibid.

Chapter 22

[1] F. Batmanghelidj, M.D. *Your Body's Many Cries For Water,* Vienna, VA: Global Health Solutions, Inc., 1992, 1995,1997, p. 115

[1a] S. Meyerowitz. *Water The Ultimate Cure,* Great Barrington, MA: S. Meyerowitz, 2000, 2001, p. 14

[2] J. Yiamouyiannis, website www.health-science.com., "Fluoride Toxicity, Immune System and Aging." Available: http://www.health-science.com/fluoride_toxicity.html, © 1995-2004 Health & Science Research Institute, U.S.A., p. 2 (accessed 2004, Nov. 9)

[3] Ibid.

[3a] Batmanghelidj, p. 179-180

[4] Ibid.

[5] Ibid., p. 10, 25, 28

[6] Ibid., p. 31-35

[6a] Ibid.

[7] Ibid.

[8] Batmanghelidj, p. 31-35

[9] Ibid., p. 41

[10] Ibid., p. 122, 166, 169

[10a] Batmanghelidg, p. 115-116

[10b] Ibid.

[11] Ibid.

[12] Ibid., p. 119

[13] M. Fox. "Multiple Sclerosis Testimonials," Dr. F. Batmanghledj's website. Available: http://www.watercure2.org, (accessed 2005, Mar. 22) Reprinted with permission from Mr. Bob Butts at above website.

[14] Batmanghelidj, p. 120

[15] Ibid., p. 120

[15a] Ibid., p. 122

[16] Ibid.

[16a] Batmanghelidj, p. 49

[17] Ibid.

[17a] Ibid.

17b M. Fox. "Multiple Sclerosis Testimonials," Dr. F. Batmanghledj's website. Available: http://www.watercure2.org, (accessed 2005, Mar. 22) Reprinted with permission from Mr. Bob Butts at above website.

17c Ibid.

17d Ibid.

18 Ibid.

18a Batmanghelidj, p. 60

19 Batmanghelidg, p. 71

20 Ibid., p. 75

21 Ibid., p. 76

21a S. Meyerowitz. *Water The Ultimate Cure*, Great Barrington, MA: S. Meyerowitz, 2000, 2001, p. 14

22 Batmanghelidj, p. 161

23 S. Meyerowitz, p. 14, 18

24 Batmanghelidj, p. 161

25 Ibid., p. 161-162

26 Meyerowitz, Ibid., p. 13

27 Ibid., p. 9 (From the introduction by Dr. Batmanghelidj in *Water The Ultimate Cure*)

28 Ibid., p. 20

28a Ibid., p. 23

29 Ibid.

29a J. F. Balch, M.D. From *The Super Anti-oxidants: Why They Will Change the Face of Healthcare in the 21st Century*, copyright © 1998, by James F. Balch. Reprinted by the permission of the publisher, M. Evans & Company, New York, p. 253-254

30 Ibid.

31 V. Saxion. *How To Feel Great All The Time*, Little Rock, AR: Lions Head Publishing, 2002, p. 58

32 Meyerowitz, p. 51

32a J. R. Lee, M.D., with Virginia Hopkins. *What Your Doctor May Not Tell You About Menopause*, New York: Warner Books, Inc., 1996, p. 297. From What Your Doctor May Not Tell You About Menopause by John Lee, M.D., Copyright © 1996 by John R. Lee, M.D., and Virginia Hopkins. By Permission of Warner Books, Inc.

33 Ibid.

34 Ibid., p. 298

Chapter 23

1 D. Colbert, M.D. *Walking in Divine Health*, Lake Mary, FL: Siloam, Strang Communications Co., 1999, p. 58

2 A. Wigmore. *The Wheatgrass Book*, (City, State, n.g.) Avery, 1985, p. 57

3 Ibid.

4 C. LeBeau. *Hydrogen Peroxide & Ozone, 13th Edition*, West Allis, WI: Vital Health Publications, 2001, p. 11

5 Ibid.

6 Ibid.

7 Ibid., p. 11

8 Ibid., p. 12, 19

[9] V. Saxion. *How To Feel Great All The Time*, Little Rock, AR: Lions Head Publishing, 2002, p. 50, 52

[10] M. Kennedy Salaman. *How To Renew You*, Menlo Park, CA: MKS, Inc., 2003, p. 177-179

[11] Ibid.

[12] J. Mercola, M.D. "Sunlight Actually Prevents Cancer," www.mercola.com. Available: http://www.mercola.com/2002/apr/3/sun_prevents_cancer.htm, p. 1 (accessed 2004, Nov. 12)

[13] Ibid.

[14] Ibid.

[15] Mercola., p. 2-3

[16] Ibid.

[17] Ibid.

[18] Mercola, p. 2

[19] Ibid., p. 3

[20] H. Winter Griffith, M.D. *Vitamins Herbs, Minerals & Supplements The Complete Guide, Revised Edition*, (City, State, n.g.) Perseus (Fisher Books), 1988, 1998, p. 42

[21] Mercola, p. 2-3

[22] Ibid.

[23] C. Ryan, BBC News, "Sunshine 'Prevents Cancer," Website: The Greatest Herbs On Earth™ Available: http://www.greatestherbsonearth.com/articles/sunshine_prevents_cancer.htm, p. 1 (2004, Nov. 12)

[24] Ibid., p. 2

[25] Ibid., p. 2

Chapter 24

[1] "Newsletter Aug 2001," Wellness Directory of Minnesota™. Available: http://www.mnwelldir.org/docs/Newsletters/01_Aug.htm (accessed 2004, Dec. 18)

[2] "Agaricus Blazei Murill," Newsletter Aug 2001. Available: http://www.mnwelldir.org/docs/Newsletters/01_Aug.htm Wellness Directory of Minnesota™ (accessed 2004, Dec. 18)

[3] "Agaricus," Alternative Cancer Therapies, Wellness Directory of Minnesota™. Available: http://www.mnwelldir.org/docs/cancer1/altthrpy.htm, (accessed 2004, Oct. 28)

[3a] Ibid.

[4] Ibid.

[4a] Ibid.

[5] Ibid.

[6] K. Gilbert Udall. *Cordyceps Sinensis Immune and Stamina Booster*, Pleasant Grove, UT: Woodland Publishing, 2000, p. 9, 11-12

[7] Ibid., p. 12-13

[7a] Reader's Digest, *The Healing Power of Vitamins, Minerals, and Herbs*, Pleasantville, New York/Montreal, 1999, 2000, p. 332-333, The Reader's Digest Association, Inc. Quoted with permission of Global Books & Home Entertainment, The Reader's Digest Association, Inc.

[8] Ibid.

[9] R. Wood, "Mushrooms Detoxify," Kitchen Coaching, Healing With Food, Food as Medicine, Mushrooms Detoxify. Available: http://www.rwood.com/Articles/Mushrooms_Detoxify.htm, p. 2 (accessed 2004, Oct. 17)

[10] G., Ph.D. *The Complete Encyclopedia of Natural Healing*, New York, N.Y., Kensington Publishing Corp, © 2000, 2001, 2002, p. 81. All rights reserved. Reprinted by arrangement with Kensington Publishing Corp., www.kensingtonbooks.com.

[11] "Hoelen," herbs2000.com. Available: http://www.herbs2000.com/herbs/herbs_hoelen.htm, p. 1-2 (accessed 2005, Jan. 22)

[12] M. Lam, M.D. "Medicinal Mushrooms," website: Dr. Lam.com, "Cancer and Immunity," Available: www.drlam.com/A3R_brief_in_doc_format/cancer_and_immunity.cfm, p. 20-21, © 2002, Michael Lam, M.D. (accessed 2004, Sept. 27)

[13] R. W. Moss, Ph.D. *Cancer Therapy: The Independent Consumer's Guide To Non-Toxic Treatment and Prevention*, New York: Equinox Press, 1992, p. 247

[14] B. Gottlieb. *Alternative Cures*, (City, State, n.g.) Rodale, Inc., 2000, p. 165

[15] S. Yeager, and the Editors of Prevention Health Books. *Doctor's Book of Food Remedies*, (City, State, n.g.) Rodale, Inc., 1998, p. 366-367

[16] Wood, p. 2

[17] R. W. Moss, Ph.D. "A Reply to Dr. Klausner: Natural Products Should be Tested First Against Cancer," from The Cancer Chronicles #29 © Sept. 1995 by Ralph W. Moss, Ph.D., "Landmark Study," Ralph Moss on Cancer - Expert Guidance for Crucial Decisions. Available: http://www.ralphmoss.com/html/try.shtml, (accessed 2005, Feb. 2)

[18] D. Tenney. *Medicinal Mushrooms, Cancer Fighters and Immunity Enhancers*, 1997, Pleasant Grove, UT: Woodland Publishing, Inc., p. 15-16

[19] Ibid, p. 18

[20] E. Mindell, R.Ph., Ph.D. *Earl Mindell's Soy Miracle*, New York, p. 106. Reprinted with permission from Simon & Schuster Adult Publishing Group, from EARL MINDELL'S SOY MIRACLE by Earl Mindell, R.Ph., Ph.D. © 1995 by Earl Mindell, R.Ph.,Ph.D, and Carol Colman.

[21] Lam, "Medicinal Mushrooms," p. 9

[22] J. Carper. *The Food Pharmacy, Dramatic New Evidence That Food Is Your Best Medicine*, New York: Bantam Books, 1988, p. 235

[23] Yeager, p. 366

[24] Moss, *Cancer Therapy*, p. 424

[25] Wood, p. 2

Chapter 25

[1] R. Morse, N.D. *The Detox Miracle Sourcebook*, Prescott, AZ: Hohm Press, 2004, p. 112

[2] F. A. Oski, M.D. *Don't Drink Your Milk! New Frightening Medical Facts About The World's Most Overrated Nutrient*, Brushton, N.Y.: Teach Services, Inc., 1996, p. 46 - Translated from the book, "Don't Drink Your Milk!" Copyright © 1996 by TEACH Services, Inc. Published by: TEACH Services, Inc. 254 Donovan Rd. Brushton, New York 12916 518/358-3494

[3] Ibid., p. 50

[4] H. Winter Griffith. *Vitamins Herbs, Minerals & Supplements The Complete Guide, Revised Edition*, (City, State, n.g.) Perseus (Fisher Books), 1988, 1998, p. 73

[5] D. Lee. *Juicing: Your Liquid Nutritional Supplement*, Pleasant Grove, UT: Woodland Publishing, 1998, p. 25

[6] M. Kennedy Salaman. *How To Renew You*, Menlo Park, CA: MKS, Inc, 2003, p. 122

[7] "Raw Dairy Sales Illegal in Manhattan," HSI Health Sciences Institute, "The Milkman Cometh," Available: http://www.hsiealert.com/ealerts/ea200412/ea20041222.html, p. 3 (accessed 2004, Dec. 30) and also rec'd as email on 12-22-04 from HSIResearch@healthiernews.com

[8] Oski, p. 51, 57

[9] Ibid., p. 53-54

[10] Ibid.

[11] Oski., p. 53-54

[12] Ibid., p. 54

[13] Ibid., p. 54-55

[14] J. R. Lee, M.D., David Zava, Ph.D., and Virginia Hopkins. *What Your Doctor May Not Tell You About Breast Cancer How Hormone Balance Can Help Save Your Life*, New York: Warner Books, 2002, p. 39-40 - From What Your Doctor May Not Tell You About ™: Breast Cancer by John R. Lee, M.D., copyright © 2002 by John R. Lee, M. D., Virginia Hopkins, M.A., and David T. Zava, Ph.D., by permission of Warner Books, Inc.

[15] M. Kennedy Salaman. *All Your Health Questions Answered Naturally*, (City, State, n.g.) MKS, Inc., 1998, p. 199

[16] Ibid.

[17] "Lactose Intake May Increase Ovarian Cancer Risk in Postmenopausal Women," HSI, Health Sciences Institute. Available: http://www.hsibaltimore.com/ealerts/ea200412/ea20041214. html p. 1-2 (accessed 2004, Dec. 30) Also rec'd. as an email alert 12/14/04 from HSI/Research@health-iernews.com

[18] Ibid.

[19] Salaman, *All Your Health Questions Answered Naturally*, p. 220

[20] J. R. Lee, M.D. with Virginia Hopkins. *What Your Doctor May Not Tell You About Menopause*, New York: Warner Books, Inc., 1996, p. 171, From What Your Doctor May Not Tell You About Menopause by John Lee, M.D., Copyright © 1996 by John R. Lee, M.D., and Virginia Hopkins. By Permission of Warner Books, Inc.

[21] R. Morse, N.D. *The Detox Miracle Sourcebook*, Prescott, AZ: Hohm Press, 2004, p. 110

[22] D. Lee. Juicing: *Your Liquid Nutritional Supplement*, Pleasant Grove, UT: Woodland Publishing, 1998, p. 23-24

[23] Ibid., p. 24

[24] Ibid., p. 25

[25] R. M. Kradjian, M.D. "The Milk Letter: A Message To My Patients," from Dr. Robert M. Kradjian, M.D. Breast Surgery Chief Div. of General Surgery, Seton Medical Centre #302 - 1800 Sullivan Ave. Daly City, CA 94015 USA. Available: http://www.notmilk.com/ Kradjian.html, "Dr. Kradjian Addresses Cow's Milk," (accessed 2005, Jan. 26)

[26] Ibid.

[27] B. Berkson, M.D., Ph.D. *From The Alpha Lipoic Acid Breakthrough*, copyright © 1998 by Burt Berkson. Used by permission of Prima Publishing, a division of Random House, Inc., p.115

[28] G. Mirkin, M.D. "Breast Milk Prevents Childhood Diabetes?" Available: http://www.drmirkin.com/diabetes/D216.htm, p. 1 (accessed 2004, Nov. 12) Copyright © 2003, www.drmirkin.com

[29] Ibid.

[30] Kradjian, M.D. "The Milk Letter: A Message To My Patients."

[31] Ibid.

[32] R. L., Blaylock, M.D. *Natural Strategies For Cancer Patients*, New York: Twin Streams, Kensington Publishing Corp., © 2003, p. 242. All rights reserved. Reprinted by arrangement with Kensington Publishing Corp. www.kensingtonbooks.com

[33] Ibid.

[34] Ibid.

[35] Ibid.

[36] Kradjian, M.D. "The Milk Letter: A Message To My Patients."

[37] "Milk and Dairy," The Food Web, "Milk and Dairy Products," Available: http;//www.anarac.com/milk_and_dairy.htm, p. 2 (accessed 2004, Nov. 12) Anarac © 2000

[37a] "Vitamin D supplements to protect against MS," 03/01/2005. NUTRAingredients.com/europe Available: http://www.nutraingredients.com/news/news-ng.asp?n=56996-vitamin-d-supplements (accessed 2005, Jun. 23)

[38] E. D. Smith, "Effects of Homogenization and Pasteurization of Milk." Available: http://www.karlloren.com/aajonus/p1.htm (accessed 2004, Dec. 5)

[39] Ibid.

[40] Ibid.

[41] R. Morse, N.D. *The Detox Miracle Sourcebook*, Prescott, AZ: Hohm Press, 2004, p. 110

[42] Ibid., p. 111

[43] D. Colbert, M.D. *What You Don't Know May Be Killing You*, Lake Mary, FL: Siloam, A Strang Co, 2000, 2004, p. 120

[44] Ibid., p. 120

[45] Ibid., p. 111

[46] G. Null, Ph.D. *The Complete Encyclopedia of Natural Healing*, Kensington Publishing Corp., New York, N. Y. © 2000, 2001, 2002, p. 87-88. All rights reserved. Reprinted by arrangement with Kensington Publishing Corp., www.kensingtonbooks.com.

[47] Kradjian, M.D. "The Milk Letter: A Message To My Patients."

[48] Ibid.

Chapter 26

[1] I. Stone, Ph.D. "Vitamin C Quotes." From Whale website. Available: http://www.whale.to/w/quotes4.html (accessed 9 Jun. 2005)

[1a] A. Hoffer, M.D., F.R.C.P.(C), with L. Pauling, Ph.D. *Healing Cancer - Complementary Vitamin & Drug Treatments*, Toronto, Ontario Canada: CCNM Press, Inc., 2004, p. 16

[2] Ibid., p. 173

[2a] R. W. Moss, Ph.D. *Cancer Therapy: The Independent Consumer's Guide To Non-Toxic Treat ment & Prevention*, New York: Equinox Press, 1992, p. 195-196

[3] Ibid.

[4] L. Keegan, Ph.D., R.N. *Healing Nutrition, 2nd edition*, Albany, N. Y. Delmar, div. of Thomas Learning, Inc., 2002, p. 176

[5] Ibid.

[6] G. Null, Ph.D. *The Complete Encyclopedia of Natural Healing. Third Edition*, © 2000, 2001, 2002, New York, N.Y. Kensington Publishing Corp., p. 81. All rights reserved. Reprinted by arrangement with Kensington Publishing Corp., www.kensington-books.com

[7] Ibid.

[8] Dr. J. Mercola, "The Benefits of Probiotics 9/29/04," Dr. Joseph Mercola. Available: http://www.mercola.com/2004/sep/29/probiotics_benefits.htm, p. 1 (accessed 2004, Dec. 31)

[9] Ibid.

[10] Ibid., p. 1

[11] M. Walker, D.P.M., "Medical Journalist Report of Innovative Biologics," from the Townsend Letter For Doctors & Patients - Feb/Mar 2001, "Homeostatic Soil Organisms for One's Primal Defense." Available; http://www.vital-nutrients.com/drwalker_on_hsos_1.htm, p. 1 (accessed) 2004, Dec. 31)

[12] Ibid.

[13] Ibid.

[14] J. S. Rubin. *The Maker's Diet*, Lake Mary, FL: Siloam, A Strang Co., 2004, p. 68

[15] C. Scott and John Lust, *Naturopath. Crude Black Molasses, The Natural "Wonder-food,"* New York, N.Y: Benedict Lust Publications, 1980, 1992, p. 20.

[16] Scott, et al., p. 23-24

[17] Ibid.

[18] Ibid.

[18a] Ibid., p. 25, 26

[19] Ibid.

[20] Ibid., p. 81-82

[21] Scott, et al., p. 73

[22] Ibid., p. 12

[23] J. Carper. *The Food Pharmacy, Dramatic New Evidence That Food Is Your Best Medicine*, New York: Bantam Books, 1988, 1989, p. 64-66,

[24] Ibid.

[25] Ibid.

[26] Ibid., p. 67

[27] Ibid., p. 70

Chapter 27

[1] H. Kroeger. *Parasites The Enemy Within*, (City, State, n.g.) Hanna Kroeger Publications, 1991, p. 29

[2] H. Regehr Clark, Ph.D., N.D. *The Cure For All Cancers*, Chula Vista, CA: New Century Press, 1993, p. 1

[3] Ibid., p. 1

[4] Ibid., p. 96, 97

[5] Ibid., p. 97

[6] S. Ziff, M. F. Ziff, D.D.S. *Dentistry Without Mercury*, Orlando, FL: Bio-Probe, Inc., 1985, p. 34

[7] Ibid., p. 39

[8] Chark, H., p. 12-13

[9] Ibid., p. 13

[10] Clark, H., Ph.D., N.D. *The Cure For All Cancers*, Chula Vista, CA: New Century Press, 1993, p. 23

[11] A. L. Gittleman, M.S. *Natural Healing For Parasites*, New York: Healing Wisdom Publications, 1995, p. 4-5

[12] Gittleman, p. 5

[13] Ibid., p. 8

[14] Ibid.

[15] "Aspilia," herbs2000.com. Available: http://www.herbs2000.com/herbs/herbs_aspilia.htm, p. 1-2, (accessed 2004, Oct. 16)

[16] H. Kroeger, Ms.D. *Free Your Body of Tumors and Cysts*, (City, State, n.g.) Hanna Kroeger Publications, p. 43.

Chapter 28

[1] C. Wade. *Carlson Wade's New Fact/Book on Bee Pollen and Your Health*, New York: the McGraw Hill Companies, 1978, 1992, p. 39. Reproduced with permission of the McGraw Hill Companies

[2] Ibid., p. 22

[2a] Ibid., p. 23, 69-70

[2b] Ibid.

[3] Ibid.

[3a] M. Stengler, N.D. *The Natural Physician's Healing Therapies* by Mark Stengler, N.D. copyright © 2001 by Mark Stengler. Used by permission of Avery Publishing, an imprint of Penguin Group (USA) Inc., p. 59-60

[4] Ibid.

[5] J. Carper., *Miracle Cures: Dramatic New Scientific Discoveries Revealing the Healing Powers of Herbs, Vitamins, and Other Natural Remedies*, New York: Harper Collins Publishers, Inc., 1997, p. 143-144

[6] Wade, p. 24

[6a] C. Leigh Broadhurst, Ph.D. *Health and Healing with Bee Products*, with permission from Alive Publishing Group, Inc., Canada. www.alive.com http://www.alive.com 2000, p. 16

[7] Ibid.

[8] Wade, p. 81-82

[9] Wade, p. 22

[10] R. Elkins, M.H. *Bee Pollen Royal Jelly Propolis and Honey*, Pleasant Grove, UT: Woodland Publishing, 1996, p. 51

[11] Broadhurst, p. 33, 38

[12] Amy Norton. "Bee Products Fight Tumors in Mice, Study Shows," from Reuters Health Information, New York, Dec. 16, 2004. Reuters content is the intellectual property of Reuters Limited. Reprinted with their permission. Reuters shall not be liable for any errors or delays in content, or for any actions taken in reliance thereon. Article from "News" at www.cancerpage.com, 2000-2005. All rights reserved. Available: http://www.cancerpage.com/news/article.asp?id=7827, p. 1 (accessed 2004, Dec. 19)

[13] Norton, p. 1

[14] Broadhurst, p. 30

[15] Elkins, p. 7, 9

[16] Ibid., p. 12

[16a] Ibid., p. 36-37, 44

[17] Ibid.

[17a] Broadhurst, p. 23

[18] Ibid.

[19] Ibid., p. 29-30

[20] Elkins, p. 42

[21] J. Carper. *The Food Pharmacy*, New York: Bantam Books, 1988, 1989, p. 216-217

[22] Ibid., p. 218-219

Chapter 29

[1] R. O. Young., Ph.D., and S. Redford Young. *The pH Miracle Balance Your Diet, Reclaim Your Health*, New York: Warner Books, Inc., 2002, pp. 15-16 - From PH Miracle, The, by Robert Young, Ph.D., Copyright © 2002 by Robert Young, Ph.D., By Permission of Warner Books, Inc.

[1a] T. A. Baroody, N.D., D.C., Ph.D. *Nutrition, C.N.C., Alkalize or Die - Superior Health Through Proper Alkaline-Acid Balance*, Waynesville, N.C: Holographic Health Press, 1991, p. 18

[2] Ibid.

[3] Ibid., p. 19

[4] Young, et al., p. 15-16

[5] Ibid.

[6] Baroody, p. 22

[7] Ibid., p. 45-53

[8] Young, p. 134-136

[9] Ibid.

[10] Ibid.

[11] Ibid.

[12] H. W. Tietze. *Papaya The Healing Fruit*, with permission from Alive Publishing Group, Inc., Canada, www.alive.com, <http://www.alive.com> 2000, p. 12

[13] "Healing Cancer," Excerpt From a book by Robert Barefoot, *Death by Diet*, Available: http://www.cancer-healing.com/met_alkalize_diet.php (accessed 2005, Jan 3)

[14] Ibid.

[15] D. Colbert, M.D. *Toxic Relief*, Lake Mary, FL: Siloam, a Strang Co., 2001, 2003, p. 50, 51

Chapter 30

[1] G. Warner. "Alternative Medical Doctor Quotes." From Whale website. Available: http://www.whale.to/m/quotes6.html (accessed 2005, Jun. 9)

[2] S. Yeager and the Editors of Prevention Health Books. *Doctors Book of FOOD REMEDIES*, (City, State, n.g.), Rodale, Inc., 1998, p. 62, 63

3 "Preserving the living and the dead," New Agriculturist on-line - Reporting Agriculture for the 21st Century, "Spice Preservatives." Available: http://www.new-agri.co.uk/02-1/focuson/focuson8.html, p. 1 (accessed 2004, Dec. 20)

3a Ibid., p. 2

4 Ibid.

5 P. Schulick. *Ginger Common Spice & Wonder Drug*, Revised Edition, Brattleboro, VT: Herbal Free Press, Ltd., 1994, p. 16

6 Ibid., p. 31

7 Ibid., p. 32

8 Schulick, p. 34

8a Ibid., p. 52

9 Ibid.

10 Schulick, p. 59

11 "Geraniol," website earthnotes.tripod.com, "Health Conditions Starting with C and herbal remedies used to treat them." Available: http://www.earthnotes.tripod.com/ckbk_c.htm, p. 2, (accessed 2004, Oct. 16)

12 J. A. Duke with Michael Castleman. *The Green Pharmacy Anti-Aging Prescriptions*, (City, State, n.g.) Rodale, Inc., 2001, p. 93

13 "Horseradish," Herbs2000.com. Available: http://www.herbs2000.com/herbs/herbs_horse-radish.htm, p. 1-2, (accessed 2004, Dec. 5)

14 "Horseradish," p. 3

15 Ibid.

16 "Oil of Oregano," Cancer Tutor™ website. Available: http://www.cancertutor.com/OtherBig_List.htm, (accessed 2004, Dec. 1)

Chapter 31

1 J. A. Duke, Ph.D. *The Green Pharmacy, The Ultimate Compendium of Natural Remedies from the World's Foremost Authority on Healing Herbs*, New York: St. Martin's Paperbacks 1998, Rodale Press, Inc. 1997, p. 22

2 R. W. Moss, Ph.D. *Cancer Therapy: The Independent Consumer's Guide To Non-Toxic Treatment & Prevention*, New York: Equinox Press, 1992, p. 137, 138

3 Ibid., p. 138

4 Moss, p.139

5 Ibid., p. 139

6 M. Nadine Antol. *Healing Teas: How to Prepare and Use Teas to Maximize Your Health*, (City, State, n.g.) Avery, Penguin Group (USA), Inc., 1996, p. 122

7 E. Mindell, R.Ph., Ph.D. *Earl Mindell's Food as Medicine*, New York, p. 126. Reprinted with permission of Simon & Schuster Adult Publishing Group, from EARL MINDELL'S FOOD AS MEDICINE by Earl Mindell, R.Ph., Ph.D. © 1994 by Earl Mindell R.Ph., Ph.D., and Carol Colman

8 J. F. Balch, M.D. *From The Super Anti-Oxidants: Why They Will Change The Face of Healthcare in the 21st Century*, copyright © 1998, by James F. Balch. Reprinted by the permission of the publisher, M. Evans & Company, New York, p. 178-179

8a Ibid.

9 Ibid.

10 Antol, p. 70, 150

11 Ibid., p. 158

[12] J. A. Duke, Ph.D. *The Green Pharmacy*, New York: St. Martin's Paperbacks, published in arrangement with Rodale Press, Inc., Emmaus, PA: 1997, 1998, p. 380

[13] Ibid., p. 380

[14] "Liver Cancer." Herbs2000.com. Available: http://www.herbs2000.com/disorders/cancer_liver.htm, p. 2 (accessed 2004, Oct. 17)

[15] Antol, p. 175, 177

[16] Ibid.

[17] Ibid.

[18] "Sir Jason Winters Story - About Sir Jason Winters," Available: http://www.sirjasonwinters.com/story.htm, (accessed 2005, Jan. 6)

[19] Ibid.

[20] Ibid., p. 2-3

Chapter 32

[1] D. Quinn. *Left For Dead*, Minneapolis, MN: R. F. Quinn Publishing Co, 1992, p. 147

[2] "Hoxsey Formula," Wellness Directory of Minnesota, Alternative Cancer Therapies. Available: http://www.mnwelldir.org/docs/cancer1/altthrpy2.htm (accessed 2004, Oct. 28)

[3] "Johanna Brandt / Fred Wortman Grape Cure For Cancer," *Cancer Tutor™*, Alternative Cancer Treatment Information Center. Available: http://www.cancertutor.com/Cancer/GrapeCure.html., p. 2 (accessed 2004, Aug 1)

[4] R. W. Moss, Ph.D. *Antioxidants against Cancer*, State College, PA: Equinox Press, 2000, 2002, p. 99

[5] T. A. M. Kramer, M.D. "Understanding Clinical Trials in Context." Available: http://www.medscape.com/viewarticle/462046 - Reprinted with permission from Medscape General Medicine 5 (4), 2003, http://www.medscape.com/viewarticle/462046 © 2003, Medscape

[6] "Cancer Cover-Up The Neal Deoul Story," by Kathleen Deoul, *Frequently Asked Questions*. Available: http://www.cancer-coverup.com/faqs/is-this-treatment-safe.htm, (accessed 2004, Dec. 26)

[7] "A Bex and a Nice Lie Down," BARISTA heartstarters for the hungry mind, June 19, 2004, Available: http://dox.media2.org/barista/archives/000781.html, p. 1 (accessed 2005, Jan 5)

[8] "Prozac: What is the Truth behind it? The Prozac Truth Exposed on this Web Site," Available: http://www.prozactruth.com, (accessed 2005, Jan. 5)

[9] Ibid.

[10] E. Shogren, "FDA kept suicide findings secret," Los Angeles Times, Published on: 04/06/04, Psych Drug Truth. Available: http://www.prozactruth.com/article_fda_secret_findings.htm, p. 1 (accessed 2005, Jan. 5)

[11] Ibid., p. 2

[12] "Drug giant accused of false claims," Psych Drug Truth, NBC NEWS, Available: http://www.prozactruth.com/article_drug_giant_accused.htm, p. 1 (accessed 2005, Jan 5)

13 T. A. M. Kramer, M.D. "Understanding Clinical Trials in Context," 10/02/03, From Medscape General Medicine™, Medscape from WebMD. Available: http://www.medscape.com/viewarticle/462046_3, "Support and Sponsorship," p. 1 (accessed 2005, Jan. 5) Reprinted with permission from Medscape General Medicine 5 (4), 2003, http://www.medscape.com/viewarticle/462046 © 2003, Medscape.

14 A. Hoffer, M.D., F.R.C.P. (C) with L. Pauling, Ph.D. *Healing Cancer - Complementary Vitamin & Drug Treatments*, Toronto, Ontario, Canada: CCNM Press, 2004, p. 77

Chapter 33

1 R. W. Moss, Ph.D. *Antioxidants against Cancer*, State College, PA: Equinox Press, Inc., 2000, 2002, p. 99

2 B. Berkson, M.D., Ph.D. *From The Alpha Lipoic Acid Breakthrough*, copyright © 1998 by Burt Berkson. Used by permission of Prima Publishing, a division of Random House, Inc., p. x

3 Ibid., p. xii

4 Ibid, p. xii, xiii

5 M. Kennedy Salaman. *Nutrition: The Cancer Answer II*, Menlo Park, CA: MKS, Inc./Statford Publishing, 1995, 2002, p. 224, 225

6 Ibid., p. 225, 226

7 M. Kennedy Salaman. *All Your Health Questions Answered Naturally*, (City, State, n.g.) MKS, Inc., 1998, p. 213

8 Ibid.

9 Salaman, *Nutrition: The Cancer Answer II*, p. 84, 85, 86

10 Ibid.

11 H. Kroeger, Ms.D. *Free Your Body of Tumors and Cysts*, (City, State, n.g.) Hanna Kroeger Publications, 1997, p. 54-55

12 Ibid.

13 R. W. Moss, Ph.D. *Cancer Therapy: The Independent Consumer's Guide To Non-Toxic Treatment & Prevention*, New York: Equinox Press, 1992, p. 269

14 Salaman, *Nutrition: The Cancer Answer II*, p. 15-16

15 Ibid., p. 15-16

16 Salaman, *Nutrition: The Cancer Answer II*, p. 22

17 "Laetrile," Alternative Health Supplies (Australia), Your Health,™ Your Choice®, "Review of Laetrile (Vitamin B17), p. 2 (accessed 2005, Jan. 5) Available: http://www.alternativehealth.com. au/articles/laetril.htm

18 Ibid., p. 2

19 A. J. Brown, "Comprehensive Cancer Therapy," The Cancer Homepage. Available: http://www.curezone.com/diseases/cancer/cancer_arlin_therapy.html, p. 8 (accessed 2004, May 18)

20 Moss, *Cancer Therapy*, p. 123

21 "Beres Drops," Over 200 Alternative Cancer Treatments Plus Other Information. Available: http://www.cancertutor.com/Other/Big_List.htm, p. 6, (accessed 2004, Oct. 17)

22 Ibid.

23 "Breuss Total Cancer Treatment," Cancer Tutor™ Alternative Cancer Treatment Information Center, Available: http://www.cancertutor.com/Cancer/Breuss.html, p. 1-2 (accessed 2004, Oct. 17)

24 Ibid.

[25] Salaman. *Nutrition: The Cancer Answer II* p. 335, 337

[26] Ibid.

[27] Ibid., p. 337

[28] Ibid.

[29] "Contortrostatin," and "C-Statin," Alternative Cancer Therapies, Wellness Directory of Minnesota™. Available: http://www.mnwelldir.org/docs/cancer1/altthrpy.htm, p. 1 (accessed 2004, Dec. 20)

[30] F. S. Markland, Ph.D., "A Snake Venom Protein with Unique Anti-tumor and Anti-angiogenic Activities." Available: http://www.calacademy.org/education/bioforum2000-2001/venoms/marklandsum...p 1, (accessed 2005, Feb. 5)

[30a] Ibid. This note was in an email that Dr. F.S. Markland sent to me on 5-22-05

[30b] S. Young, "Contortrostatin: Evaluation of Its Effect on Ovarian Tumor Growth," California State Science Fair, 2002 Project Summary, Project Number S1435. Available as a pdf document at http://www.usc.edu/CSSF/History/2002/Projects/S1435.pdf, (accessed 2005, Feb. 5)

[31] S. B. Edelson, M.D. and D. Mitchell. *What Your Doctor May Not Tell You About Immune Disorders*, New York: Warner Books, A Lynn Sonberg Book, 2003, p. 312-313, From What Your Doctor May Not Tell You About™: Autoimmune Disorders by Stephen Edelson, M.D., Copyright ©2003 by Stephen B. Edelson and Lynn Sonberg. By Permission of Warner Books, Inc.

[32] Ibid.

[33] Ibid., p. 313

[34] Ibid., p. 314

[35] "Insulin-induced Hypoglycemic Therapy (IHT)," Cancer Tutor™ website, Over 200 Alternative Cancer Treatments Plus Other Information. Available: http://www.cancer-tutor.com/Other/Big_List.htm, (accessed 2004, Dec. 11)

[36] M. Kennedy Salaman. *Nutrition: The Cancer Answer II*, Menlo Park, CA: MKS, Inc., Statford Publishing, 1995, 2002, p. 334,335

[37] Ibid., p. 335

[38] G. Null, Ph.D. *The Complete Encyclopedia of Natural Healing*, New York, N.Y. © 2000, 2001, 2002 Kensington Publishing Corp., p. 472-473. All rights reserved. Reprinted by arrangement with Kensington Publishing Corp., www.kensingtonbooks.com.

[39] Ibid.

[40] C. LeBeau. *Hydrogen Peroxide & Ozone*, 13th Edition, West Allis, WI: Vital Health Publications, 2001, p. 12-13

[41] Ibid., p. 13

[42] Moss, *Cancer Therapy*, p. 188

[43] Ibid., p. 190

[44] Ibid., p. 193

[45] Margareta-Erminia Cassani, "MGN-3: Mushroom Extract Boosts Immune System, Kills Diseased Cells," Moonbow Media, MGN-3 Disease Killing Mushrooms. Available: http://www.moonbowmedia.com/health/mgn3.htm, p. 1-2, (accessed 2005, Jan. 6)

[46] J. A. Debe, D.C., D.A.C.B.N., C.C.S.P., C.C.N., "MGN-3 - New Super Immune Stimulator." Available: http://www.drdebe.com/MGN.htm, Copyright © Nov. 9, 1998 by Joseph A. Debe, p. 1 (accessed 2004, Aug. 1)

[47] Ibid., p. 2

[48] "MSM Plus Vitamin C and B12 Cancer Treatment," Cancer Tutor™ website. Available: http://www.cancertutor.com/Cancer/MSM.html, p. 1 (accessed 2004, Dec. 1)

[49] Ibid., p. 2-3

[50] Ibid., p. 3 (The study was done by "Dr. D. McCabe, Dr. P. O. Dwyer, Dr. B. Sickle-Antanello, Dr. E. Woltering, Dr. H. Abou-Issa and Dr. A. James, published in the Archives of Surgery, 12/1986")

[51] Ibid., p. 4

[52] J. Metz, M.D. "Reduced Normal Tissue Toxicity With Proton Therapy," OncoLink, The Abramson Cancer Center of the University of Pennsylvania, posted April 28, 2002. Available: http://www.oncolink.com/treatment/article.cfm?c=9&s=70&id=211, p. 2 (accessed 2005, Jun. 1) Copyright © 1994-2005 © Trustees of the University of Pennsylvania

[53] Ibid.

[54] "Royal Rife Machine," Cancer Tutor™ website. Available: http://www.cancertutor.com/Other/Big_List.htm, p. 33 (accessed 2004, Oct. 17)

Chapter 34

[1] V. Saxion. *"How To Feel Great All The Time,"* Little Rock, AR: Lion's Head Publishing, 2002, p,. 94, 95, 96

[2] D. Colbert, M.D. *Toxic Relief,* Lake Mary, FL: Siloam A Strang Company, 2001, 2003, p. 51, 53, 54

[3] Ibid.

[4] Ibid., p. 51-52

[5] Ibid., p. 184

[6] B. Rodgers. *The 21 Day Fast,* Louisville, KY: Bob Rodgers Ministries, 2001, p. 30-37

[7] T. Evans. *Tony Evans Speaks Out On Fasting,* Chicago, IL: Moody Publishers, 2000, p. 10

[8] A. Wallis. *God's Chosen Fast,* Ft. Washington, PA: Christian Literature Crusade, p. 104. Copyright © 1968, published by CLC Publications, Fort Washington, PA. Used by permission.

[9] Colbert, *Toxic Relief,* p. 155

[10] S. Meyerowitz. *Wheatgrass Nature's Finest Medicine: The Complete Guide to Using Grasses to Revitalize Your Health,* Great Barrington, MA: Sproutman Publications, 1999, 6th edition, p. 78

[11] Colbert, *Toxic Relief,* p. 164-165

[12] Ibid., p. 165

[13] Ibid., p. 166

[14] F. Batmanghelidj, M.D. *Your Body's Many Cries For Water,* Vienna, VA: Global Health Solutions, Inc., 2nd Edition, 1992, 1995, 1997, p. 161

[15] C. Calbom and M. Keane. *Juicing For Life,* (City, State, n.g.) Avery, member of Penguin Putnam, Inc., 1992, Trillium Health Products, P. 302

Chapter 35

[1] N. Hayes. *Worship Your Foundation For The Victorious Life,* Tulsa: Harrison House Publishers, copyright 1997, p. 17

[2] Ibid, p. 22

[3] T. Law. *The Power of Praise And Worship,* Tulsa, OK: Victory House Publishers, 1985, p. 138

[4] "Cat's Claw," herbs2000.com. Available: http://www.herbs2000.com/herbs/herbs_cats_claw.htm, p. 3, (accessed 2005, Jan 11)

[5] "Bladder Cancer." Herbs2000.com. Available: herbs2000.com/disorders/cancer_bladder.htm p. 1-2, (accessed 2004, Oct. 17)

[6] M. Kennedy Salaman. *All Your Health Questions Answered Naturally*, (City, State, n.g.) MKS, Inc., 1998, p. 213

[7] "Turmeric Curcuma longa syn. C. domestica," herbs2000.com. Available: http://www.herbs2000.com/herbs/herbs_turmeric.htm, p. 3 (accessed 2005, Feb. 11)

[8] "Turmeric Curcuma longa syn. C. domestica," Herbs2000.com. Available: http://www.herbs.2000.com/herbs/herbs_turmeric.htm, p. 3 (accessed 2005, Feb. 11)

[9] Mark Stengler, N.D., p 445, *The Natural Physician's Healing Therapies* by Mark Stengler, N.D copyright © 2001 by Mark Stengler. Used by permission of Avery Publishing, an imprint of Penguin Group (USA) Inc.

[10] S. Meyerowitz. *Water The Ultimate Cure*, Great Barrington, MA: S. Meyerowitz, 2000, 2001, p. 14

[11] F. Batmanghelidj, M.D. *Your Body's Many Cries For Water*, Vienna, VA: Global Health Solutions, Inc., 1992, 1995, 1997, p. 161

AUTHOR BIO

Deanna K. Loftis resides in Louisville, Kentucky with her family. Born in Alabama, she was raised in upstate New York, graduated high school in Jasper, Alabama, married in Indiana, and settled in Kentucky, where she returned to school and earned a nursing degree. She spent several years working between med-surg and orthopedic floors in Louisville hospitals and is a licensed R.N. in both Texas and Kentucky. Deanna again returned to school for a B.B.A. (major in Managed Care), graduating Summa Cum Laude from Northwood University. She spent several years working in a Managed Care position which included following solid organ transplant patients and bone marrow (or stem cell) transplant patients for an insurance company. During this time, she also lost three family members to cancer. Because of the discouraging and horrendous side effects that her family members and patients suffered from chemo, and radiation, she started to question the appropriateness of conventional cancer treatment. As a result, Deanna began an intensive study of alternative cancer therapies which culminated in this book. Though it is already too late for some of her loved ones to benefit from the information she compiled in this book, it is not too late for you and yours!

Printed in the United States
94909LV00006B/1-3/A